W9-CGL-579

Issues & Ethics

IN THE HELPING PROFESSIONS, 10E

Gerald Corey
California State University, Fullerton
Diplomate in Counseling Psychology
American Board of Professional Psychology

Marianne Schneider Corey
Consultant

Cindy Corey
Licensed Clinical Psychologist in private practice
Multicultural Consultant

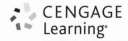

CENGAGE
Learning

Australia • Brazil • Mexico • Singapore • United Kingdom • United States

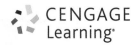
CENGAGE
Learning®

Issues and Ethics in the Helping Professions, 10th Edition
Gerald Corey, Marianne Schneider Corey, Cindy Corey

Product Director: Marta Lee-Perriard

Product Manager: Julie Martinez

Content Developer: Alexander Hancock

Product Assistant: Ali Balchunas

Marketing Manager: Zena Craft

Content Project Manager: Rita Jaramillo

Digital Content Specialist: Jennifer Chinn

Art Director: Vernon Boes

Manufacturing Planner: Karen Hunt

Intellectual Property Analyst: Deanna Ettinger

Intellectual Property Project Manager:
    Nick Barrows

Production Service/Compositor/Project
    Manager: Cenveo® Publisher Services,
    Ben Kolstad

Compositor: Cenveo® Publisher Services

XML Tagging: MPS

Text and Cover Designer: Jeanne Calabrese

Cover Image Credit: saemilee/Getty Images

For product information and technology assistance, contact us at **Cengage Learning Customer & Sales Support, 1-800-354-9706.**

For permission to use material from this text or product, submit all requests online at **www.cengage.com/permissions.** Further permissions questions can be e-mailed to **permissionrequest@cengage.com.**

Library of Congress Control Number: 2017952223

Student Edition:
ISBN: 978-1-337-40629-1

Loose-leaf Edition:
ISBN: 978-1-337-56100-6

Cengage Learning
20 Channel Center Street
Boston, MA 02210
USA

Cengage Learning is a leading provider of customized learning solutions with employees residing in nearly 40 different countries and sales in more than 125 countries around the world. Find your local representative at **www.cengage.com**.

Cengage Learning products are represented in Canada by Nelson Education, Ltd.

To learn more about Cengage Learning Solutions, visit **www.cengage.com**.

Purchase any of our products at your local college store or at our preferred online store **www.cengagebrain.com**.

Printed in the United States of America
Print Number: 06   Print Year: 2019

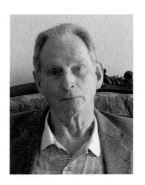

In memory of our lifelong friend and colleague, Patrick Callanan.

Patrick was a generous, honest, witty, and adventurous man who left his mark on the world through his roles as priest, father, uncle, teacher, counselor, author, mentor, and friend.

We will always remember him, as he is impossible to forget!

About the Authors

Gerald Corey is Professor Emeritus of Human Services and Counseling at California State University at Fullerton. He received his doctorate in counseling from the University of Southern California. He is a Diplomate in Counseling Psychology, American Board of Professional Psychology; a licensed psychologist; and a National Certified Counselor. He is a Fellow of the American Psychological Association (Division 17, Counseling Psychology, and also Division 49, Group Psychotherapy); a Fellow of the American Counseling Association; and a Fellow of the Association for Specialists in Group Work. He also holds memberships in the American Group Psychotherapy Association; the 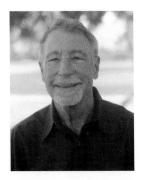 American Mental Health Counselors Association; the Association for Spiritual, Ethical, and Religious Values in Counseling; the Association for Counselor Education and Supervision; and the Western Association of Counselor Education and Supervision. Both Jerry and Marianne Corey received the Lifetime Achievement Award from the American Mental Health Counselors Association in 2011, and both of them received the Eminent Career Award from ASGW in 2001. Jerry was given the Outstanding Professor of the Year Award from California State University at Fullerton in 1991. He regularly teaches both undergraduate and graduate courses in group counseling and ethics in counseling. He is the author or coauthor of 15 textbooks in counseling currently in print, along with more than 60 journal articles and book chapters. Several of his books have been translated into other languages. *Theory and Practice of Counseling and Psychotherapy* has been translated into Arabic, Indonesian, Portuguese, Turkish, Korean, and Chinese. *Theory and Practice of Group Counseling* has been translated into Korean, Chinese, Spanish, and Russian.

During the past 40 years Jerry and Marianne Corey have conducted group counseling training workshops for mental health professionals at many universities in the United States as well as in Canada, Mexico, China, Hong Kong, Korea, Germany, Belgium, Scotland, England, and Ireland. In his leisure time, Jerry likes to travel, hike and bicycle in the mountains and the desert, and drive his grandchildren in his 1931 Model A Ford. Marianne and Jerry have been married since 1964. They have two adult daughters (Heidi and Cindy), two granddaughters (Kyla and Keegan), and one grandson (Corey).

In addition to *Issues and Ethics in the Helping Professions*, Tenth Edition (2019, with Marianne Schneider Corey and Cindy Corey), which has been translated into Japanese, Chinese, and Korean, other recent publications by Gerald Corey, all with Cengage Learning, include:

- *Groups: Process and Practice*, Tenth Edition (2018, with Marianne Schneider Corey and Cindy Corey)
- *I Never Knew I Had a Choice*, Eleventh Edition (2018, with Marianne Schneider Corey and Michelle Muratori)
- *Theory and Practice of Counseling and Psychotherapy*, Tenth Edition (and *Student Manual*) (2017)
- *Theory and Practice of Group Counseling*, Ninth Edition (and *Student Manual*) (2016)
- *Becoming a Helper*, Seventh Edition (2016, with Marianne Schneider Corey)
- *Group Techniques*, Fourth Edition (2015, with Marianne Schneider Corey, Patrick Callanan, and J. Michael Russell)

- *Case Approach to Counseling and Psychotherapy*, Eighth Edition (2013)
- *The Art of Integrative Counseling*, Third Edition (2013)

Jerry Corey is coauthor (with Barbara Herlihy) of *Boundary Issues in Counseling: Multiple Roles and Responsibilities*, Third Edition (2015) and *ACA Ethical Standards Casebook*, Seventh Edition (2015); he is coauthor (with Michelle Muratori, Jude Austin, and Julius Austin) of *Counselor Self-Care* (2018); he is coauthor (with Robert Haynes, Patrice Moulton, and Michelle Muratori) of *Clinical Supervision in the Helping Professions: A Practical Guide*, Second Edition (2010); he is the author of *Creating Your Professional Path: Lessons From My Journey* (2010). All five of these books are published by the American Counseling Association.

He has also made several educational DVD programs on various aspects of counseling practice: (1) *Ethics in Action: DVD and Workbook* (2015, with Marianne Schneider Corey and Robert Haynes); (2) *Groups in Action: Evolution and Challenges DVD and Workbook* (2014, with Marianne Schneider Corey and Robert Haynes); (3) *DVD for Theory and Practice of Counseling and Psychotherapy: The Case of Stan and Lecturettes* (2013); (4) *DVD for Integrative Counseling: The Case of Ruth and Lecturettes* (2013, with Robert Haynes); and (5) *DVD for Theory and Practice of Group Counseling* (2012). All of these programs are available through Cengage Learning.

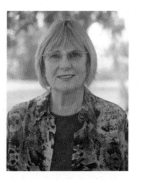

Marianne Schneider Corey is a licensed marriage and family therapist in California and is a National Certified Counselor. She received her master's degree in marriage, family, and child counseling from Chapman College. She is a Fellow of the Association for Specialists in Group Work and was the recipient of this organization's Eminent Career Award in 2001. She received the Lifetime Achievement Award from the American Mental Health Counselors Association in 2011 and is a member of the American Mental Health Counselors Association. She also holds memberships in the American Counseling Association, the American Group Psychotherapy Association, the Association for Specialists in Group Work, the Association for Multicultural Counseling and Development, the Association for Counselor Education and Supervision, and the Western Association of Counselor Education and Supervision.

Marianne has been involved in leading groups for different populations, providing training and supervision workshops in group process, facilitating self-exploration groups for graduate students in counseling, and cofacilitating training groups for group counselors and weeklong residential workshops in personal growth. Both Marianne and Jerry Corey have conducted training workshops, continuing education seminars, and personal-growth groups in the United States, Germany, Ireland, Belgium, Mexico, Hong Kong, China, and Korea.

In addition to *Issues and Ethics in the Helping Professions*, Tenth Edition (2019, with Gerald Corey and Cindy Corey), which has been translated into Japanese, Chinese, and Korean, Marianne has coauthored the following books with Cengage Learning:

- *Groups: Process and Practice*, Tenth Edition (2018, with Gerald Corey and Cindy Corey), which has been translated into Korean, Chinese, and Polish
- *I Never Knew I Had a Choice*, Eleventh Edition (2018, with Gerald Corey and Michelle Muratori), which has been translated into Chinese
- *Becoming a Helper*, Seventh Edition (2016, with Gerald Corey), which has been translated into Korean and Japanese
- *Group Techniques*, Fourth Edition (2015, with Gerald Corey, Patrick Callanan, and Michael Russell), which has been translated into Portuguese, Korean, Japanese, and Czech

Marianne has made educational video programs (with accompanying student workbooks) for Cengage Learning: *Groups in Action: Evolution and Challenges DVD and Workbook* (2014, with Gerald Corey and Robert Haynes); and *Ethics in Action: DVD and Workbook* (2015, with Gerald Corey and Robert Haynes).

Marianne and Jerry have been married since 1964. They have two adult daughters, Heidi and Cindy, two granddaughters (Kyla and Keegan), and one grandson (Corey). Marianne grew up in Germany and has kept in close contact with her family and friends there. In her free time, she enjoys traveling, reading, visiting with friends, bike riding, and hiking.

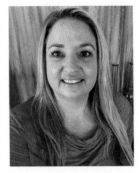

Cindy Corey is a licensed clinical psychologist in private practice in San Diego, California. She worked for over a decade as a full-time visiting professor in the Department of Counseling and School Psychology at San Diego State University in both the Community-Based Block and Marriage and Family Therapy programs. She received her master's degree in Marriage and Family Therapy from the University of San Diego and her Doctorate (PsyD) in Multicultural Community Clinical Psychology at the California School of Professional Psychology in Alhambra, California. She is a member of the American Counseling Association, the Association for Specialists in Group Work, the American Psychological Association, and the San Diego Psychological Association (SDPA). She served as the chair of the Lesbian, Gay, Bisexual, and Transgender Committee for the SDPA and has been a member of the Multicultural Committee and Women's Committee.

Cindy has focused much of her work in the area of counselor education, specializing in multicultural training, social justice, and community outreach. In addition to teaching at San Diego State University, she taught part time in the PsyD program at Alliant International University in Alhambra. Cindy has also worked as a Contracted Clinician for Survivors of Torture International, focusing primarily on helping Sudanese refugee youth adjust to life in the United States, gain employment, and attend colleges and universities.

Cindy works as a multicultural consultant and has created clinical intervention programs, training manuals, and diversity sensitive curriculum for a variety of schools, businesses, and organizations in the San Diego area. Her private practice focuses on working with women, couples, counselors, and graduate students in counseling programs.

Cindy is coauthor, with Marianne Corey and Gerald Corey of *Groups: Process and Practice,* Tenth Edition (2018).

Contents

Preface

Our friend and colleague, Patrick Callanan, died on March 17, 2017 (St. Patrick's Day). He was a coauthor with us on the previous editions of *Issues and Ethics in the Helping Professions*. For many years we enjoyed working with Patrick on various projects, and we will miss his companionship and professional involvement with us. Patrick devoted much of his life to the counseling profession as a practitioner and made a significant difference in the lives of many clients, students, and professionals.

Issues and Ethics in the Helping Professions is written for both graduate and undergraduate students in the helping professions. This book is suitable for courses in counseling, mental health counseling, human services, couples and family therapy, counseling and clinical psychology, school counseling, and social work. It can be used as a core textbook in courses such as practicum, fieldwork, internship, and ethical and professional issues or as a supplementary text in courses dealing with skills or theory. Because the issues we discuss are likely to be encountered throughout one's professional career, we strive to use language and concepts that will be meaningful both to students doing their fieldwork and to professionals interested in keeping abreast of developments in ethical, professional, and legal matters pertaining to therapeutic practice.

In this book, we want to involve our readers in learning to deal with the ethical and professional issues that most affect the actual practice of counseling and related helping professions. We address such questions as: How aware are you of how your values and life experiences affect your professional work? What are the rights and responsibilities of both the client and the counselor? How can you determine your level of competence? How can you achieve and maintain your competence? How can you provide quality services for culturally diverse populations? In what ways could you involve yourself in social justice and advocacy work? How can you go outside of the office and make a difference in the community? What major ethical issues might you encounter in couples and family therapy? in group work? in community agencies? in a school setting? in private practice? Our goal is both to provide a body of information and to teach a process for thinking about and resolving the basic issues counselors will face throughout their career. For most of the issues we raise, we present various viewpoints to stimulate discussion and reflection. We also present our personal views and commentaries, when appropriate, and challenge you to develop your own position.

The ethics codes of various professional associations offer some guidance for practice. However, these guidelines leave many questions unanswered. We believe that as a student or a professional you will ultimately struggle with the issues of responsible practice, deciding how accepted ethical principles apply in the specific cases you encounter.

Throughout this book, we aim to involve you in an active and meaningful way. We provide many opportunities for you to respond to our discussions.

Each chapter begins with Learning Objectives to guide your reading and a Self-Inventory designed to help you focus on the key topics to be discussed in the chapter. Within the chapters we frequently ask you to think about how the issues apply to you. Open-ended cases and situations are designed to stimulate thought and discussion, and we encourage you to apply the codes of ethics of the various mental health professions to the case illustrations. Reflecting on the questions following each case example will help you determine which of the therapist responses are ethically sound and which are not. We offer our commentaries after each case to guide you in the process of determining sound ethical decisions. We also cite related literature when exploring ethical, legal, professional, and clinical issues. Instructors will find an abundance of material and suggested activities, surely more than can be covered in a single course.

An *Instructor's Resource Manual* is available that contains chapter outlines, suggestions for teaching an ethics course, additional exercises and activities, a list of PowerPoint slides, and study guide questions. A Test Bank for each chapter and online quizzes are available to instructors. An electronic version of the *Instructor's Resource Manual* is available for all platforms.

Issues and Ethics in the Helping Professions comes with MindTap®. MindTap, a digital teaching and learning solution, helps students be more successful and confident in the course—and in their work with clients. MindTap guides students through the course by combining the complete textbook with interactive multimedia, activities, assessments, and learning tools. Readings and activities engage students in learning core concepts, practicing needed skills, reflecting on their attitudes and opinions, and applying what they learn. Videos of client sessions illustrate skills and concepts in action, and case studies ask students to make decisions and think critically about the types of situations they will encounter on the job. Helper Studio activities put students in the role of the helper, allowing them to build and practice skills in a nonthreatening environment by responding via video to a virtual client. Instructors can rearrange and add content to personalize their MindTap course and easily track students' progress with real-time analytics. MindTap integrates seamlessly with any learning management system.

An integrated learning package titled *Ethics in Action: DVD and Workbook* (third edition, 2015) is available to enhance the 10th edition of *Issues and Ethics in the Helping Professions*. The *Ethics in Action* DVD is designed to bring to life the ethical issues and dilemmas counselors often encounter and to provide ample opportunity for discussion, self-exploration, and problem solving of these issues and dilemmas. The vignettes on the DVD are based on a weekend workshop cofacilitated by Marianne Schneider Corey and Gerald Corey for a group of counseling students, which included challenging questions and lively discussion, role plays to bring the issues to life, and comments from the students and the Coreys. Additional material on the DVD program is designed to provide a self-study guide for students who are also reading this book. This educational program is divided into three segments: ethical decision making, values and the helping relationship, and boundary issues and multiple relationships in counseling. At the end of several chapters in this book are suggested activities and guidelines for integrating the *Ethics in Action* video program with this textbook.

What's New in the 10th Edition of *Issues and Ethics*

For the 10th edition, each chapter has been carefully reviewed and updated to present the current thinking, research, and trends in practice. The following chapter-by-chapter list of highlights outlines some sample material that has been added, updated, expanded, and revised for the 10th edition.

Chapter 1 Introduction to Professional Ethics

- Citation of updated ethics codes whenever available
- Inclusion of themes common to most codes of ethics
- Increased emphasis on positive ethics rather than rule-based ethics

Chapter 2 The Counselor as a Person and as a Professional

- Updated literature on personal therapy for trainees and for practitioners
- Updated material on sources of stress in the helping professions
- Expanded discussion of self-compassion and self-care strategies for professionals
- Updated discussions of burnout, practitioner impairment, and maintaining vitality

Chapter 3 Values and the Helping Relationship

- A new section on controversies regarding integrating personal values with a professional identity
- Increased attention to the responsibility of counselor education programs in being clear with students about managing personal values
- Increased attention to the necessity for graduate students in counseling to learn how to work within the framework of the client's value system
- More focus on avoiding value imposition by ethical bracketing
- Implications of several court cases in dismissing students unwilling to keep their personal values separate from counseling clients with a different set of values
- New section on state legislation to protect religious freedom
- New literature on the ethics of values-based referrals and discriminatory referrals
- New material on the role of spirituality and religion in counseling
- New section on ethical and clinical issues with nonreligious clients
- Description of an ethical decision-making model to determine whether religious or spiritual beliefs may be clinically salient

Chapter 4 Multicultural Perspectives and Diversity Issues

- Increased coverage of cultural pluralism and cultural competence
- Updated section on ethical issues regarding sexual orientation
- Increased and updated coverage of ethical issues and competencies required in counseling lesbian, gay, bisexual, and transgender clients

- Introduction to how a social justice orientation relates to a multicultural perspective
- Updated discussion regarding acquiring and maintaining cultural competence
- Presentation of authors' views on multicultural training

Chapter 5 Client Rights and Counselor Responsibilities

- Updated and expanded section on content of informed consent process
- Updating of all of the ethics codes on the topic of client rights and counselor responsibilities
- More attention to cultural factors related to the informed consent process
- Revised discussions of informed consent and confidentiality as it pertains to managed care
- Added literature on addressing risks of diagnosis in the informed consent process
- Expanded treatment of clinical record keeping
- Revised guidelines for keeping records with couples, families, and groups
- Updated discussion of the ethical issues involved in online counseling
- New material on alternative technologies in online counseling
- Updated material on emerging issues in online counseling
- Expanded discussion of common complaints against counselors and reasons for malpractice suits
- Revised discussion of risk management practices and implications for clinical effectiveness
- Increased focus on balancing risk management with investment in quality care of clients

Chapter 6 Confidentiality: Ethical and Legal Issues

- More emphasis on counselors having an ongoing dialogue with their clients about how, when, and with whom information will be shared
- Revised section on privacy issues with telecommunication devices
- Commentary on the use of telephone-delivered psychotherapy
- Revised discussion of confidentiality and privacy in a school setting
- New literature on duty to warn and to protect
- New section on ethical considerations with clients who self-injure
- New material on safety plans with high-risk clients
- Expansion of topic on prevention of school violence
- Expansion of discussion on predicting and preventing acts of violence
- Revision of section on dealing with dangerous clients
- Revision of risk management strategies in dealing with duty to protect situations

Chapter 7 Managing Boundaries and Multiple Relationships

- Revised discussion of how some boundary crossings can result in enhanced client care
- More attention to ways of establishing appropriate boundaries
- New section on setting appropriate boundaries outside the office

- Revised critique of the slippery slope phenomenon
- Updated literature on ways to minimize risks for those working in rural areas and in small communities
- New literature on dealing with sexual attractions

Chapter 8 Professional Competence and Training

- Increased emphasis on how competence is a significant topic for counseling students
- Expanded discussion of the gatekeeper role of faculty
- New section on training practitioners to work in a digital culture
- Expanded discussion on the role of interpersonal behavior in working with trainees and the need to have difficult conversations with trainees who manifest professional competency problems
- Updated discussion on dismissing students for nonacademic reasons
- Updated section on maintaining competence and the value of lifelong learning

Chapter 9 Ethical Issues in Supervision

- Updated coverage of informed consent in clinical supervision
- Revised material on legal aspects of supervision
- Discussion of power dynamics in the supervisory relationship
- More emphasis on the importance of a strong supervisory working alliance
- New discussion of the role of a supervision contract
- New discussion of the concept of strict liability for supervisors
- Revised material on assessment of culturally competent supervision
- Updated treatment on role of spirituality in supervision
- Expanded section on addressing gender issues in supervision
- Revised discussion of clinical supervision for school counselors
- Revised section on the ethical issues for online supervision
- Revision of multiple relationships in the supervisory process
- Updated discussion of how positive boundary crossings can enhance supervisory relationships

Chapter 10 Issues in Theory and Practice

- Updated section on assessment and diagnosis
- Updated discussion of ethical issues regarding the *DSM-5*
- Revised section on ethical and legal issues pertaining to diagnosis
- Revision of cultural considerations in assessment and diagnosis
- A critique of empirically supported treatments

Chapter 11 Ethical Issues in Couples and Family Therapy

- Expansion of the systems theory perspective
- More emphasis on the revised AAMFT code of ethics
- More attention to how a therapist's family-of-origin experiences can influence a therapist's work with families
- Updated discussion of confidentiality in couples and family therapy
- Updated discussion on dealing with secrets in working with multiple clients

Chapter 12 Ethical Issues in Group Work

- Revised and expanded discussion of training and supervision of group leaders
- Updated section on ethical issues in diversity training of group leaders
- Revised guidelines for acquiring multicultural and social justice competence in group work
- New literature on privacy and confidentiality considerations pertaining to social media in group work
- Revised section on evaluating what works in a group
- Updated material on the practice-based approach to group work

Chapter 13 Community and Social Justice Perspectives

- Additional concrete examples and cases to illustrate key concepts of social justice in community work
- Revised section on the community as client
- Updated discussion on the goals of social justice and advocacy
- New section on social justice advocacy in school counseling

Acknowledgments

We would like to express our appreciation for the suggestions given to us by reviewers, associates, students, and readers. The reviewers of this **10th edition** have been instrumental in making significant changes from the earlier editions. We especially recognize the following people who reviewed the revised manuscript of the 10th edition and offered ideas that were incorporated into this edition:

Kristen Dickens, Georgia Southern University
Maureen C. Kenny, Florida International University
Kristin Vincenzes, Lock Haven University
Julia Whisenhunt, University of West Georgia

We appreciate the feedback from the following people on selected chapters in this edition, based on their areas of special interest and expertise:

The following people provided reviews and suggestions for various aspects of Chapter 3, on dealing with values in counseling: Perry Francis, Eastern Michigan University; David Kaplan, Chief Professional Officer, American Counseling Association; and Brad Johnson, United States Naval Academy.

For Chapter 4 on ethical issues in multicultural counseling, appreciation goes to Mark Stebnicki for his contribution of a section on the culture of disability, which highlights ethical issues in counseling people with disabilities.

For Chapters 5 and 6, we thank Anne Marie "Nancy" Wheeler, JD, attorney in private practice in Maryland and the District of Columbia, affiliate faculty member at Loyola University Maryland, and consultant for the ACA Risk Management Service; and Jamie Bludworth, Assistant Professor of Counseling and Counseling Psychology at Arizona State University.

For Chapter 9 on clinical supervision, we appreciate the critique of Jamie Bludworth, Arizona State University.

For Chapter 13 on community and social justice issues, our thanks to Fred Bemak, George Mason University.

Finally, as is true of all our books, *Issues and Ethics in the Helping Professions* continues to develop as a result of a team effort, which includes the combined efforts of several people at Cengage Learning: Julie Martinez, Product Manager, Counseling, Social Work, & Human Services; Alexander Hancock, Associate Content Developer, Sociology, Counseling, and Social Work; Vernon Boes, Art Director; and Rita Jaramillo, Content Project Manager. Thanks to Ben Kolstad of Cenveo® Publisher Services, who coordinated the production of this book. Special recognition goes to Kay Mikel, the manuscript editor of this edition, whose exceptional editorial talents continue to keep this book reader friendly. Special recognition goes to Michelle Muratori of Johns Hopkins University for her work in updating literature for all of the chapters and for providing detailed input in the various aspects of this revision. We appreciate Susan Cunningham's work in creating and revising test items to accompany this text, preparing the index, updating the *Instructor's Resource Manual*, revising the PowerPoints slides, and in assisting in development of other supplements to this book. The efforts and dedication of all of these people have contributed to the high quality of this revised edition.

Gerald Corey
Marianne Schneider Corey
Cindy Corey

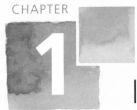

CHAPTER

Introduction to Professional Ethics

LEARNING OBJECTIVES

1. Identify common themes of ethics codes

2. Understand the limitations of codes of ethics

3. Describe three objectives fulfilled by codes of ethics

4. Explain the difference between law and ethics

5. Differentiate between aspirational ethics and mandatory ethics

6. Compare principle ethics and virtue ethics

7. Apply the six moral principles to ethical dilemmas

8. Recognize the steps in working through an ethical dilemma

9. Assess your attitudes and beliefs pertaining to a range of ethical and professional issues addressed in this book

The Focus of This Book

Working both independently and together over the years, the three of us have encountered a variety of professional and ethical issues that seem to have no clear-cut solutions. Conversations with students and colleagues reveal similar struggles. Exchanging ideas has helped us deal with these issues, and we extend this conversation to you throughout this book. We are convinced that students in the helping professions must anticipate and be prepared for these kinds of problems before their first fieldwork experience, and certainly before they begin practicing. The lack of clear-cut answers to ethical dilemmas can be frustrating, but engaging in a dialogue on these issues makes us all better clinicians and guides us toward better clinical outcomes.

We cannot dispense prescriptions or provide simple solutions to the complex situations you may encounter. Our main purpose is to facilitate critical thinking on your part and to establish a basis for you to develop a personal perspective on ethical practice within the broad limits of professional codes and divergent theoretical positions. We raise some central issues, present a range of views on these issues, discuss our position, and provide you with opportunities to refine your thinking and actively develop your own position. Many of these issues may resurface and take on different meanings at various stages in your professional life.

In this book we provide a flexible framework and a direction for working through ethical dilemmas. We have refined our ideas through our clinical experiences, our experiences teaching ethics, and by engaging in discussions with colleagues and students. We are passionate about the study of ethics because it requires that we (1) use critical thinking skills, (2) strengthen our own judgment and decision-making processes, (3) advocate for social justice issues, and (4) challenge culturally encapsulated standards in our profession.

As you read this book, you will discover our biases and viewpoints about ethical behavior. We clearly state that these represent our perspective and are not a universal standard. We offer our position not to sway you to adopt our views but to help you develop your own position. Identifying our own personal misconduct can be far more challenging than pointing out the misconduct of our colleagues, yet each of us must continually reflect on what we are doing personally and professionally. In the end, each of us is responsible for his or her own ethical practice.

You will encounter many situations that demand the exercise of sound judgment to further the best interests of your clients. Codes of ethics provide general standards, but these are not sufficiently explicit to deal with every situation. It is often difficult to interpret ethics codes, and opinions differ over how to apply them in specific cases. In all cases, the welfare of the client demands that you become familiar with the guiding principles of the ethics codes and accepted standards of practice of your profession.

The various mental health professions have developed codes of ethics that are binding for their members. Often students and practitioners confuse ethical and legal standards, or mistakenly assume that ethics are regulated by law. Ethics and the law are not synonymous (see Chapters 5 and 6). As a mental health provider, you are expected to know the ethics code of your professional organization and to be aware of the consequences of practicing in ways that are not sanctioned by the organization. Responsible practice requires that we use informed, sound, and responsible judgment. It is necessary that we demonstrate a willingness to consult with colleagues, keep up to date through reading and continuing education, and continually monitor our behavior.

We have reexamined many of the issues raised in this book throughout our professional lives. Levitt, Farry, and Mazzarella (2015) "suggest that experienced counselors still struggle with the gray areas of ethics, and what may seem like a straightforward issue rarely has clear resolutions" (pp. 94–95). Although you may think you have resolved some of these ethical and professional issues at the initial stage of your development as a counselor, these topics can take on new dimensions as you gain experience. Many students believe they should resolve all possible issues before they begin to practice, but this is an impossible task. The definition and refinement of such concerns is a developmental process that requires self-reflection, an open mind, and continual reexamination.

Some Suggestions for Using This Book

Introducing students to the many dimensions of thinking about ethical practice is essential even though our response to questions surrounding ethical issues and dilemmas often is "it depends." Although a lack of clear-cut answers can be viewed as anxiety-producing, we prefer to see it as liberating. The vast gray area within ethical decision making provides ample opportunity for creativity and empowerment as we grow as professionals.

We frequently imagine ourselves in conversations with you, our readers. We state our own thinking and offer a commentary on how we arrived at the positions we hold. We encourage you to integrate your own thoughts and experiences with the positions and ethical dilemmas we raise for consideration. In this way you will absorb information, deepen your understanding, and develop an ethical way of thinking. A main priority is to clarify your goals and to think about ways of becoming actively involved. To get the most from this book, we encourage you to focus on the following:

- *Preparation.* Prepare yourself to become active in your class by spending time reading and thinking about the questions we pose. Completing the exercises and responding to the questions and open-ended cases will help you focus on where you stand on controversial issues.
- *Expectations.* Students often have unrealistic expectations of themselves. If you have limited experience in counseling clients, think about situations in which friends sought your help and how you dealt with them. You can also reflect on the times when you were experiencing conflicts and needed someone to help you gain clarity. This is a way to relate the material to events in your own life.
- *The self-assessment survey.* The multiple-choice survey at the end of this chapter is designed to help you discover your attitudes concerning most of the issues

we discuss in the book. Take this inventory before you read the book to discover where you stand on these issues at this time. Take the inventory again after you complete the book to compare your responses to see what changes, if any, have occurred in your thinking.

- *Chapter self-inventories.* Each chapter begins with an inventory designed to encourage reflection on the issues to be explored in the chapter. Completing the inventory is a good way to focus your thinking on the topics in a chapter. Consider discussing your responses with your fellow students and peers. After reading the chapter and discussing the material in class, complete the inventory again to see if your position has changed in any way.
- *Learning objectives.* Found at the beginning of each chapter, the learning objectives guide you to focus on the main points presented in the chapter and serve as a checklist to help you assess the degree to which you have mastered these key topics.
- *Examples, cases, commentaries, and questions.* Many examples in this book are drawn from actual counseling practice in various settings with different types of clients. (Elements of these cases have been changed to protect confidentiality.) Consider how you might have worked with a given client or what you might have done in a particular counseling situation. We provide our commentary on each of the cases to guide you in clarifying the specific issues involved and in helping you think about the course of action you might take in each case. We also provide illustrations of possible therapist responses to the various ethical dilemmas in the cases, not all of which are ethical or appropriate.
- *End-of-chapter suggested activities.* These suggested activities are provided to help you integrate and apply what you have learned.
- *Code of ethics of various professional organizations.* A summary of relevant ethics codes of various professional groups is provided as boxed excerpts pertaining to the topics discussed in the chapter. You may want to visit the websites of these professional organizations and download their codes of ethics.
- *Engage in critical thinking.* Involve yourself in thinking about the issues we raise. Focus on the questions, cases, commentaries, and activities that have the most meaning for you at this time, and remain open to new issues as they assume importance for you. Develop your thoughts and positions on the ethical dilemmas presented. As you engage in discussions with your peers and faculty, be open to new perspectives on how to proceed through the ethical decision-making steps. By becoming actively involved in your ethics course, you will find additional ways to look at the process of ethical decision making.

Professional Codes of Ethics

Various professional organizations (counseling, social work, psychiatry, psychology, marriage and family therapy, human services) have established codes of ethics that provide broad guidelines for their members. The codes of these national professional organizations have similarities and also differences. Publications by the various professional organizations contain many resources to help you understand the issues underlying the ethical decisions you will be making in your professional life.

Common Themes of Codes of Ethics

Each major mental health professional organization has its own code of ethics. Obtain a copy of the ethics code of the profession you are planning to enter and familiarize yourself with its basic standards for ethical practice. You do not need to memorize every standard, but lacking knowledge of the ethics code of your profession is not an acceptable excuse for engaging in unethical behavior. The ethics codes are broad and general; they do not provide specific answers to the ethical dilemmas you will encounter. Although there are specific differences among the ethics codes of the various professional organizations, there are a number of similar themes:

- Being interested in the welfare of clients
- Practicing within the scope of one's competence
- Understanding and respecting the cultural values of clients
- Distinguishing between personal values and professional values
- Avoiding harm and exploitation
- Establishing and maintaining appropriate professional boundaries
- Protecting client's confidentiality and privacy
- Practicing within an ethical and legal framework
- Avoiding discrimination in providing services to clients
- Striving for the highest level of ethical practice
- Recognizing the importance of self-care as a basis for competent practice

Limitations of Codes of Ethics

Your own ethical awareness and problem-solving skills will determine how you translate the various ethics codes into professional behavior. The codes do not provide a blueprint for adequately dealing with all of the ethical challenges you will encounter, but they do represent the best judgment of one's peers about common ethical problems (Welfel, 2016). Codes of ethics are not cookbooks for responsible professional behavior; they do not provide recipes for effective ethical decision making. Indeed, ethics codes offer unmistakably clear guidance for only a few problems. The American Psychological Assocation's (APA) ethics code (2010) is quite clear that it neither provides all the answers nor specifically addresses every dilemma that may confront a practitioner. The ethical principles in the APA code are not enforceable rules, but they should be considered by psychologists in arriving at an ethical course of action. Pope and Vasquez (2016) remind us that ethics codes, standards, and laws are the beginning, not the end, of ethical considerations. They inform us but do not replace our effort in critically thinking through ethical issues. "Ethical decision making is a process and codes are only one part of that process" (p. 3). In short, ethics codes are necessary, but not sufficient, for exercising ethical responsibility. Ethics codes have a number of limitations (see Herlihy & Corey, 2015a; Knapp, Gottlieb, & Handelsman, 2015; Pope & Vasquez, 2016; Welfel, 2016). Problems you might encounter as you strive to be ethically responsible include the following:

- Some issues cannot be handled solely by relying on ethics codes.
- Ethics codes do not address the many situations that lie in an ethical gray zone.
- Some codes lack clarity and precision, which makes assessment of an ethical dilemma unclear.
- Simply learning the ethics codes and practice guidelines will not necessarily make for ethical practice.
- Answers to ethical dilemmas are not contained in the ethics codes.
- Conflicts sometimes emerge within ethics codes as well as among various organizations' codes.
- Ethics codes tend to be reactive rather than proactive.
- No set of rules or ethical standards can adequately guide practitioners through many of the complex situations they may encounter.
- New situations arise frequently, and no two cases are exactly the same.
- A practitioner's personal values may conflict with a specific professional value or standard within an ethics code.
- Codes may conflict with institutional policies and practices.
- Ethics codes need to be understood within a cultural framework; therefore, they need to be adapted to specific cultures.
- Codes may not align with state laws or regulations regarding reporting requirements.
- Codes of ethics are often updated and require continuing education and professional development throughout a professional's lifelong learning journey.

Using Ethics Codes as Guides

Formal ethical principles can never be substituted for an active, deliberative, and creative approach to meeting ethical responsibilities (Pope & Vasquez, 2016). Ethics codes cannot be applied in a rote manner because each client's situation is unique and may call for a different solution, which demands professional judgment. A *rule-based approach* to ethics is limited in providing meaningful assistance to clinicians who are concerned with practicing at the highest level of ethical functioning.

Becoming a professional is somewhat like learning to adjust to a different culture, and both students and professionals experience an ethical acculturation process. From our perspective, practitioners are faced with assuming the responsibility of making ethical decisions and ultimately taking responsibility for the outcomes. This process takes time, and it should include consultation. Even with many years of field experience, consultation with colleagues provides an important check on our thinking about various ethical issues.

Herlihy and Corey (2015a) suggest that codes of ethics fulfill three objectives. The first objective is to *educate professionals* about sound ethical conduct. Reading and reflecting on the standards can help practitioners expand their awareness and clarify their values in dealing with the challenges of their work. Second, ethical standards provide a *mechanism for professional accountability*. Practitioners are obliged not only to monitor their own behavior but also to encourage ethical conduct in their colleagues. One of the best ways for practitioners to guard the welfare of their clients or students and to protect themselves from malpractice suits is to practice within the spirit of the ethics codes. Third, codes of ethics serve as *catalysts for improving practice*. When practitioners interpret and apply the codes in their own practices, the questions raised help to clarify their positions on dilemmas that do not have simple or absolute answers. You can imagine the chaos if people were to practice without guidelines so that the resolution of ethical dilemmas rested solely with the individual clinician.

We must never forget that the primary purpose of a code of ethics is to safeguard the welfare of clients. Ethics codes are also designed to safeguard the public and to guide professionals in their work so that they can provide the best service possible. The *community standard* (what professionals *actually* do) is generally less rigorous than the ethical standard (what professionals *should* do). It is important to be knowledgeable of what others in your local area and subspecialties are doing in their practices.

Ethics Codes and the Law

Ethical issues in the mental health professions are regulated by both laws and professional codes. The Committee on Professional Practice and Standards (2003) of the American Psychological Association differentiates between ethics and law as follows: **ethics** pertains to the standards that govern the conduct of its professional members; **law** is the body of rules that govern the affairs of people within a community, state, or country. Laws define the minimum standards society will tolerate, which are enforced by government. An example of a minimum standard is the legal obligation mental health professionals have to report suspected child abuse. The law can also encourage us to work toward changing societal attitudes, for example, to prevent child abuse rather than merely to report it.

All of the codes of ethics state that practitioners are obligated to act in accordance with relevant federal and state statutes and government regulations. In a court case, the law generally overrules ethics. As ethical mental health practitioners, however, we can advocate for social justice both *with* and *on behalf of* our clients and the communities we serve. Practitioners should be able to identify legal problems as they arise in their work because many of the situations they encounter that involve ethical and professional judgment will also have legal implications.

Remley and Herlihy (2016) note that counselors sometimes have difficulty determining when there is a legal problem, or what to do with a legal issue once it has been identified. To clarify whether a legal issue is involved, it is important to assess the situation to determine if any of the following apply: (a) legal proceedings have been initiated, (b) lawyers are involved, or (c) the practitioner is in danger of having a complaint filed against him or her for misconduct. When confronted with a legal issue, consult a lawyer to determine which course of action to take. Remley and Herlihy do not advise consulting with counselor colleagues about how to deal with legal problems because counselors rarely have expertise in legal matters. Many professional associations have attorneys who are familiar with both legal and clinical issues, and members of these associations can use this source of consultation. Establish a working, collegial relationship with a local attorney in your state whom you can consult regarding legal issues. Some professionals have both a law degree and a mental health degree, which can be a useful resource.

Laws and ethics codes tend to emerge from what has occurred rather than from anticipating what may occur. Limiting your scope of practice to obeying statutes and following ethical standards is inadequate. We hope your behavior will not be determined by *fear-based ethics*. It is important to foster an attitude of *concern-based ethics* early in your training program, striving for the highest level of ethical care for your clients, a theme that is repeated many times throughout this book. Birrell and Bruns (2016) suggest that ethics is better viewed from a relational engagement rather than a risk management perspective. They contend that counselors need to release the fear of punishment and open themselves to authentic mutuality so that "ethics becomes relational and alive and fully integrated into each moment of the clinical encounter" (p. 396).

Ethical standards serve as a form of protection for the client, but they also help clinicians ensure their own self-care. For example, counselors sometimes struggle with setting limits around being helpful to others. Having clear guidelines in place can help you establish healthy boundaries for yourself, both personally and professionally.

At times you may encounter conflicts between the law and ethical principles, or competing ethical standards may appear to require incompatible courses of action. In these cases the values of the counselor come into play (Barnett & Johnson, 2015). Conflict between ethics codes and the law may arise in areas such as advertising, confidentiality, and clients' rights of access to their own files. If obeying one's professional code of ethics would result in disobeying the law, it is a good practice to seek legal advice. A licensed mental health professional also may contact his or her professional organization's legal department or state licensing board for consultation.

When laws and ethics collide, Knapp, Gottlieb, Berman, and Handelsman (2007) state that practitioners need first to verify what the law requires and determine the nature of their ethical obligations. Practitioners may not understand their legal requirements and may assume a conflict exists between the law and ethics when there is no such conflict. If there is a real conflict between the law and ethics, and if the conflict cannot be avoided, "psychologists should either obey the law in a manner that minimizes harm to their ethical values or adhere to their ethical values in a manner that minimizes the violation of the law" (Knapp et al., 2007, p. 55). Apparent conflicts between the law and ethics can often be avoided if clinicians anticipate problems in advance and take proactive measures.

One example of a potential conflict between legal and ethical standards involves counseling minors. This is especially true as it pertains to counseling children or adolescents in school settings. Counselors may be committed to following ethical standards in maintaining the confidentiality of the sessions with a minor, yet at times parents/legal guardians may have a legal right to information that is disclosed in these sessions. Practitioners may struggle between doing what they believe to be ethically appropriate for their client and their legal responsibilities to parents/legal guardians. When working with minors, it is necessary to be familiar both with state laws and with school policies. Some school districts may have rules regarding breaking confidentiality about substance abuse that differ from those of a private practitioner.

Mental health providers in the military are likely to experience ethical dilemmas when obligations to clients and obligations to the military organization conflict. Providers in military settings are occasionally forced to choose between client-centered therapeutic interests and organization-centered administrative interests (Johnson et al., 2010). These competing obligations can generate challenging ethical dilemmas. Information that is viewed as confidential in the civilian sector may not be protected from disclosure in a military setting. A commanding officer's need to know about the fitness of a service member may appear to conflict with the ethical values of privacy and confidentiality. Licensed health care providers in the military may struggle with apparent conflicts between their mandated and commissioned roles as military officers and their duty to their clients (Johnson & Johnson, 2017). Strategies for successfully managing these situations can be found, and Johnson, Grasso, and Maslowski (2010) state that "genuine conflict between an ethical and legal course of action—when abiding by law will automatically violate the code of ethics or vice versa—are infrequent occurrences" (p. 552).

In ethical dilemmas involving legal issues, a wise course is to seek advice from legal counsel and to discuss the situation with colleagues familiar with the law. When neither the law nor an ethics code seems to resolve an issue, therapists are advised to consider other professional and community standards and their own conscience as well. This subject is addressed more fully in Chapters 5 and 6.

Evolution of Ethics Codes

Codes of ethics are established by professional groups for the purpose of protecting consumers, providing guidelines for practitioners, and clarifying the professional stance of the organizations. Ethics codes undergo periodic revisions and are best viewed as living documents responsive to the needs of counselors, the clients they serve, and society in general. For example, the revised *Code of Ethics* of the American Counseling Association (ACA, 2014) addresses evolving ethical issues pertaining to ethical decision making, professional values, managing and maintaining boundaries, technology, the nonimposition of counselor personal values, counselor education, and legal issues, to mention a few—all of which were in response to recent developments in the field (Kaplan et al., 2017). A new section of the code covers informed consent, privacy, and security of electronic communications, distance counseling, online and research maintenance, and social media. Most professional associations revise their ethics codes every 5 to 10 years. It is necessary that the standards reflect changes in the profession and evolving social trends.

However useful the ethics codes may be, they can never replace the informed judgment and goodwill of the individual counselor. We emphasize again the need for a level of ethical functioning higher than merely following the letter of the law or the code. For instance, you might avoid a lawsuit by not paying attention to cultural diversity, but many of your ethnically diverse clients would likely suffer from your insensitive professional behavior.

Professional Monitoring of Practice

The legal and ethical practice of most mental health professionals is regulated in all 50 states. State licensing laws establish the scope of practice of professionals and how these laws will be enforced by licensing boards. Some psychotherapy professions are regulated through registration and certification; others, such as social workers, marriage and family therapists, professional counselors, and psychologists, are regulated through licensure. The major duties of regulating boards are (1) to determine standards for admission into the profession, (2) to screen applicants applying for certification or licensure, (3) to regulate the practice of psychotherapy for the public good, and (4) to conduct disciplinary proceedings involving violations of standards of professional conduct as defined by law. Mental health professionals can lose their certification or license if their state regulating board finds that they have engaged in unethical practice or illegal behavior, whether personally or professionally. The topic of licensure is treated in more detail in Chapter 8.

In addition to state regulatory boards, most professional organizations have ethics committees—elected or delegated bodies that oversee the conduct of members of the organization. The main purposes of ethics committees are to educate the association's membership about ethics codes and to protect the public from unethical practices. These committees meet regularly to process formal complaints against individual members of the professional organization, and they also revise and update their organization's code of ethics.

When necessary, practitioners must explain to clients how to lodge an ethical complaint. When a complaint is lodged against a member, the committee launches an investigation and deliberates on the case. Eventually, a disposition is reached. The complaint may be dismissed, specific charges within the complaint may be dismissed, or the committee may find that ethical standards have been violated and impose sanctions. Possible sanctions include a reprimand; a recommendation that a specific course of remedial action be taken, such as obtaining ongoing supervision or personal therapy; probation or suspension for a specified period of time; a recommendation that the member be allowed to resign from the organization; or a recommendation that the member be expelled.

Expulsion or suspension of a member is a major sanction. Members have the right to appeal the committee's decision. Once the appeals process has been completed or the deadline for appeal has passed, the sanctions of suspension and expulsion are communicated in writing to the members of the professional organization. Practitioners who are expelled from the association also may face the loss of their license or certificate to practice, but only if the state board conducts an independent investigation. Cases that result in expulsion are often serious enough to involve law enforcement and criminal charges. Many cases also result in civil court proceedings, which are usually published in the local press. Mental health professionals facing ethics violations may believe they were not given fair treatment by the ethics committee, and in such cases they can respond with their perspective.

Ethical Decision Making

Some Key Terms

Professional mental health workers are designated by a variety of terms: *mental health professional, practitioner, therapist, counselor, social worker, school counselor, rehabilitation counselor, addictions counselor, community worker, couples and family therapist, helper,* and *clinician*. Throughout this book, we generally use these terms interchangeably, reflecting the differing nomenclature of the various professions.

Although values and ethics are frequently used interchangeably, the two terms are not identical. **Values** pertains to beliefs and attitudes that provide direction to everyday living, whereas **ethics** pertains to the beliefs we hold about what constitutes right conduct. Ethics are moral principles adopted by an individual or group to provide rules for right conduct. **Morality** is concerned with perspectives of right and proper conduct and involves an evaluation of actions on the basis of some broader cultural context or religious standard.

Ethics represents aspirational goals, or the maximum or ideal standards set by the profession, practiced through your professional behavior and interactions (Remley & Herlihy, 2016). Codes of ethics are conceptually broad in nature and generally subject to interpretation by practitioners. Although these minimum and maximum standards may differ, they are not necessarily in conflict.

Community standards (or *mores*) vary on interdisciplinary, theoretical, and geographical bases. The standard for a counselor's social contact with clients may be different in a large urban area than in a rural area, or between practitioners employing a humanistic versus a behavioral approach. Community standards often become the ultimate *legal* criteria for determining whether practitioners are liable for damages. Community standards define what is considered reasonable behavior when a case involving malpractice is litigated. Courts have consistently found that mental health care providers have a duty to exercise a reasonable degree of skill, knowledge, and care. **Reasonableness** is usually defined as the care that is ordinarily exercised by others practicing within that specialty in the professional community.

Professionalism has some relationship to ethical behavior, yet it is possible to act unprofessionally and still not act unethically. For instance, not returning a client's telephone calls promptly might be viewed as unprofessional, but it would probably not be considered unethical unless the client were in crisis.

Some situations cut across these concepts. For example, sexual intimacy between counselors and clients is considered unethical, unprofessional, immoral, and illegal. Keep the differences in the meanings of these various concepts in mind as you read.

Levels of Ethical Practice

One way of conceptualizing professional ethics is to contrast mandatory ethics with aspirational ethics. **Mandatory ethics** describes a level of ethical functioning wherein counselors act in compliance with minimal standards, acknowledging the basic "musts" and "must nots." The focus is on behavioral rules, such as providing for informed consent in professional relationships. **Aspirational ethics** describes the highest standards of thinking and conduct professional counselors seek, and it requires that counselors do more than simply meet the letter of the ethics code. It entails an understanding of the spirit behind the code and the principles on which the code rests. Each section in the ACA's *Code of Ethics* (2014) begins with an introduction, which sets the tone and addresses what counselors should aspire to with regard to ethical practice. Practitioners who comply at the first level, *mandatory ethics*, are generally safe from legal action in courts of law or professional censure by state licensure boards. At the higher level of ethical functioning, *aspirational ethics*, practitioners go further and reflect on the effects their interventions may have on the welfare of their clients. An example of aspirational ethics is providing services for no fees (pro bono) for those in the community who cannot afford needed services.

Positive ethics focuses not only on how professionals can harm clients but on how therapists can do better at helping clients. Instead of focusing on a remedial approach to dealing with an ethical matter, positive ethics requires "anchoring all professional behavior and decisions in an overarching ethical philosophy of what psychologists can be, not simply avoiding what they should not do" (Knapp et al., 2015, p. 7). The goal of positive ethics shifts the emphasis of mental health providers away from a focus on wrongdoing and disciplinary actions and toward an articulated vision of the highest level of practice (Knapp & Vande-Creek, 2012).

When the word **unethical** is used, people think of extreme violations of established codes. In reality, most violations of ethics probably happen quite inadvertently in clinical practice. The ethics codes of most professional organizations require practitioners to engage in self-monitoring and to take responsibility for misconduct. Welfel (2005) indicates that the professional literature focuses on preventing misconduct and on responding to serious ethical violations. However, the literature has not offered much guidance regarding minor infractions committed by professionals. Welfel states that by taking minor ethical violations seriously and by seeking honest ways to remediate such infractions, counselors can demonstrate their professionalism and personal commitment to benefiting those they serve.

Welfel's (2005) model progresses from awareness, through reflection, to a plan of action whereby counselors can ethically repair damage when they recognize they have violated ethics codes in minor ways. She emphasizes that the first step in recovering from an ethical violation is for the practitioner to recognize that he or she has acted in a way that is likely to be ethically problematic. If a practitioner is not aware of the subtle ways his or her behavior can adversely affect the client, such behavior can go unnoticed, and the client will suffer. For instance, a professional who is struggling financially in her private practice may prolong the therapy of her clients and justify her actions on theoretical grounds. She is likely to ignore the fact that the prolongation of therapy is influenced by her financial situation.

Practitioners can easily find themselves in an ethical quagmire based on competing role expectations. The best way to maintain a clear ethical position is to focus on your clients' best interests. School counselors may be so focused on academic and scheduling issues that they do not reach out to the community and develop the network with other helping professionals needed to make productive referrals for families and students in crises. In school systems teachers and others sometimes label students and families as dysfunctional or unmotivated. The counselor needs to advocate and help others look for strengths and reframe limitations if progress is to be made. The counselor can be an ethical model in a system where ethics is not given much consideration.

Clients' needs are best met when practitioners monitor their own ethics. Ethical violations may go undetected because only the individual who committed the violation knows about it. Rather than just looking at others and proclaiming "That's unethical!" we encourage you to honestly examine your own thinking and apply guidelines to your behavior by asking yourself, "Is what I am doing in the best interests of my clients? Would the codes of my professional organization agree? Am I practicing my own self-care and maintaining healthy boundaries in the decisions I am making with my clients?" Self-evaluation and reflection is an ongoing process that both benefits our clients and enriches our personal and professional growth.

Principle Ethics and Virtue Ethics

Several writers have developed models for ethical decision making, including Barnett and Johnson (2008, 2015), Cottone (2001), Cottone and Tarvydas (2016), Forester-Miller and Davis (2016), Frame and Williams (2005), Kitchener (1984), Knapp and colleagues (2015), Knapp and VandeCreek (2012), Koocher and Keith-Spiegel (2016), Meara, Schmidt, and Day (1996), Welfel (2016), and Wheeler and Bertram (2015). This section is based on an amalgamation of elements from these various models and our own views.

In a key article titled "Principles and Virtues: A Foundation for Ethical Decisions, Policies, and Character," Meara and colleagues (1996) differentiate between principle ethics and virtue ethics. **Principle ethics** is a set of obligations and a method that focuses on moral issues with the goals of (a) solving a particular dilemma or set of dilemmas and (b) establishing a framework to guide future ethical thinking and behavior. Principles typically focus on acts and choices, and they are used to facilitate the selection of socially and historically acceptable answers to the question "What shall I do?"

A thorough grounding in principle ethics opens the way for another important perspective, virtue ethics. **Virtue ethics** focuses on the character traits of the counselor and nonobligatory ideals to which professionals aspire rather than on solving specific ethical dilemmas. Simply stated, principle ethics asks "Is this situation unethical?" whereas virtue ethics asks "Am I doing what is best for my client?" Even in the absence of an ethical dilemma, virtue ethics compels the professional to be conscious of ethical behavior. Meara and her colleagues maintain that it is not a question of subscribing to one or the other form of ethics. Rather, professional counselors should strive to integrate virtue ethics and principle ethics to reach better ethical decisions and policies.

Some mental health practitioners concern themselves primarily with avoiding malpractice suits. They tend to commit themselves to a rule-bound approach to ethics as a way to stay out of trouble. Other professionals, although concerned with avoiding litigation, are first and foremost interested in doing what is best for their clients. These professionals would consider it unethical to use techniques that might not result in the greatest benefit to their clients or to use techniques in which they were not thoroughly trained, even though these techniques might not lead to a lawsuit.

Meara and colleagues (1996) identify four core virtues—prudence, integrity, respectfulness, and benevolence—that are appropriate for professionals to adhere to in making ethical decisions. They also describe five characteristics of virtuous professionals, which they see as being at the heart of virtue ethics:

- Virtuous agents are motivated to do what is right because they judge it to be right, not just because they feel obligated or fear the consequences.
- Virtuous agents rely on vision and discernment, which involve sensitivity, judgment, and understanding that lead to decisive action.
- Virtuous agents have compassion and are sensitive to the suffering of others. They are able to take actions to reduce their clients' pain.
- Virtuous agents are self-aware. They know how their assumptions, convictions, and biases are likely to affect their interactions with others.
- Virtuous agents are connected with and understand the mores of their community and the importance of community in moral decision making, policy setting, and character development. They understand the ideals and expectations of their community.

Virtue ethics focuses on ideals rather than obligations and on the character of the professional rather than on the action itself. To meet the goals, ideals, and needs of the community being served, consider both principles and virtues because both are important elements in thinking through ethical concerns.

A Case of Positive Ethics

Your client, Kevin, is making good progress in his counseling with you. Then he informs you that he has lost his job and will not be able to continue seeing you because of his inability to pay your fees. Here is how four different therapists handled a similar situation.

Therapist A: I'm sorry but I can't continue seeing you without payment. I'm giving you the name of a local community clinic that provides low-cost treatment.

Therapist B: I don't usually see people without payment, but I appreciate the difficulty you find yourself in. I'll continue to see you, and you pay whatever portion of my fee you can afford.

Therapist C: I suggest that you put therapy on hold until you can financially afford it.

Therapist D: I can't afford to see you without payment, but I am willing to suggest an alternative plan. Continue writing in your journal, and once a month I will see you for half an hour to discuss your journal. You pay what you can afford for these sessions. When your financial situation has been corrected, we can continue therapy as usual.

- How do you react to the various therapists' responses?
- Which response appeals to you and why?
- Can you think of another response?

- Would you be willing to see this client without payment? Why or why not?
- Would you consider bartering in place of charging a fee? Why or why not?
- Would you consider a sliding scale for this client?
- Do you have concerns about the responses of any of these therapists?

In considering what you might do if you were the therapist in this case, reflect on the standards pertaining to **pro bono services** found in the ethics codes of National Association of Social Workers (NASW, 2008), ACA (2014), and APA (2010). All three codes encourage practitioners to contribute to society by devoting a portion of their professional time and skills to services for which there is no expectation of significant financial return.

Commentary. This case is a good example of how positive ethics can become operational. A counselor operating from the framework of positive ethics is motivated to look for ways to be of the greatest assistance possible to clients. Positive ethics is concerned with how exemplary behavior can be applied to a difficult situation, such as a client no longer able to afford psychological services (Knapp & VandeCreek, 2012). You could continue to see Kevin as part of your pro bono services, or, as therapists B and D suggested, you might find a creative strategy to help Kevin remain in counseling while changing your fee or the frequency of counseling.

There is no simple solution to this case. It involves the therapist, the client, the setting, and the situation, all of which need to be considered in context. When a client can no longer pay for services, the therapist must not abandon the client. If treatment is to be terminated, at least a few sessions should be offered to assist Kevin in working through termination issues and this loss of support. In addition, you could refer Kevin to an agency that would see him without a fee, such as a qualified counselor in a community mental health center, or to a professional who uses a sliding fee scale, or to a beginning therapist who is building his or her practice. There are many appropriate ways to deal with this situation. The ACA (2014) *Code of Ethics* states that counselors may adjust fees if the usual charge creates an undue hardship for the client (Standard A.10.c.). Although it is important to take care of your clients, you do not want to do so at the expense to yourself, which could lead to resentment that negatively affects your treatment of this client. If you adjust your fee by using a sliding scale, it needs to be done with consideration to your financial needs and responsibilities. In response to Kevin's job loss, you must still promote his best interests and minimize harm, while simultaneously remaining realistic about your own financial situation and the realities of your work setting. Bartering with your client for services is another alternative. This choice is generally not clinically or ethically advisable, but it may be an appropriate and culturally relevant solution with some clients. Ethical and practice guidelines for bartering are addressed in Chapter 7. •

Moral Principles to Guide Decision Making

Building on the work of others, especially Kitchener (1984), Meara and colleagues (1996) describe six basic moral principles that form the foundation of functioning at the highest ethical level as a professional: *autonomy, nonmaleficence, beneficence, justice, fidelity,* and *veracity.* Applying these ethical principles and the related ethical standards is not as simple as it may seem, especially when dealing with culturally diverse populations and social justice concerns. (See Chapters 4 and 13 for more on these issues.) These moral principles involve a process of striving that is never fully complete. We describe each of these six basic moral principles, cite a specific ethical guideline from the ACA, APA, or NASW, and provide a brief discussion of the cultural implications of using each principle.

- **Autonomy** refers to the promotion of self-determination, or the freedom of clients to be self-governing within their social and cultural framework. Respect for autonomy entails acknowledging the right of another to choose and act in accordance with his or her wishes and values, and the professional behaves in a way that enables this right of another person. Practitioners strive to decrease client dependency and foster client empowerment. The ACA's (2014) introduction to Section A states it this way:

> Counselors facilitate client growth and development in ways that foster the interest and welfare of clients and promote formation of healthy relationships.
>
> Trust is the cornerstone of the counseling relationship, and the counselors have the responsibility to respect and safeguard the client's right to privacy and confidentiality. Counselors actively attempt to understand the diverse cultural backgrounds of the clients they serve. Counselors also explore their own cultural identities and how these affect their values and beliefs about the counseling process.

The helping services in the United States are typically based on traditional Western values of individualism, independence, interdependence, self-determination, and making choices for oneself. It often appears as though Western cultures promote individualism above any other cultural value. However, many cultures follow a different path, stressing decisions with the welfare of the family and the community as a priority. As the ACA standard described here implies, ethical practice involves considering the influence of cultural variables in the counseling relationship.

We cannot apply a rigid yardstick of what is a value priority in any culture without exploring how a particular client views priorities. For instance, what are the implications of the principle of autonomy when applied to clients who do not place a high priority on the value of being autonomous? Does it constitute an imposition of values for counselors to steer clients toward autonomous behavior when such behavior could lead to problems with others in their family, community, or culture?

- **Nonmaleficence** means avoiding doing harm, which includes refraining from actions that risk hurting clients. Professionals have a responsibility to minimize risks for exploitation and practices that cause harm or have the potential to result in harm. The APA (2010) principle of beneficence and nonmaleficence states,

> Psychologists strive to benefit those with whom they work and take care to do no harm.

What are the cultural implications of the principle of nonmaleficence? Traditional diagnostic practices can be inappropriate for certain cultural groups. For instance, a therapist may assign a diagnostic label to a client based on a pattern of behavior the therapist judges to be abnormal, such as inhibition of emotional expression, hesitation to confront, being cautious about self-disclosing, or not making direct eye contact while speaking. Yet these behaviors may be considered normal in certain cultures. Another example may be a school counselor who inappropriately labels a boy ADHD, which may color the perceptions of other staff members in a negative way so they pressure the parents to put the boy on medication. Practitioners need to develop cultural awareness and sensitivity in using assessment, diagnostic, and treatment procedures.

- **Beneficence** refers to doing good for others and to promoting the well-being of clients. Beneficence also includes concern for the welfare of society and doing good for society. Beneficence implies being proactive and preventing harm when possible (Forester-Miller & Davis, 2016). Ideally, counseling contributes to the growth and development of clients within their cultural context. Whatever practitioners do can be judged against this criterion. The following ACA (2014) guideline illustrates beneficence:

> The primary responsibility of counselors is to respect the dignity and to promote the welfare of clients. (A.1.a.)

Consider the possible consequences of a therapist encouraging an Asian client to behave more assertively toward his father. The reality of this situation may be that the father would refuse to speak again to a son who confronted him. Even though counselors may be operating with good intentions and may think they are being beneficent, they may not always be doing what is in the best interest of the client. Is it possible for counselors to harm clients unintentionally by encouraging a course of action that has negative consequences? How can counselors know what is in the best interest of their clients? How can counselors determine whether their interventions will work for their clients? As we have previously stated, there are no simple answers to complex questions.

- **Justice** means to be fair by giving equally to others and to treat others justly. Practitioners have a responsibility to provide appropriate services to all clients and to treat clients fairly. Everyone, regardless of age, sex, race, ethnicity, disability, socioeconomic status, cultural background, religion, or sexual orientation, is entitled to equal access to mental health services. An example might be a social worker making a home visit to a parent who cannot come to the school because of transportation, child care matters, or poverty. NASW's (2008) guideline illustrates this principle:

> Social workers pursue social change, particularly with and on behalf of vulnerable and oppressed individuals and groups of people. Social workers' social change efforts are focused primarily on issues of poverty, unemployment, discrimination, and other forms of social injustice. These activities seek to promote sensitivity to and knowledge about oppression and cultural and ethnic diversity. Social workers strive to ensure access to needed information, services, and resources; equality of opportunity; and meaningful participation in decision making for all people. (Ethical Principles, Social Justice.)

Traditional mental health services may not be just and fair to everyone in a culturally diverse society. If intervention strategies are not relevant to some segments of the population, justice is being violated. How can practitioners adapt the techniques they use to fit the needs of diverse populations? How can new helping strategies be developed that are consistent with the worldview of culturally different clients?

- **Fidelity** means that professionals make realistic commitments and do their best to keep these promises. This entails fulfilling one's responsibilities of trust in a relationship. Fidelity involves loyalty to clients and to making their welfare of primary concern. ACA's (2014) *Code of Ethics* encourages counselors to inform clients about counseling and to be faithful in keeping commitments made to clients:

> Clients have the freedom to choose whether to enter into or remain in a counseling relationship and need adequate information about the counseling process and the counselor. Counselors have an obligation to review in writing and verbally with clients the rights and responsibilities of both counselors and clients. Informed consent is an ongoing part of the counseling process, and counselors appropriately document discussions of informed consent throughout the counseling relationship. (A.2.a.)

Fidelity involves creating a trusting and therapeutic relationship in which people can search for solutions. However, what about clients whose culture teaches them that counselors are experts whose job is to provide answers for specific problem situations? What if a client expects the counselor to behave in this way? If the counselor does not meet the client's expectations, is trust being established?

- **Veracity** means truthfulness, which involves the practitioner's obligation to deal honestly with clients. Unless practitioners are truthful with their clients, the trust required to form a good working relationship will not develop. Veracity encompasses being truthful in all of our interactions, not just with our clients but also with our colleagues (Kaplan et al., 2017).

The six principles discussed here are a good place to start in determining the degree to which your practice is consistent with promoting the welfare of the clients you serve. To this list, Wise and Barnett (2016) add **self-care**, which involves taking adequate care of ourselves so that we are able to implement the moral principles and virtues that are fundamental ethical concepts. If mental health professionals do not practice self-care, they will be unable to effectively implement these moral principles. Self-care is an ethical imperative and is vital to gaining and maintaining competence as a counselor (Wise, Hersh, & Gibson, 2012). It is often difficult for counselors to shift their focus from clients to themselves; however, self-care is a prerequisite to being able to take care of others.

Counselors may be faced with a conflict between certain ethical principles such as the client's autonomy and self-determination versus the counselor's duty to take action to protect the client from harm. For example, hospitalizing a client against his or her wishes is a restriction of freedom, yet not taking action could result in the client's death (Wheeler & Bertram, 2015). At times, therapists may need to balance other ethical principles (especially nonmaleficence) with autonomy. Rosenfeld (2011) has written about problems associated with overly respecting client self-determination and autonomy when harmful religious beliefs and practices are not challenged. Rosenfeld's point may be well-taken, yet it does raise the fundamental question, "Who decides what constitutes harmful religious beliefs and practices?"

Steps in Making Ethical Decisions

When making ethical decisions, ask yourself these questions: "Which values do I rely on and why?" "How do my values affect my work with clients?" "Do my personal values have a place in my professional work?" When making ethical decisions, the National Association of Social Workers (2008) cautions you to be aware of your clients' as well as your own personal values, cultural and religious beliefs, and practices. Acting responsibly implies recognizing any conflicts between personal and professional values and dealing with them effectively. The American Counseling Association's (2014) *Code of Ethics* states that when counselors encounter an ethical dilemma, they are expected to carefully consider an ethical decision-making process. To make sound ethical decisions, it is necessary to slow down the decision-making process and engage in an intentional course of ethical deliberation, consultation, and action (Barnett & Johnson, 2015). Furthermore, when engaging in an ethical decision-making process, documentation of this process is important in case you are questioned about your choices, actions, and behaviors. Although no one ethical decision-making model is most effective, mental health professionals need to be familiar with at least one of the models or an amalgam that best fits for them.

Ethical decision making is *not* a purely cognitive and linear process that follows clearly defined and predictable steps. Indeed, it is crucial to acknowledge that emotions play a part in how you make ethical decisions. As a practitioner, your feelings will likely influence how you interpret both your client's behavior and your own behavior. Furthermore, if you are uncomfortable with an ethical decision and do not adequately deal with this discomfort, it will certainly influence your future behavior with your client. An integral part of recognizing and working through an ethical concern is discussing your beliefs and values, motivations, feelings, and actions with a supervisor or a colleague.

In the process of making the best ethical decisions, it is also important to *involve your clients* whenever possible. Because you are making decisions about what is best for their welfare, it is appropriate to discuss the nature of the ethical dilemma that pertains to them. For instance, ethical decision making from a feminist therapy perspective calls for involving the client at every stage of the therapeutic process, which is based on the feminist principle that power should be equalized in the therapeutic relationship (Brown, 2010).

Consulting with the client fully and appropriately is a fundamental step in ethical decision making, for doing so increases the chances of making the best possible decision. Walden (2015) suggests that important therapeutic benefits can result from inclusion of the client in the ethical decision-making process, and she offers some strategies for accomplishing this goal at both the organizational and individual levels. When we make decisions about a client *for* the client rather than *with* the client, Walden maintains that we rob the client of power in the relationship. When we collaborate with clients, they are empowered. By soliciting the client's perspective, we stand a good chance of achieving better counseling results and the best resolution for any ethical questions that arise. Potential therapeutic benefits can be gained by including clients in dealing with ethical concerns, and this practice represents functioning at the aspirational level. In fact, Walden questions whether it is truly possible to attain the aspirational level of ethical functioning *without* including the client's voice in ethical concerns. By adding the voice and the unique perspective of the consumers of professional services, we indicate to the public that we as a profession are genuinely interested in protecting the rights and welfare of those who make use of our services. Bringing the client into ethical matters entails few risks, and both the client and the professional may benefit from this collaboration.

The **social constructionist model** of ethical decision making shares some aspects with the feminist model but focuses primarily on the social aspects of decision making in counseling (Cottone, 2001). This model redefines the ethical decision-making process as an interactive rather than an individual or intrapsychic process and places the decision in the social context itself, not in the mind of the person making the decision. This approach involves negotiating, consensualizing, and when necessary, arbitrating.

Garcia, Cartwright, Winston, and Borzuchowska (2003) describe a **transcultural integrative model** of ethical decision making that addresses the need for including cultural factors in the process of resolving ethical dilemmas. They present their model in a step-by-step format that counselors can use in dealing with ethical dilemmas in a variety of settings and with different client populations. Frame and Williams (2005) have developed a model of ethical decision making from a multicultural perspective based on universalist philosophy. In this model cultural differences are recognized, but common principles such as altruism, responsibility, justice, and caring that link cultures are emphasized.

Many of the ethical dilemmas we will encounter are not likely to have a readily apparent answer. Birrell and Bruns (2016) assert that answers to ethical matters are not contained in the code of ethics, no matter how detailed. The ethical encounter and ethical moments cannot be codified or reified or legalized. Relational ethics is about learning how to tolerate ambiguity and uncertainty. "Counselors can only struggle toward answers in the shared search toward mutuality and interdependence, which has the capacity to bring healing to the individuals they serve" (p. 396). Keeping in mind the feminist model of ethical decision making, Walden's (2015) views on including the client's voice in ethical concerns, a social constructionist approach to ethics, and a transcultural integrative model of ethical decision making, we present our approach to thinking through ethical dilemmas. Following these steps may help you think through ethical problems.

1. *Identify the problem or dilemma.* It is important to determine whether a situation truly involves ethics. To determine the nature of the problem or dilemma, gather all the information that sheds light on the situation. Clarify whether the conflict is ethical, legal, clinical, cultural, professional, or moral—or a combination of any or all of these. The first step toward resolving an ethical dilemma is recognizing that a problem exists and identifying its specific nature. Because ethical decision making in practice is a complex and multifaceted process, it is useful to look at the problem from many perspectives and to avoid relying on a simple solution (Levitt et al., 2015). Consultation with your client begins at this initial stage and continues

throughout the process of working toward an ethical decision, as does the process of documenting your decisions and actions. Frame and Williams (2005) suggest reflecting on these questions to identify and define an ethical dilemma: What is the crux of the dilemma? Who is involved? What are the stakes? What values of mine are involved? What cultural and historical factors are in play? What insights does my client have regarding the dilemma? How is the client affected by the various aspects of the problem? What are my insights about the problem? Taking time to engage in reflection is a basic first step.

2. *Identify the potential issues involved.* After the information is collected, list and describe the critical issues and discard the irrelevant ones. Evaluate the rights, responsibilities, and welfare of all those who are affected by the situation. Consider the cultural context of the situation, including relevant cultural dimensions of the client's situation such as culture, race, socioeconomic status, and religious or spiritual background. Other relevant variables include the client's age and the client's relationship with other family members. It is important to consider the context of power and privilege and also to assess acculturation and racial identity development of the client (Frame & Williams, 2005). Part of the process of making ethical decisions involves identifying and examining the ethical principles that are relevant in the situation. Consider the six fundamental moral principles of autonomy, nonmaleficence, beneficence, justice, fidelity, and veracity and apply them to the situation, including those that may be in conflict. It may help to prioritize these ethical principles and think through ways in which they can support a resolution to the dilemma. Reasons can be presented that support various sides of a given issue, and different ethical principles may sometimes imply contradictory courses of action. When it is appropriate, and to the degree that it is possible, involve your client in identifying potential issues in the situation.

3. *Review the relevant ethics codes.* Consult available guidelines that could apply in your situation. Ask yourself whether the standards or principles of your professional organization offer a possible solution to the problem. Consider whether your own values and ethics are consistent with, or in conflict with, the relevant codes. If you are in disagreement with a particular standard, do you have a rationale to support your position? It is imperative to document this process to demonstrate your conscientious commitment to solving a dilemma. You can also seek guidance from your professional organization on any specific concern relating to an ethical or legal situation. Most of the national professional organizations provide members with access to a telephone discussion of ethical and legal issues. These consultations focus on giving members guidance in understanding and applying the code of ethics to a particular situation and in assisting members in exploring relevant questions. However, these consultations do not tell members what to do, nor does the organization assume responsibility for making the decision.

4. *Know the applicable laws and regulations.* It is necessary that you keep up to date on relevant state and federal laws that might apply to ethical dilemmas. In addition, be sure you understand the current rules and regulations of the agency or organization where you work. This is especially critical in matters of keeping or breaching confidentiality, reporting child or elder abuse, dealing with issues

pertaining to danger to self or others, parental rights, record keeping, assessment, diagnosis, licensing statutes, and the grounds for malpractice. However, realize that knowledge of the laws and regulations are not sufficient in addressing a dilemma. As Welfel (2016) aptly puts it, "rules, laws, and codes must be fully understood to act responsibly, but they are the starting point of truly ethical action, not the end point" (p. 24).

5. *Obtain consultation.* You do not have to make ethical decisions alone, but it is important to maintain client confidentiality when consulting others. It is generally helpful to consult with several trusted colleagues to obtain different perspectives on the area of concern and to arrive at the best possible decision. Consultation can uncover ideas that you have not considered, and it can also help you gain objectivity. As a counselor, it is expected that you will seek consultation and supervision, even if these sources are not available in your work setting (Levitt et al., 2015). Wheeler and Bertram (2015) suggest that two heads are better than one, and that three heads are often even better! Do not consult only with those who share your viewpoint. If there is a legal question, seek legal counsel. If the ethical dilemma involves working with a client from a different culture or who has a different worldview than yours, it is prudent to consult with a person who has expertise in this culture. If a clinical issue is involved, seek consultation from a professional with appropriate clinical expertise. After you present your assessment of the situation and your ideas of how you might proceed, ask for feedback on your analysis. Are there factors you are not considering? Have you thoroughly examined all of the ethical, clinical, and legal issues involved in the case? It is always wise to document the nature of your consultation, including the suggestions provided by those with whom you consulted. In court cases, a record of consultation illustrates that you have attempted to adhere to community standards by finding out what your colleagues in the community would do in the same situation. In an investigation the "reasonable person" standard may be applied: "What would a professional in your community with 3 years' experience have done in your situation?"

6. *Consider possible and probable courses of action.* At this point, take time to think about the range of courses of actions. Brainstorm to identify multiple options for dealing with the situation. Generate a variety of possible solutions to the dilemma (Frame & Williams, 2005). Consider the ethical and legal implications of the possible solutions you have identified. What do you think is likely to happen if you implement each option? By listing a wide variety of courses of action, you may identify a possibility that is unorthodox but useful. Be creative and list as many options as you can think of, even if you are not sure an option will work (Forester-Miller & Davis, 2016). Of course, one alternative is that no action is required. As you think about the many possibilities for action, discuss these options with your client as well as with other professionals and document these discussions.

7. *Enumerate and consider the possible consequences of various decisions.* Consider the implications of each course of action for the client, for others who will be affected, and for you as the counselor (Forester-Miller & Davis, 2016). Examine the probable outcomes of various actions, considering the potential risks and benefits of each

course of action. Again, collaboration with your client about consequences for him or her is most important, for doing this can lead to your client's empowerment. Use the six fundamental moral principles (autonomy, nonmaleficence, beneficence, justice, fidelity, and veracity) as a framework for evaluating the consequences of a given course of action. Realize that there are likely to be multiple outcomes rather than a single desired outcome in dealing with an ethical dilemma. Continue to reflect on other options and consult with colleagues who may see possibilities you have not considered.

8. *Choose what appears to be the best course of action.* To make the best decision, carefully consider the information you have received from various sources. The more obvious the dilemma, the clearer the course of action; the more subtle the dilemma, the more difficult the decision will be. After deciding, try not to second-guess your course of action. You may wonder if you have made the best decision in a given situation, or you may realize later that another action might have been more beneficial. Hindsight does not invalidate the decision you made based on the information you had at the time. Once your decision has been enacted, follow up to assess whether your actions had the desired outcomes (Forester-Miller & Davis, 2016). Evaluate your course of action by asking these questions (Frame & Williams, 2005): How does my action fit with the code of ethics of my profession? To what degree does the action taken consider the cultural values and experiences of the client? How might others evaluate my action? What did I learn from dealing with this ethical dilemma? Once you have decided on a course of action, remain open to the possibility that circumstances may require that you make adjustments to your plan. Wheeler and Bertram (2015) recommend careful documentation of the ethical decision-making process you used in arriving at a course of action, including the options you considered and ruled out. It is important to document the outcome and to include any additional actions that were taken to resolve the issue. We also recommend documenting any consultations you had to help in the decision-making process. Review your notes and follow up to determine the outcomes and whether further action is needed. To obtain the most accurate picture, involve your client in this process.

The goal of any ethical decision-making process is to help you take into account all relevant facts, use any resources available to you, and reason through the dilemma in a way that points to the best possible course of action. Clinicians have different perspectives and values, which are a part of their decision-making process, and ethical issues can have diverse outcomes. Reflecting on your assessment of the situation and on the actions you have taken is essential. By following a systematic model, you can be assured that you will be able to provide a rationale for the course of action you chose (Forester-Miller & Davis, 2016). The procedural steps we have listed here should not be thought of as a simple and linear way to reach a resolution on ethical matters. However, we have found that these steps do stimulate self-reflection and encourage discussion with clients and colleagues. Using this process, we are confident that you will find a solution that is helpful for your client, your profession, and yourself.

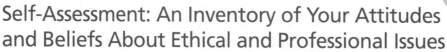

Self-Assessment: An Inventory of Your Attitudes and Beliefs About Ethical and Professional Issues

This inventory surveys your thoughts on various professional and ethical issues in the helping professions. It is designed to introduce you to issues and topics presented in this book and to stimulate your thoughts and interest. You may want to complete the inventory in more than one sitting, giving each question full concentration.

This is not a traditional multiple-choice test in which you must select the "one right answer." Rather, it is a survey of your basic beliefs, attitudes, and values on specific topics related to the practice of therapy. For each question, write in the letter of the response that most clearly reflects your view at this time. In many cases the answers are not mutually exclusive, and you may choose more than one response if you wish. In addition, a blank line is included for each item so you can provide a response more suited to your thinking or to qualify a chosen response.

Notice that there are two spaces before each item. Use the space on the left for your answer at the beginning of the course. At the end of the course, take this inventory again, placing your answer in the space on the right. Cover your initial answers so as not to be influenced by how you originally responded. Then you can see how your attitudes have changed as a result of your experience in the course. Engaging in open and honest discussions with your peers and faculty surrounding your answers both before and after your course will further aid in your self-reflection and growth.

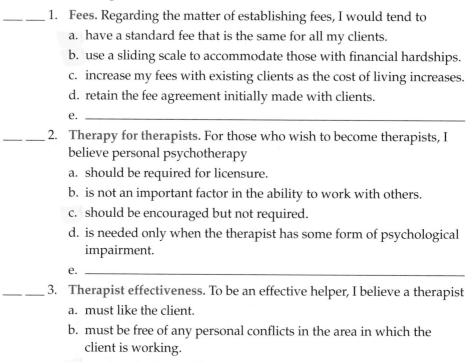

___ ___ 1. **Fees.** Regarding the matter of establishing fees, I would tend to

     a. have a standard fee that is the same for all my clients.

     b. use a sliding scale to accommodate those with financial hardships.

     c. increase my fees with existing clients as the cost of living increases.

     d. retain the fee agreement initially made with clients.

     e. _____

___ ___ 2. **Therapy for therapists.** For those who wish to become therapists, I believe personal psychotherapy

     a. should be required for licensure.

     b. is not an important factor in the ability to work with others.

     c. should be encouraged but not required.

     d. is needed only when the therapist has some form of psychological impairment.

     e. _____

___ ___ 3. **Therapist effectiveness.** To be an effective helper, I believe a therapist

     a. must like the client.

     b. must be free of any personal conflicts in the area in which the client is working.

     c. needs to be licensed by the state.

d. needs to have experienced feelings or situations similar to those being experienced by the client, but not necessarily the same problem.

e. _____

____ ____ 4. **Ethical decision making.** If I were faced with an ethical dilemma, the first step I would take would be to

a. review the relevant ethics codes.

b. consult with an attorney.

c. identify the problem or dilemma.

d. decide on what appears to be the best course of action.

e. _____

____ ____ 5. **Being ethical.** For me, being an ethical practitioner *mainly* entails

a. acting in compliance with mandatory ethical standards.

b. reflecting on the effects my interventions are likely to have on the welfare of my clients.

c. avoiding obvious violations of my profession's ethics codes.

d. thinking about the legal implications of everything I do.

e. _____

____ ____ 6. **Unethical supervisor.** If I was an intern and was convinced that my supervisor was encouraging trainees to participate in unethical behavior in an agency setting, I would

a. first discuss the matter with the supervisor.

b. report the supervisor to the director of the agency.

c. ignore the situation for fear of negative consequences.

d. report the situation to the ethics committee of the state professional association.

e. _____

____ ____ 7. **Multicultural knowledge and skills.** Practitioners who work with culturally diverse groups without having multicultural knowledge and skills

a. may be insensitive to their clients.

b. may be guilty of unethical behavior.

c. should realize the need for specialized training.

d. may be acting illegally.

e. _____

____ ____ 8. **Feelings toward clients.** If I had strong feelings, positive or negative, toward a client, I would most likely

a. discuss the feelings with my client.

b. keep my feelings to myself.

c. discuss my feelings with a supervisor or colleague.

d. accept my feelings unless they began to interfere with the counseling relationship.

e. _____

_____ _____ 9. **Being ready.** I won't be ready to counsel others until
   a. my own life is free of major problems.
   b. I have experienced counseling as a client.
   c. I feel confident and know that I will be effective.
   d. I have developed the ability to examine my own life and relationships.
   e. _____

_____ _____ 10. **Client's feelings.** If a client expressed strong feelings of attraction or dislike for me, I would
   a. help the client work through these feelings and understand them.
   b. enjoy these feelings if they were positive.
   c. refer my client if these feelings were negative.
   d. direct the sessions into less emotional areas.
   e. _____

_____ _____ 11. **Dealing with diversity.** Practitioners who counsel clients whose sex, race, age, social class, or sexual orientation is different from their own
   a. will most likely not understand these clients fully.
   b. need to be sensitive to the differences between their clients and themselves.
   c. should refer the client to someone who is more culturally competent.
   d. will probably not be effective with such clients because of these differences.
   e. _____

_____ _____ 12. **Ethics versus law.** If I were faced with a counseling situation in which it appeared that there was a conflict between an ethical and legal course to follow, I would
   a. immediately consult with an attorney.
   b. always choose the legal path first and foremost.
   c. strive to do what I believed to be ethical, even if it meant challenging a law.
   d. refer my client to another therapist.
   e. _____

_____ _____ 13. **Values.** In terms of appreciating and understanding the value systems of clients who are culturally different from me, I would
   a. not impose my cultural values on them.
   b. refer them to another therapist.
   c. attempt to modify my counseling procedures to fit their cultural values.
   d. familiarize myself with the specific cultural values of my clients.
   e. _____

_____ _____ 14. **Objectivity.** If a client came to me with a problem and I could see that I would not be objective because of my values, I would

    a. respect my client's values, even though I have different values.

    b. tell the client at the outset about my fears concerning our conflicting values.

    c. refer the client to someone else.

    d. attempt to understand my need to impose my values.

    e. _____

_____ _____ 15. **End-of-life decisions.** With respect to a client's right to make his or her own end-of-life decisions, I would

    a. use the principle of a client's self-determination as the key in any dilemma of this sort.

    b. tell my client what I would do if I were in this situation.

    c. suggest that my client see a clergy person.

    d. encourage my client to find meaning in life, regardless of his or her psychological and physical condition.

    e. _____

_____ _____ 16. **When to refer.** I would tend to refer a client to another therapist

    a. if I had a strong dislike for the client.

    b. if I did not have much experience working with the kind of problem the client presented.

    c. if I saw my own needs and problems getting in the way of helping the client.

    d. if I had strong value differences with my client.

    e. _____

_____ _____ 17. **Role of values.** My ethical position regarding the role of values in therapy is that, as a therapist, I should

    a. never impose my values on a client.

    b. expose my values, without imposing them on the client.

    c. challenge my clients to find other ways of viewing their situation.

    d. keep my values out of the counseling relationship.

    e. _____

_____ _____ 18. **Sexual orientation.** If I were to counsel lesbian, gay, bisexual, and transgender clients, a major concern of mine would be

    a. accepting them as clients because of my personal values or internalized homophobia.

    b. not knowing and understanding enough about their sexual orientation or overidentifying because of my own identity.

    c. establishing a positive therapeutic relationship and deciding whether to disclose my own sexuality identity.

    d. making mistakes that could damage the therapy process.

    e. _____

_____ _____ 19. **Unethical behavior.** Of the following, I consider the most unethical form of therapist behavior to be

   a. promoting dependence in the client.

   b. becoming sexually involved with a client.

   c. breaking confidentiality without a good reason to do so.

   d. accepting a client who has a problem that goes beyond my competence.

   e. _____

_____ _____ 20. **Counseling friends.** Regarding the issue of counseling friends, I think

   a. it is seldom wise to accept a friend as a client.

   b. it should be done rarely, and only if it is clear that the friendship will not interfere with the therapeutic relationship.

   c. friendship and therapy should not be mixed.

   d. it should be done only when it is acceptable to both the client and the counselor.

   e. _____

_____ _____ 21. **Confidentiality.** Regarding confidentiality, I believe it is ethical to break confidence

   a. when there is reason to believe a client may do serious harm to him- or herself.

   b. when there is reason to believe that a client will do harm to someone else.

   c. when the parents of a client ask for certain information.

   d. and inform the authorities when a client is breaking the law.

   e. _____

_____ _____ 22. **Termination.** A therapist should terminate therapy with a client when

   a. the client decides to do so.

   b. the therapist judges that it is time to terminate.

   c. it is clear that the client is not benefiting from the therapy.

   d. the client reaches an impasse.

   e. _____

_____ _____ 23. **Sex in therapy.** A sexual relationship between a *former* client and a therapist is

   a. always ethically problematic because of the power imbalance.

   b. ethical only 5 years after termination of therapy.

   c. ethical only when client and therapist discuss the issue and agree to the relationship.

   d. never ethical, regardless of the time that has elapsed.

   e. _____

_____ _____ 24. **Touching.** Concerning the issue of physically touching a client, I think touching

     a. is unwise because it could be misinterpreted by the client.

     b. should be done only when the therapist genuinely thinks it would be appropriate.

     c. is an important part of the therapeutic process.

     d. is ethical when the client requests it.

     e. _____

_____ _____ 25. **Sex in supervision.** A clinical supervisor has initiated sexual relationships with former trainees (students). He maintains that because he no longer has any professional responsibility to them this practice is acceptable. In my view, this behavior is

     a. clearly unethical because he is using his position to initiate contacts with former students.

     b. not unethical because the professional relationship has ended.

     c. not unethical but is unwise and inappropriate.

     d. somewhat unethical because the supervisory relationship is similar to the therapeutic relationship.

     e. _____

_____ _____ 26. **Spirituality and religion.** Regarding the role of spiritual and religious values, as a counselor I would be inclined to

     a. ignore such values out of concern that I would impose my own beliefs on my clients.

     b. actively strive to get my clients to think about how spirituality or religion could enhance their lives.

     c. avoid bringing up the topic unless my client initiated such a discussion.

     d. conduct an assessment of my client's spiritual and religious beliefs during the intake session.

     e. _____

_____ _____ 27. **Family therapy.** In the practice of family therapy, I think the

     a. therapist's primary responsibility is to the welfare of the family as a unit.

     b. therapist should focus primarily on the needs of individual members of the family.

     c. therapist should attend to the family's needs and, at the same time, be sensitive to the needs of the individual members.

     d. therapist has an ethical obligation to state his or her bias and approach at the outset.

     e. _____

_____ _____ 28. **Managed care.** The practice of limiting the number of therapy sessions a client is entitled to under a managed care plan is

    a. unethical as it can work against a client's best interests.

    b. a reality that I expect I will have to accept.

    c. an example of exploitation of a client's rights.

    d. wrong because it takes away the professional's judgment in many cases.

    e. _____

_____ _____ 29. **Gift-giving.** If a client were to offer me a gift, I would

    a. accept it cheerfully.

    b. never accept it under any circumstances.

    c. discuss the matter with my client.

    d. attempt to figure out the motivations for the gift.

    e. _____

_____ _____ 30. **Bartering.** Regarding bartering with a client in exchange for therapy services, my position is that

    a. it all depends on the circumstances of the individual case.

    b. I would consider this practice if the client had no way to pay for my services.

    c. the practice is unethical.

    d. before agreeing to bartering I would always seek consultation.

    e. _____

_____ _____ 31. **Diagnosis.** Concerning the role of diagnosis in counseling, I believe

    a. diagnosis is essential for planning a treatment program.

    b. diagnosis is counterproductive for therapy because it is based on an external view of the client.

    c. diagnosis can be harmful in that it tends to label people, who then are limited by the label.

    d. the usefulness of diagnosis depends on the theoretical orientation and the kind of counseling a therapist does.

    e. _____

_____ _____ 32. **Testing.** Concerning the place of testing in counseling, I think tests

    a. generally interfere with the counseling process.

    b. can be valuable tools if they are used as adjuncts to counseling.

    c. are essential for people who are seriously disturbed.

    d. can be either used or abused in counseling.

    e. _____

_____ _____ 33. **Risks of group therapy.** Regarding the issue of psychological risks associated with participation in group therapy, my position is that

    a. clients should be informed at the outset of possible risks.

    b. these risks should be minimized by careful screening.

c. this issue is exaggerated because there are very few real risks.

d. careful supervision will offset some of these risks.

e. _____

_____ 34. **Internet or technology-enhanced counseling.** Regarding the practice of counseling via the Internet, I believe

a. the practice is fraught with ethical and legal problems.

b. technology offers real promise for many clients who would not, or could not, seek out face-to-face counseling.

c. it is limited to dealing with simple problems because of the inability to make an adequate assessment.

d. I would never provide distance counseling without having some personal contact with the client.

e. _____

_____ 35. **Inadequate supervision.** As an intern, if I thought my supervision was inadequate, I would

a. talk to my supervisor about it.

b. continue to work without complaining.

c. seek supervision elsewhere.

d. question the commitment of the agency toward me.

e. _____

_____ 36. **Supervision.** My view of supervision is that it is

a. a place to find answers to difficult situations.

b. an opportunity to increase my clinical skills.

c. valuable to have when I reach an impasse with a client.

d. a way for me to learn about myself and to get insights into how I work with clients.

e. _____

_____ 37. **Social justice counseling.** Counseling from a social justice perspective involves addressing the realities of oppression, privilege, and social inequities. This means that I

a. need to be aware of sociopolitical forces that have influenced my clients.

b. need to teach my clients how to become advocates for themselves.

c. will assist people in gaining full participation in society.

d. need to be an advocate beyond the office if I am to make a difference.

e. _____

_____ 38. **Advocacy competence.** To become a competent client advocate, a counselor must

a. gain awareness of his or her own beliefs, attitudes, and biases as they relate to the impact social and political factors have on marginalized and underserved populations.

b. have the courage to speak out against injustices.

c. engage in considerable reflection before taking action.

d. assess whether to engage in social advocacy action, and if so, what kinds of actions are practical and appropriate.

e. _____

___ ___ 39. **Community responsibility.** Concerning responsibility of mental health professionals to the community, I believe

a. practitioners should educate the community concerning the nature of psychological services.

b. professionals should attempt to change patterns that need changing.

c. community involvement falls outside the proper scope of counseling.

d. practitioners should empower clients in the use of the resources available in the community.

e. _____

___ ___ 40. **Role in community.** If I were working as a practitioner in the community, the major role I would expect to play would be that of

a. a change agent.

b. an adviser.

c. an educator or a consultant.

d. an advocate.

e. _____

A Suggestion for Using This Inventory This self-inventory is an engaging way to assist students in thinking about a wide range of ethical issues they will be exploring during the semester. The inventory is a comprehensive look at key issues addressed throughout the book. Create an interactive exercise by asking students to bring their completed inventories to class to compare their views. Such a comparison can stimulate debate and help the class understand the complexities in this kind of decision making. Ask students to circle the items they felt most strongly about, and ask others how they responded to these items in particular. Toward the end of the course, ask students about any shifts in their thinking that resulted from their reading and discussions in class.

Professional Organizations and Codes of Ethics

You can obtain particular codes of ethics by contacting the organizations directly or by downloading these ethics codes from the organizations' websites. Visit their website for more information on any of these organizations.

1. **American Counseling Association (ACA)**
   Code of Ethics, ©2014
   www.counseling.org

2. **National Board for Certified Counselors (NBCC)**
   Code of Ethics, ©2012
   www.nbcc.org

3. **Commission on Rehabilitation Counselor Certification (CRCC)**
   Code of Professional Ethics for Rehabilitation Counselors, ©2010
   www.crccertification.com

4. **Association for Addiction Professionals (NAADAC)**
   Code of Ethics, ©2008
   www.naadac.org

5. **Canadian Counselling and Psychotherapy Association (CCPA)**
   Code of Ethics, ©2007
   www.ccpa-accp.ca

6. **American School Counselor Association (ASCA)**
   Ethical Standards for School Counselors, ©2016
   www.schoolcounselor.org

7. **American Psychological Association (APA)**
   Ethical Principles of Psychologists and Code of Conduct, ©2010
   www.apa.org

8. **American Psychiatric Association**
   The Principles of Medical Ethics With Annotations Especially Applicable to Psychiatry, ©2013
   www.psych.org

9. **American Group Psychotherapy Association (AGPA)**
   Ethical Guidelines for Group Therapists, ©2006
   www.groupsinc.org

10. **American Mental Health Counselors Association (AMHCA)**
    Code of Ethics, ©2015
    www.amhca.org

11. **American Association for Marriage and Family Therapy (AAMFT)**
    Code of Ethics, ©2015
    www.aamft.org

12. **International Association of Marriage and Family Counselors (IAMFC)**
    Ethical Code, ©2011
    www.iamfc.com

13. **Association for Specialists in Group Work (ASGW)**
    Best Practice Guidelines, ©2008
    www.asgw.org

continued

Professional Organizations and Codes of Ethics *continued*

14. **National Association of Social Workers (NASW)**
    Code of Ethics, ©2008
    www.socialworkers.org

15. **National Organization for Human Services**
    Ethical Standards for Human Service Professionals, ©2015
    www.nationalhumanservices.org

16. **American Music Therapy Association (AMTA)**
    Code of Ethics, ©2015
    www.musictherapy.org

17. **British Association for Counselling and Psychotherapy (BACP)**
    Ethical Framework for Good Practice in Counselling and Psychotherapy, ©2013
    www.bacp.co.uk

Additional Resources Some professional organizations also provide casebooks, which interpret and explain various ethical standards contained in the code. The *ACA Ethical Standards Casebook* (Herlihy & Corey, 2015a) describes each of the standards in the ACA's (2014) *Code of Ethics*, and features contributors giving their perspectives on the key themes. A useful work to gain an understanding of the practical application of the American Psychological Association's ethics code is *Practical Ethics for Psychologists: A Positive Approach* (Knapp & Vande-Creek, 2012). Two excellent desk reference manuals are *Ethics Desk Reference for Psychologists* (Barnett & Johnson, 2008), which interprets the APA code and provides guidelines for ethical and effective practice; and *Ethics Desk Reference for Counselors* (Barnett & Johnson, 2015), which interprets the ACA 2014 *Code of Ethics* and offers recommendations for preventing ethical problems.

Chapter Summary

This introductory chapter focused on the foundations of creating an ethical stance and explored various perspectives on teaching the process of making ethical decisions. Professional codes of ethics are indeed essential for ethical practice, but merely knowing these codes is not enough. The challenge comes with learning how to think critically and knowing ways to apply general ethical principles to particular situations. Realize that various courses of action may be acceptable and that generally there is no single right answer to a complex ethical dilemma (Forester-Miller & Davis, 2016). Become active in your education and training (see the "Professional Organizations and Codes of Ethics" box for information on joining a professional association). We also suggest that you try to keep an open mind about the issues you encounter during this time and throughout your professional career. An important part of this openness is a willingness to focus on yourself as a person and as a professional.

Suggested Activities

Note to the student. At the end of each chapter we have provided a range of activities for instructors and students to choose from. The questions and activities are intended to stimulate you to become an active learner. We invite you to personalize the material and develop your own positions on the issues we raise. We suggest that you choose those activities that you find the most challenging and meaningful.

1. As a practitioner, how will you determine what is ethical and what is unethical? How will you develop your guidelines for ethical practice? Make a list of behaviors that you judge to be unethical. After you have thought through this issue by yourself, you may want to explore your approach with classmates.

2. Take the self-assessment survey of your attitudes and beliefs about ethics in this chapter. After completing the survey, circle the five items you had the strongest reactions to or had the hardest time answering. Bring these items to class for discussion.

3. Look over the codes of ethics of the professional organizations. What are the major benefits of having a code of ethics? What are your impressions of each of these codes? To what degree do they provide you with the needed guidelines for ethical practice? What limitations do you see in them? What do the various codes have in common?

4. Check out at least one of the websites of the professional organizations listed in the "Professional Organizations and Codes of Ethics" box. Answer the following questions for each organization you investigate: What is the main mission of the organization? What does the organization offer you as a student? What are the benefits of being a member? What kinds of professional journals and publications are available? What information can you find about conferences?

5. The University of Holy Cross in New Orleans, Louisiana, hosts the *Law and Ethics in Counseling Conference* early each year. Counselors, counselor educators, counseling graduate students, and scholars gather to discuss contemporary topics in legal and ethical issues in counseling. You can find information about this conference at http://uhcno.edu/academics/continuing-studies. For questions, contact the conference director, Dr. Ted Remley, at tremley@uhcno.edu. Check the link to see what papers and handouts may be available from this conference.

Ethics in Action Video Exercises

Ethics in Action is a 2-hour video program available at the online premium website or as a DVD/Workbook. The program consists of 22 vignettes role-played by students and discussions with the students facilitated by Gerald and Marianne Corey. The program is divided into three parts: (1) ethical decision making; (2) values and the helping relationship; and (3) boundary issues and multiple relationships. This is an interactive program, whether students are using the online version or the DVD/Workbook version. Both versions call on students to write responses to questions for each of the vignettes.

The *Ethics in Action* video program and this text deal with the topic of ethical decision making—with emphasis on the eight steps in making ethical decisions. Also explored in the first part of the video is the role of codes of ethics in making decisions.

In Part 1 of the video program, six role plays provide concrete examples of applying the steps in making ethical decisions described in this chapter. The role plays illustrate ethical dilemmas pertaining to teen pregnancy, interracial dating, culture clash between client and counselor, counselor competence, giving advice, and multicultural issues. After viewing each of these six vignettes, we encourage you to complete the exercises that pertain to each role-play situation, either in the online program or the workbook that accompanies the DVD.

To make the fullest use of this integrated learning package, conduct small group discussions in class and engage in role-playing activities. Students can take on the role of counselor for the vignette and demonstrate how they would deal with the dilemma presented by the client. For those not using either the online or DVD program, descriptive summaries of the vignettes are provided with these exercises to facilitate role plays and class discussions at the end of relevant chapters in this textbook. We hope the material in the video program, and in this text, will be a catalyst for students to try out alternative approaches to dealing with each ethical challenge presented.

MindTap for Counseling

Go to MindTap® for digital study tools and resources that complement this text and help you be more successful in your course and career. There's an interactive eBook plus videos of client sessions, skill-building activities, quizzes to help you prepare for tests, apps, and more—all in one place. If your instructor *didn't* assign MindTap, you can find out more about it at CengageBrain.com.

CHAPTER

2

The Counselor as a Person and as a Professional

LEARNING OBJECTIVES

1. Appreciate the role of counselor self-awareness in ethical practice

2. Provide a rationale for the importance of personal therapy for counselors

3. Clarify how countertransference can be an ethical concern

4. View client dependence as a potential ethical problem

5. Describe the main sources of stress that counselors must address

6. Understand how stress can lead to therapist impairment

7. Develop a personal strategy for ongoing self-care

SELF-INVENTORY

The self-inventories will help you to identify and clarify your attitudes and beliefs about the issues to be explored in the chapter. Select the one answer that best expresses your thoughts at this time. Complete the inventory before reading the chapter. After reading the chapter and discussing the material in class, complete the inventory again to see if your position has changed in any way.

Directions: For each statement, indicate the response that most closely identifies your beliefs and attitudes. Use the following code:

5 = I *strongly agree* with this statement.

4 = I *agree* with this statement.

3 = I am *undecided* about this statement.

2 = I *disagree* with this statement.

1 = I *strongly disagree* with this statement.

_____ 1. Unless therapists have a high degree of self-awareness, there is a real possibility that they will use their clients to satisfy their own needs.

_____ 2. Before therapists begin to practice, they should be free of personal problems and conflicts.

_____ 3. Therapists should be required to undergo their own therapy before they are licensed to practice.

_____ 4. Mental health practitioners who satisfy personal needs through their work are behaving unethically.

_____ 5. Many in the helping professions face a high risk of burnout because of the demands of their job.

_____ 6. Clinicians who are self-aware are more likely to avoid experiencing overidentification with their clients.

_____ 7. If I have strong feelings about a client, I could profit from personal therapy.

_____ 8. Feelings of anxiety in a beginning counselor indicate unsuitability for the counseling profession.

_____ 9. A competent professional can work with any client.

_____ 10. I fear that I will have difficulty challenging my clients.

_____ 11. Ethics codes apply to the professional role behaviors of members, but it is difficult to distinguish between the personal and the professional.

_____ 12. The person and the professional are often inseparable.

_____ 13. Real therapy does not occur unless a transference relationship is developed.

_____ 14. When therapists are not aware of their own needs, they may misuse their power in the therapeutic situation.

_____ 15. An experienced and competent clinician has little need for either periodic or ongoing psychotherapy.

Introduction

A primary issue in the helping professions is the role of the counselor *as a person* in the therapeutic relationship. As counselors we ask clients to look honestly at themselves and to decide what they want to change or improve upon. It is important for us to be willing to challenge ourselves as we do our clients. Some questions we might ask ourselves include the following: "What strengths do I have that assist me in helping others as well as myself?" "Do I possess any qualities that are barriers for me in being helpful to others or myself?" "How might I create a plan to address these barriers?" "Am I doing in my own life what I ask others to do in their life?" When we invite our clients to change, we must be willing to do the same in our lives.

Counselors in training acquire an extensive theoretical and practical knowledge as a basis for their practice. They also bring their human qualities and life experiences to every therapeutic session. Being willing to live in accordance with what we teach is a major component of what makes us effective change agents. Compassion for others and dedication to serving others are the hallmarks of being able to make a difference.

In this chapter we deal with some of the ways therapists' personal needs and problems can present ethical issues for the client–therapist relationship. It is difficult to talk about the counselor *as a professional* without considering the counselor's personal qualities because a practitioner's personal life affects his or her professional behavior. A clinician's beliefs, values, personal attributes, level of personal functioning, and ways of living inevitably influence the way he or she carries out a professional role, which to us is central to ethical practice. We also address topics that are closely linked to the counselor's personal life and professional identity: self-awareness, influence of counselor's personality traits, goals, personal needs, transference, countertransference, personal dynamics, job stress, balancing life roles, and therapist self-care.

LO1

Self-Awareness and the Influence of the Therapist's Personality and Needs

Professionals who work intimately with others have a responsibility to be committed to awareness of their own life issues. Without a high level of self-awareness, mental health professionals can obstruct the progress of their clients as the focus of therapy shifts from meeting the client's needs to dealing with the inadequacies of the therapist. Consequently, practitioners must be aware of their own needs, areas of "unfinished business," personal conflicts, defenses, and vulnerabilities and how these influence their therapeutic work. In this section we consider two specific areas we think you need to examine if you are going to be a helping professional: personal needs and unresolved conflicts.

Motivations for Becoming a Counselor

Ask yourself these two questions: "What motivates me to become a counselor?" and "What are my rewards for counseling others?" There are many answers to these questions. You might experience a sense of satisfaction from being with people who are struggling to achieve self-understanding and who are willing to experience pain as they seek a healthier lifestyle. Addiction counselors who are themselves in recovery, for example, may appreciate being part of the process of change for others with substance abuse problems. Indeed, many counselors have been motivated to enter the field because of their own struggles in some aspect of living. It is crucial to be aware of your motivations and to recognize that your way of coping with life's challenges may not be appropriate for your clients. In many ways therapeutic encounters serve as mirrors in which therapists can see their own lives reflected. As a result, therapy can become a catalyst for change in the therapist as well as in the client.

Of course, therapists *do* have their own personal needs, but these needs cannot assume priority or get in the way of a client's growth. Therapists need to be aware of the possibility of working primarily to be appreciated by others instead of working toward the best interests of their clients. Therapeutic progress can be blocked if therapists use their clients, even unconsciously, to fulfill their own needs. Although therapists may meet some of their needs through their work, this should be a by-product rather than a primary aim.

Out of an exaggerated need to nurture others or to feel powerful, professional helpers may come to believe that they know how others ought to live. Some counselors may be tempted to use their value system as a template for their clients, but giving advice and directing another's life encourages dependence and promotes a tendency for clients to look to others instead of to themselves for solutions. Part of the therapist's job is to empower clients so they can function independently and discover their own unique solutions. Therapists who need to feel powerful or important may begin to think that they are indispensable to their clients or, worse still, try to *make* themselves so.

The goals of therapy also suffer when therapists with a strong need for approval focus on trying to win the acceptance, admiration, and even awe of their clients. When we are unaware of our needs and personal dynamics, we are likely to satisfy our own unmet needs or perhaps direct clients away from exploring conflicts that we ourselves fear. Some clients may feel a need to please their therapist, and they are easily drawn into taking care of their therapist's psychological needs. Relying too heavily on personal self-disclosure when working with clients moves the focus away from our clients and puts the spotlight on the therapist.

Some therapists feel ill at ease if their clients fail to make immediate progress; consequently, they may push their clients to make premature decisions or may make decisions for them. As a way of understanding your needs and their possible influence on your work, ask yourself these questions:

- How will I know when I'm working for my own benefit at the expense of my client's benefit?
- If I have personal experience with a problem a client is having, how can I work to be objective enough to relate to this person professionally and ethically?

- How much do I depend on being appreciated by others in my own life? Do I depend primarily on sources outside of myself to confirm my worth?
- Am I getting my needs for nurturance, recognition, and support met from those who are significant in my life?
- Do I feel inadequate when clients don't make progress? If so, how could my attitude and feelings of inadequacy adversely affect my work with these clients?
- Do I have healthy boundaries in place and set limits for myself both personally and professionally?

Personal Problems and Conflicts

Mental health professionals can and should be *aware* of their unresolved problems and conflicts. Personal therapy may reduce the intensity connected with these problems, yet it is not realistic to believe that such problems are ever fully resolved. Clearly, then, we are not implying that therapists should have resolved all their personal difficulties before they begin to counsel others. Indeed, such a requirement would eliminate most of us from the field. In fact, a counselor who rarely struggles may have real difficulty relating to a client who feels desperate or is caught in a hopeless conflict. The critical point is not *whether* you happen to be struggling with personal problems but *how* you are dealing with problems you face.

Reflect on the following questions: Do you recognize and try to deal with your problems, or do you invest a lot of energy in denying that you have problems? Do you find yourself blaming others for your problems? Are you willing to consult with a therapist, or do you tell yourself that you can handle it, even when it becomes obvious that you are not doing so?

When you are in denial of your own problems, you will most likely be unable to pay attention to the concerns of your clients, especially if their problem areas are similar to yours. Suppose a client is trying to deal with feelings of hopelessness and despair. How can you explore these feelings if in your own life you are denying them? Or consider a client who wants to explore her feelings about her sexual orientation. Can you facilitate this exploration if you feel uncomfortable talking about sexual identity issues and do not want to deal with your discomfort? Sometimes it can be difficult to identify strengths and weaknesses. We encourage you to ask colleagues, peers, and your personal counselor for honest feedback as to how they perceive you and what they see as your strengths and areas needing further work for you as a person and a professional. Asking for this type of feedback requires courage, yet doing so can be an illuminating experience and well worth the effort. When engaged in this discussion, willingly suspend any tendency to be defensive. Reflect on the information shared and create a plan to learn from it, integrate it, make changes, and move forward.

You will have difficulty helping a client in an area that you are reluctant to look at in your own life. It is important to recognize the topics that make you uncomfortable, not just with clients, but in your personal life as well. Knowing that your discomfort will most probably impede your work with a client can supply the motivation for you to change and to realize that you also have an ethical responsibility to be present with your clients. One of the gifts of being a counselor is that it is a career choice that can lead us to becoming better versions of ourselves.

Personal Therapy for Counselors

Throughout this chapter we stress the importance of counselors' self-awareness. A closely related issue is whether those who wish to become counselors should experience their own personal psychotherapy, and also whether continuing or periodic personal therapy is valuable for practicing professionals. We strongly support the value of personal therapy for counselors in training because it provides a window into what counseling might be like for clients. Wise and Barnett (2016) identify engaging in personal psychotherapy on a periodic basis as a self-care strategy and as a form of positive self-development. Personal therapy can be one of the ways to maintain self-care and competence throughout one's career. We recommend that you involve yourself in therapeutic experiences that increase your availability to your clients. There are many ways to accomplish this goal: individual therapy, group counseling, consultation with trusted colleagues, continuing education (especially of an experiential nature), keeping a personal journal, and reading. Other less formal avenues to personal and professional development are reflecting on and evaluating the meaning of your work and life, remaining open to the reactions of significant people in your life, traveling to experience different cultures, taking a yoga or a meditation class, practicing mindfulness in daily living, engaging in spiritual activities, enjoying physical exercise, spending time with friends and family, and being involved with a hobby. The common theme throughout these activities is that they focus on your own self-care and physical and emotional health. Taking care of yourself is paramount in helping you guide others through their therapeutic journey.

Experiential Learning Toward Self-Understanding

Experiential learning is a basic component of many counseling programs, providing students with the opportunity to share their values, life experiences, and personal concerns in a peer group. Many training programs in counselor education recognize the value of having students participate in personal-awareness groups with their peers. Such a group experience does not necessarily constitute group therapy; however, it can be therapeutic in that it provides students with a framework for understanding how they relate to others and can help them gain a deeper insight into their shared concerns. A group can be set up specifically for the exploration of personal concerns, or such exploration can be made an integral part of training and supervision. Whatever the format, students will benefit most if they are willing to focus on themselves personally and not merely on their clients. Beginning counselors tend to focus primarily on client dynamics, as do many supervisors and counselor educators. Being in a group affords students the opportunity to explore questions such as these: "How am I feeling about being a counselor?" "How do I assess my relationships with my clients?" "What reactions are being evoked in me as I work with clients?" "Can I be open with my own reactions as a counselor?" "Am I willing to appropriately self-disclose in my work as a counselor?" By being personally invested in their own therapeutic process, students can use the training program as an opportunity to expand their abilities to be helpful.

It is important for counselor educators and supervisors to clarify the fine line between training and therapy in the same way that fieldwork agencies must maintain the distinction between training and service. Although these areas overlap, it is clear that the emphasis for students needs to be on training in both academic and clinical settings, and it is the educator's and supervisor's responsibility to maintain that emphasis. It is essential that students be informed at the outset of the program of any requirement for personal exploration and self-disclosure. Students have a right to know about the nature of courses that involve experiential learning. The informed consent process is especially important in cases where the instructor also functions in the role of the facilitator of a group experience. We discuss this topic at greater length in Chapters 7, 8, and 9.

The Case of a Required Therapeutic Group

Miranda is a psychologist in private practice hired by the director of a graduate program in counseling psychology to lead an experiential group. She assumes that the students have been informed about this therapeutic group, and she is given the impression that students are eagerly looking forward to it. When she meets with the students at the first class, however, she encounters a great deal of frustration. They express resentment that they were not told that they would be expected to participate in a therapeutic group. Some students fear negative consequences if they do not participate.

- If you were a student in this group, how might you feel and react?
- Is it ever ethical to mandate self-exploration experiences?
- The students knew from their orientation and the university's literature that this graduate program included some form of self-exploration. In your opinion, was this disclosure sufficient for informed consent?
- If you were Miranda, what would you do in this situation? How would you deal with the students' objections?

Commentary. Informing students prior to entering the program that self-exploration will be part of their training only minimally satisfies the requirement for informed consent. Students have a right to be informed about every aspect of the experiential group: the rationale for the group, issues pertaining to confidentiality, and their rights and responsibilities regarding participation in experiential activities. Shumaker, Ortiz, and Brenninkmeyer (2011) recommend that experiential groups include a detailed informed consent process and teach students what constitutes appropriate self-disclosure in such a group. Clear guidelines must be established so students know what their rights and responsibilities are. In addition to this general orientation by the program, each instructor (in this case, Miranda) has an obligation to ensure that students have been properly informed about these expectations and requirements. Miranda has an obligation to ensure that group participation is genuinely voluntary and, if not, that the experience is clearly related to program training objectives. Miranda could explain to trainees the value of an experiential group in terms of gaining insights into their personal dynamics, such as potential areas of countertransference. By identifying areas that can lead to countertransference, trainees are in a position to do further work in their own therapy outside of the group. In our view, Miranda needs to provide an opportunity for students to share their concerns at the initial group meeting. She needs to provide a rationale for experiential learning and explore with students how participation in an experiential group can equip them with the awareness and skills to become effective group facilitators.

Personal Therapy During Training

Studies on Personal Therapy for Trainees Personal therapy can be a valuable component for the growth of clinicians. In many theoretical traditions, and particularly in the psychodynamic tradition, personal therapy is deemed essential in the development of therapists (Ronnestad, Orlinsky, & Wiseman, 2016). An assumption of many training programs is that personal counseling should be a requirement for students planning to go into the counseling profession. Gold and Hilsenroth (2009) demonstrated that graduate clinicians who had personal therapy felt more confident in their role and delivered treatments that were twice as long as those of graduate clinicians who did not experience personal therapy. Their study also found that graduate clinicians who had experienced personal therapy developed strong agreement with their clients on the goals and tasks of treatment. Dearing, Maddux, and Tangney (2005) emphasized the responsibility of faculty, supervisors, and mentors in educating trainees about appropriate pathways to self-care and prevention of impairment. Students are more likely to seek personal therapy when faculty members convey favorable and supportive attitudes about student participation in therapy. Faculty can provide modeling for students by appropriately sharing their own experiences with therapy during their training and later. Dearing and colleagues indicate that confidentiality issues, general attitudes about therapy, and the importance of personal therapy for professional development were key predictors for trainees seeking their own therapy. They suggest that students consider the potential benefits, both personally and professionally, of psychotherapy during their training, including alleviation of personal distress, a means of gaining insight into being an effective therapist, and development of healthy and enduring self-care habits. Ronnestad and colleagues (2016) report that studies pertaining to the influence of psychotherapy on *therapists as people* include "positive increments in self-awareness, self-knowledge, self-understanding, self-care, and self-acceptance as well as reduction in symptoms and improved relationships and personal growth generally" (p. 230). Furthermore, personal therapy can teach us more about the profession as we observe and learn new strategies by participating as a client. Our capacity for empathy increases as we begin to understand how challenging it may be for clients to come to us and the courage it takes to share intimate details with a helping professional.

Counselor education programs would do well to work with therapy providers outside the program or at their university's counseling center to offer psychological services to graduate students in their programs. Because of the ethical problems of counselor educators and supervisors providing therapy for their students and supervisees, faculty members have an obligation to become advocates for their students by identifying therapeutic resources students can afford. Some training programs provide a list of practitioners who are willing to see students at a reduced fee. There are both practical and ethical reasons to prefer professionals who are not part of a program and who do not have any evaluative role in the program when providing psychological services for trainees. Practitioners from the community could be hired by a counselor-training program to conduct therapeutic groups, or students might take advantage of either individual or group counseling from a community agency, a college counseling center, or a private practitioner.

Reasons for Participating in Personal Psychotherapy In your own therapy you can take an honest look at your motivations for becoming a helper. You can explore how your needs influence your actions, how you use power in your life, and what your values are. Your appreciation for the courage your clients show in their therapeutic journey will be enhanced through your own experience as a client. In addition, we believe personal therapy is a valuable form of ongoing self-care. As therapists, we are often in the role of giver; to preserve our vitality, we need to create spaces in which the "giver" can be supported. Personal therapy affords opportunities for you to learn how to establish and maintain a working alliance and how to deal with the challenges and uncertainties involved in therapeutic work (Ronnestad et al., 2016). As Wise and Barnett (2016) state: "Good personal therapy is good not only for therapists as clients but also, in the long run, for the therapists' clients" (p. 231).

When students are engaged in practicum, fieldwork, and internship experiences and the accompanying individual and group supervision sessions, the following personal themes may surface:

- A tendency to tell people what to do
- A strong need to alleviate clients' pain
- Discomfort with intense emotion
- A need for quick solutions
- A fear of making mistakes
- An intense need to be recognized and appreciated
- A tendency to assume too much responsibility for client change
- A fear of doing harm, however inadvertently
- A tendency to deny or not recognize client problems when they activate your own problems
- A preoccupation with winning approval and for clients and supervisors to like you
- An internal focus on what you *should* say or do next rather than on what the client is saying and experiencing

When trainees begin to practice psychotherapy, they sometimes become aware that they are taking on a professional role that resembles the one they played in their family. They may recognize a need to preserve peace by becoming caretakers. When trainees become aware of concerns such as these, therapy can provide a safe place to explore them. Trainees are likely to struggle with creating a sustainable balance between caring for clients and caring for others. Personal therapy can help trainees become aware of the interplay between *care of the self* and *care of the other* (Wise, Hersh, & Gibson, 2012). It is important for graduate programs to provide a safe context for training, and the rights and welfare of students must be considered. However, we believe counselor educators can go too far in the direction of protecting the rights of counselor trainees, for example, by not requiring any form of self-exploratory experience as part of their training program. Educators must also be concerned about protecting the public. In Chapter 8 we provide some real cases that elaborate on this point. One way to ensure that clients will get the best help available is to prepare students both academically and personally for the tasks they will face as practitioners.

The ethics codes of various professions state that it is *not* appropriate for supervisors to function as therapists for their supervisees. However, good supervision is therapeutic in the sense that the supervisory process involves assisting supervisees in identifying their personal problems so that clients are not harmed. Both trainees and experienced therapists must recognize and deal effectively with their countertransference, which can be explored in personal therapy.

Consider the situation of a therapist who himself is a veteran with a disability working with other disabled veterans. He may be experiencing a great deal of anger and frustration over the lack of attention to the basic needs of his clients, but he may be suffering from the same neglect. As a result, the therapist's personal problems may get in the way of focusing on his clients' needs. Countertransference reactions also need to be considered for addiction therapists, especially for therapists who are in recovery themselves. For example, in inpatient substance abuse treatment programs, the daily intensity of treatment may affect both client and therapist. In this kind of environment, ongoing supervision is required. Participating in one's own recovery group is often expected, and personal therapy can be most useful.

When practitioners have been found guilty of a violation, some licensing boards require therapy as a way for practitioners to recognize and monitor their countertransference. We think this provides a rationale for psychotherapy for both trainees and practitioners as a way of reducing the potential negative consequences of practicing psychotherapy. On an ongoing basis, therapists must recognize and deal with their personal issues and their potential impact on clients. Therapists should seek personal therapy before distressing life situations lead to burnout and harm to clients (Barnett, Johnston, & Hillard, 2006).

Ongoing Therapy for Practitioners

Experienced practitioners can profit from therapy that provides them with opportunities to reexamine their beliefs and behaviors, especially as these factors pertain to their effectiveness in working with clients. In a study examining the personal therapy experiences of more than 4,000 psychotherapists of diverse theoretical orientations in more than a dozen countries, Orlinksy and Ronnestad (2005) found that more than 88% rated the experience as positive. Another large-scale study (3,995 psychotherapists in six English-speaking countries) found that personal therapy among therapists is a common practice and that it is considered beneficial (Orlinsky, Schofield, Schroder, & Kazantzis, 2011). In a meta-analysis, more than three-quarters of therapists across multiple studies believed that their personal therapy had a strong positive influence on their development as clinicians (Orlinsky, Norcross, Ronnestad, & Wiseman, 2005). Norcross (2005) has gathered self-reported outcomes of personal therapy that reveal positive gains in multiple areas, including self-understanding, self-esteem, work functioning, social life, emotional expression, and intrapersonal conflicts. The most frequent long-lasting benefits to practitioners pertained to interpersonal relationships and the dynamics of psychotherapy. Some of the lessons learned are the centrality of warmth, empathy, and the personal relationship; having a sense of what it is like to be a therapy client; the need for patience in psychotherapy; and learning how to deal with transference and countertransference.

Transference and Countertransference

Although the terms *transference* and *countertransference* derive from psychoanalytic theory, they are universally applicable to many other approaches to counseling and psychotherapy, and to relationships in general. These concepts refer to the client's general reactions to the therapist and to the therapist's reactions to the client. The therapeutic relationship can intensify the reactions of both client and therapist, and how practitioners handle both their own feelings and their clients' feelings will have a direct bearing on therapeutic outcomes. If a therapist's own feelings are not attended to, the client's progress will most likely be impeded. Therefore, this matter has implications from both an ethical and a clinical perspective.

Transference: The "Unreal" Relationship in Therapy

Transference is the process whereby clients project onto their therapists past feelings or attitudes they had toward their caregivers or significant people in their lives. Transference is understood as having its origins in early childhood and constitutes a repetition of past themes in the present. How the clinician deals with a client's transference is crucial. If therapists are unaware of their own dynamics, they may miss important therapeutic issues and be unable to help their clients resolve the feelings they are bringing into the therapeutic relationship.

The client's feelings are rooted in past relationships, but those feelings are now felt and directed toward the therapist. This pattern causes a distortion in the way clients perceive and react to the therapist. By bringing these early memories to the relationship with the therapist, clients are able to gain insight into how their past relationships with significant others have resulted in unresolved conflicts that influence their present relationships. Safran and Kriss (2014) explain how therapists can assist clients in understanding how their past plays out in the present: "Because transference involves a type of reliving of clients' early relationships in the present, the therapist's observations and feedback can help them to see, understand, and appreciate their own contributions to the situation" (p. 36).

Transference is not a catch-all concept intended to explain every feeling clients express toward a therapist. Many reactions clients have toward counselors are based on the here-and-now style the counselor exhibits. If a client expresses anger toward you, it may or may not be transference. If a client expresses positive reactions toward you, likewise, these feelings may or may not be genuine; dismissing them as infantile fantasies can be a way of putting distance between yourself and your client. It is possible for therapists to err in either direction—being too quick to explain away negative feelings or too willing to accept positive feelings. To understand the real import of clients' expressions of feelings, therapists have to actively work at being open, vulnerable, and honest with themselves. Although ethical practice implies that therapists are aware of the possibility of transference, they also need to be aware of the potential of discounting the genuine reactions their clients have toward them.

Let's examine two brief, open-ended cases in which we ask you to imagine yourself as the therapist. How do you think you would respond to each client? What are your own reactions?

The Case of Jasmine

Jasmine is extremely dependent on you for advice in making even minor decisions. It is clear that she does not trust herself and often tries to figure out what you might do in her place. She asks you personal questions about your marriage and your family life. She has elevated you to the position of someone who makes wise choices, and she is trying to emulate you. At other times she tells you that her decisions typically turn out to be poor ones. Consequently, when faced with a decision, she vacillates and becomes filled with self-doubt. Although she says she realizes that you cannot give her the answers, she keeps asking you what you think about her decisions.

- How would you deal with Jasmine's behavior?
- How do you interpret Jasmine's attachment to you?
- How would you respond to her questions about your private life?
- Can you normalize what Jasmine is feeling without directly self-disclosing?
- If many of your clients expressed the same thoughts as Jasmine, is there anything in your counseling style that you may need to examine?
- Would you consider any cultural factors in evaluating Jasmine's behavior?

Commentary. When clients ask you questions about your private life, consider what has prompted these inquiries. The client's reasons for asking the questions may be more important than your answers and can offer useful clinical material to be explored. You may not be inappropriately fostering dependence in Jasmine, but you will want to explore the dynamics of Jasmine's need to get your opinion. Consider looking at any potential cultural influences in Jasmine's style of relating to you as a person of authority. Above all, therapists are ethically obligated to promote client autonomy. If you find yourself offering Jasmine advice, it is time to look within yourself and examine your possible contribution to her dependency. •

The Case of Marisa

Marisa informs you that she terminated therapy with a prior therapist "because he was unable to understand or help her." She tends to project blame on others and does not take responsibility for her problems. Marisa tells you that she is disappointed in the way her counseling is going with you. She doesn't know if you care very much about her. She would like to be special to you, not "just another client."

- How would you deal with Marisa's expectations?
- Would you explore with Marisa her experience with her prior therapist? Explain.
- Can you see a potential ethical issue in the manner in which you would respond to her?
- Would you tell Marisa how she affects you? Why or why not?
- How could you address the issues underlying Marisa's comments without responding directly to what she is asking?

Commentary. Marisa's desire to redefine the therapy process and become special in your eyes should be explored. A therapist with a strong need to please or to be a caretaker may inadvertently promote dependence or role-blurring. If you go out of your way to make Marisa feel special, consider your reasons for doing so. Marisa's desire to feel special with you likely has roots in other relationships in her life. It is crucial to assist Marisa in exploring why feeling "special" is a particular need for her interpersonally rather than being too quick to reassure her. •

Countertransference: Ethical Implications LO3

So far we have focused on the transference feelings of clients toward their counselors, but counselors also have emotional reactions to their clients, some of which may involve their own projections. It is not possible to deal fully here with all the possible nuances of transference and countertransference. Instead, we focus on the ethical implications of improperly handling these reactions in the therapeutic relationship.

In the past, **countertransference** was considered as any projections by therapists that distort the way they perceive and react to a client. This phenomenon occurs when there is inappropriate affect, when clinicians respond in highly defensive ways, or when they lose their objectivity in a relationship because their own conflicts are triggered. In other words, the therapist's reaction to the client is intensified by the therapist's own experience. Freud considered a therapist's countertransference as an obstacle to therapy; the therapist's task was to work through these reactions in supervision and personal therapy. In current practice, countertransference is viewed differently. It refers to all of the therapist's reactions, not only to the client's transference reactions. In this broader perspective, countertransference involves the therapist's total emotional response to a client including feelings, associations, fantasies, and fleeting images (Safran & Kriss, 2014; Wolitzky, 2011). Examples of countertransference reactions include the arousal of guilt from unresolved personal problems, inaccurate interpretations of the client's dynamics because of projection on the therapist's part, experiencing an impasse with a client and frustration over not making progress, and impatience with a client (Norcross & Guy, 2007).

Manifestations of Countertransference Countertransference can show itself in many ways, as has been described by Watkins (1985) in his classic thought-provoking article. Each example in the following list presents potential ethical and clinical issues because the therapist's clinical work can be obstructed by countertransference reactions if these reactions are not managed:

1. *Being overprotective with a client* can reflect a therapist's fears. A counselor's unresolved conflicts can lead him or her to steer a client away from those areas that open up the therapist's own pain. Such counselors may treat those clients as fragile and infantile.

- In your personal life, are you aware of reacting to certain people in overprotective ways?
- Do you find that you allow others to experience their pain, or do you have a tendency to want to move away from their pain very quickly or offer advice to relinquish their pain?

2. *Treating clients in benign ways* may stem from a counselor's fear of clients' anger. To guard against this anger, the counselor creates a bland counseling atmosphere. This tactic results in superficial exchanges.

- Are you aware of how you typically react to anger directed at you?
- What do you need to do when you become aware that your exchanges are primarily superficial?

3. *Rejecting a client* may be based on the therapist's perception of the client as needy and dependent. Instead of moving toward the client to work with him or her, the counselor may back away from the client.

- How do you react to unmotivated clients?
- Do you find yourself wanting to create distance from certain types of behavior in people?
- Do you find yourself clinging to clients with certain types of behavior?
- What can you learn about yourself by looking at those people whom you are likely to reject?

4. *Needing constant reinforcement and approval* can be a reflection of countertransference. Just as clients may develop an excessive need to please their therapists, therapists may have an inordinate need to be reassured of their effectiveness. When therapists do not see immediate positive results, they may become discouraged, angry, ambivalent, or anxious.

- Do you need to have the approval of your clients? How willing are you to challenge clients even at the risk of being disliked?
- How effectively are you able to challenge others in your own personal life? What does this behavior tell you about you as a therapist?

5. *Seeing yourself in your clients* can be another form of countertransference. This is not to say that feeling close to a client and identifying with that person's struggle is necessarily countertransference. However, beginning therapists often identify with clients' problems to the point that they lose their objectivity and become overly compassionate, which has ethical and clinical implications. Therapists may become so lost in the client's world that they are unable to separate their own feelings or to create healthy boundaries between work and their personal life. If the counselor becomes too emotionally engaged when experiencing the client's emotions during session, the client may try to take on the caregiver role for the therapist.

- In your personal life, have you ever found yourself so much in sympathy with others that you could no longer be of help to them? What does that tell you about you?
- From an awareness of your own dynamics, list some personal traits of clients that could elicit overidentification on your part.

6. *Developing sexual or romantic feelings* toward a client can exploit the vulnerable position of the client. Seductive behavior on the part of a client can easily lead to the adoption of a seductive style by the therapist, particularly if the therapist is

unaware of his or her own dynamics and motivations. It is natural for therapists to be more at ease with some clients than others, and these feelings do not necessarily mean therapists cannot counsel these clients effectively. More important than the mere existence of such feelings is the manner in which therapists deal with them. The possibility that therapists' sexual feelings and needs might interfere with their work is one important reason therapists should experience their own therapy when starting to practice and should consult other professionals when they encounter difficulty due to their feelings toward certain clients.

- How would you handle sexual feelings toward a client?
- What would you do if you found yourself frequently being sexually attracted to your clients?

7. *Giving advice* can easily happen with clients who seek answers. The opportunity to give advice places therapists in a superior position, and they may delude themselves into thinking that they do have answers for their clients. Some therapists experience impatience with their clients' struggles toward autonomous decision making. Such counselors may engage in excessive self-disclosure, especially by telling their clients how they have solved a particular problem for themselves. In doing so, the focus of therapy shifts from the client's struggle to the needs of the counselor. Providing advice as a regular intervention can be counterproductive. Even if a client has asked for advice, there is every reason to question whose needs are being served when a therapist falls into advice giving.

- With family members and friends do you succumb to advice giving? If so, how does this affect your relationships with them?
- Are there times when advice is warranted? If so, when? How would a client's culture need to be considered regarding the practice of giving advice?

8. *Developing a social relationship with clients* may stem from countertransference, especially if it is acted on while therapy is taking place. Clients occasionally let their therapist know that they would like to develop a closer relationship than is possible in the limited environment of the office. Mixing personal and professional relationships can destroy the therapeutic relationship and could lead to a malpractice suit. Ask yourself these questions:

- Will my own needs for preserving these friendships with clients interfere with my therapeutic responsibilities and defeat the purpose of therapy?
- Will I be able to remain objective and continue to challenge my clients if I develop a friendship with them?
- Will my client be able to return to therapy if we form a social relationship after termination?

Effective Management of Countertransference Reactions Countertransference can be either a constructive or a destructive element in the therapeutic relationship. A therapist's countertransference may illuminate some significant dynamics of a client. A client may actually be stimulating reactions in a therapist by the ways in which he or she makes the practitioner into a key figure from the past. The fact that the client may have stimulated the countertransference in the therapist does not make this a client's problem. The key here is how the therapist responds. Clinicians who recognize these patterns and are able to manage their own countertransference reactions can eventually help the client change old dysfunctional themes. Hayes, Gelso, and Hummel (2011) present the following guidelines for therapeutic practice for working effectively with countertransference:

- Countertransference can greatly benefit the therapeutic work if clinicians monitor their feelings and use their responses as a source for understanding clients and helping clients to understand themselves.
- The ability of therapists to gain self-understanding and establish appropriate boundaries with clients is fundamental to managing and effectively using their countertransference reactions.
- Personal therapy and clinical supervision can be especially helpful to therapists in understanding how their internal reactions influence the therapy process and how to use these countertransference reactions to assist clients.

Therapists must develop some level of objectivity and guard against reacting defensively and subjectively when they encounter intense feelings expressed by their clients.

Countertransference: Clinical Implications

Countertransference becomes problematic when it is not recognized, monitored, and managed. Destructive or harmful countertransference occurs when a counselor's own needs or unresolved personal conflicts become entangled in the therapeutic relationship, obstructing or destroying a sense of objectivity. In this way, countertransference becomes an ethical issue, as is illustrated in the following cases.

The Case of Lucia

Lucia is a Latina counselor who has been seeing Thelma, who is also a Latina. Thelma's presenting problem was her depression related to an unhappy marriage. Her husband, an alcoholic, refuses to come to counseling with Thelma. She works full time in addition to caring for their three children. Lucia is aware that she is becoming increasingly irritated and impatient with her client's "passivity" and lack of willingness to take a strong stand with her husband. During one of the sessions, Lucia says to Thelma: "You are obviously depressed, yet you seem unwilling to take action to change your situation. You have been talking about the pain of your marriage for several months and tend to blame your husband for how you feel. You keep saying the same things, and nothing changes. Your husband refuses to seek treatment for himself or to cooperate with your therapy, yet you are not doing anything to change your life for the better." Lucia says this with a tinge of annoyance. Thelma seems to listen but does not respond. When Lucia reflects on this session, she becomes aware that she has a tendency to be more impatient and harsh with female clients from her own culture, especially over the issue of passivity. She realizes that she has not invited Thelma to explore ways that her cultural background and socialization have influenced her decisions. In talking about this case with a supervisor, Lucia explores why she seems to be triggered by women like Thelma.

She recognizes that she has a good deal of unfinished business with her mother, whom she experienced as extremely passive.

- If you were Lucia's supervisor, what would you most want to say to her?
- Both the therapist and the client share a similar cultural background. To what extent does that need to be explored?
- If you were Lucia's supervisor, would you suggest self-disclosure as a way to help her client? What kind of therapist disclosure might be useful? Do you see any drawbacks to therapist self-disclosure in this situation?
- Because of Lucia's recognition of her countertransference with passive women, would you suggest that she refer Thelma to another professional? Why or why not?
- What reactions do you have to the manner in which Lucia dealt with Thelma? Could any of Lucia's confrontation be viewed as therapeutic? What would make her confrontation nontherapeutic?
- Was Lucia remiss in not attending to the alcohol problem of the husband?
- Could Lucia's recognition of her own struggles with her mother facilitate her work with women like Thelma?
- What are the ethical ramifications in this case?
- If your unresolved personal problems and countertransference reactions were interfering with your ability to work effectively with a particular client, what actions would you take?

Commentary. Regardless of how self-aware and insightful counselors are, the demands of practicing therapy are multifaceted. The emotionally intense relationships counselors develop with clients can be expected to tap into their own unresolved conflicts. Because countertransference may be a form of identification with the client, the counselor can easily get lost in the client's world and be of little therapeutic value. In the case of Lucia, the ethical course of action we suggest would be for Lucia to involve herself in personal therapy to deal with her own unresolved personal issues. Supervision would enable her to monitor her reactions to certain behaviors of clients that remind her of aspects in herself that she struggles with.

When countertransference interferes with good counseling work, ethical practice requires that practitioners pay attention to their emotional reactions to their clients, that they attempt to understand such reactions, and that they do not inflict harm because of their personal problems and conflicts. Personal therapy can provide us with a deeper self-understanding, which increases our ability to stay focused on the needs of our clients. •

The Case of Ruby

Ruby is counseling Henry, who expresses extremely hostile feelings toward homosexuals and toward people who have contracted AIDS. Henry is not coming to counseling to work on his feelings about gay people; his primary goal is to work out his feelings of resentment over his wife, who left him. In one session he makes derogatory comments about gay people. He thinks they are deviant and that it serves them right if they do get AIDS. Ruby's son is gay, and Henry's prejudice affects her emotionally. She is taken aback by her client's comments, and she finds that his views are getting in the way as she attempts to work with him. Her self-dialogue has taken the following turns:

- I should tell Henry how he is affecting me and let him know I have a son who is gay. If I don't, I am not sure I can continue to work with him.
- I think I will express my hurt and anger to a colleague, but I surely won't tell Henry how he is affecting me. Nor will I let him know I am having a hard time working with him.

- Henry's disclosures get in the way of my caring for him. Perhaps I should tell him I am bothered deeply by his prejudice but not let him know that I have a gay son.

- Because of my own countertransference, it may be best that I refer him without telling him the reason I am having trouble with him.

- I want to explore why Henry continues to bring up his reactions to gay people rather than addressing the personal concerns he said brought him to therapy.

Which of Ruby's possible approaches to Henry do you find yourself most aligned with? If Ruby came to you as a colleague and wanted to talk about her reactions and the course she should take with Henry, what would you say to her? In reflecting on what you might tell her, consider these issues:

- Is it ethical for Ruby to work on a goal that her client has not brought up?

- To what degree would you encourage Ruby to be self-disclosing with Henry? What should she reveal of herself to him? What should she not disclose? Why?

- Is it ethical for Ruby to continue to see Henry without telling him how she is affected by him?

Commentary. All of Ruby's self-dialogue statements are potential avenues for productive exploration. Because of her own countertransference, Ruby is experiencing difficulty in refocusing Henry on his stated goal for therapy. If she cannot get beyond her reactions, it will be difficult for her to be therapeutic with him. Ruby may or may not choose to tell Henry, without going into too much detail, that he is having an effect on her personally. Such self-disclosures should always be for the client's benefit, not the therapist's. Ruby can acknowledge her reactions without indulging herself in them. If Henry's comments become abusive, or if Ruby feels she can no longer be therapeutic, Ruby should consider an appropriate referral. If Henry were our client, we would approach him with a sense of interest over his focusing his resentment on gay people when he declared that his goal for therapy is to deal with his resentment toward his ex-wife. •

Client Dependence

Many clients experience a period of dependence on counseling or on their counselor. This temporary dependence is not necessarily problematic, especially during the early phase of therapy. Some clients see the need to consult a professional as a sign of weakness. When these clients finally allow themselves to need others, their dependence does not necessarily mean that the therapist is unethical. There are ethical implications, however, when counselors *encourage* and promote dependency. This may happen for any number of reasons. Counselors may keep clients longer than necessary for financial reasons. Some therapists in private practice fail to challenge clients who show up and pay regularly, even though they appear to be stymied. Clinicians can foster dependence in their clients in subtle ways. When clients insist on answers, these counselors may readily tell them what to do. Dependent clients can begin to view their counselors as having great wisdom; therapists who have a need to be perceived in this way collude with their clients in keeping them dependent.

When therapists offer quick solutions to clients' problems, they could impede clients' empowerment. With the growth of managed care in the United States as an alternative to traditional fee-for-service delivery systems, the client–counselor relationship is changing in many ways. In the relatively brief treatment and the restricted number of sessions allowed in most managed care plans, client dependence is often less of an issue than it might be with long-term therapy. However, even in short-term, problem-oriented therapy aimed at solutions, clients can develop an unhealthy dependence on their therapist. When this happens, it is the therapist's duty to deal with it therapeutically and not to blame the client.

Whether therapists are encouraging dependence in clients is often not clear-cut. To help you to think of possible ways that you might foster dependence or independence in your clients, consider the following case.

The Case of Blake

Blake, a young counselor, encourages his clients to text him at any time. He expects to be on call at all times. He frequently lets sessions run overtime, lends money to clients when they are destitute, and devotes many more hours to his job than are required. He says the more he can do for people, the better he feels.

- How might Blake's style of counseling either help or hinder a client?
- Do you see any potential ethical issues in the way Blake treats his clients?
- In what ways could Blake's style be keeping his clients dependent on him?
- Can you identify with Blake in any ways? Do you see yourself as potentially needing your clients more than they need you?
- In what cultural contexts might Blake's style be viewed positively?

Commentary. From our perspective, the overriding ethical question is whether Blake's behaviors toward clients demonstrate beneficence or maleficence. In other words, is Blake really helping his clients? We also wonder about Blake's boundaries with his clients. Some of Blake's behaviors are inconsistent with promoting client autonomy and seem aimed more at meeting Blake's own needs. We want to be careful not to judge Blake's enthusiasm and devotion to his work in a negative way, but Blake could be at high risk for burnout or empathy fatigue based on this high level of involvement with his clients. •

Delaying Termination as a Form of Client Dependence

Most professional codes have guidelines that call for termination whenever further therapy will not bring significant gains, but some therapists have difficulty doing this. They run the risk of unethical practice because of either financial or emotional needs. Therapists who become angry with clients when they express a desire to terminate therapy are showing signs of problematic countertransference. Obviously, termination cannot be mandated by ethics codes alone; it rests on the honesty of the therapist and the willingness to include the client in a collaborative discussion about the client's readiness for ending therapy. Termination of a professional relationship can be a complex process, and problems often occur during termination. A successful termination calls for a blending of clinical, practical, and ethical factors that become the foundation for the termination process (Davis & Younggren, 2009).

Rather than viewing termination as a discrete event that marks the end of therapy, it is best viewed as a process for ending therapy over a period of time. Open-ended treatments over a long period of time without clear and identifiable goals are especially difficult to end. In our view, the ultimate sign of an effective therapist is his or her ability to help clients reach a stage of self-determination wherein they no longer need a therapist. Essentially, it is our goal to work ourselves out of a job by empowering our clients and helping them achieve their goals in therapy.

Most of the ethics codes state that practitioners should terminate services to clients when such services are no longer required, when it becomes reasonably clear that clients are not benefiting from therapy, or when the agency or institution limits do not allow provision of further counseling services. Apply the general spirit of these codes to these questions:

- How would you know when services are no longer required?
- What criteria would you use to determine whether your client is benefiting from therapy?
- What would you do if your client feels he or she is benefiting from therapy, but you don't see any signs of progress?
- What would you do if you are convinced that your client is coming to you seeking friendship and not really for the purpose of changing?
- What are the ethical ramifications if your agency limits the number of sessions yet your client is clearly benefiting from counseling? What if termination is likely to harm the client?

Imagine yourself as the therapist in the following two cases. Ask yourself what you would do and why if you were confronted with the problems described.

The Case of Jiwoo

After five sessions Jiwoo asks: "Do you think I'm making any progress in solving my problems? Do I seem any different to you now than I did 5 weeks ago?" Before you give him your impressions, you ask him to answer his own questions. He replies: "Well, I'm not sure whether coming here is doing that much good. I suppose I expected resolutions to my problems before now, but I still feel anxious and depressed much of the time. It feels good to come here, and I usually continue thinking about what we discussed after our sessions, but I'm not coming any closer to decisions. Sometimes I feel certain this is helping me, and at other times I wonder whether I'm just fooling myself."

- What are some pros and cons of your answering Jiwoo's question?
- What criteria can you employ to help you and your client assess the value of counseling for him? Are there techniques from specific theories that could help Jiwoo measure his growth? What clinical assessments might assist in measuring his growth?
- Does the fact that Jiwoo continues to think about his session during the rest of the week indicate that he is probably getting something from counseling? Why or why not?

Commentary. The fact that Jiwoo asks this question is a positive sign for us because it shows that he is involved in the outcomes of his own therapy. This is an opportunity for you to explore Jiwoo's expectations and his goals for treatment. Avoid being defensive with him and explain how the therapeutic process works. Ask about specific aspects of his therapy that he has found helpful and not helpful. Informed consent as an ongoing process rather than a one-time event, and Jiwoo's question provides another opportunity for you to extend his knowledge about the therapeutic process. •

The Case of Enjolie

Enjolie has been coming to counseling for some time. When you ask her what she thinks she is getting from the counseling, she answers: "This is really helping. I like to talk and have somebody listen to me. You are the only friend I have and the only one who really cares about me. I suppose I really don't do that much outside, and I know I'm not changing that much, but I feel good when I'm here."

- Is it ethical for you to continue the counseling if Enjolie's main goal seems to be the "purchase of friendship"? Why or why not?
- Would it be ethical to terminate Enjolie's therapy without exploring her need to see you?
- How do you imagine Enjolie would perceive your suggestions to terminate therapy? What clinical issues would you need to keep in mind?
- Would it be ethical for you to continue to see Enjolie if you were convinced that she was not making any progress?

Commentary. We might ask Enjolie to describe what brought her to therapy and help her to define her current goals for treatment. We would point out that therapy is not the place to make friends with us; it is a chance for her to learn how to make friends in her outside life. We could explore with her what she is doing to find people who will listen to her and what she could do to establish friendships. We would encourage Enjolie to focus on the extent to which she is achieving her goals outside of therapy. If we were convinced that Enjolie was not benefiting from individual therapy, we would consider referring her to a therapy group as the focus of this modality is on interpersonal relationships. •

Stress in the Counseling Profession

The Hazards of Helping

Helping professionals engage in work that can be demanding, challenging, and emotionally taxing. Students often are not given sufficient warning about the hazards of the profession they are about to enter. Many counselors in training look forward to a profession in which they can help others and, in return, feel a deep sense of self-satisfaction. Students may not be told that the commitment to self-exploration and to inspiring this search in clients can be fraught with difficulties. The counselor, as a partner in the therapeutic journey, can be deeply affected by a client's pain. Effective practitioners use their own life experiences and personal reactions to help them understand their clients and as a method of working with them. As you will recall, the process of working therapeutically with people can open up personal issues in the therapist's life, and countertransference may result. If you find yourself struggling, seek consultation to ensure that the client's best interests are at the forefront and that your practice is ethically sound.

Graduate training programs in the helping professions need to prepare students for the work that lies ahead for them. Self-care education should start at the beginning of a graduate program to prevent future problems in students' careers. Emphasize the importance of self-care and encourage students to create a self-care action plan for their graduate school journey. This action plan could be revisited throughout their program of study and again when students begin their clinical experience and prepare to enter the profession. Self-care principles and practices extend beyond graduate school to encompass the entire span of one's career (Wise & Barnett, 2016). If students are not adequately prepared, they may be especially vulnerable to early disenchantment, distress, and burnout due to unrealistic expectations. Training programs have an ethical responsibility to design strategies to assist students in dealing effectively with job stress, in preventing burnout, and in emphasizing the role of self-care as a key factor in maintaining vitality. Ideally, the faculty in graduate training programs will model self-care attitudes and practices for students. Newsome, Waldo, and Gruszka (2012) state that learning to deal with stress to prevent burnout and compassion fatigue is a critical aspect of professional development. They contend that training programs do not do enough to educate trainees about the negative effects of job-related stress, how to prevent burnout, or how to develop self-compassion. Newsome and colleagues' study offers compelling evidence for including mindfulness groups as part of the training program for counseling students: "Significant and sustained gains in stress reduction, mindfulness, and self-compassion argue that mindfulness groups offer significant benefits for future helping professionals" (p. 309).

Stress Caused by Being Overly Responsible

When therapists assume full responsibility for their clients' lack of progress, they are not helping clients to be responsible for their own therapy. Practitioners who accept too much responsibility sometimes experience their clients' stress as their own. It is important to recognize when this is happening. Signs to look for are irritability and emotional exhaustion, feelings of isolation, abuse of alcohol or drugs, having a relapse from recovery, reduced personal effectiveness, indecisiveness, compulsive work patterns, drastic changes in behavior, and concerned feedback from friends or partners. Stress is an event or a series of events that leads to strain, which can result in physical and psychological health problems. To assess the impact of stress on you both personally and professionally, reflect on these questions:

- To what degree are you able to recognize your problems?
- What steps do you take in dealing with your problems?
- Do you practice strategies for managing your stress?
- To what degree are you taking care of your personal needs in daily life?
- Do you listen to your family, friends, and colleagues when they tell you that they are seeing signs of severe stress?
- Are you willing to ask for help? If so, from whom?
- Are you willing to make changes to more effectively manage your stress?

Sources of Stress

In his book *Empathy Fatigue,* Stebnicki (2008) writes about the stress generated by listening to the multiple stories of trauma that clients bring to therapy. These stories are saturated with themes of grief, loss, anxiety, depression, and traumatic stress. When these stories mirror therapists' own personal struggles too closely, **empathy fatigue** may result, which shares some similarities with other fatigue syndromes such as compassion fatigue, secondary traumatic stress, vicarious traumatization, and burnout. The symptoms of empathy fatigue are common to professionals who treat survivors of stressful and traumatic events; who treat people with mood, anxiety, and stress-related disorders; and who work in vocational settings with people with mental and physical disabilities. Stebnicki believes that monitoring our empathy fatigue is critical for maintaining our emotional, physical, and spiritual well-being.

Linnerooth, Mrdjenovich, and Moore (2011) contend that human service professionals who experience and demonstrate empathy toward their clients are at greater risk for compassion fatigue, a condition that escalates when professionals fail to recognize and attend to their own needs. They add, "paradoxically, the more empathic providers are toward their clients, the more likely they are to internalize their clients' trauma" (p. 88). Skovholt (2012) suggests that counselors need "to learn to be both present and separate and also to be able to strategically attach, detach, and reattach" (p. 128). Skovholt and Trotter-Mathison (2016) write about **empathy balance,** which involves being able to enter the client's world without getting lost in that world. Too little empathy results in the absence of caring, but too much empathy may result in practitioners losing themselves in the stories of their clients. The challenge is learning to balance caring for others with caring for self.

The work of professional counselors can lead to significantly increased levels of stress, which is often manifested in physical, mental, emotional, and spiritual fatigue. Clearly, the stress that clients experience and talk about in their therapy can have a major impact on therapists' experience of stress, especially if they are not practicing self-care.

Other sources of stress are associated with working in managed care and educational systems. For mental health professionals who deal with managed care, pressures involve getting a client's treatment approved, justifying needed treatment, quickly alleviating a client's problem, dealing with paperwork, and the anxiety of being put in an ethical dilemma when clients are denied further clinically necessary treatment. For school counselors, in addition to the expectation that they can immediately solve the behavioral problems of children, there is the added stress of dealing with the frustrations of the family, the teachers, and the administrators in the school system. Although a multiplicity of demands are placed on school counselors, they often must function alone with little opportunity for their own supervision or for talking about how their work is affecting them personally.

This is equally true for clinicians in private practice who practice in isolation and do not have the benefits of working with colleagues. Therapists in private practice can connect with other colleagues in the field at regularly scheduled consultations or supervision groups. Even if you work in an office with other therapists, you may not see them often because they are busy with clients, which leaves little time for interacting on a personal or professional basis. Therapists who work with violent and suicidal clients are particularly vulnerable to stress, and it is essential that they develop self-care strategies to avoid burnout. At times, demands may be placed on clinicians that are contrary to their training. Probation officers, the courts, and other stakeholders may view therapists treating sex offenders as an extension of the law enforcement team, creating particular expectations and some role ambiguity. A stressful work environment may not only lead to burnout among the staff but also have a negative impact on clients.

If you fail to recognize the sources of stress that are an inevitable part of helping, you will not have developed effective strategies to combat these stresses. You cannot expect to eliminate all the strains of daily life, but you can develop practical strategies to recognize and cope with them. Doing so is a key part of being an ethical practitioner. Some professional organizations and state licensing boards have impaired professional or peer support programs. These programs can be a significant resource for dealing with the impacts of stress.

Counselor Burnout and Impairment

Stress, distress, burnout, and vicarious traumatization are ongoing challenges associated with the work of helping professionals (Galek, Flannelly, Greene, & Kudler, 2011; Skovholt, 2012; Skovholt & Trotter-Mathison, 2016; Smith & Moss, 2009; Wise & Barnett, 2016). It is essential for therapists to practice self-care to protect their effective functioning and provide clients with the competent services they deserve (Wise & Barnett, 2016). Clinicians who do not engage in self-care practices are at risk of not being able to competently fulfill their professional duties. Neglecting self-care "can undermine our confidence and hurt our ability to practice ethically. It can sink us in discouragement, compassion fatigue, and burnout" (Pope & Vasquez, 2016, p. 114). **Burnout** is a state of physical, emotional, intellectual, and spiritual depletion characterized by feelings of helplessness and hopelessness. Maslach (2003) identifies burnout as a type of job stress that results in a condition characterized by physical and emotional exhaustion, depersonalization, and a reduction of personal accomplishments. Long work hours, seeing difficult clients, heavy involvement in administrative duties, and the perception of having little control over work activities can place practitioners at high risk for emotional exhaustion and depersonalization (Stevanovic & Rupert, 2009). Although some level of involvement with clients provides a sense of personal accomplishment, overinvolvement requires extra time and depletes emotional energy, which puts clinicians at risk for experiencing the negative components of burnout (Rupert, Miller, & Dorociak, 2015).

In recent years Fried and Fisher (2016) have found that clinicians and researchers are calling attention to the negative consequences of prolonged and extreme emotional stress among practitioners who work with vulnerable and at-risk populations. Professional work with people who are diagnosed with mental health conditions can be rewarding, yet it is highly stressful as well. In a study of the antecedents and consequences of burnout in psychotherapists, Lee, Lim, Yang, and Lee (2011) found that emotional exhaustion was most closely related to job stress and excessive involvement with clients. Vilardaga and his colleagues (2011) list some difficult conditions that lead to burnout among addiction and mental health counselors: funding cuts, restrictions on the delivery of services, changing certification and licensure standards, mandated clients, special needs clients, low salaries, staff turnover, agency upheaval, and limited career opportunities.

If practitioners do not take steps to remedy burnout or make changes in how they deal with stress, the eventual result is likely to be impairment. **Impairment** is the presence of a chronic illness or severe psychological depletion that can prevent a professional from being able to deliver effective services and often results in consistently functioning below acceptable practice standards. A number of factors can negatively influence a counselor's effectiveness, both personally and professionally, including substance abuse, chronic physical illness, and burnout. Impaired professionals are unable to effectively cope with stressful events and are unable to adequately carry out their professional duties. Therapists whose inner conflicts are consistently activated by client material may respond by distancing themselves, which clients may interpret as a personal rejection.

In a survey of work–family conflict and burnout among practicing psychologists, Rupert, Stevanovic, and Hunley (2009) found evidence supporting the interdependence of family- and work-life domains. Family support is related to well-being at work and to lower levels of burnout. Conflict between the work and family domains has a significant impact on how psychologists feel about their work. Rupert and colleagues (2009) contend that strategies to reduce burnout among psychologists must extend beyond the work setting to consider the quality of family life and the integration of work and family life. Rupert and colleagues (2015) report that minimizing conflict between the demands of work and family life is of central importance in reducing the risk of burnout. They note that the positive psychology movement focuses less on negative aspects of stress and more on building job engagement and positive attitudes toward work. This positive focus is a primary prevention approach that rests on internal and external resources. To prevent burnout, Rupert and colleagues "encourage taking a proactive approach and striving to maximize a fit between work demands and personal strengths, to develop resources at work and at home, and to establish a balance between work and personal lives" (pp. 172–173).

We ask you to reflect on the sources of stress in your life. What patterns do you see? How do you manage your stress? What steps are you taking to prevent burnout?

- Do you ask peers, colleagues, or supervisors for help?
- Are you willing to make time outside of your regular school or work hours to seek supervision?

- Do you seek personal therapy, body work (massage, yoga, Pilates), and spiritual practices when doing so might be beneficial?
- Do you have a passion in your life other than your work?
- Are you able to create space in your life for the things you value such as family, friendships, and personal hobbies or interests?

Take action now to guard against burnout. Consider these strategies for self-care:

- Schedule time for yourself.
- Find a hobby that you can do regularly.
- Make time to be with family and friends.
- Consult with colleagues and seek peer support.
- Avoid making your work the center of your life.
- Maintain a balance between work and leisure.
- Balance other-care with self-care.

To learn more about stress in the helping professions, preventing compassion fatigue and burnout, and self-care strategies, we recommend *The Resilient Practitioner* by Skovholt and Trotter-Mathison (2016).

ETHICS CODES: Professional Impairment

American Association for Marriage and Family Therapy (2015)
Marriage and family therapists seek appropriate professional assistance for issues that may impair their work performance or clinical judgment. (3.3.)

National Organization for Human Services (2015)
Human services professionals strive to develop and maintain healthy personal growth to ensure that they are capable of giving optimal services to clients. When they find that they are physically, emotionally, psychologically, or otherwise not able to offer such services they identify alternative services for clients. (Standard 35.)

American Psychological Association (2010)
When psychologists become aware of personal problems that may interfere with their performing work-related duties adequately, they take appropriate measures, such as obtaining professional consultation or assistance, and determine whether they should limit, suspend, or terminate their work-related duties. (2.06.b.)

American Counseling Association (2014)
Counselors monitor themselves for signs of impairment from their own physical, mental, or emotional problems and refrain from offering or providing professional services when impaired. They seek assistance for problems that reach the level of professional impairment, and, if necessary, they limit, suspend, or terminate their professional responsibilities until it is determined that they may safely resume their work. Counselors assist colleagues or supervisors in recognizing their own professional impairment and provide consultation and assistance when warranted with colleagues or supervisors showing signs of impairment and intervene as appropriate to prevent imminent harm to clients. (C.2.g.)

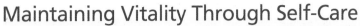

Maintaining Vitality Through Self-Care

Self-care refers to positive actions that promote wellness and effective coping. Stated broadly, "self-care includes routine positive practices and mindful attention to one's physical, emotional, relational, and spiritual selves in the context of one's personal and professional lives" (Wise & Barnett, 2016, p. 210). Professional work suffers when self-care is neglected, which makes self-care a basic tenet of ethical practice. Competence is an ethical obligation and provides a major link between ethics and self-care (Wise et al., 2012). To work in a competent and ethical manner, clinicians need to acquire and regularly practice self-care and wellness strategies. Ongoing self-care is an essential part of a therapist's professional competence and personal wellness program (Barnett et al., 2006; Wise & Barnett, 2016; Wise et al., 2012). Awareness of our current wellness state is a fundamental component in maintaining personal wellness and promoting wellness in others. Our ability to serve others as counselors is connected to our ability to promote wellness in our own life (Blount, Lambie, & Kissinger, 2016). People who take care of themselves and maintain social and personal networks are more likely to demonstrate concern for others. Good self-care is associated with improved ethical behavior (Knapp et al., 2015). If we take care of ourselves, we are more able to take care of our clients (Barnett, 2017a). If we do not practice self-care, eventually we will not have the stamina required to be present with our clients. "Becoming and being a resilient practitioner is about wellness. Our own wellness is necessary so we can marshal the enormous energy necessary for the work with our clients" (Skovholt, 2012, p. 140).

A proliferation of recent literature emphasizes that it is critical for mental health professionals to incorporate proactive self-care strategies in their life. In a key article in the *American Psychologist*, Walsh (2011) outlined a comprehensive review of therapeutic lifestyle changes (TLCs) to promote wellness for clients. Walsh's self-care strategies are an extremely useful wellness approach for mental health practitioners as well. Considerable research and clinical evidence supports these **therapeutic lifestyle changes**: exercise, nutrition and diet, time in nature, relationships, recreation, relaxation, stress management, religious or spiritual involvement, and service to others. Walsh states that TLCs are sometimes as effective as either psychotherapy or pharmacotherapy, and they offer significant therapeutic advantages such as enhancing health and well-being. Although there is evidence for the efficacy of therapeutic lifestyle changes, Walsh contends that TLCs are insufficiently appreciated, taught, or used. This model specifically incorporates elements of mindfulness, spirituality, and positive psychology as ways to promote physical and psychological health.

Mindfulness, acceptance and commitment therapy, and positive psychology all stress positive principles and practices for self-care (Wise et al., 2012). Mindfulness refers to a way of being aware of our thoughts, emotions, and sensations as they arise in us. A nonstriving attitude, which is accessible through various mindfulness techniques, reduces reactivity to distressing emotions and thoughts, leading to a more adaptive mode of consciousness (Brown, Marquis,

& Guiffrida, 2013). Mindfulness practices helped counselor trainees relate to themselves and others with increased authenticity, acceptance, and empathy, and these practices fostered compassion for self and empathy for others (Campbell & Christopher, 2012). Clients can benefit from a counselor's mindfulness practices even though clients are not practicing mindfulness themselves and are unaware that the counselor is practicing mindfulness (Brown et al., 2013). Through the practice of mindfulness, counselors learn the pathway to compassion, which embodies the personal characteristics associated with therapeutic presence.

Patsiopoulos and Buchanan (2011) point out that little research addresses self-compassion, which involves developing attitudes of caring, being nonjudgmental, being accepting, and being kind to ourselves. Self-compassion can enhance counselor well-being, counselor effectiveness in the workplace, and therapeutic relationships with clients. Patsiopoulos and Buchanan conclude: "Our hope is that the practice of self-compassion by counselors will facilitate compassionate and healing workplace environments, in which counselors care for themselves and each other, while providing quality client care" (p. 306). Neff's (2011) work on self-compassion strongly suggests that people who are more self-compassionate lead healthier, more productive lives than those who are self-critical. Neff's research shows that self-compassion enables us to see ourselves clearly and to make changes that lead to fulfillment. If we are able to create a compassionate way of being for ourselves, we stand a good chance of demonstrating compassion toward our clients. If you are interested in reading more on self-compassion, we recommend *Self-Compassion: Stop Beating Up on Yourself and Leave Insecurity Behind* by Kristin Neff (2011).

Chapter Summary

The life experiences, attitudes, and caring that we bring to our practice are crucial factors in establishing an effective therapeutic relationship. If we are willing to engage in self-exploration, it is likely that understanding our fears, personal conflicts, and personal needs will enhance our ability to be present for our clients. Although knowledge and technical skill are crucial, establishing a good working relationship is of paramount importance in effective helping.

Personal therapy during training and throughout therapists' professional careers can enhance counselors' ability to focus on the needs and welfare of their clients. Therapists probably cannot take clients any further than they have taken themselves; therefore, ongoing self-exploration is critical. By focusing on your own personal development, you will be better equipped to deal with the range of transference reactions your clients are bound to have toward you. You also will be better able to detect potential countertransference and have a basis for managing your reactions in a therapeutic manner. Because there is a potential for unethical behavior in mismanaging countertransference, you may find some form of personal therapy useful and that you need to review your personal concerns periodically throughout your career. This honest self-appraisal will assist you in being an effective helper.

Stress and the inevitable burnout that typically results from inadequately dealing with chronic sources of stress also raise ethical questions. Therapists who are psychologically and physically exhausted can rarely provide effective assistance to their clients. Mental health professionals who have numbed themselves to their own pain are ill equipped to deal with the pain of their clients. Impaired practitioners may do more harm than good for clients. There are no simple answers to the question of how to maintain your vitality, but from an ethical perspective, it is critical that you find your own answers to caring for yourself both personally and professionally.

Suggested Activities

These activities and questions are designed to help you apply your learning. Many of them can be done alone or with another person; others are designed for discussion either with the whole class or in small groups. Select those that seem most significant to you and write on these issues in your journal.

1. In small groups, explore your motivations for wanting to pursue a career as a helper. What personal needs do you expect to meet through your professional work?
2. In small groups, explore the following questions: To what degree might your personal needs get in the way of your work with clients? How can you recognize and meet your needs without having them interfere with your work with others?
3. In small groups share your concerns over becoming a counselor. What problems do you expect to face as a beginning counselor? What are your greatest fears? At the conclusion of this exercise, identify what you learned about yourself through disclosing your concerns.
4. In groups of three, take turns stating the personal qualities that you can offer people as a counselor. What talents, skills, and gifts do you possess that will be an asset to you in your work as a counselor?
5. Think of the type of client you might have the most difficulty working with. Then become this client in a role play with one other student. Have your partner attempt to counsel you. After you have had a chance to be the client, reverse roles and you become the counselor.
6. In small groups discuss any possible experiences you have had with burnout, what contributed to it, and what helped you to address this condition. Discuss some possible causes of professional burnout, and brainstorm ways of preventing or minimizing it.
7. Reflect on the benefits of seeking personal therapy as a helper. If you were to seek therapy at this point in time, what issues or concerns would be most pressing for you to explore? Are there particular family-of-origin issues that might affect your work with clients that you need to address in therapy?
8. Make a realistic appraisal of how well you take care of yourself in all areas of your life. Would you benefit from making changes in your diet/nutrition, exercise regime, sleep, or work–leisure balance? To what extent do you take time to attend to the dimensions of your life that are important to you? Identify areas that need improvement and create a self-care plan. If you choose, share your plan with another person.

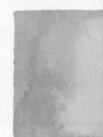

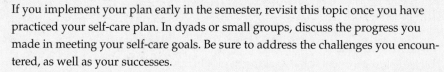

If you implement your plan early in the semester, revisit this topic once you have practiced your self-care plan. In dyads or small groups, discuss the progress you made in meeting your self-care goals. Be sure to address the challenges you encountered, as well as your successes.

- What are some of the barriers that prevent you from practicing self-care?
- Who might you be able to ask for support in reaching your self-care goals?
- If time, money, or excessive responsibilities keep you from self-care, how might you address these issues?

Ethics in Action Video Exercises

9. In video role play 2, Dealing With Anger: A Protective Brother, the client (Richard) reports that his sister is dating an Asian man. Richard is angry and says that he is not going to let that happen. He adds that his sister is not going to mess with his family like that. The counselor (Nadine) asks Richard if he thinks his sister should live to make him happy. He says, "My sister is going to do what I say and that's just it!"

    This vignette shows how a counselor's own unfinished personal issues can get in the way of counseling a client who is expressing anger. Identify and discuss the ethical issues you see played out in this vignette. Reenact the role play by having several students take the role of counselor to show alternative perspectives.

10. Video role play 5, Giving Advice: Take Charge, illustrates how a counselor's lack of self-awareness can be problematic. In this situation, the counselor (Nadine) is giving an abundance of advice, which may be a countertransference issues on her part. She is telling her client (John) how he needs to take charge and decide what is the right way to treat his children. When counselors focus on telling clients what they should be doing, this might be a clue to the counselor's unresolved issues. Role-play how you might deal with John's concerns about how he is making decisions about treating his children. Show how you might deal with a client who asks for your advice.

MindTap for Counseling

Go to MindTap® for digital study tools and resources that complement this text and help you be more successful in your course and career. There's an interactive eBook plus videos of client sessions, skill-building activities, quizzes to help you prepare for tests, apps, and more—all in one place. If your instructor *didn't* assign MindTap, you can find out more about it at CengageBrain.com.

Values and the Helping Relationship

LEARNING OBJECTIVES

1. Clarify how therapist values operate in the counseling process

2. Better understand the ethical issues involved in imposing therapist values

3. Identify appropriate reasons for a referral of a client to another professional

4. Describe what is meant by discriminatory referrals

5. Comprehend the implications of recent court cases addressing discriminatory referrals

6. Recognize when supervision may be needed to address value concerns

7. Assess value conflicts regarding sexual attitudes and behavior

8. Reflect on values pertaining to abortion

9. Critically examine a variety of case examples on value situations

10. Understand the role of spiritual/religious values in counseling

11. Explore values pertaining to end-of-life decisions

Directions: For each statement, indicate the response that most closely identifies your beliefs and attitudes. Use the following code:

5 = I *strongly agree* with this statement.

4 = I *agree* with this statement.

3 = I am *undecided* about this statement.

2 = I *disagree* with this statement.

1 = I *strongly disagree* with this statement.

_____ 1. It is both possible and desirable for counselors to remain neutral to prevent their values from influencing clients.

_____ 2. It is sometimes appropriate for counselors to influence clients to adopt values that seem to be in the best interests of clients.

_____ 3. It is acceptable for counselors to express their values as long as they do not try to impose them on clients.

_____ 4. It is appropriate for counselors to challenge clients to make an evaluation of their values.

_____ 5. Before I can effectively counsel a person, I have to decide whether my life experiences and values are similar enough for me to understand that person.

_____ 6. Clarifying values is a major part of the counseling process.

_____ 7. I would not influence my clients to accept my values.

_____ 8. I am aware of my values and where I acquired them.

_____ 9. I tend to have difficulty with people who think differently from the way I do.

_____ 10. Ultimately, the choice of living or dying rests with my clients, and therefore I do not have the right to persuade them to make a different choice.

_____ 11. I have an ethical obligation to ask myself why I would want to refer a client because of a value conflict.

_____ 12. To be helpful to a client, a practitioner must accept and approve of the client's values.

_____ 13. Ethical practice demands that counselors address a client's spiritual or religious background.

_____ 14. It is important to include a client's spiritual/religious background in the assessment process.

_____ 15. If a client complained of a lack of meaning in life, I would be inclined to introduce a discussion of spirituality or religion as a way to find meaning.

Introduction

The question of values permeates the therapeutic process. In this chapter we ask you to think about your values and life experiences and the influence they can have on your work. We ask you to consider the possible impact of your values on your clients, the effect your clients' values may have on you, the possible conflicts that can arise if you and your clients have different values, and the importance of learning to manage these conflicts in an effective way. We also hope to bring attention to the central role culture plays in determining the values we hold, both personally and professionally.

Can therapists keep their values out of their counseling sessions? The belief that practitioners can be completely objective and value-free is no longer a dominant perspective in the field of psychology (Shiles, 2009). Levitt and Moorhead (2013) contend that values not only enter the counseling relationship but can significantly affect many facets of the relationship. Counselors need to understand how their own values can permeate their work with clients for good or ill, perhaps unconsciously and unintentionally. Francis and Dugger (2014) emphasize that counselors are ethically responsible to monitor the various ways they may communicate their values to clients "and be aware of how the power differential that exists within each counseling relationship may result in the imposition of their values" (p. 132). Hancock (2014) cautions therapists about letting personal beliefs assume priority: "When the therapist's personal beliefs—no matter how deeply held—interfere with the ethical obligations of the profession, the beliefs become more important than the client" (p. 7). Hancock argues that "personal beliefs can and do inform the lives of practitioners; however, they cannot trump the ethical principles and standards of the profession—not when serving the welfare of the client" (p. 8).

Although clinicians may not agree with the values of some clients, mental health practitioners are expected to respect the rights of clients to hold their own views. By demonstrating a nonjudgmental attitude toward clients with different values, we can remain invested in the work our clients are doing. For example, a counselor can help a client who is deciding whether or not to leave a committed relationship by exploring the client's motivations and the possible consequences of either decision, but pressuring the client to choose a particular outcome would be unethical. By honoring the client's self-determination, we help to empower the client.

Controversies Regarding Integrating Personal Values With a Professional Identity

Counselors must respect the values of their clients and have the ability to work with a range of clients with diverse worldviews and values. Your clients have the right to live by their personal values even if those values conflict with your personal values. Wise and her colleagues (2015) state: "Ultimately, all trainees (and trainers) must develop the cognitive complexity and flexibility to hold their own personal beliefs in a way that allows them to be able to serve a diverse clientele in a beneficial, nonharmful manner" (p. 265). Sells and Hagedorn (2016) suggest that it is possible for students to integrate their personal values and religious identity with a new professional identity. This can be done by introducing a student who is struggling with a value conflict to a mentor who is a faculty member or a working professional who shares common values with the student and who is able to integrate personal values with ethical practice. The mentor can demonstrate "to a student how he or she can embrace religious faith and professional ethical obligations simultaneously" (p. 271). Students also have some responsibility, in collaboration with faculty and supervisors, to find a suitable values mentor when they are struggling with a conflict between their personal and professional values (Brad Johnson, personal communication, August 14, 2016).

The religious values of some counselors are in conflict with the affirmation of diverse sexual orientations, and some counseling programs are in institutions that disaffirm or disallow diverse sexual orientations. Smith and Okech (2016a) asked: "How does CACREP simultaneously honor both religious diversity and sexual orientation diversity in its accrediting practices" (p. 252)? Smith and Okech (2016a) identified 15 CACREP-accredited programs in faith-based institutions that have anti-LGBT codes or disaffirming codes of conduct and doctrinal statements that are informed by a conservative Christian religious doctrine. Clearly, the mission and policies of these institutions are in conflict with the ACA's (2014) nondiscrimination standard. Counseling students in such programs may feel justified in exposing their clients to their own personal religious beliefs regarding sexual morality and what kind of relationships are acceptable because those beliefs are espoused by their faculty and enshrined in institutional policy.

Smith and Okech (2016a) also identified 17 CACREP-accredited programs in faith-based institutions with LGBT-affirming codes or nondiscriminatory policies and codes of conduct. The differences between programs with disaffirming codes of conduct and programs that affirm sexual diversity demonstrates a need for increased dialogue in the counseling profession and a "call upon counselor educators to develop empirically informed best practice to guide faculty who must navigate such discriminatory institutional norms" (p. 258). Smith and Okech (2016b) contend that "it is time for the field to provide clarification on the systemic issue of how to negotiate accreditation practices related to religious institutions that disaffirm or disallow LGB-identified students and faculty" (p. 283). It should be noted that institutions that are not LGBT-affirming, regardless of the mission or policies of the institution, must abide by all CACREP standards.

Hancock (2014) asserts that it is the mission of education and training institutions to provide a context in which students can acquire the attitudes, knowledge, and skills essential for providing diversity-competent mental health services. Counselors' personal beliefs and values must not supersede professional mandates to serve the best interests of their clients. Phan, Hebert, and DeMitchell (2013) contend that the profession should define the responsibilities that must be met by all counselors: "A profession by its very nature requires its members to set aside their personal preferences to serve the needs and interests of the person receiving their service" (p. 62).

Clarifying Your Values and Their Role in Your Work

Counselors must develop the ability to manage their personal values so that they do not unduly influence the counseling process. Kocet and Herlihy (2014) describe this process as **ethical bracketing**: "intentional setting aside of the counselor's personal values in order to provide ethical and appropriate counseling to all clients, especially those whose worldviews, values, belief systems, and decisions differ significantly from those of the counselor" (p. 182). Setting aside our personal values does not mean that we must give up or change our values (Kaplan et al., 2017). Counselors do not have to like or agree with their clients' choices to fulfill their ethical obligation to help those seeking their assistance. Many clients will have a worldview different from that of the counselor, and clients bring to us a host of problems. They may have felt rejected by others or suffered from discrimination. Clients should not be exposed to further discrimination by counselors who refuse to render services to them because of differing values.

In our ethics courses, students sometimes ask, "Can I put a values statement in my informed consent document that communicates the nature of my personal values so prospective clients can make an informed decision about whether to enter a professional relationship with me?" If you were to incorporate a personal values statement in your informed consent materials, what would you include? Would you identify specific areas you have difficulty maintaining objectivity about because of the values you hold? Would you include your position on any of the value areas we address in this chapter? Although perhaps well intentioned, such disclosures put the emphasis in the wrong place—on the counselor's values. This can easily convey a judgmental attitude to clients about issues with which they may be struggling. Clients often come to therapy in search of a safe and supportive environment in which they can share secrets and unburden themselves of shame or guilt. Clients are in a vulnerable position and need understanding and support from a counselor, not judgment.

In counseling, your clients struggle to make changes in their lives. We question the underlying assumption that counselors have greater wisdom than their clients and can prescribe better ways of being happier. Unquestionably, psychoeducation is a part of counseling, and counselors do facilitate a process of helping clients gain a fuller understanding of their problems. However, the process of counseling is meant to help clients discover their own resources for dealing with problems rather than listening to advice from others. Counseling is a dialogue between therapist and client that is meant to further the client's goals and empower the client to make choices that are in his or her best interest.

The following questions may help you begin to think about the role your values will play in your work with clients:

- Do you think it is ever justified to influence a client's set of values? If so, when and in what circumstances?

- In what ways could discussing your values with clients unduly influence the decisions they are making?
- Can you interact honestly with your clients without making value judgments?
- If you were convinced that your client was making a self-destructive decision, would you express your concerns?
- Do you think therapists are responsible for informing clients about a variety of value options?
- How are you affected when your clients adopt your beliefs and values?
- Are you able to allow your clients to select their own values and live by their beliefs, even if they differ from yours?
- Do you think a referral is ever justified on the basis of a conflict of values between a counselor and client? If so, in what instances?
- Do you believe certain values are inherent in the therapeutic process? If so, what are these values?
- How does exposing your clients to your viewpoint differ from subtly influencing them to accept your values?
- What are some potential advantages and disadvantages in having similar life experiences with your client?
- In what ways are challenging clients to examine their values different from imposing values on them?

Because your values can significantly affect your work with clients, you must clarify your assumptions, core beliefs, and values and the ways in which they may influence the therapeutic process. If counselors have a strong commitment to values they rarely question, whether these values are conventional or unconventional, may they be inclined to promote these values at the expense of their clients' exploration of their own attitudes and beliefs? If counselors rarely reflect on their own values, it is unlikely that they can provide a climate in which clients can examine their values. Exploring values is at the heart of why many counselor education programs encourage personal therapy for counselors in training. Personal therapy sessions provide an opportunity to examine your beliefs and values and to explore your motivations for wanting to share or impose these beliefs. Clinical supervision sessions are another arena in which the impact of values when working with clients can be examined. Ongoing clinical supervision throughout one's professional career is also encouraged.

In the following sections we examine some sample cases and issues to help you clarify what you value and how this might influence the goals of counseling and the interventions you make with your clients. As you read these examples, keep the following questions in mind:

- What is my position on this issue?
- Where did I develop my views?
- Am I open to being challenged by others?
- Under what circumstances would I disclose my values to my clients? Why? What are my reasons for wanting to reveal my values to a client?
- Do my actions respect the principle of clients' self-determination that is consistent with their culture?

The Ethics of Imposing Your Values on Clients

The imposition of values by the counselor is an ethical issue in counseling individuals, couples, families, and groups. **Value imposition** refers to counselors directly attempting to influence a client to adopt their values, attitudes, beliefs, and behaviors. It is possible for mental health practitioners to do this either actively or passively, and with or without awareness. Jadaszewski (2016) contends that mental health practitioners and consumers of psychotherapy services often lack awareness of the role values play in the psychotherapeutic endeavor. At times, therapists may unintentionally influence clients to change some of their values and behaviors in certain directions. Jadaszewski suggests that a key aspect of informed consent is clarifying with clients some potential ways that values can influence psychotherapy. Informing clients about the role of values in therapy can guard against undue influence by the therapist. For example, a key element in some addiction treatment programs is that clients accept that there is a power higher than themselves. Although clients are encouraged to define for themselves what this higher power is, some addiction counselors may be tempted to impose their own personal beliefs of what the higher power is, which raises ethical issues. Counselors are cautioned about this kind of value imposition in their professional work in this ACA (2014) standard:

> Counselors are aware of—and avoid imposing—their own values, attitudes, beliefs, and behaviors. Counselors respect the diversity of clients, trainees, and research participants, and seek training in areas in which they are at risk of imposing their values onto clients, especially when the counselor's values are inconsistent with the client's goals or are discriminatory in nature. (A.4.b.)

School counselors receive a similar caution in the ASCA (2016) code:

> [School counselors] respect students' and families' values, beliefs, sexual orientation, gender identification/expressions and cultural background and exercise great care to avoid imposing personal beliefs or values rooted in one's religion, culture or ethnicity. (A.1.f.)

A school counselor violated these ethical standards and imposed her personal beliefs for a preference of sexual abstinence at her school. A South Shore Public School District counselor, Grossman claimed she was following her fundamental Christian beliefs when she removed the pamphlets on instruction in the use of condoms and replaced them with literature advocating abstinence. When her contract was not renewed, she brought suit against the school district, contending that the district was hostile to her religious beliefs (*Grossman v. South Shore Public School District*, 2007). The Seventh Circuit Court of Appeals took the position that religious beliefs do not trump the policies and requirements of the employing school district. Grossman acted unethically in disregarding the curriculum of the school and advocating her own personal beliefs about abstinence. The court concluded that the nonrenewal of her contract was based on her actions rather than on her personal beliefs (Phan et al., 2013).

In group work, values imposition may come from both the leader and the members in the group. The group leader should not short-circuit members' exploration of issues by providing answers. Some members may inappropriately respond by giving advice to another member. Value clashes often occur between members, and leaders have a responsibility to intervene so that no member can impose his or her values on others in the group. The group leader's central function is to help members find answers that are congruent with their own values, and these answers will not be the same for all group members.

Value Conflicts: To Refer or Not to Refer

LO3

David Kaplan, chief professional officer at the American Counseling Association, states that the lack of competence across sexual orientations cannot be used as an excuse to refuse to counsel an LGBT client (personal communication, August 6, 2016). All counselors are expected to have basic competencies across race, ethnicity, gender, sexual orientation, and all other characteristics listed in the nondiscrimination statement of the ACA's (2014) *Code of Ethics*. Farnsworth and Callahan (2013) state that values are intrinsic to the process of psychotherapy, and value conflicts will occasionally pose challenges for conducting therapy, regardless of how accepting and compassionate the trainee may be.

Merely disagreeing with a client's value system is not ethical grounds for a referral; it is possible to work through value conflicts successfully. Consider a referral only when you clearly lack the necessary skills to deal with the issues presented by the client. Do not try to convince yourself that you are working in a client's best interest by referring a person because of your discomfort with their beliefs and actions. Farnsworth and Callahan (2013) believe referrals are appropriate when they reflect self-awareness on the part of the trainee that the client's goal is beyond the scope of the trainee's competence. Farnsworth and Callahan (2013) suggest that trainees who experience discomfort with certain clients should honestly consider the degree to which prejudice may be biasing their evaluation of a situation. "Because value conflicts are an inescapable element of psychotherapy, the best protection that can be afforded to clients is for all trainee clinicians to develop greater personal and professional awareness of their own values and recognize the impact that those values have on the services they provide" (p. 205). To competently deal with value conflicts, trainees must maintain awareness of potential conflict areas with clients and their own internal reactions to clients throughout the duration of the therapy process. The counseling process is not about your personal values; it is about the values and needs of your clients. Your task is to help clients explore and clarify their beliefs and apply their values to solving their problems. If clients conclude that their lives are not fulfilled, they can use the counseling relationship to reexamine and modify their values or their actions, and they can explore the range of options open to them.

Hancock (2014) provides a core principle in managing value conflicts: "When there is a conflict between a student's 'sincerely held' religious beliefs and the needs of that client, without question the client's needs must come first" (p. 6). Referring a client because his or her religious beliefs conflict with your values can and does lead to feelings of abandonment and violates the ethical principle of "do no harm" (David Kaplan, personal communication, August 6, 2016). Before considering a referral, explore your part of the difficulty through consultation or supervision. What barriers within you would make it difficult for you to work with a client who has a different value system? When you recognize instances of such value conflicts, ask yourself these questions: "Who's comfort is paramount in the client–counselor relationship?" "Why is it necessary that there be congruence between my value system and my client's value system?" "Have I considered the potential for harm to my client in making a referral?"

It can be burdensome for clients to be saddled with your disclosure of not being able to get beyond value differences. Clients may interpret this as a personal rejection and suffer harm as a result. Counseling is about working with clients within the framework of *their* value system. If you experience difficulties over conflicting personal values, the ethical course of action is to seek supervision and learn ways to effectively manage these differences. Linde (2016) points out that the 2014 *ACA Code of Ethics* makes it clear that counseling is about the client, not the counselor.

Value conflicts may become apparent only after a client has been working with you for some time. Consider this scenario. You believe you would have difficulty counseling a woman who is considering an abortion. You have been counseling a woman for several months on other concerns, and one day she discloses that she is pregnant. She wants to explore all of her options because she is uncertain about what to do. Would you tell your client that you needed to refer her because of your values pertaining to abortion? Could such a referral be considered client abandonment? Would it be ethical for you to offer advice from your value position if she asks for your advice? What are the ethical and legal aspects of imposing your values on this client? If you cannot maintain objectivity regarding a certain value, this is your dilemma to struggle with and is not the client's problem. Your ethical responsibility is to seek supervision or consultation. If you were to refer this client, you still have the obligation to understand how this conflict of values may be influencing the direction of therapy and why you considered a referral to be necessary (Farnsworth & Callahan, 2013).

Discriminatory Referrals

Many people think the mandate to avoid discriminatory referrals is a new directive. However, this mandate is consistent with Carl Rogers's concept of *unconditional positive regard*, which has influenced the counseling profession for more than 50 years. Person-centered theory rests on the foundation of acceptance, respect for a client's autonomy, and avoidance of judgment. These core principles are infused in the ACA's *Code of Ethics* (David Kaplan, personal communication, August 6, 2016).

It is understandable that students often wrestle with the question of when to refer a client. Professional associations do not present a uniform theme, and different professions have different positions on the justification for referral due to a clinician–client value conflict. If ethics scholars and professional associations have differing perspectives, counselor education faculty and students also may be unclear about the circumstances determining the ethics of referrals.

Insufficient training is sometimes used as an excuse or a cover for the real reason for making a referral—the counselor's difficulty with the client's values. Beginning counselors often have not had enough time or experience to feel competent across a wide range of client problems. When faced with a topic you know little about, good first steps are to educate yourself, seek supervision, and obtain further training. It may seem that you are only one step ahead of your client in terms of knowing how to help this person, but the impulse to refer can hurt the client. It also will significantly inhibit your growth as an effective counselor.

Shiles (2009) notes that far too little has been written about situations in which referring a client is inappropriate, unethical, and may constitute an act of discrimination. Shiles asserts that inappropriate referrals have been made for clients with differing religious beliefs, sexual orientations, or cultural backgrounds. Counselors often rationalize these referrals as a way to provide the client with the best services; however, such practices may ultimately be discriminatory. Shiles makes the following observations:

- Referrals have become common practice among mental health service providers at the expense of exploring other possibilities. Mental health providers may not be aware of the potential ethical violation in their referral decision because this topic is not highlighted in the professional literature.
- The overuse of client referral among mental health providers often involves discriminatory practices that are rationalized as ways to avoid harming the client and practicing beyond one's level of competence. Discriminatory referrals have gone unnoticed and unchallenged far too often.
- The psychological community needs to critically examine why mental health practitioners may refer clients over value conflicts and why these practitioners assume that such practices are appropriate, reasonable, and acceptable.

The *Code of Ethics* of the American Association for Marriage and Family Therapy (2015) has this nondiscrimination standard: "Marriage and family therapists provide professional assistance to persons without discrimination on the basis of race, age, ethnicity, socioeconomic status, disability, gender, health status, religion, national origin, sexual orientation, gender identity or relationship status" (1.1). The AAMFT code also addresses referrals: "Marriage and family therapists respectfully assist persons in obtaining appropriate therapeutic services if the therapist is unable or unwilling to provide professional help" (1.10). We have difficulty with the concept of a therapist being *unable* or *unwilling* to work with a client. This vague wording can be used to discriminate and seems to open the door to referral based primarily on a therapist's values or personal beliefs and preferences. What does *unable* mean? What are the implications of being *unwilling*? These two AAMFT standards seem to contradict each other, and clarification is sorely needed.

McGeorge, Carlson, and Farrell (2016) studied family therapists' beliefs and practices related to the referral of lesbian, gay, and bisexual clients and found that the majority of participants believed it is ethical to refer LGB clients based on counselors' (a) values and religious beliefs, (b) negative beliefs about LGB people and relationships, and (c) lack of competence in working with LGB individuals. This result surprised McGeorge and her colleagues because the preponderance of the literature concludes that referral based on sexual orientation is a discriminatory practice that harms LGB individuals. They take the position that "training programs need to communicate that students are expected to develop clinical competence to work with LGB clients, which teaches students that they cannot ethically make the choice to avoid working with this or any other population" (p. 15).

We tell our students who want to make a referral based on a value conflict to ask themselves these questions:

- What skills am I lacking in counseling a client struggling with a critical life decision?
- Is this my issue and feelings of discomfort or are these my client's feelings?
- Can I obtain the knowledge necessary to acquire competence through continuing education, consultation, or supervision?
- How quickly can I gain the knowledge necessary to be of service to my client?
- What is stopping me from gaining that knowledge, supervision, or consultation?
- How can I determine what would ethically justify a referral?

A related key question is, "When does an individual become a client?" Kaplan's (2014) answer is that "the counselor's ethical obligations to an individual start at first contact or assignment, not at the first session" (p. 146). For example, a counselor in private practice who does not have any openings cannot dismiss a person who calls inquiring about services. The counselor has an ethical obligation to provide alternative options, such as other practitioners in the area. This ethical obligation is present even though the counselor will never provide any counseling services to the individual.

LO5

The Legal Framework Regarding Values Discrimination

Counselors are sometimes too eager to suggest a referral rather than explore how they could work with a client's problem. In two recent court cases, Christian students filed suit against their public universities over the requirement that students avoid imposing their moral values on clients.

Julea Ward was enrolled in a counseling program at Eastern Michigan University. She frequently expressed a conviction that her Christian faith prevented her from affirming a client's same-sex relationship or a client's heterosexual extramarital relationship. During the last phase of her program in 2009, Ward was enrolled in a practicum that involved counseling clients and was randomly assigned to counsel a gay client. Ward asked her faculty supervisor either to refer the client to another student or to allow her to begin counseling and make a referral if the counseling sessions involved discussion of his relationship issues.

Ward was told that refusing to see a client on the basis of sexual orientation was a violation of the ethics code for the counseling profession and was therefore not acceptable. The counseling program initiated an informal and then a formal review process into Ward's request for a referral. The program offered her a plan for remediation, which she refused. Ward was dismissed from the program because of her refusal to counsel gay clients and her unwillingness to participate in a remediation plan that would help her manage her personal values in such a way as to avoid imposing her beliefs and values on clients.

Ward sued the university in U.S. District Court, claiming that her dismissal violated her religious freedom and her civil rights. The district court ruled that the university was justified in dismissing Ward for violating provisions of the code of ethics that prohibit discrimination based on race, religion, national origin, age, sexual orientation, gender, gender identity, disability, marital status/partnership, language preference, or socioeconomic status. The court also ruled that the university was justified in enforcing a legitimate curricular requirement, specifically that counseling students must learn to work with diverse clients in ways that are nondiscriminatory.

The Alliance Defending Freedom (ADF) is a legal organization that defends individuals and organizations whose conservative religious views or actions are challenged in various arenas of public life. It was founded and funded in 1994 by several key evangelical Christian leaders and has since taken on many conservative religious causes (Perry Francis, personal communication, September 25, 2016). With help from the ADF, Ward appealed her case to the United States Court of Appeals for the Sixth Circuit, which sent the case back to district court for a jury trial. To avoid a costly trial, the case was settled out of court. As part of the settlement, the ADF dropped their demands that the university's curriculum, policies, and practices be changed (Eastern Michigan University, 2012).

A second related court case had a similar outcome. Jennifer Keeton, enrolled in a counseling program at Augusta State University, actively sought to impose her religious and moral values on clients whose behavior she deemed to be morally wrong. Keeton stated that her intention was to recommend "conversion therapy" to gay clients and to inform them that they could choose to be straight. She was dismissed from the program when she declined to participate in a remedial program designed to assist her in managing to keep her personal values separate from those of a client. The federal appeals court upheld the right of the university to enforce standards expected of students in a counseling program, even when a student objects on religious grounds. Keeton asked the court to order her reinstatement in the program, but the court dismissed her case, stating that the university was justified in enforcing ethical standards for its students (Rudow, 2012).

Some key lessons can be learned from analyzing the Ward and Keeton cases. The courts recognized the right of university programs to adopt policies that prohibit discrimination based on a professional association's code of ethics. The courts agreed that training programs can prohibit students from imposing their values on clients (Behnke, 2012). Counselor education programs have an ethical responsibility and a legal right to ensure the appropriate treatment of clients who are under the care of their supervisees (Julie Whisenhunt, personal communication, October 5, 2016).

State Legislation to Protect Religious Freedom

In some states "freedom of conscience" clauses are being inserted into legislation in an attempt to protect religious freedom. For example, Arizona's Senate Bill 1365 ensures that mental health professionals will not put their licensure status in jeopardy by denying services to clients on the basis of sincerely held religious beliefs. This bill was signed into law by the governor of Arizona in May 2012.

The state of Tennessee passed controversial legislation in 2016 that would allow therapists in that state with "sincerely held principles" to deny services to potential clients who identify as lesbian, gay, bisexual, or transgender without risk of legal consequences. This discriminatory bill under the guise of "religious freedom" seeks to protect conservative therapists from certain 2014 changes in the American Counseling Association's *Code of Ethics*. As long as reluctant practitioners refer the client to another qualified professional, the bill states that they will be protected from licensure suspensions and any legal penalties. Supporters claim the bill protects the rights of therapists by allowing them to refer individuals to more appropriate professionals. Opponents claim that this legislation is part of a wave of bills around the country that legalizes discrimination against lesbian, gay, bisexual, and transgender people. The American Counseling Association's CEO, Richard Yep (2016), contends that denying services based on a counselor's personal beliefs could harm access to professional care for many of the most vulnerable individuals. We agree with Yep's position: "These so-called 'religious freedom' bills set a dangerous precedent and send a harmful message that fairness and equality are secondary to personal opinion" (p. 7). Meyers (2016a) writes that discriminatory attitudes and policies seem to be on the increase since the Supreme Court's decision in June 2015 requiring states to recognize the validity of same-sex marriages. "Currently, there are nearly 200 pieces of proposed anti-LGBT legislation in the United States" (p. 25). Wise and her colleagues (2015) believe that these legislative initiatives (such as the bills enacted in Arizona and Tennessee) limit the ability of educators to train students to provide competent care to a diverse public. Such legislative actions are potentially in conflict with the ethical commitment to nondiscrimination outlined in the ethical standards for the APA and the ACA.

We find it disconcerting that in some states students and practitioners in the helping professions are being given the legal right to refuse to offer counseling services to a client who does not share their religious beliefs and moral convictions. Mental health professionals should be able to work effectively with the diversity of worldviews, beliefs, and cultural identities they will encounter; conscientious objection acts clearly violate the letter and spirit of the ethics codes of the helping professions. If counseling students are not willing to learn to work with the wide range of clients they will encounter, we suggest that they reconsider whether counseling is the right profession for them.

Informed Consent on Managing Personal Values

Prior to enrollment, prospective students must be informed about what is expected of them as ethical practitioners, especially their ethical responsibilities when working with clients who have diverse value systems. Counselor education programs have a responsibility to clearly and comprehensively inform incoming students about the ethical aspects of managing their values and what is expected of them as ethical practitioners. Bieschke and Mintz (2012) have proposed that training programs use a **Values Statement** to inform prospective students about the competencies they will be expected to develop during their training program.

> The Values Statement offers a path in which trainees can simultaneously maintain their values and offer competent care to diverse others. The Values Statement does this by outlining the competencies expected of trainees in regard to working with clients whose worldviews differ markedly from their own. (p. 198)

It is recommended that this statement appear on the program's website as well as in the student handbook, and that students be required to sign and date their acknowledgment that they have read and understood the statement.

Students have a right to maintain their personal values; they are not asked to change those values and beliefs. However, they have an ethical responsibility to acquire and use professional knowledge and skills in serving the diverse range of clients that they are likely to encounter in their practice. Personal values and professional values and skills can coexist even when they are in tension (Pipes, Holstein, & Aguirre, 2005).

Prior to admission students should be told that they cannot *ethically* discriminate against clients because of a difference in values or refuse to work with a general category of clients. In light of the contentious court cases and legislative actions, Wise and her colleagues (2015) call for training programs to take a proactive approach to conscience clauses rather than assume a reactive stance. They recommend that students who are entering a program indicate explicit agreement with nondiscrimination policies. According to Bieschke and Mintz (2012), use of a Values Statement helps training programs prevent future legal and legislative battles. When potential counseling students are informed of the expectations of the program early in the admissions process, they have time to decided whether they want to enroll in the program. Students need to be aware of the fundamental aspects of the code of ethics because these requirements will influence their development as mental health professionals and will affect their participation in the program.

Seeking Supervision Regarding Your Values

We have emphasized that it is not ethical to refer clients based solely on a difference of values and beliefs between the counselor and the client. Through supervision, counselors in training can learn how to manage their values and how to avoid using their professional role to influence clients in a given direction or to make decisions for clients about how to live. In addition, counselors in training can explore their values and beliefs and increase their self-awareness and identify potential future or current value discrepancies in personal therapy. By being proactive, counselors in training can guard against unintentionally imposing their values on clients. It is the professional responsibility of the counselor to be invested in the *process* of a client's decision making rather than directing the person toward *outcomes* that the counselor deems "right." When counselors enter a professional relationship, they take on the values of the profession as expressed in the code of ethics and are expected to bracket off personal values as they enter the world of the client (Sells & Hagedorn, 2016).

Consider the following list of potential clients and indicate whether you believe you could work with them or would be challenged in doing so because of your countertransference or your own values. When would you need to consider supervision to stay neutral or to work effectively with the client? You may think it unlikely that you will encounter some of these situations, but you need to be prepared to deal with them if and when they do arise. Use this code in the following examples:

A = I *could* work with this person effectively.

B = I *would be personally challenged* in working with this person.

C = I *would need to seek supervision* to explore how my values or countertransference could affect my work with the person.

_____ 1. A woman who is considering an abortion and wants help in making her decision

_____ 2. A teenager who is having unsafe sex and sees no problem with this behavior

_____ 3. A person who shows little conscience development, who is strictly interested in his or her own advancement, and who uses others to achieve personal aims

_____ 4. A gay or lesbian couple wanting to work on conflicts in their relationship

_____ 5. A person who wants to leave a partner and children to pursue a sexual affair

_____ 6. A person with strongly held religious beliefs that differ from your own

_____ 7. A woman who says that if she could turn her life over to a higher power she would find peace

_____ 8. A couple who comes for couples counseling while maintaining an affair

_____ 9. An interracial couple coming for premarital counseling

_____ 10. A high school student who thinks she may be bisexual and wants to explore her feelings around coming out

_____ 11. A same-sex couple wanting to adopt a child

_____ 12. An investment counselor who misleads clients to get a commission and who is not held accountable

_____ 13. An interracial couple wanting to adopt a child and being faced with their respective parents' opposition to the adoption

_____ 14. A client from another culture who has values very different from yours (such as arranging the marriage of their children)

_____ 15. A transgender person seeking support for coping with societal pressures and discrimination

_____ 16. An undocumented worker seeking assistance in coping with severe discrimination by an employer

_____ 17. A couple that has an "open marriage" and regularly engages in swinging

_____ 18. A person with very strong political opinions that differ vastly from your own

_____ 19. Parents who want your help in changing a child's behavior because it does not conform with their religious or cultural beliefs

_____ 20. A mandated client who has no intention of changing and who is convinced he does not have a problem

Look back over the list, and pay particular attention to the items you marked "B" or "C." What are some of the difficulties that come up for you in these situations? If you were seeking supervision, what questions would you ask? Do any of these situations have legal implications? As you reflect on your responses, think about your ethical responsibilities as a counselor. What underlying beliefs do you have that may make it difficult to help certain clients? What might you need to shift in your thinking to effectively work with clients that trigger you?

Values Conflicts Regarding Sexual Attitudes and Behavior

Mental health practitioners may be working with clients whose sexual values and behaviors differ sharply from their own. Examine your values with respect to sexual attitudes and behavior. Do you see them as being restrictive or permissive? Think about each of the following statements and mark "A" in the space provided if you mostly agree and "D" if you mostly disagree with the statement.

_____ 1. Internet sex talk can be a creative way to express sexuality.

_____ 2. Sex is most meaningful as an expression of love and commitment.

_____ 3. Recreational sex is healthy if it is consensual.

_____ 4. Sex with multiple partners is not okay unless you know your partners well.

_____ 5. Safe sexual practices are essential throughout your life.

_____ 6. Sex with multiple partners while in a committed relationship is acceptable if the partners agree with such an arrangement.

_____ 7. Same-gender sex or exploration is the right choice for some people.

_____ 8. Hooking up is an acceptable means of sexual expression and meeting people.

_____ 9. Adolescents should avoid becoming sexually intimate because they cannot deal with the consequences.

_____ 10. Internet infidelity is not as serious as actual infidelity.

_____ 11. Women should be as free as men to express themselves in sexual ways.

_____ 12. Sexting should be engaged in only by adults.

_____ 13. A person's sexual practices are acceptable if they are within his or her cultural norms.

_____ 14. A person's gender identity and expression does not necessarily define his or her sexual orientation.

_____ 15. I can accept that some people enjoy watching pornography.

_____ 16. We are sexual beings no matter what our age.

_____ 17. Being asexual is a legitimate form of sexual expression for some people.

_____ 18. Each spouse in a marriage has the right to demand sexual activities at any time, even if the other individual is not interested.

Can you counsel people who are experiencing conflict over their sexual choices if their values differ dramatically from your own? If you have liberal attitudes about sexual behavior, will you be able to respect the conservative views of some of your clients? If you think their moral views are giving them difficulty, will you try to persuade your clients to adopt a more liberal view? How will you deal with the guilt clients may experience? Will you treat it as an undesirable emotion that they need to overcome? Conversely, if you have strict sexual guidelines for your own life, will the more permissive attitudes of some of your clients be a problem for you? Who has influenced your choices pertaining to sexual practices? In general, how comfortable would you be discussing sexual practices and concerns with your clients? How willing or able are you to talk about sexual practices with clients whose sexual orientation is different from your own? Ignoring talk of sexuality with clients can lead to unintended harm and negative outcomes. In our experience, both counselors in training and licensed professionals may experience personal discomfort and lack professional competence when talking about issues of sexuality with clients. Harris and Hays (2008) found that "therapists' perceived sexual knowledge, and their comfort with sexual material, influenced their willingness to engage in sexuality-related discussions with their clients" (p. 239). We find that the more experience students have in talking openly about sexuality in their training and supervision, the greater the likelihood that they will raise relevant issues of sexuality with their clients.

Consider the following case as a way to clarify how your values would influence your interventions with this couple.

The Case of Lee and Juan

During the past few years Lee and Juan have experienced many conflicts in their relationship. Although they have made attempts to resolve their problems by themselves, they have finally decided to seek the help of a counselor. Even though they have been thinking about separating with increasing frequency, they still have some hope that they can achieve a satisfactory relationship.

Three couples counselors, each holding a different set of values pertaining to intimate relationships, describe their approach to working with Lee and Juan. As you read these responses, think about the degree to which each represents what you might say and do if you were counseling this same-sex couple.

Counselor A. This counselor believes it is not her place to bring her values pertaining to the relationship into the sessions. She is fully aware of her biases regarding the preservation of long-term relationships, and she does not impose nor expose these values. Her primary interest is to help Lee and Juan discover what is best for them as individuals and in their relationship. She sees it as unethical to push her clients toward a definite course of action, and she lets them know that her job is to help them be honest with themselves.

- What are your reactions to this counselor's approach?
- What values of yours could interfere with your work with Lee and Juan?

Counselor B. This counselor has been married three times herself. She maintains that far too many couples stay in their marriages or long-term relationships and suffer unnecessarily. She explores with Lee and Juan the conflicts that they bring to the sessions. The counselor's interventions are leading them in the direction of separation as the desired course of action, especially after they express this as an option. She suggests a trial separation and states her willingness to counsel them individually, with some joint sessions. When Lee brings up his guilt and reluctance to separate because of the commitment they made to each other, the counselor confronts him with negative consequences to each of them by staying in an unsatisfactory relationship.

- What, if any, ethical issues do you see in this counselor's work? Is this counselor exposing or imposing her values?
- What interventions made by the counselor do you agree with? What are your areas of disagreement?

Counselor C. At the first session this counselor states his belief in the preservation of long-term relationships. He believes that many couples give up too soon in the face of difficulty. He says that most couples have unrealistically high expectations of what constitutes a "healthy relationship." The counselor lets it be known that his experience continues to teach him that separation rarely solves any problems but instead creates new problems that are often worse. He tells the couple of his bias toward saving their relationship so they can make an informed choice about initiating counseling with him.

- What are your personal reactions toward the orientation of this counselor?
- Do you agree with him stating his bias?
- If he kept his bias and values hidden and accepted this couple into therapy, do you think he could work objectively with them? Why or why not?

Commentary. This case shows how the value system of the counselor can determine the direction of counseling. The counselor's attitudes come into play in working with Lee and Juan. The counselor who is dedicated to preserving a committed relationship is bound to function differently from the counselor who puts primary value on the welfare of the individual. What might be best for one person in this relationship is not necessarily in their best interests as a couple. It is essential, therefore, for counselors who work with couples to be aware of how their values influence the goals and procedures of therapy. Counselors B and C let their values control the process of therapy. It is not the counselor's responsibility to decide about the quality of the relationship or whether the relationship is worth saving. In ethical practice, clients are encouraged to look at their own values and to choose a course of action that is best for them. •

Value Conflicts Pertaining to Abortion

LO8

People's views about abortion are emotionally charged, and counselors may experience a value clash with their clients on this issue. Clients who are exploring abortion as an option often present a challenge to clinicians, both legally and ethically. From a legal perspective, mental health professionals are expected to exercise "reasonable care," and if they fail to do so, clients can take legal action against them for negligence.

Counselors are clearly obligated to familiarize themselves with the legal requirements in their state that relate to abortion, especially if they are counseling minors considering an abortion. Laws, regulations, and policies vary widely; consult with an attorney when necessary. The matter of parental consent in working with minors varies from state to state. For example, in 1987 Alabama enacted the Parental Consent for Abortion Law, requiring physicians to have parental consent or a court waiver before performing an abortion on an unemancipated woman. Consider the situation of a young woman under the age of 18 who tells her school counselor that she is planning to get an abortion and does not want her parents to know about this. In Alabama this counselor is expected to explain this law to the young woman (including the option of a court waiver of parental consent) and advise her that the counselor is obliged to comply with this law, and not encourage any violation of it.

In the following vignette, we present the case of Brooke. What value conflicts, if any, might you face with Brooke? What issues do you find most challenging, and how might you deal with them? Review the eight steps in making an ethical decision outlined in Chapter 1. What steps would you take in dealing with this case in an ethical manner?

The Case of Brooke

Brooke is a 14-year-old student sent to you because of her problematic behavior in the classroom. Her parents have recently separated, and Brooke is having difficulty coping with the breakup. Eventually, she tells you that she is having sexual relations with her boyfriend without using any form of birth control.

- What are your reactions to Brooke's sexual activity?
- What would you want to know about her boyfriend?
- If you sense that her behavior is an attempt to overcome her feelings of isolation, how would you deal with it?
- Would you try to persuade her to use birth control and practice safer sex? Why or why not? If you did, would this constitute an imposition of your values?

You have been working with Brooke for several sessions now, and she discovers that she is pregnant. Her boyfriend is 15 and declares that he is in no position to support her and a child.

She has decided to have an abortion but feels anxious about following through with it. To clarify how you might respond if Brooke was your client, read the following statements and put an "A" in the space provided if you agree more than disagree with the statement; put a "D" in the space if you mainly disagree.

_____ 1. I would explore Brooke's ambivalence relative to the abortion.

_____ 2. I would encourage Brooke to consider other options, such as adoption, keeping the child as a single parent, or marrying.

_____ 3. I would reassure Brooke about having an abortion, telling her that many women make this choice.

_____ 4. I would consult with a supervisor or a colleague about the possible legal implications in this case.

_____ 5. I would consult with an attorney for legal advice.

_____ 6. If I worked in a school setting, I would familiarize myself with the policies of the school, as well as any possible state law pertaining to minors considering an abortion.

_____ 7. I would attempt to arrange for a session with Brooke and her parents as a way to open communication on this issue.

_____ 8. I would encourage Brooke to explore all the options and consequences of each of her choices.

_____ 9. I would inform Brooke's parents, because I believe they have a right to be part of this decision-making process.

_____ 10. I would attempt to arrange for a couples session with Brooke and her partner as a way of helping them discuss their options.

_____ 11. I would refer Brooke to an outside agency or practitioner because her problems are too complex for counseling in a school setting.

_____ 12. I would pay particular attention to helping Brooke clarify her value system; I would be sensitive to her cultural, religious, and moral values and the possible implications of specific choices she might make.

_____ 13. I would refer Brooke to another professional because of my opposition to abortion.

_____ 14. I would tell Brooke that I will support whatever decision she makes for herself.

As you examine your own values pertaining to abortion as they may apply to the practice of counseling, reflect on these questions:

• What would you do if you find it difficult to be objective due to your personal views on abortion?

• If you were to consider referring Brooke, how might she be affected by this action?

• If you chose to refer Brooke, what would your reasons be for doing so?

• Other than a referral, what could you do outside of your counseling sessions with Brooke to work through your own value conflict with her?

• If you are firmly opposed to abortion, how could you bracket off your personal values and work within the framework of Brooke's values?

• Which of your values are triggered by Brooke's case, and how could these values either help or hinder you in working with her?

Commentary. Brooke's case illustrates several complex problems. In working with clients who are facing choices around unplanned pregnancy, it can be useful to ask them to talk about the value systems they hold and in what ways these values support or conflict with the choices they are considering. In situations such as this that are often highly value laden, it is crucial for the counselor to help the client explore his or her options while being sure to use the client's frame of reference for the discussion.

If you determine that you could not work effectively with Brooke, explore your reasons for making this decision with a supervisor, but not necessarily with the client. We would not want to burden Brooke with our struggle pertaining to our values. We would seek consultation as a way of learning how to manage our personal values so that they would not have a negative impact when working with Brooke.

Case Study of Other Possible Value Conflicts

In this section we present a case study that highlights value conflicts. Try to imagine yourself working with Reggie. How do you think your values would affect your work with him?

The Case of Reggie

Reggie comes to see Savannah, who has been a practicing therapist for 2 years. Reggie is in a long-term relationship and he has had several affairs, which he blames mostly on his partner. His goal in therapy is to find some way to ameliorate his guilt. After a few sessions, Savannah suggests he consider couples therapy because much of the content of his sessions has had to do with his relationship with his partner. He refuses this referral. She then tells him that she cannot, in good conscience, continue to see him because his behavior bothers her and she sees no way to help him obtain his goal of alleviating his guilt and continuing his affairs. Savannah suggests that he seek another therapist and offers him three referrals.

- What is your reaction to Savannah's refusal to continue counseling Reggie?
- Is this a case of a therapist exposing or imposing her values on a client?
- Reggie's goals for counseling are different from Savannah's goals for Reggie. Should she discuss this conflict with Reggie, and if so, how?
- What are the ethical considerations in this case?
- How would you deal with Reggie if he were your client?

Commentary. Savannah is not being therapeutic by imposing her value system pertaining to affairs on Reggie. This issue is not about her but about her client. On the other hand, Reggie creates an impossible situation for himself by blaming his partner for his affairs and being unwilling to do couples therapy. It is the counselor's job to explore the meaning of the client's behaviors rather than rendering judgment. Savannah can point out the ways in which Reggie's choices appear to be creating difficulties for him without treating him as though he is a "bad" person. Depending on how Savannah handles termination and referral, her client may feel that she has abandoned him. Reggie seems more than willing to talk about his relationship, and this discussion may eventually lead toward a recommendation for couples counseling.

Striving for Openness in Discussing Values

Beginning counselors may experience discomfort in working with clients for a variety of reasons. Their task is to learn to address this discomfort and see what it may be about. When you experience discomfort due to a client's very different system of values, challenge yourself to develop ways of working with this client. Ask yourself why a client's different values cause you discomfort and are problematic for you. Try to work collaboratively to identify and clarify the client's value system and to determine the degree to which the client is living in accordance with *his or her* core beliefs and values. Your task is to discover what is problematic for the client and to explore this with the client. The emphasis should be on the client's problem, and not on *your problem* with a client.

If you feel secure in your own values, you will not be threatened by really listening to, and deeply understanding, people who think differently or people who do not share your worldview. Listen to your clients with the intent of understanding what their values are, how they arrived at them, and the meaning these values have for them. Being open to your clients can significantly broaden you as a person, and it will enhance your ability to work ethically and effectively with clients.

The Role of Spiritual and Religious Values in Counseling

Addressing spiritual and religious values in the practice of counseling encompasses particularly sensitive, controversial, and complex concerns. As you read the following section, clarify your spiritual or religious values and think about how your views might either enhance or interfere with your ability to establish meaningful contact with certain clients. It is important to be aware of and understand your own spiritual or religious attitudes, beliefs, values, and experiences if you hope to facilitate an exploration of these matters with clients. "Spirituality is often defined as a more personal quest for transcendence and meaning, [whereas] religion is often linked with dogma and ritual" (Barnett & Johnson, 2011, p. 148). We concur with Barnett and Johnson's view that these constructs are related, and we use the terms interchangeably.

In our early years of practicing, the role of spirituality and religion in counseling was not considered an appropriate topic for discussion. A shift has occurred over time, and today there is a growing awareness and willingness to explore spiritual and religious beliefs and values within the context of the practice of counseling and counselor education programs (Barnett & Johnson, 2011; Dobmeier & Reiner, 2012; Hagedorn & Moorhead, 2011; Johnson, 2013). The topic of integrating spirituality and religion into the practice of counseling and psychotherapy has received increasing attention in the literature since the 1970s. Survey data of both practicing counselors and counselor educators indicate that spiritual and religious matters are therapeutically relevant, ethically appropriate, and potentially significant topics for the practice of counseling in secular settings (Delaney, Miller, & Bisono, 2007; Dobmeier & Reiner, 2012; Francis, 2016; Walker, Gorsuch, & Tan, 2004; Young, Wiggins-Frame, & Cashwell, 2007). However, controversy remains over how to address and use spiritual and religious interventions and the ethical implications of such interventions in therapeutic practice (Francis, 2016). Smith and Okech (2016a) state that the ACA and CACREP should continue to acknowledge the role of spirituality and religion in counseling and point out that the ACA has endorsed the Association for Spiritual, Ethical, and Religious Values in Counseling's (2009) *Competencies for Addressing Spiritual and Religious Issues in Counseling*. We encourage you to review these competencies.

Worthington (2011) believes the increased openness of therapists to clients' spiritual and religious concerns has been fueled by the multicultural movement. People have been empowered to define themselves from a cultural perspective, which includes their spiritual, religious, and ethnic values. Spirituality and religion exist in all cultures. If therapists are to include spirituality in therapy, they must be comfortable with spiritual concerns as a topic of discussion in therapy. Johnson (2013) views spiritually informed therapy as a form of multicultural therapy. When the client is interested in talking about these matters, the first step is for the therapist to be sincerely interested in the client's spiritual beliefs and experiences and how he or she finds meaning in life. Johnson believes that a client-defined and life-affirming sense of spirituality can be a significant avenue for connecting with the client and can be an ally in the therapeutic change process. However, the emphasis is on what the client wants, not on the therapist's spiritual experiences or agenda for the client.

In the course of counseling, practitioners ask many questions about a client's life, yet they sometimes omit inquiring about what gives meaning to a client's life and what beliefs have provided support for the client in difficult times. Spiritual assessment provides insight into how a client relates to spirituality and religion and how this may be affecting the client (Dailey, 2012). Asking questions about a client's religious or spiritual background at the outset of the professional relationship conveys their potential relevance to the therapeutic process (Barnett & Johnson, 2011). If counselors do not include questions about a client's spiritual or religious values and concerns during assessment, the client may be hesitant to bring up these concerns in their treatment.

For many clients, spirituality or religion are core aspects of their sense of self, worldview, and value system. Religious or spiritual concerns may be relevant to the motivation of some clients who seek therapy, either as areas of conflict for them or as sources of strength and support that can enhance the therapy process (Barnett & Johnson, 2011). Francis (2016) claims that clients' core beliefs and values are often used as ways of coping and gaining support in times of challenge. "These beliefs and values are part of what makes up the cultural picture of the client and can be used by the skillful and sensitive counselor to help the client navigate the counseling process toward healing and wholeness" (p. 563). Meditation, prayer, being in nature, mindfulness, connecting with others, enjoying the arts, and yoga are some ways spirituality is used as a resource. The key is to find out what works for the client (Johnson, 2013). Some clients do not talk explicitly about spirituality but existential themes tend to emerge in therapy. Listen for how clients talk about their concerns regarding meaning, values, mortality, and being in the world. It is important to attend to how clients define, experience, and access whatever helps them stay connected to their core values and their inner wisdom.

Spiritual and Religious Values in Assessment and Treatment

Assessment is a process of looking at all the potential influences on a client's problem to form a holistic picture of the client's current level of functioning. The exploration of spirituality or religious influences can be just as significant as exploring family-of-origin influences. During the intake and assessment process, the counselor will gather information on many aspects of a client's life. Practitioners should remain finely tuned to their clients' stories and to the reasons clients seek professional assistance.

Frame (2003) presents many reasons for conducting assessments in the area of spirituality in counseling, some of which include understanding the worldview and the contexts in which clients live; assisting clients in grappling with questions regarding the purpose of living and what they most value; exploring religion and spirituality as client resources; uncovering religious and spiritual problems; and determining appropriate interventions. Assessment gives a counselor an opportunity to identify possible influences that spirituality or religion may have on a client's presenting problem. Francis (2016) points out that "if it is determined that a client's religious or spiritual issues are having an impact on the creation, maintenance, or resolution of his or her problems, a more comprehensive assessment of that interaction needs to be undertaken" (pp. 561–562). Based on the results of a comprehensive assessment, a determination can be made about the appropriateness of incorporating the client's religious and spiritual beliefs and practices as part of the therapeutic process.

When clients indicate they are concerned about any of their religious beliefs or spiritual concerns or practices, the therapist needs to be capable of working at this level. However, counselors must be mindful of how this topic is introduced into the therapy process. It is not appropriate to urge clients to explore religion and spirituality if they do not see these as relevant factors in their lives. Therapists can unduly influence clients by bringing up matters of religion and spirituality when clients have indicated they are not interested in exploring these issues. Barnett and Johnson (2011) caution that "practitioners must avoid making religion a preeminent focus when it is not a significant concern for the client" (p. 153). For a more detailed discussion on spiritual assessment, see Cashwell and Young (2011b).

Ethical and Clinical Considerations With Nonreligious Clients

We also must honor the beliefs and concerns of individuals who identify as nonreligious. Sahker (2016) focuses on ethical and clinical considerations in providing therapy with people who are nonreligious and estimates that between 16% and 23% of American adults and 33% of adults under the age of 30 claim to be nonreligous. Individuals experiencing spiritual struggles may seek therapy when deciding to leave the religion of their family of origin. These clients may be seeking a safe place to discuss their doubts and distress related to internal conflicts involving nonbelief. Some who have left the religion of their family of origin experience rejection by family members, and clients often want to express and explore the pain they experience as a result of their choice. To practice ethically and effectively with these clients, therapists must gain competence in making assessments and in providing treatment for these people. The assessment process is crucial in identifying any religious or spiritual concerns, both positive and negative, that an individual may have and assessing whether these beliefs, past or present, provide them with meaning or with distress. If clients say they want to talk about religious or nonreligious matters, these concerns should be addressed in their therapy. Sahker (2016) provides a theoretical model of assessment, conceptualization, and intervention that can be an effective clinical tool in working with the nonreligious.

Religious Teachings and Counseling

Religious beliefs and practices affect many dimensions of human experience, both positively and negatively. At their best, both counseling and religion are able to foster healing through an exploration of self by learning to accept oneself; by giving to others; by forgiving others and oneself; by admitting one's shortcomings; by accepting personal responsibility; by letting go of hurts and resentments; by dealing with guilt; and by learning to let go of self-destructive patterns of thinking, feeling, and acting.

Although religion and counseling are comparable in a number of respects, some key differences exist. For example, counseling does not involve the imposition of counselors' values on clients, whereas religion mostly involves teaching doctrines and beliefs that individuals are expected to accept and practice. Ethically, it is important to monitor yourself for subtle ways that you might be inclined to introduce your values in your counseling practice. For instance, you might influence clients to embrace a religious perspective, or you might influence them to give up certain beliefs that you think are no longer functional for them. Keep in mind that it is the client's place to determine what specific values to retain, replace, or modify.

Personal Beliefs and Values of Counselors

As we have mentioned, if mental health practitioners are to competently and ethically serve the diverse needs of clients, they must be capable and prepared to look at spirituality and religion when these are important to their clients. Johnson (2013) believes that therapists would do well to spend time reflecting on their own spiritual identity and journey, especially on experiences that were emotionally intrusive and fostered reactivity. If therapists understand and have worked through their spiritual emotional baggage, they can listen to their clients' spiritual experiences, values, and practices without becoming emotionally reactive and imposing their personal agenda on clients.

Your Personal Stance As you examine your own position on the place of spiritual and religious values in the practice of counseling, reflect on these questions:

- What connection, if any, do you see between spirituality, religion, and the problems of the client?
- Do you think it is ever justified for clinicians to introduce or teach their religious or spiritual values to clients and to base their clinical practice on these values? Explain.

- How would you describe the influence of religion or spirituality in your life? What relevance might this have to the way you practice counseling?
- How would you manage situations in which your beliefs about religion or spirituality conflict with those of your client?
- Are therapists forcing their values on their clients when they decide what topics can be discussed? Explain.
- If you have no religious or spiritual convictions, how would you work with clients who hold strong views in these areas?
- Is there an ethical issue when a counseling agency that is attached to a church imposes the church's teachings or religious dogma as part of their counseling practices? Explain.
- To what degree are you willing to collaborate with clergy or indigenous healers if it appears that clients have questions you are not qualified to answer?
- How does a counselor in a public school deal with spiritual or religious issues that students may bring up? Do parents need to be informed that spiritual issues may be discussed in counseling?

An Ethical Decision-Making Process Model

Barnett and Johnson (2011) describe an ethical decision-making process model to determine whether religious or spiritual beliefs may be clinically salient, and if so, to identify ethical principles and standards in determining how to proceed. These key points of their model can be applied when dealing with ethical dilemmas pertaining to a client's religious or spiritual beliefs and concerns in the therapeutic context:

- Respectfully assess a client's religious or spiritual beliefs at the beginning of the counseling relationship. Tailor this assessment to the individual client, the psychotherapy context, and the client's preference for considering these concerns.
- Carefully assess any connection between a client's presenting problem and religious or spiritual beliefs. Be aware of the wide range of religious and spiritual beliefs and practices in various cultural groups by engaging in both didactic and experiential learning.
- Weave the results of an initial assessment into the informed consent process. If religious or spiritual concerns will be explicitly addressed in therapy, develop a treatment plan that incorporates this focus and obtain your client's informed consent.
- Honestly consider your potential countertransference to a client's religious beliefs and practices. If your countertransference might undermine the therapeutic endeavor or harm the client, seek consultation.
- Evaluate your competence in a given case by reviewing the professional literature, practice guidelines, laws, and ethics standards pertinent in working with a client's religious concerns.
- Consult with experts in the area of religion and spirituality in the practice of psychotherapy. Colleagues with expertise in religion and spirituality can help you explore your countertransference involving a client's spirituality or religion.

- If appropriate and clinically indicated, and with a client's consent, consider consulting with a client's own clergy.
- Evaluate the potential benefits and risks of integrating religious or spiritual interventions into treatment and decide whether to treat a client or make a referral. If you are making a referral, document the reasoning and steps you took to enhance your own knowledge and experience.
- Assess outcomes and make necessary adjustments to a client's treatment plan.

Training in Dealing With Spiritual and Religious Concerns

Spiritual and religious aspects of living may be as much a part of the context of the presenting problem as are issues of gender, race, or culture. In one survey, 73% of therapists reported that it was important to address spiritual issues in therapy, but most did not believe they possessed the necessary competence to do so (Hickson, Housley, & Wages, 2011). Practitioners should reach out to members of the religious community and indigenous healers with whom they can collaborate on behalf of the client when it is appropriate and when written consent is given.

The Association for Spiritual, Ethical, and Religious Values in Counseling (ASERVIC, 2009) developed a set of competencies in spirituality. These competencies outline the knowledge and skills counselors need to master to effectively engage clients in the exploration of their spiritual and religious lives (Robertson & Young, 2011).

In a national survey of student perceptions, 84% of the interns indicated they were introduced to spirituality and religion in their CACREP-accredited program through their coursework (Dobmeier & Reiner, 2012). Most of these counseling interns believed they were prepared to deal with spiritual issues in their practice. More than half of the respondents identified wellness, meaning, faith, hope, and forgiveness as topics addressed in their coursework. Dobmeier and Reiner conclude that counselor education programs need to inform students of the ASERVIC competencies so students have a framework for evaluating their readiness to apply these competencies in their work with clients.

Educational programs can encourage students to look at what they believe and how their beliefs and values might influence their work. Just as it is not possible to know every aspect of all cultures, the same is true of religion. Even though counselors cannot know about all religions or all aspects of spirituality, they can work effectively when clients introduce religious or spiritual concerns. Therapists can invite clients to explain and explore the areas of spiritual or religious concerns that are problematic for them.

The Case of Rory

Rory, who has been in counseling for some time with Fiona, sees himself as a failure and cannot move past his guilt. He insists that he cannot forgive himself for his past. He is in great turmoil and berates himself for his aberrant ways. Fiona is an atheist, but she knows that Rory is a profoundly religious man and asks during one of the sessions, "How would you view and react to a person with a struggle similar to yours? What kind of God do you believe in? Does your God offer judgments or grace? What does your religion teach you about forgiveness?" Fiona is attempting to use Rory's convictions to reframe his thinking. Once he begins to look at his behavior through the eyes of his religious beliefs, his attitudes toward his own behavior change dramatically. Because Rory believes in a loving God, he finally learns to be more forgiving of himself.

- How do you react to how Fiona worked with Rory?
- Would you use Rory's religious beliefs as an intervention? Why or why not?
- Do you see Fiona's interventions as inauthentic or culturally sensitive? Explain.

Commentary. Fiona noticed a discrepancy between Rory's religious beliefs and his assessment of his behaviors. By using the client's own belief system, she assisted him in reframing his self-assessment and in the process helped him to be true to his own belief system. •

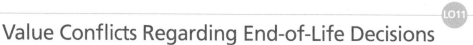

Value Conflicts Regarding End-of-Life Decisions

Many aspects must be considered when it comes to end-of-life care, not just decisions that may affect the timing of death. As the U.S. population ages, many counselors will assist clients in making end-of-life decisions, including decisions about taking active steps toward hastening death. With growing public support and continuing efforts by states to legalize physician-assisted suicide, it is very likely that an increasing number of clients will seek professional assistance in making end-of-life decisions.

Bevacqua and Kurpius (2013) believe counselors in training should be prepared to deal professionally with value-laden end-of-life decisions. Their study of counseling students showed interesting results with regard to age of clients, clinical experience, and religious affiliation of student trainees. There was much more support for a 77-year-old client seeking active euthanasia than for a 25-year-old client doing so. Students' clinical experience was positively related to their support of client autonomy. A negative relationship was found between a trainee's religiosity and respecting a client's right to consider euthanasia. These findings suggest that counselors' personal religious values may affect their therapeutic work with clients, either directly or indirectly. Bevacqua and Kurpius recommend close clinical supervision as a way to ensure that counseling students foster a client's autonomy rather than allowing their own values to influence a client's end-of-life decision.

Withholding and withdrawing treatment is legal in all 50 states, so all of us have some choices regarding our own death. End-of-life decisions that involve physician-assisted suicide have become an increasingly controversial issue since the Death With Dignity Act became law in Oregon in 1997. Washington's voter referendum in 2008 was similar to the Oregon act and became law in 2009, and in 2013 Vermont became the first state to pass a Death With Dignity act through legislation. Montana has physician-assisted suicide by way of a court ruling (*Baxter v. State of Montana*, 2009). More than 30 states have specific laws prohibiting physician-assisted suicide, and 4 states have no specific laws regarding physician-assisted suicide (Kristen Dickens, personal communication, October 15, 2016). Other states are considering legislation as well. Signed into law October 5, 2015, and in effect from June 9, 2016, the **California End-of-Life Option Act** is a physician-assisted suicide law modeled on the Oregon **Death With Dignity Act**. An interesting map that tracks legislation can be found at https://www.deathwithdignity.org/take-action/.

If you will be working with clients concerned about end-of-life care, it is essential to know the laws in your jurisdiction and in your state and to be familiar with the ethical guidelines of your professional organization concerning an individual's freedom to make end-of-life decisions. It is essential that you seek legal consultation in cases involving a client's request for more explicit assistance with hastened death. Some key questions are: Do people who are terminally ill, have an incurable disease, or are in extreme pain, have a right to choose the time and the means of their own death by seeking aid-in-dying? What is the appropriate role for counselors in dealing with clients who are making end-of-life decisions? Werth and Holdwick (2000) provide the following definitions for some key concepts related to end-of-life matters:

- **Rational suicide** means that a person has decided—after going through a decision-making process and without coercion from others—to end his or her life because of extreme suffering involved with a terminal illness.
- **Aid-in-dying** consists of providing a person with the means to die; the person self-administers the death-causing agent, which is a lethal dose of a legal medication.
- **Hastened death** means ending one's life earlier than would have happened without intervention. It involves speeding up the dying process, which can entail withholding or withdrawing treatment or life support.

Mental health professionals who are involved in end-of-life care decisions need to be knowledgeable about the implications of advance directives and their involvement with the client. **Advance directives** contain decisions people make about end-of-life care that are designed to protect their self-determination when they reach a point in their lives when they are no longer able to make decisions of their own about their care. The two main forms of advance directives are a Living Will and a Durable Power of Attorney for Health Care. In a Living Will the person specifies the conditions under which he or she wishes to receive certain treatment or to refuse or discontinue life-sustaining treatment. A Durable Power of Attorney for Health Care enables a person to identify one or more individuals who are empowered to speak for the ill person if this individual becomes unable or unwilling to speak for him- or herself. Some consider the Durable Power of Attorney to be more important because without having someone to speak on behalf of a dying person, the Living Will may be fairly ineffective. The Living Will can be helpful in guiding decisions but may be more powerful in providing evidence to other people about the ill person's wishes (James Werth, personal communication, May 7, 2013).

One of the continuing education workshops we attended was on "End-of-Life Decisions." The program consisted of a panel of presenters from different disciplines including clinical psychology, philosophy, medicine, psychiatry, social work, and law. What struck us was the complexity of this topic in practice. Although many health providers search for the best answers to difficult life-and-death situations, there are few simple answers. We came away from the conference with an increased awareness and appreciation of the difficult and complex nature of working with people who are dying. It reinforced our belief in how critical it is for helping professionals to be clear about their own values on a range of issues pertaining to end-of-life care.

Mental health counselors must understand their own values and attitudes about end-of-life options (such as clients' autonomy and their right to participate in hastening their own death). In addition, counselors need to understand their role in the decision-making process of clients who may choose to hasten their dying process (Bevacqua & Kurpius, 2013). Although there are no easy answers to questions about end-of-life care, mental health professionals are likely to face these situations with their clients. Gamino and Bevins (2013) identify a host of ethical challenges and dilemmas that counselors may need to consider: respecting client autonomy; assessing an individual's capacity for decision making; honoring advance directives; respecting an individual's cultural values; maintaining confidentiality; dealing with medical futility; establishing and maintaining appropriate boundaries; and including families in the scope of care. In addressing these ethical issues, practitioners should assist their clients in making decisions within the framework of their clients' own beliefs and value systems. Counselors must struggle with the ethical quandaries of balancing the need to protect client rights to autonomy and self-determination with meeting their ethical and legal responsibilities regarding end-of-life care. They must be prepared to work with both those who are dying and their family members. Indeed, they must develop *death competence*, a term proposed by Gamino and Ritter (2012) that refers to "specialized skill in tolerating and managing clients' problems related to dying, death, and bereavement" (pp. 29–30).

At this point in time, consider the following questions:

- What is your position on an individual's right to decide matters pertaining to living and dying? Does your position vary based on the person's physical health?
- How might your beliefs and values help or hinder your work with a client in making his or her own decision about end-of-life care?

Preserving and promoting a client's self-determination is a fundamental aspect of ethical care at the end of life. When people enter into a therapeutic relationship, they retain the right to determine what is done to them and for them, which captures the essence of the principle of autonomy. People from non-Western cultures may value autonomy differently, placing more value on the individual's role within the family or community than on the individual's personal interests (Gamino & Bevins, 2013).

Codes of Ethics Regarding End-of-Life Decisions

The National Association of Social Workers' (2003) policy statement pertaining to client self-determination in end-of-life decisions is based on the premise that choice should be intrinsic to all aspects of life and death, including decisions individuals with terminal conditions make regarding their continuing care or treatment options. These options include aggressive treatment of the medical condition, life-sustaining treatment, medical intervention intended to alleviate suffering (but not to cure), withholding or withdrawing life-sustaining treatment, voluntary active euthanasia, and physician-assisted suicide. A terminal condition is one in which there is no reasonable chance of recovery and in which the application of life-sustaining procedures would serve only to postpone the end of life. The *NASW Standards for Social Work Practice in Palliative and End of Life Care* (NASW, 2004) provides useful specific guidelines for any mental health professional who is working with clients on end-of-life care issues.

The American Psychological Association has been active in end-of-life care issues. APA has convened four groups to examine end-of-life issues, developed fact sheets for the general public, issued a comprehensive report on the topic, and passed two resolutions related to end-of-life issues. The APA has had continuing education programs on end-of-life issues at the national convention for many years (Werth & Crow, 2009) and now has a series of online modules regarding end-of-life topics.

In its *Code of Ethics*, AMHCA (2015) addresses end-of-life care for terminally ill clients. Regarding quality of care, AMHCA offers this guideline:

> Mental health counselors ensure that clients receive quality end-of-life care for their physical, emotional, social, and spiritual needs. This includes providing clients with an opportunity to participate in informed decision making regarding their end-of-life care, and a thorough assessment, from a qualified end-of-life care professional, of clients' ability to make competent decisions on their behalf. (I.8.a.)
>
> Mental health counselors are aware of their own personal, moral, and competency issues as it relates to end-of-life decisions. When mental health counselors assess that they are unable to work with clients on the exploration of end-of-life options, they make appropriate referrals to ensure clients receive appropriate help. (I.8.b.)

The policy statement of NASW (2003), the standards on end-of-life care of NASW (2004), and the end-of-life care standards of AMHCA (2015) provide social workers and mental health counselors with some general guidelines by which they can examine the ethical and legal issues pertaining to end-of-life decisions.

The American Counseling Association (2014) removed the specific reference to end-of-life care during the most recent revision of their *Code of Ethics*. The previous version of the code (ACA, 2005) allowed counselors to refer these clients based on, among other issues, moral and values conflicts for the counselor. This change was made by the ACA (2014) to remain internally consistent with the prohibition of referring clients solely due to a values conflict (A.11.b.) and reflects prioritizing clients' needs over counselors' values (Francis, 2014). The AMHCA's (2015) code differs on this issue and allows referrals based on the counselor's own personal, moral, or values issue. The ACA (2014) standard states that professional counselors must be aware of and "avoid imposing" the values they hold when working with all clients (A.4.b.). In addition, the laws of each state guide counselors' actions as they seek to provide the most competent care to clients who struggle with these monumental issues (Perry Francis, personal communication, August 15, 2016).

From an ethical and a legal standpoint, conducting a thorough assessment is critical in situations pertaining to end-of-life decisions. This assessment should consider matters such as diagnosable mental disorders, psychological factors that may be causing distress, quality of relationships, and spiritual concerns (Werth & Crow, 2009). The NASW (2004) standards for end-of-life care specifically address the importance of conducting a comprehensive assessment as a basis for developing interventions and designing treatment plans with dying persons. Some areas for consideration in this assessment are relevant past and current health situation, family structure and roles, stage in the life cycle, spirituality and faith, cultural values and beliefs, client's and family's goals in palliative treatment, social supports, and mental health functioning.

Role of Professionals in Helping Clients With End-of-Life Decisions

As a counselor, you need to be willing to discuss end-of-life decisions when clients bring such concerns to you. If you are closed to any personal examination of this issue, you may interrupt these dialogues, cut off your clients' exploration of their feelings, or attempt to provide clients with your own solutions based on your values and beliefs.

Some end-of-life decisions are made more broadly than is the case with physician-assisted suicide. One path is refusing all treatment as a choice of ending one's life. This option should not be considered as a passive approach because some action must be taken or not taken to allow death to occur. A question to address is, "Does a therapist have an ethical responsibility to explore the client's decision to refuse treatment?" Even though it is not against the law to refuse treatment, the client may have made this decision based on misinformation or a misunderstanding. Thus, a counselor could help the client assess the nature of the information upon which this decision was based. It is also necessary to assess for depression when clients decide to forgo treatment.

Psychological services are useful for healthy individuals who want to make plans about their own future care. Mental health practitioners need to acquire knowledge about the psychological, ethical, and legal considerations in end-of-life care. They can have a key role in helping people make choices regarding how they will die and about the ethical issues involved in making those choices (Kleespies, 2004). As a counselor, you are obligated to assist clients in an informed decision-making process, regardless of your personal beliefs about the outcome (Werth & Crow, 2009). It is the client's beliefs that must be understood and considered, not the counselor's values and beliefs pertaining to end-of-life decisions.

The mental health professions face the challenge of formulating ethical and procedural guidelines on right-to-die issues, especially in light of advances in medical technology and the aging of the population. In addition, in all states patients are free to refuse treatment to prolong life. Now let's examine some specific cases involving end-of-life decisions.

The Case of Fernando

A counselor has been seeing a client named Fernando who has been diagnosed with an aggressive and painful cancer. After a series of chemotherapy treatments and pain medication, Fernando tells the counselor that nothing seems to work and that he has decided to end his life. They discuss his decision for several sessions, examining all aspects, and Fernando becomes even clearer about his decision to end his life. Here are four counselors' responses to the decision Fernando has made.

Counselor A: Have you thought about a specific way you would end your life? If so, I have a duty to prevent you from carrying out an actual suicide by encouraging you to seek hospitalization or your giving me a written *no-suicide* contract.

Counselor B: I have a great deal of difficulty accepting your decision. I am asking you not to take any action for at least 3 weeks to give us time to talk about this further. Are there possibly ways for you to find meaning in your life in spite of your suffering?

Counselor C: Our relationship has come to mean a lot to both of us, especially at a time like this. I will continue to see you as long as you choose to come, and I will help you deal with your pain in any way that I can.

Counselor D: I need to consider what you are telling me. I want to continue working with you at this crucial point; however, I would like to consult with my attorney to make sure that I am fulfilling my legal obligations.

Counselor E: Could I contact your physician to discuss your medical status. Would you agree to my making this contact?

Consider each of these approaches, and then clarify what you would do in this situation by answering these questions:

- What are your thoughts about each counselor's response? Which one comes closest to your thinking?
- What would you want to say to Fernando?
- Is it ethical to impose your values on Fernando in this case? Why or why not?
- Do you think the state has the right to decide how individuals with terminal illnesses will die?

Commentary. We are not aware of any statute that imposes a reporting duty on mental health professionals when clients have a life-threatening condition and express thoughts of self-harm. However, state laws are not uniform with regard to reporting and protecting in the case of suicidal threats, so it is imperative that you become familiar with the law in your state or jurisdiction. According to James Werth, who coedited a book on the duty to protect, the laws of the majority of states and all ethics codes *allow,* but do not mandate, intervention with respect to danger to self (personal communication, May 7, 2013). Mental health professionals would not typically be found negligent for failing to take steps to protect a client who is considering hastening his or her own death if that person is in the final stages of a terminal illness. If a client is suffering from severe depression, yet is not facing a life-threatening disease, therapists may have an obligation to take steps to prevent suicide or self-harm.

In the case of Fernando, Counselor A suggested a "no-suicide" contract. This contract is only one factor in assessing whether the therapist went far enough in trying to protect Fernando. Although some consider this type of contract to be a useful clinical intervention, this approach is legally problematic. A therapist who is put on the stand by an attorney could be made to look negligent by relying on such a contract. Rather than rely on a no-suicide contract, a better approach is to develop a safety plan with a client. Counselor D tells Fernando that he wants to consult with an attorney to make sure he is attending to the legal aspects involved in this case, which can be considered as mainly a risk management intervention. Counselor E asks permission of Fernando to contact his physician to discuss his medical status, which seems like a useful strategy.

When you encounter this kind of case, the proper ethical and legal course is not always clear. If you do not report, you may be thinking of your client's autonomy, self-determination, and welfare. If your client is of sound mind, you may believe that he has a right to decide not to live in extreme pain. By providing him with the maximum degree of support as long as he wants this, you may think you have discharged your duty to this client. However, if you do not attempt to prevent his suicide and he does end his life, the family could sue you for breach of your professional duty. If you take measures to protect him from ending his life, and if he terminates his therapy because of your interventions, you will not be in a position to offer support or to help him in other ways.

Given the ethical, legal, and clinical complexity present with a terminally ill client who is contemplating hastening his or her own death, we encourage you to develop competence in managing end-of-life issues if you plan to work with this population. Also, be quick to pursue legal and collegial consultation when this issue emerges in your practice and document those consultations. •

The Case of Bettina

Bettina lives at boarding school and has made several suicide attempts. Because these attempts were judged to be primarily attention-getting gestures, her counselor feels manipulated and does not report them to Bettina's parents. During the last of these attempts, however, Bettina seriously hurts herself and ends up in the hospital.

- Do you see any conflict between what is ethically right and what is legally right in this situation?

- At what point in the client–counselor relationship is the counselor obligated to report Bettina's harm to self to the proper authorities?

- Did the counselor take the "cry for help" too lightly? Explain.

- What are the ethical and legal implications for the counselor in deciding that Bettina's attempts were more manipulative than serious and therefore should be ignored?

- If the counselor told Bettina that she was going to inform the girl's parents about these suicide attempts and Bettina had responded by saying that she would quit counseling if the counselor did so, what do you think the counselor should do?

Commentary. A client may use suicidal behaviors as a means of gaining attention, which complicates matters clinically, but this does not relieve the therapist from the obligation to treat the client's threats and actions seriously. Active measures were not taken by this counselor to protect the client from self-harm. Even one suicidal attempt demands a comprehensive assessment of the client's risk for suicide. This was not done, which resulted in the client's injury and hospitalization. The counselor was vulnerable to an accusation of serious negligence, which could have ended in Bettina's death.

For a comprehensive discussion of the issues associated with end-of-life decisions, we highly recommend *Counseling Clients Near the End of Life: A Practical Guide for Mental Health Professionals* by Werth (2013a). •

Chapter Summary

This chapter has addressed a variety of value-laden counseling situations and issues. We have focused our attention on the ways your values and those of your clients, the codes of ethics, and the legal system are interrelated in your counseling relationships.

Recent court cases have supported the right of counseling programs to enforce requirements that counseling students refrain from imposing their personal values on their clients. Some states have added freedom of conscience clauses to legislation to ensure that the licensure status of mental health professionals will not be in jeopardy should they deny services to clients on the basis of sincerely held religious beliefs. We have stressed that students need to be clearly informed before they enroll in a program about what is expected of them academically and personally. We all have a right to embrace our own personal and moral values, but it is crucial that students do not use their personal values as a yardstick by which to measure the values of clients. Counselors in training must understand and be prepared to follow the ethics codes of their profession.

It is important for clinicians to be open to addressing spiritual and religious concerns in the assessment process. Spiritual and religious values can play a vital role in the lives of many who seek counseling, and these values may be a valuable resource in therapy. In short, spirituality is a major source of strength for many clients and an important factor in promoting healing and well-being. Counselor education programs have an obligation to incorporate information about spiritual and religious competencies so that counselors will have a framework for addressing these concerns when clients are interested in doing so. A counselor's role is not to prescribe a particular pathway to clients in fulfilling their spiritual needs, but to help clients clarify their own pathway.

End-of-life decisions are another area in which counselors need to clarify their values. Mental health professionals have the challenge of clarifying their own beliefs and values pertaining to end-of-life decisions so that they can assist their clients in making decisions within the framework of clients' beliefs and value systems. In this matter, the counselor's role is to assist clients in making the best possible decisions in their situation. However, professionals must to be aware of state laws and professional codes of ethics concerning an individual's freedom to make certain kinds of end-of-life decisions.

Suggested Activities

1. Have a panel discussion on the topic "Is it possible for counselors to remain neutral with respect to their clients' values?" The panel can also discuss different ways in which counselors' values may affect the counseling process.
2. Invite several practicing counselors to talk to your class about the role of values in counseling. Invite counselors who have different theoretical orientations. For example, you might ask a behavior therapist and a humanistic therapist to talk to your class at the same time, if it is feasible, on the role of values.
3. In pairs discuss counseling situations that might involve a conflict of values. Then choose a specific situation to role-play, with one student playing the part of the client and the other playing the part of the counselor. Be sure to leave adequate time at the end to process the experience.

4. The case examples given in this chapter address a wide variety of value issues. In small groups, select two or three of these vignettes and discuss how you, as a group, might address the ethical issues raised in each of these cases.

5. Discuss this statement: "It is sometimes appropriate for counselors to influence clients to adopt values that seem to be in the best interests of clients."

   - In what ways do you agree or disagree with this statement?
   - How is the "best interest of the client" determined in counseling?
   - Under what circumstances would it be a good idea for the counselor to influence the client's values?
   - Under what circumstances might it be harmful for the counselor to influence the client's values?

6. Set up a debate with one side arguing for and the other side against this premise: A counselor should expose his or her values at the beginning of a therapy relationship. After the debate, have the entire group share their reactions and identify points that were most persuasive for them as observers.

7. Review the ASERVIC "Competencies for Addressing Spiritual and Religious Issues in Counseling" described in this chapter. How well has your program prepared you to deal with spiritual and religious concerns of clients you may see? What are your specific areas of strength? What are some areas you need to develop?

8. Some counselors believe terminally ill clients have the ultimate right to determine if, how, and when they will end their life. Other counselors believe their obligation is to assist clients in finding meaning in life regardless of a particular set of circumstances. In two groups, argue for and against rational suicide, addressing both ethical and legal issues. (Note: A good website to check out is www.deathwithdignity.org/acts.)

9. In this exercise one student acts as the counselor and the other as the client. The task of the counselor is to try to persuade the client to do what the counselor thinks would be best for the client. Then switch roles. Discuss your reactions to each role. In the role of counselor, what potential problems could emerge by imposing your agenda on clients, even if you think it is in their best interest? In the role of client, how did you feel when the counselor tried to persuade you to follow a particular course of action?

Ethics in Action Video Exercises

10. In video role play 7, Family Values: The Divorce, the client (Janice) has decided to leave her husband and get a divorce. She tells her counselor (Gary) that she doesn't want to work on her marriage anymore. Janice says that she is tired of her husband's anger and moods. The counselor responds: "I hate to hear that. What about your kids? Who will be the advocate for them?" She says, "If I am happy, they will be happy. I will take care of my kids." The counselor concludes by asking, "Is divorce the best way to take care of your children?" It is clear that the counselor has an agenda for the client. The counselor's focus is on the welfare of her children. The client feels misunderstood and does not think the counselor is helping her.

In small groups, discuss the main ethical issues in this case. If you were Janice's counselor, how do you imagine you would respond? What kind of questions would you ask of Janice, if any? Put yourself in this situation with a client similar to Janice. Assume that your client is experiencing a great deal of ambivalence about getting a divorce, even though she tells you she is convinced that her marital situation is hopeless. She pleads with you to tell her whether she should remain married or get a divorce. What approach might you take? If your client expects you to provide her with an answer, because she is coming to you as the expert, what would you do? Have one student role-play the confused client who is searching for an answer and ask several students to give different ways of proceeding with this client.

11. In video role play 8, Sexuality: Promiscuity, the client (Suzanne) is having indiscriminate sexual encounters, and her counselor (Richard) expresses concern for Suzanne when he learns about her sexual promiscuity. Richard then focuses on how Suzanne's behavior plays out the recurring theme of abandonment by her father, but she thinks there is no connection. If you were Suzanne's counselor, how would you deal with the situation as she presents it? What main ethical issues do you think this role play illustrates and what is your stance on these? Is it ethically appropriate for you to strongly influence your client to engage in safer sex practices, even if she did not ask for this? Demonstrate how you would approach Suzanne through role-playing.

12. In video role play 9, Being Judgmental: The Affair, the client (Natalie) shares with her counselor that she is struggling with her marriage and is having a long-term affair. The counselor (Janice) says, "Having an affair is not a good answer for someone—it just hurts everyone. I do not think it is a good idea." How would your values influence your interventions in this situation? In what value areas pertaining to relationships might you have difficulty maintaining objectivity? Are there situations in which you might want to get your client to adopt your values? This vignette can be useful in small group discussions, and also in role-playing. Have one student role-play the counselor and show how he or she might work with Natalie. In a second role play, have one student become the counselor's supervisor and demonstrate what issues you might explore with Janice.

13. Video role play 10, Imposing Values: Religion as an Answer, portrays a conflict of values between the client and the counselor. The client, LeAnne, thinks prayer should be her answer to her personal problems. She doesn't believe she is hearing the Lord clearly. Her counselor, Suzanne, has some trouble understanding what her client's religion means to her and how to work within LeAnne's religious framework in the counseling relationship. Instead, Suzanne comments that she feels that she is in competition with God and the client's religion. Suzanne wants her client to put more faith in the counseling process as an answer to her problems rather than relying on her religion.

In small groups discuss some of these questions: Is it ethical for you to challenge your client's belief in the power of prayer and her reliance on God to solve her problems? Explain. What ethical issues do you see if a client introduces spiritual or religious concerns and the counselor does not want to explore these with the client? If LeAnne were your client, how might you proceed with her? What concerns do you have, if any, about your ability to remain objective with LeAnne if she wants to talk about finding her answers in her religion?

14. In video role play 11, Value Conflicts: Contemplating an Abortion, there is a value clash between the client and the counselor. The client (Sally) is considering an abortion, and the therapist has difficulty with this possible decision. Lucia, the counselor,

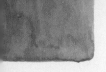

says that she is feeling uncomfortable because of her belief that life begins at conception. Lucia tells Sally that she will have to get some consultation so that she can sort out her thinking.

In small groups, discuss the ethical issues involved in this situation. How do you imagine the client feels about her counselor's responses? What are your thoughts about a counselor disclosing his or her beliefs about abortion so the client knows where the counselor stands? What are your thoughts from an ethical perspective if the counselor were to suggest a referral because of a value conflict? This would be a good case to role-play and show various ways of dealing with the client. When should a counselor seek supervision and consultation if his or her values conflict with those of the client?

15. In video role play 12, Counselor Disapproval: Coming Out, the client (Conrad) discloses his homosexual orientation. Conrad states that this is something he is struggling with, mainly because it is not accepted in his culture or in his religion. The client admits that he trusts his counselor (John) and it feels good to be able to make this disclosure. Conrad wants his counselor's help in coming out to his friends and family. So, it appears that the client wants to explore his thoughts and feelings about his sexual orientation in light of his cultural and religious values.

Conrad finds the counselor is unreceptive, and John says, "Are you sure this is the best thing for you?" Then John discloses that he does not approve of homosexuality, emphasizing that he does not see this as "being very healthy." Conrad has negative reactions to John's judgmental attitude and lack of acceptance of who he is as a person. In small groups discuss some of these questions: How does John's disclosure of his values affect the client–counselor relationship? If you were John's supervisor, what would you want him to look at? If you were the counselor in this situation, how would you respond to Conrad? If the counselor were to refer Conrad because of a value conflict, this would be a discriminatory referral, which is unethical. What steps can the counselor take, short of referral, to work effectively with this client?

16. In video role play 13, An Ethical and Legal Issue: End-of-Life Decision, the client (Gary) tells his counselor that he just found out he is HIV-positive and is seriously considering ending his life. The counselor (Natalie) tells Gary that she can't believe what she is hearing. Natalie is doing her best to persuade him not to take his life. She tells him that he is taking the easy way out if he chooses to end his life. She asks him if he has a plan. Natalie suggests to him that he think about his family and other options. She lets Gary know that he may be in a crisis state and not able to make a good decision.

What are the ethical and legal issues involved in this case? Can you see any potential conflict between the ethical and legal issues in this situation? If you were Gary's counselor, would you respect his decision to end his life, or would you attempt to influence him to search for alternatives to suicide? After discussing the issues involved in this case, practice role-playing the way you might deal with Gary.

MindTap for Counseling

Go to MindTap® for an eBook, videos of client sessions, activities, practice quizzes, apps, and more—all in one place. If your instructor didn't assign MindTap, you can find out more information at CengageBrain.com.

Multicultural Perspectives and Diversity Issues

LEARNING OBJECTIVES

1. Understand basic terminology related to multiculturalism and diversity

2. Identify how cultural encapsulation is an ethical matter

3. Examine ethics codes from a multicultural/diversity and social justice perspective

4. Evaluate a range of cultural values and assumptions in therapy

5. Explore ethical issues pertaining to sexual orientation

6. Understand ethical issues in working with people with disabilities

7. Clarify when matching of client and counselor is important

8. Explain how unintentional racism and microaggressions affect clients

9. Discuss what is involved in developing multicultural competence

SELF-INVENTORY

Directions: For each statement, indicate the response that most closely identifies your beliefs and attitudes. Use the following code:

5 = I *strongly agree* with this statement.

4 = I *agree* with this statement.

3 = I am *undecided* about this statement.

2 = I *disagree* with this statement.

1 = I *strongly disagree* with this statement.

_____ 1. To counsel effectively, I must be of the same ethnic background as my client.

_____ 2. Basically, all clients are multicultural.

_____ 3. Being culturally competent is an ongoing learning journey; I will never know everything about every culture.

_____ 4. I will be able to examine my behavior and attitudes to determine the degree to which cultural bias influences the interventions I make with clients.

_____ 5. Whether we are aware of it or not, culture influences our lives and defines reality for each of us.

_____ 6. Counselors should advocate on behalf of oppressed clients and empower them to find their voice.

_____ 7. An effective mental health practitioner facilitates assimilation of culturally diverse clients into society.

_____ 8. Ethical practice requires that counselors become familiar with the value systems of diverse cultural groups.

_____ 9. I would have no trouble working with someone from a culture very different from mine because we would be more alike than different.

_____ 10. If I just listen to my clients, I will know all I need to know about their cultural background.

_____ 11. Establishing a trusting relationship is more difficult when the counselor and the client come from different cultures.

_____ 12. Unless practitioners have been educated about cultural differences, they cannot determine their competency to work with diverse populations.

_____ 13. As a condition for licensure, all counselors should have specialized training and supervised experience in multicultural/diversity counseling.

_____ 14. At this point in my educational career, I feel well prepared to counsel culturally diverse client populations.

_____ 15. All mental health professionals need to appreciate the ways that diversity influences the client–counselor relationship and the counseling process itself.

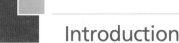

Introduction

In this chapter we examine the cultural values, beliefs, and assumptions of helping professionals and their clients and discuss how these values may influence therapeutic outcomes. We emphasize the ethical dimensions of becoming aware of our own values and potential biases, as well as understanding the client's worldview and tailoring the therapeutic process to the client's cultural context. Our cultural experiences, values, and assumptions are the basis of our worldview and possible biases, so it is important to be aware of how they influence our practice. We also discuss sexual orientation and gender identity, and the values surrounding these topics.

One of the major challenges facing mental health professionals is understanding the complex role cultural diversity and similarity play in therapeutic work. Clients and counselors bring a wide variety of attitudes, values, culturally learned assumptions, biases, beliefs, and behaviors to the therapeutic relationship. Some counselors may deny the importance of these cultural variables in counseling; others might overemphasize the importance of cultural differences, lose their spontaneity, and thus may lose contact with their clients. Because each of us comes from a unique blend of cultures and identities, all counseling interactions can be seen as multicultural events. Working effectively with cultural diversity in the therapeutic process is a requirement of good ethical practice.

Duran, Firehammer, and Gonzalez (2008) assert that culture is part of the soul: "When the soul or culture of some persons are oppressed, we are all oppressed and wounded in ways that require healing if we are to become liberated from such oppression. When discussing these issues, it is important to realize that we have all been on both sides of the oppression/oppressor coin at different points in our lives" (p. 288). Mental health practitioners must avoid using their own group as the standard by which to assess appropriate behavior in others. In addition, greater differences may exist within the same cultural group than between different cultural groups, and we need to be intraculturally sensitive as well as multiculturally sensitive. Cultural sensitivity is not limited to one group but applies to all cultures. There is no sanctuary from cultural bias.

Cultural diversity, as well as cultural prejudice, is a fact of life in our world. Yet it is only within the past couple of decades that helping professionals have realized that they can no longer ignore the pressing issues involved in serving culturally diverse populations. To the extent that counselors are focused on the values of the dominant culture and unaware of variations among groups and individuals, they are at risk for practicing unethically. We need to be mindful of how diversity plays out in all counseling interactions if we are to practice ethically, competently, and effectively.

In this chapter we focus on the ethical implications of a multicultural perspective or lack thereof in the helping professions. To ensure that the terms we use in this chapter have a clear meaning, we have provided specific definitions in the box titled "Multicultural Terminology."

Multicultural Terminology

The word **culture,** interpreted broadly, is associated with a racial or ethnic group as well as with gender, age, religion or spirituality, economic status, nationality, physical capacity or disability, and affectional or sexual orientation. Pedersen (2000) describes culture as including demographic variables such as age, gender, and place of residence; status variables such as social, educational, and economic background; formal and informal affiliations; and the ethnographic variables of nationality, ethnicity, language, and religion. Considering culture from this broad perspective provides a context for understanding that each of us is a member of many different cultures. Culture can be considered as a lens through which life is perceived. Each culture, through its differences and similarities, generates a phenomenologically different experience of reality (Diller, 2015). Choudhuri, Santiago-Rivera, and Garrett (2012) define culture as a "total way of life held in common by a group of people who share similarities in speech, behavior, ideology, livelihood, technology, values, and social customs" (p. 34).

Ethnicity is a sense of identity that stems from common ancestry, history, nationality, religion, and race. This unique social and cultural heritage provides cohesion and strength. It is a powerful unifying force that offers a sense of belonging and sharing based on commonality (Lum, 2004; Markus, 2008).

An **oppressed group** refers to a group of people who have been singled out for differential and unequal treatment and who regard themselves as objects of collective discrimination. These groups have been characterized as subordinate, dominated, and powerless.

Multiculturalism is a generic term that indicates any relationship between and within two or more diverse groups. A multicultural perspective takes into consideration the specific values, beliefs, and actions influenced by a client's ethnicity, gender, religion, socioeconomic status, political views, sexual orientation, physical and mental/cognitive abilities, geographic region, and historical experiences with the dominant culture. Multiculturalism provides a conceptual framework that recognizes the complex diversity of a pluralistic society, while at the same time suggesting bridges of shared concern that bind culturally different individuals to one another (Pedersen, 1991, 2000).

Multicultural counseling "can be operationally defined as the working alliance between counselor and client that takes the personal dynamics of the counselor and client into consideration alongside the dynamics of the cultures of both of these individuals" (Lee & Park, 2013, p. 5). From this perspective, counseling is a helping intervention and process that defines contextual goals consistent with the life experiences and cultural values of clients, balancing the importance of individualism versus collectivism in assessment, diagnosis, and treatment (Sue & Sue, 2013).

Cultural diversity refers to the spectrum of differences that exists among groups of people with definable and unique cultural backgrounds (Diller, 2015).

Diversity refers to individual differences on a number of variables that can potentially put clients at risk for discrimination based on age, gender, gender identity, race, ethnicity, culture, national origin, religion, sexual orientation, disability, language, or socioeconomic status. Both multiculturalism and diversity have been politicized in the United States in ways that have often been divisive, but these terms can equally represent positive assets in a pluralistic society.

Cultural pluralism is a perspective that recognizes the complexity of cultures and values the diversity of beliefs and values. Lee and Park (2013) add that "counselors must provide services that help people to solve problems or make decisions in the midst of such sweeping demographic and sociological change" (p. 5).

Cultural diversity competence refers to a practitioner's level of awareness, knowledge, and interpersonal skills needed to function effectively in a pluralistic society and to intervene on behalf of clients from diverse backgrounds (Sue & Sue, 2013).

Cultural empathy pertains to therapists' awareness of clients' worldviews, which are acknowledged in relation to therapists' awareness of their own personal biases (Pedersen, Crethar, & Carlson, 2008).

Culture-centered counseling is a three-stage developmental sequence, from multicultural awareness to knowledge and comprehension to skills and applications. The individual's or group's culture plays a central role in understanding their behavior in context (Pedersen, 2000).

Cultural awareness includes a compassionate and accepting orientation that is based on an understanding of oneself and others within one's culture and context (Crethar & Winterowd, 2012).

Social justice work in counseling involves the empowerment of individuals and family systems to better express their needs as well as to advocate on their behalf to address inequities and injustices they encounter in their community and in society at large (Toporek, Lewis, & Crethar, 2009). Counseling from a social justice perspective involves being aware of and addressing the realities of oppression, privilege, and social inequities.

Cultural tunnel vision is a perception of reality based on a very limited set of cultural experiences. *Culturally encapsulated counselors* define reality according to a narrow set of cultural assumptions and fail to evaluate other viewpoints, making little attempt to understand and accept the behavior of others.

Globally literate counselors display a cultural curiosity that is characterized by an openness to engaging in new cultural experiences. Global literacy goes beyond tolerance of diverse cultures and worldviews; it promotes mutual respect and understanding (Lee, 2013b).

Stereotypes are oversimplified and uncritical generalizations about individuals who are identified as belonging to a specific group. Such learned expectations can influence how counselors see the client.

Racism is any pattern of behavior that, solely because of race or culture, denies access to opportunities or privileges to members of one racial or cultural group while perpetuating access to opportunities and privileges to members of another racial or cultural group (Ridley, 2005). Racism can operate on individual, interpersonal, and institutional levels, and it can occur intentionally or unintentionally.

Unintentional racism is often subtle, indirect, and outside our conscious awareness; this can be the most damaging and insidious form of racism (Sue, 2005). Practitioners who presume that they are free of any traces of racism seriously underestimate the impact of their own socialization. Whether these biased attitudes are intentional or unintentional, the result is harmful for both individuals and society.

Cultural racism is the belief that one group's history, way of life, religion, values, and traditions are superior to others. This allows for an unequal distribution of power to be justified a priori (Sue, 2005).

Microaggressions are persistent verbal, behavioral, and environmental assaults, insults, and invalidations that often occur subtly and are difficult to identify (Choudhuri et al., 2012). They usually involve demeaning implications and may be perpetrated against others on the basis of their race, gender, sexual orientation, or ability status.

There is some concern about how to refer appropriately to certain racial and ethnic groups as preferred names tend to change. For instance, some alternate names for one group are Hispanic, Latino (Latina), Mexican American, or Chicana (Chicano). Practitioners can show sensitivity to the fact that a name is important by asking their clients how they would like to be identified and by listening for the words clients themselves use.

In our discussions as coauthors and in our classrooms with students, we have debated the pros and cons of including cases that identify specific cultures and issues of difference. Although it is useful to challenge readers to wrestle with cultural specifics, we share a concern with our students that we not perpetuate stereotypes of any specific cultural group. We hope that the benefits of including specific cultural identities in this textbook and case examples helps to facilitate meaningful reflection on complex ethical, legal, clinical, and cultural issues. We hope this chapter will inspire and motivate you as a developing clinician to see the many ways culture enhances our lives, the lives of our clients, and the therapeutic alliance we establish as we engage with clients.

The Problem of Cultural Tunnel Vision

Cultural pluralism is a perspective that recognizes the complexity of cultures and values the diversity of beliefs and values. To operate as if all our clients are the same is simplistic and can result in unethical and ineffective practice. Lum (2011) maintains that the route to cultural competence begins with an understanding of our own personal and professional cultural awareness. It is critical to develop an understanding of our personal and cultural values and beliefs and to examine our personal assumptions, biases, and values. Our cultural self-awareness can have a direct influence on our practice and our relationships with clients. For example, if we value autonomy and independence, yet have never reflected on or examined our own values, assumptions, and biases, we may inadvertently impose this value on a client who prizes interdependence and collectivism. From Lum's perspective, cultural awareness alone is not sufficient; it is the first step leading to cultural sensitivity and to achieving cultural competence.

Issues pertaining to culture often are complex and multilayered, which can leave a clinician feeling overwhelmed and tempted to ignore or oversimplify the presenting issues. This can lead to **cultural tunnel vision,** a perception of reality based on a very limited set of cultural experiences. Trainees could unwittingly impose their values on unsuspecting clients by assuming that everyone shares these values. Students are faced with the challenge of exploring their attitudes and fears about people who are different from them. At times, student helpers from privileged backgrounds have expressed the attitude, explicitly or implicitly, that clients from other racial and ethnic groups are unresponsive to professional psychological intervention and lack the motivation to change, which these student helpers label as "resistance." Students need to be trained to ask themselves if what they call resistance may be a healthy response on the part of the client to the helper's cultural and theoretical bias. Students are not alone in their susceptibility to cultural tunnel vision. It is important for both counselors in training and practicing mental health professionals to continuously examine their potential for cultural tunnel vision.

Sue, Capodilupo, Nadal, and Torino (2008) suggest that many White Americans have difficulty acknowledging race-related issues because they stir up guilt feelings about their privileged status and threaten their self-image as moral, fair, and decent human beings. As they point out, "to accept the racial reality of [People of Color] inevitably means confronting one's own unintentional complicity in the perpetuation of racism" (p. 277). Similarly, an American person of color may assume that all White Americans view the world through a privileged status. We need to examine any generalization that rules out differences among groups.

In the 1960s Gilbert Wrenn (1962), one of the pioneers in the counseling profession, characterized a **culturally encapsulated counselor** as having some of the following traits:

- Defines reality according to one set of cultural assumptions
- Shows insensitivity to cultural variations among individuals
- Accepts unreasoned assumptions without proof or ignores proof because that might disconfirm one's assumptions
- Fails to evaluate other viewpoints and makes little attempt to accommodate the behavior of others
- Is trapped in one way of thinking that resists adaptation and rejects alternatives

Years later Wrenn (1985) maintained that cultural encapsulation continues to be a problem for counseling professionals, and we believe Wrenn's observations of decades ago remain relevant today. A good way to begin to develop a multicultural perspective is by becoming more aware of our own culturally learned assumptions, some of which may be culturally biased. This provides a context for understanding how diverse cultures share common ground and also how to recognize areas of similarity and uniqueness. Pedersen (2008) reminds us that the complexity of culture can be viewed as friend rather than foe because it helps us avoid searching for easy answers to hard questions. Pedersen has long maintained that it is no longer possible for effective counselors to ignore their own cultures or the cultures of their clients through encapsulation. Whether we are aware of it or not, culture controls our lives and defines reality for each of us. Cultural factors are an integral part of the helping process, and these factors influence the interventions we use with our clients.

Social justice moves beyond cultural awareness and focuses on active support and advocacy, including promoting equality and justice for underserved and oppressed groups of people (Crethar & Winterowd, 2012). Cultural competence involves having an understanding of how social systems operate with respect to the treatment of culturally diverse groups. This entails understanding the impact of systemic forces such as racism, sexism, heterosexism, classism, and ableism on the psychosocial development of individuals (Lee & Park, 2013).

Lee (2013b) makes a case for becoming a globally literate person, "a lifelong process that is rooted in a commitment to living one's life in a manner that makes cultural diversity a core principle.... Embracing a globally literate lifestyle also involves a commitment to social justice and social responsibility" (p. 311). Globally literate counselors are committed to expanding their comfort zone throughout their careers. Lee emphasizes that global literacy is not mainly learned in the classroom; rather, it is "the result of one's attempt to become a lifelong student of cultural diversity and a true citizen of the world" (p. 312). This concept is in stark contrast to counselors who are culturally encapsulated and believe that their culture represents the "best way" to live.

The Challenges of Reaching Diverse Client Populations

The *Multicultural and Social Justice Counseling Competencies* developed by the Association for Multicultural Counseling and Development (AMCD, 2015) provides a framework for the effective delivery of services to diverse client populations. Another useful resource is the APA's (1993a) "Guidelines for Providers of Psychological Services to Ethnic, Linguistic, and Culturally Diverse Populations." The APA's guidelines challenge practitioners to respect the roles of family members and the community structures, hierarchies, values, and beliefs that are an integral part of the client's culture. Providers should identify resources in the client's family and the larger community and use them in delivering culturally sensitive services. For example, an entire Native American family may come to a clinic to provide support for an individual in distress because many of the healing practices found in Native American communities are centered on the family and the community.

Psychology has traditionally been based on Western assumptions, which have not always considered the influence and impact of racial and cultural socialization (APA, 2003a). Many clients have come to distrust helpers associated with the establishment or with social service agencies because of a history of unequal treatment. Clients from oppressed groups may be slow to form trusting relationships with counselors, and mental health professionals may have difficulty identifying with these clients if they ignore the history behind this distrust. Helpers from all cultural groups need to honestly examine their own assumptions, expectations, and attitudes about the helping process.

The medical model of clinical counseling often is not a good fit for people of lower socioeconomic status. Child care and transportation difficulties are insurmountable economic barriers for many. In addition, taking time off from work for medical appointments may mean loss of pay. Therapists must be willing to go outside of the office to deliver services in the community. Home-based therapy has been used extensively with ethnic minority clients and families, mainly because many people in the community do not trust traditional mental health professionals (Zur, 2008). Zur comments that making a home visit with these clients can be a way to get a firsthand view of their home, rituals, neighborhood, community, and support system. Going outside the office can decrease suspicion and enhance trust; however, it is important to consider ethical considerations when using nontraditional modalities of therapy. Delivering helping services in nontraditional ways is discussed in detail in Chapter 13.

Sometimes cultural traditions contribute to the underutilization of traditional psychotherapeutic services by clients from diverse groups. Cultural beliefs and norms may stop some people from seeking professional help when faced with a problem. For example, consider Jiwoo's experience of being torn between marrying a person selected by his parents and marrying a woman of his choice. He might first look for a solution within himself through contemplation. If he were unable to resolve his dilemma, he might seek assistance from a family member or from a religious or spiritual adviser. Then he might look to some of his friends for advice and support in making the best decision. If none of these approaches resulted in a satisfactory resolution of his problem, Jiwoo might then reach outside his cultural community for an "outside expert" as a last resort. The fact that he did not seek counseling services sooner has little to do with resistance or with insensitivity on the part of counselors; Jiwoo was following a route congruent with his cultural background.

Some argue that ethnic minority clients who use counseling resources may lose their cultural values in the process. Some culturally encapsulated helpers mistakenly assume that a lack of assertiveness is a sign of dysfunctional behavior that should be changed. Labeling this behavior dysfunctional reflects the counselor's value orientation and also may result in microaggressions. Practitioners need to consider whether passivity is a problem from the client's culturally learned perspective and whether assertiveness is a useful behavior that the client hopes to acquire.

Ethics Codes From a Diversity Perspective

Most ethics codes mention the practitioner's responsibility to recognize the needs of diverse client populations. Gallardo, Johnson, Parham, and Carter (2009) develop the theme that integrating culturally responsive practices with more traditional models of therapy is of major importance when we consider the diverse client populations that mental health professionals serve. They add that it is not enough for therapists to simply practice within the framework of the ethics codes. Gallardo and colleagues take the position "that if we begin with a cultural framework at the outset, the lens by which we view our ethics codes, and minimum standards, also evolves to more accurately reflect the cultural realities inherent in our services" (p. 427). Culture influences every facet of our existence, so it is necessary that culturally responsive practice be central in all that we do.

Take the time to review the ethics codes of one or more professional organizations to determine for yourself the degree to which such codes take multicultural dimensions into account. Then consider how you could increase your multicultural competencies beyond what is suggested by these codes. The Ethics Codes box titled "Addressing Diversity" provides an overview of how the various codes address these issues.

ETHICS CODES: Addressing Diversity

The **Canadian Counselling Association's** (2007) code of ethics calls for members to respect diversity:

> Counselors actively work to understand the diverse cultural background of the clients with whom they work, and do not condone or engage in discrimination based on age, color, culture, ethnicity, disability, gender, religion, sexual orientation, marital, or socio-economic status. (B.9.)

continued

ETHICS CODES: Addressing Diversity *continued*

In the Preamble of the **Code of Professional Ethics for Rehabilitation Counselors** (CRCC, 2010), the following statement recognizes the value of diversity:

> Rehabilitation counselors are committed to facilitating the personal, social, and economic independence of individuals with disabilities. In fulfilling this commitment, rehabilitation counselors recognize diversity and embrace a cultural approach in support of the worth, dignity, potential, and uniqueness of individuals with disabilities within their social and cultural context. They look to professional values as an important way of living out an ethical commitment.

The *ASCA Ethical Standards for School Counselors* (ASCA, 2016) offers the following guideline regarding the social justice mandate:

> School counselors monitor and expand personal multicultural and social justice advocacy awareness, knowledge and skills to be an effective culturally competent school counselor. Understand how prejudice, privilege and various forms of oppression based on ethnicity, racial identity, age, economic status, abilities/disabilities, language, immigration status, sexual orientation, gender, gender identity expression, family type, religious/spiritual identity, appearance and living situations (e.g., foster care, homelessness, incarceration) affect students and stakeholders. (B.3.i.)

The *Code of Ethics of the American Mental Health Counselors Association* (AMHCA, 2015) emphasizes self-awareness on the part of the counselor:

> Mental health counselors have a responsibility to educate themselves about their own biases toward those of different races, creeds, identities, orientations, cultures, and physical and mental abilities; and then to seek consultation, supervision and/or counseling in order to prevent those biases from interfering with the counseling process. (C.2.c)

The **ACA** (2014) ethics code infuses issues of multiculturalism and diversity throughout the document, including sections dealing with the counseling relationship, informed consent, bartering, accepting gifts, confidentiality and privacy, professional responsibility, assessment and diagnosis, supervision, and education and training programs.

> Multicultural/Diversity Considerations: Counselors maintain awareness and sensitivity regarding cultural meanings of confidentiality and privacy. Counselors respect differing views toward disclosure of information. Counselors hold ongoing discussions with clients as to how, when, and with whom information is to be shared. (B.1.a.)

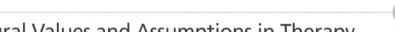

Cultural Values and Assumptions in Therapy

Cultural conflicts sometimes occur between the values inherent in traditional approaches to counseling and the values of culturally diverse groups. Counselors who operate from culturally biased views of mental health and who use intervention strategies that are not congruent with the values of culturally diverse people perpetuate forms of injustice and institutional racism (Duran et al., 2008).

Chung and Bemak (2012) believe clinicians must be willing to redefine their professional roles and adapt their practices to better suit the client's worldview, life experiences, and cultural identity. "Western skills, techniques, interventions, models, and theories need to be aligned to be culturally sensitive" (p. 72). Chung and

Bemak also contend that counselors cannot ignore the impact of racism, sexism, and other forms of discrimination and oppression on the well-being of their clients, nor the negative impact these "isms" may have on families and communities. Ivey, D'Andrea, and Ivey (2012) state that traditional approaches to counseling theory and skills may be inappropriate and ineffective with some groups. Special attention must be given to how socioeconomic factors, sexism, heterosexism, and racism influence a client's worldview. Ivey and colleagues note that traditional counseling strategies are being adapted for use in a more culturally respectful manner. In working with diverse clients, mental health professionals need to expand their perception of mental health practices to include support systems such as family, friends, community, self-help programs, and occupational networks.

Cultural differences are real, and they influence all human interactions (Lee & Park, 2013). Clinicians may misunderstand clients of a different sex, race, ethnicity, age, social class, or sexual orientation. If practitioners fail to integrate these diversity factors into their practice, they are infringing on the client's cultural autonomy and basic human rights. Without awareness, the counselor's ability to be helpful is limited. For instance, a clinician may misinterpret a client's close relationships with extended family members to be indicative of enmeshment and pathologize her behavior as being overly dependent. Ethical practice requires that practitioners be trained to address diversity factors when they become relevant in the therapy process. In the cases that follow, the therapists imposed their values in ways that significantly detracted from the value of therapy and may have resulted in significant harm to the clients. The imposition of values can be transparent—as in these cases—or more subtle, but in both cases it is unethical.

The Case of Hanh

Stacy is a high school counselor. A Vietnamese student, Hanh, is assigned to her because of academic difficulties. Stacy observes that Hanh is slow and deliberate in his conversational style, and she immediately assigns him to a remedial speech class. In the course of their conversations, Hanh discloses to Stacy that his father wants him to apply to college and major in pre-med. Hanh is not sure that he even wants to attend college. Stacy gives Hanh a homework assignment, asking him to tell his father that he no longer wants to pursue college plans and wants to follow a direction that appeals to him.

- Was the fact that Hanh spoke slowly and deliberately an indication that he needed a remedial speech class? Can you offer other explanations for Hanh's slow and deliberate speech?

- If you were Hanh's therapist, how would you deal with the conflict between Hanh's goals and his father's expectations?

- Was Stacy culturally sensitive when asking Hanh to directly confront his father? What other alternatives were available?

- Was Stacy too quick in making her assessments, considering that Hanh was sent to the school counselor by a teacher? Would it have made a difference if he had come voluntarily for guidance?

- Would you recommend family counseling? If so, how would you present this to Hanh and his parents?

Commentary. When there is a cultural difference between counselor and client, counselors must familiarize themselves with how the client approaches counseling and avoid imposing their worldview on the client. Although we hope the counselor would explore with Hanh his choice of a major in college and the conflict with his father over his educational and career plans, it is inappropriate for the counselor to tell Hanh what to do. Suggesting that Hanh directly confront his father has serious implications; Hanh's father may never speak to him again if Hanh is confrontational. Our assessment skills need to encompass the cultural context and the consequences of proposed interventions on the client's life. •

The Case of Cynthia

Sage has recently set up a private practice in a culturally diverse neighborhood. Cynthia comes to Sage for counseling. Cynthia is depressed, feels that life has little meaning, and feels trapped by the needs of her husband and small children. When Sage asks about any recent events that could be contributing to her depression, she tells him that she has discussed with her husband her desire to return to school and pursue a career of her choosing. Her husband threatened a divorce if she followed through with her plans. Cynthia then consulted with her pastor, who pointed out her obligations to her family. Sage is aware of his own cultural biases, which include a strong commitment to family and to the role of the man as the head of the household. Although he feels empathy for Cynthia's struggle, he persuades her to postpone her own aspirations until her children have grown up. She agrees to this because she feels guilty about asserting her own needs, and she is also fearful of being left alone. Sage then works with her to find other ways to add meaning to her life that would not have such a dramatic impact on the family.

- List the potential gender and cultural issues in this case. How might you have addressed each of them?

- Sage did not explore the lack of meaning in Cynthia's life until after he persuaded her to give up her aspirations. What ethical issue does this raise?

- If Cynthia had shared Sage's family values, would his approach have been appropriate?

Commentary. Cynthia spoke with two significant people regarding her aspirations, and both of them rejected her goals. The therapist also ignored her aspirations. A more ethical approach would be to provide a supportive environment in which Cynthia could explore her struggles without the therapist imposing his agenda on her. Cynthia should not feel pressured to adopt the therapist's value system, nor let her actions be determined by her need to please the therapist. Sage's ethical duty is to listen to Cynthia's aspirations without judgment and to respect her struggle in her journey toward finding her own answers. •

Individualistic Versus Collectivistic Cultural Values

Writers in the field of multicultural counseling allege that most contemporary theories of therapy and therapeutic practices are grounded in individualistic assumptions frequently associated with the values of mainstream U.S. culture (Duran et al., 2008; Sue & Sue, 2013). These values include autonomy, independence, self-determination, and becoming your own person. According to Johnson, Barnett, Elman, Forrest, and Kaslow (2012), Western cultures tend to promote independent models of the self that emphasize personal control and the preeminence of individual rights and responsibilities. Feminist and multicultural scholars are critical of this model and emphasize the salience of mutual interdependence, connection to others, communal responsibilities, and emotional responsiveness in leading a moral life. The broader social contexts of families, groups, and communities are often important to clients who value the interdependent self more than the independent self. Duran and colleagues (2008) claim that Western (individualistic) counseling interventions have at times been used to promote social control and conformity rather than the psychological well-being of people in diverse groups.

Practitioners who draw from any of the contemporary therapeutic models would do well to reflect on the underlying values of their theoretical orientation. Many of the therapy systems reflect core value orientations of mainstream American culture. Hogan (2013) characterizes these underlying values as emphasizing the patriarchal nuclear family; keeping busy; measurable and visible accomplishments; individual choice, responsibility, and achievement; self-reliance and self-motivation; change and novel ideas; competition; direct communication; materialism; and equality, informality, and fair play. The degree to which these value orientations fit clients from other cultures needs to be carefully considered by practitioners.

Challenging Stereotypical Beliefs and Cultural Bias

Counselors may think they are not culturally biased, yet may continue to hold stereotypical beliefs and cultural biases that could affect their practice. Some examples include these statements: "Failure to change stems from a lack of motivation." "People have choices, and it is up to them to change their lives." To assume that what people lack is motivation is simplistic and judgmental and does not encourage exploration of their struggles. Furthermore, many people do not have a wide range of choices due to environmental and multisystemic factors beyond their control.

Practitioners who counsel people in diverse groups without an awareness of their own stereotypical beliefs, cultural biases, and faulty assumptions can cause harm to their clients. Cross-culturally competent practice requires that mental health practitioners be aware of the unique cultural realities of their clients. Culturally competent counselors are engaged in an aspirational practice and are continually developing attitudes and beliefs, knowledge, and skills that enable them to work effectively with diverse clients. They realize that they can never say they have arrived at a final state of competency.

Examining Some Common Assumptions

Unexamined assumptions of therapists can be harmful to clients, especially assumptions based on one's own cultural biases. Becoming a culturally competent clinician involves acknowledging that we bring our cultural biases, assumptions, stereotypes, and life experiences to our work with clients. When we are helped to recognize our cultural biases and assumptions, we are less likely to act against the best interests of clients from diverse groups and backgrounds. Crethar and

Winterowd (2012) show how counselors with a *social justice orientation* are aware of their assumptions and how these views influence the therapeutic process:

> When counselors work from the assumption that their clients have the same needs, desires, values, and perspectives as they do, they are likely to make errors based on differences in culture and context. Counselors with multicultural competence take the time to co-develop goals with clients and their communities that prioritize the clients' values, culture, and context. Goals and therapeutic approaches that emerge as a result of such collaboration ultimately serve clients best. (pp. 5–6)

Mental health practitioners need to examine how privilege operates in the therapeutic relationship. Certain groups have more privileges and entitlements than others; examples include White, male, and middle-class privilege. It is important to examine the economic privilege that we may have as counselors that can prevent us from fully understanding the everyday struggles and worldviews of clients who are from lower socioeconomic backgrounds. People who face homelessness, poverty, and extreme financial burdens are often filled with feelings of shame and are the recipients of judgment, ridicule, and blame in society. A counselor's economic privilege might lead to misunderstanding in the following ways:

- Labeling clients as resistant or unmotivated if they are not able to arrive for appointments on time, are absent from sessions, or are unable to pay for sessions
- Challenging clients to take steps to improve their economic conditions without addressing or validating sociocultural restrictions that affect a client's disadvantaged position in society
- Assuming clients from lower socioeconomic status groups are less intelligent, less effective as parents, or less educated

Gerald Monk (2013), who works with counselor trainees in community settings, says "it is easy to overlook the constraining social factors that affect our clients pertaining to class and socioeconomic status" (p. 105). It is crucial that trainees acknowledge their privileged background, monitor how their own socioeconomic status differs from that of their clients, and become aware of how this difference affects the therapeutic relationship. Monk tells his economically privileged students that being privileged is not wrong. The key issue is not *being* privileged, but how this privilege is *used*. He states: "Our trainee therapists need to develop a consciousness of their own social class influences and refrain from imposing their own class-related assumptions on their clients' particular life challenges" (p. 105).

The following sections examine some commonly held beliefs and assumptions about the therapeutic environment that have implications for effectively working with clients from diverse cultural backgrounds.

Assumptions About Self-Disclosure Therapists may assume that clients will be ready to talk about their intimate personal issues, or that self-disclosure is essential for the therapeutic process to work. Sue and Sue (2013) point out that most forms of contemporary therapy place value on one's ability to self-disclose by sharing intimate personal material. The assumption is that self-disclosure is a characteristic of a healthy personality. The converse is that individuals who are reluctant to self-disclose in therapy possess negative traits such as being guarded and mistrustful. However, it is unacceptable in some cultures to reveal personal problems because it not only reflects on the person individually but also on the whole family. Some clients may view self-disclosure and interpersonal warmth as inappropriate in a professional relationship with an authority figure (Barnett & Johnson, 2015). There are strong pressures on many Asian American clients not to reveal personal concerns to strangers or outsiders. Similar pressures have been reported for Latino, American Indian, and African American clients, military clients, as well as those from various other cultures. Therapists need to realize that cultural forces may be operating when clients are slow to disclose personal details. Indeed, for many clients it seems strange for them to talk about themselves personally to a professional therapist whom they do not know. This is illustrated in Alberto's case.

The Case of Alberto

Alberto, a Latino client, comes to a community college counseling center on the recommendation of his physician, who found no organic basis for his symptoms of depression, chronic sleep disturbance, and the imminent threat of failing his classes. As you begin your initial session with Alberto, you recognize that he is extremely guarded, revealing little about himself or how he is feeling. You believe that self-disclosure and openness to the expression of feelings are necessary for change to occur. In trying to help Alberto, you challenge him to be more self-disclosing.

- To what areas of your client's sense of privacy and culture might you want to be sensitive?

- If you were to encourage Alberto to be more self-disclosing, what possible consequences might there be in his outside life? Explain.

- Can you think of some reasons Alberto's cautiousness may be more adaptive than maladaptive?

- What cultural norms about gender and self-disclosure do you bring to your work with Alberto that may help or inhibit your work with him?

Commentary. It is important not to pathologize a client who is cautious during the early phase of therapy. Be aware of and respect the differences that exist among different cultures and people in establishing trust, especially in the beginning of a therapeutic relationship. For some, it is very foreign to speak to a stranger without first developing a rapport with the person. Some clients have a greater need than others to develop a relationship with a therapist before they make themselves vulnerable. The fact that Alberto followed through on his physician's recommendation is a sign that he is open to help, and your task is to provide the structure that allows him to feel safe enough to express his concerns. It would be especially useful for you to explain to Alberto how the therapeutic process works. By acknowledging how difficult it is to open up to strangers, Alberto is likely to feel understood by you. The case of Alberto reminds us that counselors must ensure their own competence—in this case cultural competence—before launching into therapy work with culturally different clients. •

The Case of Lily

Lily, a licensed professional counselor, has come to work in a family-life center that deals with many immigrant families. She often reacts impatiently with the pace of her clients' disclosures. Lily decides to teach her clients by modeling self-disclosure for them. With one of her reticent couples she says: "My husband and I fight and disagree a lot. We express our feelings openly and clear the air. I believe it is my ability to vent my anger and express my hurt that allows me to work through difficult times."

- How do you evaluate Lily's self-disclosure? Would such a disclosure be useful to you if you were her client?

- Would you be inclined to make a similar type of disclosure to your clients? Why or why not?

- What values are being imposed on Lily's clients? How might they react to or interpret her self-disclosure?

Commentary. Therapist self-disclosure can serve a therapeutic purpose, but the client's needs and concerns should guide such disclosures. Self-disclosure that is done for the benefit of the therapist, that burdens the client with unnecessary information, or that creates a role reversal where a client takes care of the therapist can be considered a boundary violation (Zur, 2009). Self-disclosure should never be used to meet the clinician's personal needs at the expense of the client's treatment needs. In this case, without taking the time to really know her clients, Lily burdened them with self-disclosures in her impatience and her rush to find a solution. Lily's disclosure seems designed to justify her own behavior rather than to help the couple. •

Assumptions About Directness and Respect Traditional therapeutic approaches tend to stress directness and assertiveness, yet in some cultures directness is perceived as rudeness and something to be avoided. Americans generally want to get to the "bottom line" and tend to get impatient when that does not happen. People from many cultures value less direct styles of communication. For example, Latinos may engage in *platica* (small talk) before beginning to address their concerns, and this talk may be totally unrelated to their reason for seeking your services. The counselor could assume that this lack of directness is evidence of pathology, or at least a lack of assertiveness, rather than a sign of respect. Many Asian Americans, Latinos, and Native Americans have been brought up not to speak until spoken to, especially when they are with older people or with authority figures. A counselor may interpret the client's hesitancy to speak as resistance when it is really a sign of respect.

If therapists cannot connect to clients using the techniques in which they were trained, it is incumbent on them to find other ways to connect with their clients. Simply put, when therapists have trouble understanding and working with a client, the client is not the problem. The problem rests with the therapist's inability to come up with a way to facilitate the client's exploration of his or her problem. Consulting with a colleague who is familiar with the client's culture may provide a new perspective on why the client is reticent to talk. The case of Miguel provides another example of a therapist's assumptions about directness.

The Case of Miguel

Miguel, a Latino born in the United States, has completed his PhD and is working at a community clinic in family therapy. In his training he has learned about the concepts of directness, assertiveness, and triangulation (the tendency of two people who are in conflict to involve a third person in their emotional system to reduce the stress). Miguel is watching for evidence of these tendencies. While he is counseling a Latino family, the father says to his son, "Your mother expects you to show her more respect than you do and to obey her." Miguel says to the mother, "Can you say this directly to your son rather than allowing your husband to speak for you?" The room falls silent, and there is great discomfort.

- What might account for the discomfort in the room?
- How could Miguel have handled this situation differently?
- What were Miguel's assumptions?

Commentary. As with many vignettes in this book, we cannot emphasize enough the need for cultural sensitivity. The "great discomfort in the room" was evidence that something had gone astray. To intervene in a respectful and helpful way, Miguel could have begun by acknowledging the patriarchal communication mode common to many Latino families. By asking the mother to directly address the son, Miguel reduced the father's role in a way that was culturally inappropriate. By focusing on the variables of directness and triangulation, Miguel missed other aspects of the moment. His intervention was ill timed because he had not established a strong connection with the family. Miguel's response to what occurred in this session could be the deciding factor in whether the family returns for another session.

Clinicians may assume that being assertive is better than being nonassertive and that clients are better off if they can tell people directly what they think and what they want. However, every culture deals with interpersonal situations in a unique way. It is critical to recognize that there are different perspectives on the value of being direct and assertive; therapists should avoid assuming that assertive behavior is the norm and is desirable for everyone. •

Assumptions About Self-Actualization and Trusting Relationships Many mental health professionals assume that it is important for the individual to become a self-actualizing person. Counselors may focus on self-actualization for the individual without regard for the impact of the individual's change on the significant people in that person's life or the impact of those significant people on the client. A creative synthesis between self-actualization and responsibility to the group may be a more realistic goal for many clients.

Most therapeutic approaches emphasize the importance of the relationship between client and counselor. When joining with clients, the counselor needs to take into account the culture from which a client comes and consider how trust is built from the client's perspective. Whether the client and the counselor come from a similar background or a different one, the process of building rapport and trust are closely linked to cultural norms and intercultural experiences. It is the counselor's responsibility to ensure that these conversations about culture take place and that cultural differences are approached in a respectful way.

Assumptions About Nonverbal Behavior Many cultural expressions are subject to misinterpretation, including appropriate personal space, eye contact, handshaking, dress, formality of greeting, perspective on time, and so forth. People from Western countries often feel uncomfortable with periods of silence and tend to talk to ease their tension. In some cultures silence may be a sign of respect and politeness rather than a lack of a desire to continue to speak. Silence may be a reflection of fear or confusion, or it may be a cautious expression and reluctance to do what the counselor is expecting of the client.

Students in the helping professions are often systematically trained in a range of microskills that include attending, open communication, observation, hearing clients accurately, noting and reflecting feelings, and selecting and structuring, to mention a few (Ivey, Ivey, & Zalaquett, 2018). Although these behaviors are aimed at creating a positive therapeutic relationship, individuals from certain ethnic groups may have difficulty responding positively or understanding the intent of the counselor's instructions and behavior. The counselor whose confrontational style involves direct eye contact, physical gestures, and probing personal questions could be seen as intrusive by clients from another culture.

As we mentioned earlier, in some cultures direct eye contact is considered a sign of interest and presence, and a lack thereof can be viewed as being evasive. However, in any culture an individual may maintain more eye contact while listening and less while talking. Research indicates that some African Americans may reverse this pattern by looking more when talking and looking slightly less when listening. Among some Native American and Latino groups, eye contact by the young is a sign of disrespect. Some cultural groups tend to avoid eye contact when talking about serious subjects (Ivey et al., 2018). Clinicians need to acquire sensitivity to cultural differences to reduce the probability of miscommunication, misdiagnosis, and misinterpretation of behavior.

A Personal Case History Some time ago Marianne Corey and Jerry Corey conducted a training workshop with counselors from Mexico. Marianne was perceived by a male participant as being too direct and assertive. He had difficulty with Marianne's active leadership style and indicated that it was her place to defer to Jerry by letting him take the lead. Recognizing and respecting our cultural differences, we were able to arrive at a mutual understanding of different values.

Jerry had difficulty with the participants showing up after the scheduled time and had to accept the fact that we could not follow a strict time schedule. Typically we have thought that if people were late or missed a session, group cohesion would be difficult to maintain. Because the issue was openly discussed in this situation, however, the problem did not arise. We quickly learned that we had to adapt ourselves to the participants' view of time and they to us as well. To insist on interpreting such behavior as resistance would have been to ignore the cultural context.

Addressing Sexual Orientation

LO5

Most of the previous discussion on multiculturalism has focused on issues of culture and ethnicity. However, the concept of human diversity encompasses much more than racial and ethnic factors; it encompasses multiple forms of oppression, discrimination, and prejudice, including those directed toward age, gender, ability, religious affiliation, and sexual orientation. In 1973 the American Psychiatric Association stopped labeling **homosexuality,** a sexual orientation in which people seek emotional and sexual relationships with same-gendered individuals, as a form of mental illness. In 1975 the American Psychological Association endorsed this move by recommending that psychologists actively work to remove the stigma that had been attached to homosexuality. Along with these changes came the assumption that therapeutic practices would be modified to reflect this viewpoint: The mental health system had finally begun to treat the *problems* of gay, lesbian, bisexual, and transgender people rather than treating *them* as the problem.

The ethics codes of the ACA (2014), the APA (2010), the AMHCA (2015), the AAMFT (2015), the CCA (2007), the CRCC (2010), and the NASW (2008) clearly state that **discrimination,** or behaving differently and usually unfairly toward a specific group of people, is unethical and unacceptable. As an example of a non-discrimination policy, consider this standard of the *Code of Professional Ethics for Rehabilitation Counselors* (CRCC, 2010):

> Rehabilitation counselors do not condone or engage in discrimination based on age, color, culture, disability, ethnicity, gender, gender identity, race, national origin, religion/spirituality, sexual orientation, marital status/partnership, language preference, socioeconomic status, or any basis proscribed by law. (A.2.b.)

The Supreme Court declared same-sex marriage to be legal in all 50 states in 2015, but discrimination against same-sex couples continues today. Therapists are faced with various clinical and ethical issues in working with **lesbian, gay, bisexual,** and **transgender** (LGBT) people, and this work needs to include a recognition of the societal factors that contribute to oppression and discrimination based on sexual orientation or gender identity.

One of these ethical issues involves therapists confronting their own values regarding same-sex or bisexual desire and behavior. Working with lesbian, gay, bisexual, and transgender individuals presents a challenge to mental health providers who hold strong personal values regarding sexual orientation and gender identity. Given the current sociopolitical climate, some LGBT clients may not feel comfortable disclosing their sexual orientation. Mental health professionals who have negative reactions to LGBT people may be inclined to impose their own values and attitudes, or at least to convey strong disapproval, or they may want to refer these people to another professional.

Counselors must examine their own views regarding heterosexuality, racism, and sexism to better understand and deal with any biases they may have toward working with LGBT clients (Ferguson, 2016). Unless mental health providers become conscious of their own assumptions and possible counter-transference, they may project their misconceptions and their fears onto their clients. Therapists are challenged to confront these personal prejudices, myths, fears, and stereotypes regarding sexual orientation. This is particularly important when a client discloses his or her sexual orientation well into an established therapeutic relationship. In such situations, prejudicial or judgmental attitudes and behaviors on the part of the therapist can do serious damage to the client. We highlight this topic because it illustrates not only the ethical problems involved in imposing values but also the problems involved in effectively addressing the mental health concerns of gay, lesbian, bisexual, and transgender clients.

Heterosexism is a worldview and a value system that can undermine the healthy functioning of the sexual orientations, gender identities, and behaviors of LGBT individuals. Practitioners need to understand that heterosexism pervades the social and cultural foundations of many institutions and often contributes to negative attitudes toward people who are not heterosexual or do not meet the socially accepted standards of stereotypical gender roles and behaviors.

A therapist who works with LGBT people has a responsibility to understand the special concerns of these individuals and is ethically obligated to develop the knowledge and skills to competently deliver services to them. The Association for Lesbian, Gay, Bisexual, and Transgender Issues in Counseling (ALGBTIC, 2008) has developed a set of competencies for counselors in training to help them examine their personal biases and values pertaining to sexual orientation. Competent counselors will develop appropriate intervention strategies that ensure effective service delivery. Among the specific competencies listed are the following:

- Competent counselors recognize the societal prejudice and discrimination experienced by LGBT individuals and assist them in overcoming internalized negative attitudes toward their sexual and gender identities.
- Counselors strive to understand how their own sexual orientation and gender identity influences the counseling process.
- Counselors seek consultation or supervision to ensure that their own biases or knowledge deficits do not negatively influence their relationships with LGBT clients.
- Counselors understand that attempting to change the sexual orientation or gender identity of LGBT individuals is not supported by research and is unethical.

The ALGBTIC (2009) has also developed competencies geared toward counselors who work with transgender individuals, families, groups, or communities. These competencies are based on a wellness, resilience, and strength-based approach. The authors who developed the *Competencies for Counseling With Transgender Clients* believe counselors are in a unique position to make institutional change that can result in a safer environment for transgender people. This begins with counselors creating a welcoming and affirming environment for transgender individuals and their loved ones. Counselors must respect and attend to the whole individual, and should not simply focus on gender identity issues. Counselors who work with transgender people are expected to seek professional development opportunities to enhance their knowledge and skills related to their clients. For a complete list of the specific competencies in working with transgender individuals, see ALGBTIC (2009).

One way to increase your awareness of ethical and therapeutic considerations in working with LGBT clients is to take advantage of continuing education workshops sponsored by national, regional, state, and local professional organizations. By participating in such workshops, you can learn specific interventions and strategies appropriate for LGBT clients. From an advocacy perspective, it is important to familiarize yourself with LGBT resources in your local community. You may not know the sexual orientation of a client until the therapeutic relationship develops, thus, you need to have a clear idea of your own assumptions, attitudes, and values relative to this sexual orientation. Take a moment to consider the questions in the box titled "Assess Your Competence to Counsel LGBT Clients."

Assess Your Competence to Counsel LGBT Clients

The ALGBTIC (2008) competencies have relevance to all mental health professionals. Consider these questions:

- Do you hold any specific attitudes, beliefs, assumptions, and values that could interfere with your ability to effectively counsel lesbian, gay, bisexual, and transgender clients?
- What competencies do you most need to develop in working effectively with sexual orientation and gender identity issues?
- How would you react if 3 months into the therapeutic relationship you learned that your client was attracted to same-sex partners?
- How open are you to counseling a same-sex couple who want to explore their difficulties in the area of intimate relationships?
- To what degree are you familiar with the specific issues of discrimination facing many LBGT people?
- What steps can you take to learn more about the LGBT community and mental health issues that pertain to this group?

The Role of Counselor Educators and Therapists in Challenging "Isms"

In our profession it is not uncommon to have multiple professional identities, such as therapist, consultant, and educator. On occasion these roles are blended, and at other times we wear only one professional hat at a time. As agents of social change, we work diligently to prevent and reduce prejudice in many forms. In our work as counselor educators, we take an active role in challenging students around their "isms" for the purpose of making them more effective counselors.

As clinicians, however, we encounter clients who express racist, sexist, and homophobic remarks, but we do not automatically challenge these statements. We have to ask ourselves whether it is within our role as counselors to challenge clients' beliefs and to share our reactions of feeling offended. Is this a reflection of our own agenda and not that of our clients? We do not aspire to always keep these roles completely separate, but as counselors we have a responsibility to examine with great thoughtfulness our intentions, our actions, and their consequences for our clients.

Sometimes it is beneficial to draw attention to a client's prejudicial beliefs in the context of the issues the client is working on in treatment. For example, when counseling a woman who recognizes her rigid thinking and wants to examine this, we were able to connect her racist remarks to an all-or-nothing way of seeing the world and others. This connection helped the client increase her awareness of how this contributed to her relational difficulties. In another instance, when working with middle school children, we were able to use their discriminatory remarks as a catalyst for a discussion on difference, empathy, and power. What roles or professional identities do you hold that you think would be difficult for you to put aside in the face of a values clash?

Value Issues of Lesbian, Gay, Bisexual, and Transgender Clients

Like any other oppressed group, LGBT individuals experience discrimination, prejudice, and oppression when they seek employment or a place of residence. Given the stresses they encounter, they often have special counseling needs that may raise ethical and social justice issues.

It is a mistake to assume that lesbians or gay men who come to counseling want to explore matters pertaining to their sexual orientation or that their depression is related to sexual orientation. An array of problems unrelated to sexual orientation may be of primary concern. In short, therapists need to listen carefully to their clients and be willing to explore whatever concerns they bring to the counseling relationship, as the following case shows.

The Case of Chandler and Karlo

Karlo, a licensed professional clinical counselor, was sought out by Chandler, a 26-year-old woman who identified as lesbian and is a devout Catholic. Chandler heard Karlo speak at a continuing education class on multiple identities and believes he will be understanding of her situation. Chandler appreciated that Karlo is an advocate for the LGBTQ community as well as someone who spoke about "respecting the religious beliefs of all of his clients." During their first session, Chandler shares with Karlo the reasons she chose him as her counselor. She also discloses that she wants his help in living as a heterosexual woman. Chandler feels she cannot be a "good Catholic" if she continues to "live in sin" as a lesbian. She knew Karlo did not believe a person chooses his or her identity, but she felt that he would respect her belief system.

Use the eight steps for ethical decision making (see Chapter 1) outlined here to solve this ethical dilemma:

- Identify the problems or dilemmas that you see in this case.
- Identify the potential issues involved (legal, ethical, clinical, cultural).
- Review and identify the relevant ethics codes.
- Review and identify the applicable laws and regulations.
- Obtain consultation (and practice self-reflection). What questions would you ask your supervisor, your colleagues, and yourself about this case?
- Consider possible and probable courses of action.
- Enumerate the consequences of various decisions.
- Choose what appears to you to be the best course of action.

What reactions do you have to this case and how would you handle them? Do your personal reactions align or contrast with your sense of professional obligation in any way?

- If you held Karlo's worldview, how would you respond if Chandler came to you with her request?
- Would you agree to work with Chandler? If so, how would you proceed? Would you tell her if you disagreed with her? Why or why not? Could you work with her even if you disagreed with her?
- If you chose not to work with Chandler, what reasons would you give her? What types of referrals would you make? If Chandler chose to go to a "camp" that advertises being able to change a person's sexual orientation through religious counsel, how would you feel about refusing to accept her as your client?

Commentary. Karlo's personal beliefs and professional ethics were at odds. He felt strongly that being lesbian was not a sin, and he did not believe people can turn their sexual orientation on and off. However, Karlo was committed to honoring his client's belief system; Chandler ultimately had the right to live in a way that was congruent with her own moral code. Karlo chose to work with Chandler in part because he feared she might seek a therapist who practiced conversion therapy, which Karlo felt would be detrimental to her well-being. Karlo was open about the fact that he did not see being gay as a sin or as being at odds with a religious practice. They decided that his role would be to focus on helping Chandler think critically and deeply about her decision rather then pushing her toward a specific outcome.

In examining this case, what stands out for us is that the client was experiencing an intolerable dilemma. She could not find a way to tolerate being gay and being religious. In choosing Karlo, she consciously or unconsciously handed her struggle over to him. By accepting Chandler as a client, Karlo had to wrestle with an ambivalence similar to that of his client. An advocate of the LGBTQ community, he felt guilty for "supporting" Chandler's journey to change her sexual identity, but he also felt a professional obligation to respect his client's deepest wishes. Karlo might explain to Chandler that conversion therapy has been found to be harmful to clients. He does not practice it, nor would he recommend a therapist who does so. Karlo could make Chandler aware of the standard in the ACA (2014) *Code of Ethics* concerning harmful practices: "Counselors do not use techniques/procedures/modalities when substantial evidence suggests harm, even if such services are requested" (C.7.c.). Both the client and the therapist need to make sure they have the same goals for treatment. •

A Court Case Involving a Therapist's Refusal to Counsel Homosexual Clients

In their article, "Legal and Ethical Issues in Counseling Homosexual Clients," Hermann and Herlihy (2006) describe the case of *Bruff v. North Mississippi Health Services, Inc.* (2001). This interesting case illustrates the complexity counselors confront when their value system and religious beliefs conflict with their client's issues. This section is based largely on Hermann and Herlihy's provocative article.

In 1996 Jane Doe initiated a counseling relationship with Sandra Bruff, a counselor employed at the North Mississippi Medical Center, an employee assistance program provider. After several sessions, Jane Doe informed Bruff that she was a lesbian and wanted to explore her relationship with her partner. Bruff refused on the basis of her religious beliefs, but offered to counsel her in other areas. Jane Doe discontinued counseling, and her employer filed a complaint with Bruff's agency. Bruff again repeated her reason for refusing to work with Jane Doe and added that she would be willing to work with clients on any areas that did not conflict with her religious beliefs.

Eventually, Bruff was dismissed by her employer. Bruff appealed to an administrator of the medical center who asked her to clarify the situations in which she could not work with a client. She reiterated that she would "not be willing to counsel anyone on any subject that went against her religion" (cited in Hermann & Herlihy, 2006). She was offered a transfer to a Christian counseling center, which she refused on the basis that the director of the center was too liberal. She was given another opportunity for a position in the agency, but lost to a more qualified candidate. Another position in the agency became available, but she did not apply, and eventually she was terminated. Bruff filed suit, and a jury trial in a federal court ruled in her favor. However, on appeal the court reversed the jury's findings and found that there was no violation of Bruff's rights. The court noted that the employer had made several attempts to accommodate Bruff but that Bruff remained inflexible.

Hermann and Herlihy (2006) summarize some of the legal aspects of the *Bruff* case:

- The court held that the employer did make reasonable attempts to accommodate Bruff's religious beliefs.

- Bruff's inflexibility and unwillingness to work with anyone who has conflicting beliefs is not protected by the law.

- A counselor who refuses to work with LGBT clients can cause harm to them. The refusal to work on an LGBT client's relationship issue constitutes discrimination, which is illegal in most states. As you may recall from Chapter 3, Tennessee passed controversial legislation in 2016 that allows a therapist to deny service to LGBT individuals on the grounds of "religious freedom."

- Counselors cannot use their religious beliefs to justify discrimination based on sexual orientation, and employers can terminate counselors who engage in this discrimination.

Hermann and Herlihy believe the *Bruff* case sets an important legal precedent. They assert that the appeals court decision is consistent with the Supreme Court's precedent interpreting employers' obligations to make reasonable accommodations for employees' religious beliefs. From a legal perspective, the court case clarifies that refusing to counsel homosexual clients on relationship matters can result in the loss of a therapist's job. A homosexual client who sues a counselor for refusing to work with the client on issues related to sexual orientation is also likely to prevail in a malpractice suit as the counselor could be found in violation of the standard of care in the community.

In discussing the ethical implications of the *Bruff* case, Hermann and Herlihy (2006) emphasize the importance for counselors to develop nonjudgmental and accepting attitudes, regardless of their own value system. In short, counselors who discriminate based on sexual orientation are violating ethical standards.

Consider these questions as you think about the issues involved in this case:

- How would you deal with client's issues that conflict with your moral beliefs?

- Is it possible to provide clients with services consistent with an ethical standard of care if counselors conceal their beliefs that homosexuality is wrong?

- If your moral beliefs are substantially different from your client, is this equivalent to your not being competent to work effectively with this client? Are referrals ever justified because of major value conflicts?

- How do you determine that your referral will benefit or harm your client?

- Do counselors have an ethical obligation to reveal their religious beliefs prior to the onset of a professional relationship?

- If you fully disclose your limitations and own them as your problem, are you behaving ethically and legally?

- To what degree does your informed consent document protect you from an ethical or legal violation?

- How would you apply the basic moral principles addressed in Chapter 1 to making ethical decisions in this case?

Commentary. We find this case very challenging; the ethical issues exposed have no easy answers and require a great deal of discussion. An inability to discuss the problem precludes finding a solution. The *Bruff* case illustrates both ethical and legal issues related to value imposition and conflict of values between counselor and client (see Chapter 3). In a counseling relationship, it is not the client's place to adjust to the therapist's values, yet this counselor maintained that she could not work with clients whose beliefs went against her religious views.

Bruff demonstrates a lack of understanding that counseling is not about her but about the client's needs and values.

Although we do not question Bruff's right to possess her own personal values, we do have concerns about the manner in which she dealt with the client involved in this case. We expect counselors to avoid using their personal value system as the criteria against which they judge how their clients should think and act. Counselors must develop the capacity to put their values aside (or bracket them) and focus on the needs of the client, which is a mark of a true professional.

We also question whether it was appropriate for this counselor to have a position in a public counseling agency given her inexperience and ineffectiveness working with diverse client populations. Bruff showed inflexibility both in dealing with her clients and in her response to the agency's attempts to accommodate her values by transferring her to another position. •

The Culture of Disability*

People with chronic medical, physical, and mental disabilities represent the largest minority and disadvantaged group in the United States. Disability has become a natural and ordinary part of life (Smart, 2016). Yet people with disabilities are part of a misunderstood culture because they do not conform to the socially determined and accepted standards of normalization, beauty, physical attractiveness, and being able-bodied.

The number of people with disabilities across the life span is steadily growing. This can be seen in part by the rise of childhood disabilities such as autism, attention deficit and hyperactivity disorders, and by the cumulative lifestyle factors that lead to obesity, diabetes, heart disease, and cancers. Disabilities in U.S. society are even more prevalent as a result of prolonged and sustained military action in war zones around the world. This has resulted in catastrophic physical injuries (traumatic brain injury, spinal cord injury, chronic pain, and amputations) and serious mental health concerns (posttraumatic stress, depression, substance abuse, and addictions) among men and women who have placed their lives in harm's way on our behalf (Jackson, Thoman, Suris, & North, 2012; Stebnicki, 2016). To serve this growing population, counselors must acquire unique cultural attributes that are foundational in cultivating an ethical, competent, multicultural practice. Counselors must acquire a basic awareness and knowledge of working with those in the **disability community** and understand some of the ethical dilemmas and concerns that may arise with this unique and diverse group of individuals.

The Disability Community

Understanding the unique cultural attributes of the disability community is essential in gaining a therapeutic alliance with individuals who may or may not identify themselves as part of the disability community. Although accurate statistical incidence and prevalence of all categories of disability are difficult to acquire,

*We are indebted to Mark A. Stebnicki, PhD, LPC, DCMHS, CRC, CCM, professor and coordinator of the Military and Trauma Counseling Certificate, Department of Addictions and Rehabilitation, East Carolina University, for contributing this section on counseling people with disabilities.

disability researchers generally accept that there are somewhere between 36 million and 54 million Americans with disabilities. Included in the definition of disability are people with medical, physical, mental health, substance use disorders, and psychiatric disabilities.

The foundational principle in counseling people with disabilities is treat the person first rather than treat the disability. It is also foundational to understand the continuum model of disability, which illustrates that there is no superhuman or perfect earthly being. Rather, we are all made up of differing abilities along a theoretical continuum. At one end of the continuum is the theoretical superhuman, and at the other end is the person who is near death. Helping professionals should focus therapy on the person's current functional abilities and capabilities, which lie somewhere along the continuum of disability. Achieving optimal levels of psychosocial functioning with the individual based on his or her *abilities* defines best practices in working with people with disabilities.

Stephen Hawking, a renowned British theoretical physicist, provides one example of a person with a disability (amyotrophic lateral sclerosis [ALS]) who transcends the typical course and prognosis of his disease and exhibits extraordinary *differing abilities*. The uninformed observer may look at this individual as a person in a wheelchair who has severe physical and communication deficits, and some practitioners may feel compelled to "treat the disability," or the person's deficits. This would be considered working within the *biomedical model* of disease, disability, and illness. A culturally competent practitioner acting in an ethical manner would acknowledge and embrace Professor Hawking's *abilities* rather than his *disabilities*. Working in new paradigms of disability such as the holistic and psychosocial models of *health and wellness* (Nosek, 2005) is a good starting point for approaching therapy embracing the client's unique and diverse cultural attributes. Understanding the individual's cultural identity and how the client perceives his or her abilities is key. Allowing clients to express and communicate their experience of disability and how it may (or may not) hinder their day-to-day functioning is also essential in establishing a strong rapport and working toward an optimal working alliance.

Understanding disability from the disability community's perspective has been the life work of Livneh (2012) as well as many others. Livneh's exhaustive work in psychosocial rehabilitation suggests that the disability community as a whole has historically been marginalized and segregated in multiple life areas (for example, schools, employment, housing, and transportation). It is important for counselors to understand this because they may be dealing with clients who have low self-esteem or perhaps have identified with a particular societal stereotype of disability created by their experience of discrimination. Indeed, there are distinct attitudinal differences in society between people with and without disabilities. Some of the major influences on the treatment and individual responses to disability include (a) our sociocultural conditioning; (b) our childhood influences; (c) various psychodynamic mechanisms that cultivate cultural tunnel vision; (d) the perception that disability is seen as a punishment for sin; (e) our existential anxiety and aesthetic aversion toward people who have disfigurement, physical limitations, and perceptions toward what "normal" is; and (f) other disability-specific related factors.

The ethical and cultural issues of disability are wide-reaching and are of paramount concern, especially for those who do not have a voice to express themselves due to cognitive or communication deficits and for those with severe psychiatric disabilities. Having a disability in the United States can lead to even more intense levels of social isolation, discrimination, stereotypes, poverty, and dependence on public/government assistance. People who lack the mental capacity to consent to their medical or mental health treatment, or those not capable of handling their financial affairs, are particularly vulnerable and are easily manipulated by others. People with disabilities often are not provided with equivalent services or are denied services or programs available to others. Historically, many individuals within the disability community comment that attitudinal barriers are more of a hindrance than the disability itself (Hahn & Belt, 2004; McCarthy, 2003; Nosek, 2005; Wright, 1983).

Ethical Concerns in the Role of Client Advocate

Given the decreased functional capacity and severity of some disabilities, many counselors take on the natural role of **client advocate**. Many times, counselors justify their actions by acting in a beneficent and nonmaleficent manner. In most cases, counselors truly believe they are working for their clients' best interests. Accordingly, our colleagues often observe us doing good work *for* rather than *with* our clients. Some of us may enjoy the image of being *the expert* with all the knowledge and resources for our clients. However, the most helpful role of the counselor is to form a collaborative relationship with clients. Consider the following questions:

- How does our own worldview influence what we believe to be the best treatment practices for our clients with severe disabilities?
- What measures have we taken with our clients to ensure that we are working in a professional role to help protect our clients' autonomy?
- Do we treat clients with severe disabilities differently from those considered able-bodied?

Indeed, the role as client advocate raises potential ethical concerns because of the intense emotional nature of the work we do. This is especially relevant for clients who do not have a voice for themselves due to cognitive, communication, or psychiatric disabilities. The disability community more than other groups is prey to manipulation, wrong-doing, and human rights violations. Thus client advocate is a natural role for the counselor, but counselors must be mindful to approach clients with disabilities with empathy and not sympathy.

Acting as client advocate involves the integration of a variety of professional activities facilitating empowerment strategies critical to ensure client independence. Counselors who act in the role of client advocate engage in socially conscious, action-oriented behaviors considered to be ethically responsible. Some counselors may work to help remove institutional, attitudinal, and sociocultural barriers by raising awareness of certain risk factors for disease such as HIV/AIDS. Other counselors focus on prevention activities with high-risk populations such as adolescent substance abuse and addictions. Other counselors regularly use state or regional protection and advocacy services to help clients being discriminated against in a variety of employment, education, housing, public transportation, or independent living settings.

Competent and ethical counselors acting as client advocates know how to balance the multiple roles and responsibilities across a continuum of services offered to clients. Assisting clients to cultivate higher levels of independence will strengthen the therapeutic alliance and cultivate client-based skills of problem solving, healthy risk-taking, and other therapeutic tasks. Some in the disability community argue that counselors acting as client advocates can foster dependency. Indeed, there are multiple concerns surrounding this issue, and counselors must carefully monitor themselves or consult with a qualified and competent clinical supervisor. The ethical principles of beneficence and nonmaleficence, if not carefully monitored, can indeed compromise client autonomy.

Blending the roles of consultant, adviser, and cultural facilitator combines traditional counseling and psychotherapy strategies with person-centered approaches to client advocacy. Role blending can assist counselors to ameliorate the consequences of acting purely in the role of client advocate. Many professional counselors recognize the ethical complexity of these issues and understand the potential benefits in cultivating culturally centered therapeutic relationships for people with disabilities. In thinking about the ethical complexity of issues in working with people with disabilities, consider the case of Melvin.

The Case of Melvin

Melvin, a 23-year-old Army veteran, was injured in an explosion while deployed to Afghanistan. Three members of his platoon died in this explosion and several others were injured. Melvin sustained a crushing injury that required an emergency above the knee amputation. He spent about 3 months at an Army hospital in a postacute rehabilitation unit after major surgery and has been assigned to a Wounded Warrior Battalion at his home garrison. You meet Melvin for the first time during the intake interview and have begun treatment planning for therapeutic engagement. Melvin's treatment plan includes individual counseling once a week with a primary emphasis on the psychosocial adjustment needs of his newly acquired traumatic amputation. Melvin will continue in outpatient physical therapy with the goals of ambulation, balance, and strength conditioning using his new prosthetic leg. During your second session as Melvin's counselor, you notice how emotionally detached he is. He talks at a very low volume, rarely makes eye contact, and appears highly anxious, nervous, and hypervigilant at times. In addition, Melvin seems reluctant to disclose anything about his combat experience and his multiple overseas deployments while in the Army. He does, however, tell you that he is angry with the Army hospital system and his program of physical therapy: "I hate this place ... I've lost everything in life ... no one understands what I've been through ... my new leg doesn't fit properly, I am in constant pain ... people just treat me like a patient ... sometimes I feel the world would be better off without me."

- Do you have an ethical obligation to further evaluate Melvin's possible suicide ideation related to his statement "the world would be better off without me"? What specific level of lethality is Melvin inferring?

- How can you advocate on behalf of Melvin as it relates to his statements that "my new leg doesn't fit properly ... I am in constant pain"?

- What specific cultural attributes (i.e., military and disability culture) are of concern during your therapeutic interactions with Melvin?
- How do Melvin's traumatic amputation and posttraumatic stress symptoms hinder his psychosocial adjustment to his newly acquired disability?

Commentary. It is critical to follow up with an assessment of Melvin's level of suicide ideation. However, Melvin has multiple issues to address beyond the immediate mental health concerns. It is important to understand that Melvin is a member of two distinct cultural groups: the military culture (Army) and a person with a disability (traumatic amputation). Skilled and competent counselors understand the unique cultural characteristics of clients like Melvin. Melvin is just beginning to adjust to his newly acquired disability (3 to 4 months postinjury). His traumatic physical disability is complicated by the psychological trauma of the memory of the explosion, and he exhibits a range of posttraumatic stress symptoms. Working with Melvin requires the counselor to treat more than just the mental health condition. Melvin had a traumatic amputation, and the psychosocial adjustment issues related to his traumatic physical injury should be addressed along with the complex issues of PTSD and how that affects Melvin's active duty status. Eventually, Melvin will be medically separated from active duty and will have to transition to civilian life as an Army veteran. Therapeutic interventions should consider both Melvin's mental health and his psychosocial adjustment needs. •

Matching Client and Counselor

Diversity includes factors such as culture, religion, race, ability, age, gender, sexual orientation, education, and socioeconomic level. Is matching client and counselor on these various aspects of diversity desirable or possible? Does the clinician have to share the experiential world of the client to be effective? It is impossible to match client and therapist in all areas of potential diversity, which means that all encounters with clients are diverse, at least to some degree. Some argue that successful multicultural counseling is highly improbable due to the barriers between groups. Others argue that well-trained practitioners, even though they differ from their clients, are capable of providing effective counseling.

Shared Life Experiences With Your Clients

Must you have similar life experiences to work effectively with clients? Counselors do not necessarily need to have experienced each of the struggles of their clients to be effective in working with them. When the counselor and the client connect at a certain level, cultural and age differences can be transcended. Consider for a moment the degree that you can communicate effectively with the following clients:

- A person significantly older or younger than you
- A person of a different racial, ethnic, or cultural group
- A person with a disability
- A person with a criminal record
- A person who is abusing alcohol or drugs
- A person who is in recovery from an addiction
- A person with strong political beliefs that differ greatly from your own
- Parents struggling with child behavior issues

It is possible for a relatively young clinician to work effectively with an elderly client. For example, the client may be experiencing feelings of loss, guilt, sadness, and hopelessness. The young counselor can empathize with these feelings even though they come from a different source. However, it is essential that counselors develop sensitivity to the differences in their background and experiences from those of their clients.

To facilitate your reflection on whether you need to have life experiences similar to those of your client, assess the degree to which you think you could establish a good working relationship with Sylvia.

The Case of Sylvia

At a community clinic, Sylvia, who is 38, tells you that she is an alcoholic. During the intake interview she says, "I feel bad because I've tried to stop my drinking and haven't succeeded. I am fine for a while, and then I begin to think that I could do a lot better. I see all the ways in which I do not measure up—how I let my kids down, the many mistakes I've made with them, the embarrassment I've caused my husband—and then I get so down I start drinking again. I know that what I am doing is self-destructive, but I'm not able to stop. I very much want your advice on what I should do."

- What experiences have you had with alcoholism or its treatment, and how important is that?

- If you do not have competence in dealing with substance abuse, how could you acquire the knowledge and skills to effectively work in this area?

- In what ways does Sylvia's gender affect your view of her problem?

- Would you refer Sylvia to a substance abuse treatment program, either inpatient or outpatient? Explain.

- Is it ethical to treat Sylvia's psychological problems without first attending to her addiction problem? Explain.

- Sylvia wants your advice. What advice might you offer? What danger, if any, do you see in offering advice in this kind of situation?

Commentary. We support the thinking that the addiction must be treated before attempting to deal with Sylvia's other psychological difficulties, which brings up the issue of advice giving. When is it appropriate for the therapist to provide advice to a client? There are at least two kinds of advice. One form of advice could be a part of the treatment recommendations. For example, the therapist might suggest that Sylvia consult a physician or attend AA meetings. This form of advice is common and can provide necessary adjuncts to therapy. Furthermore, some racial/cultural minorities often seek solid "advice" from therapists and find the lack of concrete suggestions to be disconcerting (Sue & Sue, 2013).

Another form of advice would be to tell a client like Sylvia specific things she should do, such as turn to religion, start an exercise program, or move to a new area. Telling a client specific actions to take in the face of major life events tends to be counterproductive and should generally be avoided. This kind of advice often backfires. If Sylvia does agree with the advice given, or if she has not followed the advice, she may not return for further therapy sessions. Counselors can assist their clients by brainstorming with them about possibilities leading to solutions for their problems, but they should resist the temptation to provide specific actions in the form of giving advice. •

How to Address Differences in Therapeutic Relationships

Cultural differences are subjective, complex, and dynamic. Some therapists wonder whether differences should be addressed, and if they are, should the clinician or the client initiate this? The crucial factor is the client's perception of difference in the therapeutic process. Assuming that there is a standard way to work with clients of a certain cultural background is a mistake. Instead, practitioners need to explore the meanings clients ascribe to these cultural differences. Some writers maintain that most clients will not initiate discussions of cultural differences due to the power differential that exists, which suggests that the therapist can directly take responsibility to address these differences. Other writers take the position that it is more appropriate to wait for the client to bring up cultural differences. Lee (2013a) observes that "what is clearly evident in cross-cultural encounters is that the cultural differences between counselor and client, when not fully appreciated or understood, can be a significant impediment to the counseling process" (p. 14). Lee recommends that the counselor "acknowledge the wall and decrease the cultural distance between the counselor and client" (p. 14).

We take the position that clinicians can learn to work with clients who differ from them in gender, race, culture, religion, socioeconomic background, physical ability, age, or sexual orientation. But our stance is tempered by certain reservations and conditions. First, clinicians need to have training in multicultural and social justice perspectives, both academic and experiential. Second, as in any other counseling situation, it is important that the client and the practitioner agree to develop a working therapeutic relationship. Third, helpers are advised to be flexible in applying theories and techniques to specific situations. The counselor who has an open stance has a greater likelihood of success than someone who rigidly adheres to a single theoretical system. Fourth, the mental health professional should be open to being challenged and tested. In multicultural counseling, clients are more likely to exhibit caution and may use a variety of defenses as survival strategies to protect their true feelings. A counselor may be perceived to be a symbol of the establishment. If helpers act defensively, clients may feel that the clinician's values or solutions are being imposed on them and harm may come to these clients. Some clients believe that a professional who is not part of the solution to their problem is really part of the problem.

Addressing Unintentional Racism and Microaggressions

It is especially important in multicultural counseling situations for counselors to be aware of their own value systems, of potential stereotyping, any traces of prejudice, and of their cultural countertransference. Earlier we described those culture-bound counselors who are unintentionally racist. In some ways, such counselors can be more dangerous than those who are more open with their prejudices. The concepts of unintentional racism and microaggressions are related and usually involve demeaning implications perpetrated against clients on the basis of their race, gender, sexual orientation, or ability status. Sue and colleagues (2007) describe **racial microaggressions** as "brief and commonplace daily verbal, behavioral, or environmental indignities, whether intentional or unintentional, that communicate hostile, derogatory, or negative racial slights and insults toward people of other races" (p. 271). Perpetrators of these offenses are frequently unaware of what they are communicating. Sue and colleagues describe three forms of this insidious type of oppression: microassault, microinsult, and microinvalidation. A *microassault* is an explicit derogation characterized by either a verbal or nonverbal attack that is designed to hurt the victim through name-calling, avoidance, or intentional discriminatory acts. *Microinsults* are rude and insensitive comments that demean a person's heritage and identity. *Microinvalidations* are characterized by communications that negate, exclude, or nullify the thoughts, feelings, or realities of a person.

Microaggressions in the counseling relationship can be subtle; here are a few examples:

- A couples counselor refers to the female client in a heterosexual couple as a wife, rather than using the woman's name.
- A male therapist asks his female client who is a mother of three children if she has a job.
- A school counselor discourages her students of color from taking college preparatory courses or tells them they should apply for jobs that are more "realistic" for someone from their background.
- During an intake session a counselor comments to her African American male client that he "speaks so eloquently."
- During an intake a counselor says to his plus-sized client, "Obviously your weight is a problem as well."
- A counselor asks his new client if he has a girlfriend or a wife, without knowing the client's sexual orientation.

The key to changing unintentional racism lies in examining our basic assumptions. Two forms of covert racism that Ridley (2005) identifies are color blindness and color consciousness. The counselor who says, "When I look at you, I see a person, not a Black person" may encounter mistrust from clients who have difficulty believing that. Likewise, a therapist is not likely to earn credibility by saying, "If you were not Black, you wouldn't have the problem you're facing." These examples of color blindness and color consciousness are rather extreme, but there are many more subtle variations on these themes.

Sue and Sue (2013) regard **color blindness** as a racial microaggression. When a client reports feeling alienated in the workplace because she is the only person of color employed there, a color-blind counselor might minimize her concerns and say, "I think you are being too paranoid. We should emphasize similarities not people's differences" (Sue & Sue, 2013, p. 170). This statement conveys the message that race is not a critical variable that affects people's lives and that it has no sociopolitical relevance. People who say they are color blind usually are trying to communicate that they do not discriminate and that they treat others equally; however, in doing so, they are ignoring a vital part of that person's identity. The statement "I don't see color" can be interpreted as "I don't see *your* color." The statement gives the impression that those who benefit from racial privilege are closing their eyes to the experiences of others and do not acknowledge the privileges they automatically receive as a product of their race. This notion of color blindness can be extended to dimensions of culture other than race. Whether the result is overlooking a client's gender, sexual orientation, ethnicity, or any other important dimension of his or her life, *cultural blindness* will surely detract from one's effectiveness as a helper.

Increasing Your Sensitivity to Cultural Diversity

Try to identify your own assumptions as you think about these questions:

- Does a counselor need to share the cultural background of the client to be effective?
- If you were to encounter considerable "testing" from a client who is culturally different from you, how do you think you would react? What are some ways in which you could work with testing behavior?
- How might your own experiences with discrimination help or hinder you in working with clients who have been discriminated against?
- What stereotypes are you aware of having?

When counselors identify "unusual behavior" in a client, it is important to determine whether such behavior is unusual within the client's cultural context. Clients may become suspicious if they sense the therapist has already come to a conclusion. Rather than suffering from clinical paranoia, these clients may be reacting to the realities of an environment in which they have suffered oppression and prejudice. In such cases, clients' responses may make complete sense. Practitioners who appreciate the context of such perceptions are less likely to pathologize clients and are able to begin working with clients from their experiential framework.

LO9

Multicultural Training for Mental Health Workers

Although referral is sometimes an appropriate course of action, it should not be viewed as a solution to the problem of inadequately trained helpers. Many agencies have practitioners whose cultural backgrounds are less diverse than the populations they serve. With the increasing number of culturally diverse clients seeking counseling, we recommend that all counseling students, regardless of their racial or ethnic background, receive training in multicultural counseling and therapy (MCT). This didactic training can be paired with experiential learning opportunities in which students intentionally immerse themselves in another culture.

The standards established by the Council for Accreditation of Counseling and Related Educational Programs (CACREP, 2016) require that programs provide curricular and experiential offerings in multicultural and pluralistic trends, including characteristics within and among diverse groups nationally and internationally. CACREP standards call for supervised practicum experiences that include people from the environments in which the trainee is preparing to work. It is expected that trainees will study ethnic groups, subcultures, the changing roles of women, sexism, urban and rural societies, cultural mores, spiritual issues, and differing life patterns. The Council on Rehabilitation Education (CORE, 2009) also has accreditation standards that address these issues. It is not realistic to develop expertise with every culture or subculture. However, trainees should take active steps to increase their competence with those groups they plan to serve (Barnett & Johnson, 2015).

Characteristics of the Culturally Skilled Counselor

Part of multicultural competence entails recognizing our limitations and is manifested in our willingness to (a) seek consultation and supervision, (b) participate in continuing education, and (c) when appropriate, make referrals to a professional who is competent to work with a particular client population. Acquiring cultural competence is an active and lifelong learning process that may include formal training, critical self-evaluation, and questioning of what is occurring in cross-cultural therapeutic partnerships. Lee and Park (2013) state that multicultural competency must be acquired and maintained by all counselors. Cultural competency involves more than self-awareness and knowledge; it entails acquiring skills for effective multicultural intervention. Culturally competent therapists are able to adapt and incorporate various therapeutic approaches to address multiple facets of each client's unique needs and life experiences. They also are attuned to both interpersonal and intrapersonal factors for fostering the therapeutic relationship (Chu, Leino, Pflum, & Sue, 2016). Ivey and colleagues (2018) emphasize that awareness, knowledge, and skills are meaningless unless we take action. Counselors who are committed to taking action are willing to work and practice at reducing the gap between knowledge and doing. Comas-Diaz and Brown (2016) predict that in the coming decades "cultural competence will become a required core competence to be demonstrated in the supervision, licensing, and advanced certification of clinical psychologists" (p. 265).

A major contribution to the counseling profession has been the development of **multicultural competencies,** a set of knowledge and skills that are essential to the culturally skilled practitioner. Clinicians do not have to master all of these competencies before they begin to see clients, but gaining proficiency should be an ongoing process. Initially formulated by Sue and colleagues (1982), these competencies were later revised and expanded by Sue, Arredondo, and McDavis (1992). Arredondo and her colleagues (1996) updated and operationalized these competencies, and Sue and his colleagues (1998) extended multicultural counseling competencies to individual and organizational development. The most recent version of the competencies, *Multicultural and Social Justice Counseling Competencies* (MSJCC), was developed by the Association for Multicultural Counseling and Development (2015). Ratts, Singh, Butler, Nassar-McMillan, and McCullough (2016) provide a summary of the MSJCC, which has been endorsed by both the AMCD and the ACA. This endorsement supports the integration of multicultural and social justice competencies across aspects of the counseling profession. Ratts and colleagues (2016) contend that both counselors and clients bring to the therapeutic relationship a constellation of identities, privileged and marginalized statuses, and cultural values, beliefs, and biases that must be recognized and addressed. The MSJCC calls for counselors to address issues of power, privilege, and oppression that affect clients. "The MSJCC require counseling professionals to see client issues from a culturally contextual framework and recommend interventions that take place at both individual and system levels" (p. 41).

The essential attributes of culturally competent counselors, compiled from the sources cited above, are listed in the box titled "Multicultural Counseling Competencies."

Multicultural Counseling Competencies

I. Counselor Awareness of Own Cultural Values and Biases

A. With respect to *attitudes and beliefs,* culturally competent counselors:
- are sensitive to cultural group differences because they possess self-awareness of their own cultural heritage and identity.
- are aware of how their personal attitudes and beliefs about people from different cultural groups may facilitate or hamper effective counseling.
- are aware of their own racist, sexist, heterosexist, or other detrimental attitudes and beliefs.
- are able to recognize the limits of their multicultural competencies and expertise.
- recognize their sources of discomfort with differences that exist between themselves and clients in terms of race, ethnicity, culture, gender, sexual orientation, and other sociodemographic variables.

B. With respect to *knowledge,* culturally competent counselors:
- have specific knowledge about their own racial and cultural heritage and how it personally and professionally affects their definitions of and biases about normality/ abnormality and the process of counseling.
- possess knowledge and understanding about how oppression, racism, discrimination, and stereotyping affect them personally and in their work.
- possess knowledge about their social impact on others. They are knowledgeable about communication style differences, how their style may clash or foster the counseling process with persons of color or others different from themselves, and how to anticipate the impact it may have on others.
- consider clients as individuals within a cultural context.

C. With respect to *skills,* culturally competent counselors:
- seek out educational, consultative, and training experiences to improve their understanding and effectiveness in working with culturally different populations.
- are constantly seeking to understand themselves as racial and cultural beings and are actively seeking a nonracist identity.

II. Understanding the Client's Worldview

A. With respect to *attitudes and beliefs,* culturally competent counselors:
- are aware of their negative and positive emotional reactions toward other racial and ethnic groups that may prove detrimental to the counseling relationship. They are willing to contrast their own beliefs and attitudes with those of their culturally different clients in a nonjudgmental fashion.
- are aware of stereotypes and a monolithic perspective they may hold toward other racial and ethnic minority groups.

continued

B. With respect to *knowledge,* culturally competent counselors:
  - possess specific knowledge and information about the particular client group with whom they are working.
  - understand how race, culture, ethnicity, and so forth may affect personality formation, vocational choices, manifestation of psychological disorders, help-seeking behavior, and the appropriateness or inappropriateness of counseling approaches.
  - understand and have knowledge about sociopolitical influences that impinge on the lives of racial and ethnic minorities.

C. With respect to *skills,* culturally competent counselors:
  - familiarize themselves with relevant research and the latest findings regarding mental health and mental disorders that affect various ethnic and racial groups. They should actively seek out educational experiences that enrich their knowledge, understanding, and cross-cultural skills for more effective counseling behavior.
  - become actively involved with minority individuals outside the counseling setting so that their perspective of minorities is more than an academic or helping exercise.

III. Developing Culturally Appropriate Intervention Strategies and Techniques

A. With respect to *attitudes and beliefs,* culturally competent counselors:
  - respect clients' religious and spiritual beliefs and values, including attributions and taboos, because these affect worldview, psychosocial functioning, and expressions of distress.
  - respect indigenous helping practices and respect help-giving networks among communities of color.
  - value bilingualism and do not view another language as an impediment to counseling.

B. With respect to *knowledge,* culturally competent counselors:
  - have a clear and explicit knowledge and understanding of the generic characteristics of counseling and therapy and how they may clash with the cultural values of various cultural groups.
  - are aware of institutional barriers that prevent minorities from using mental health services.
  - have knowledge of the potential bias in assessment instruments and use procedures and interpret findings in a way that recognizes the cultural and linguistic characteristics of clients.
  - have knowledge of family structures, hierarchies, values, and beliefs from various cultural perspectives. They are knowledgeable about the community where a particular cultural group may reside and the resources in the community.
  - are aware of relevant discriminatory practices at the social and the community level that may affect the psychological welfare of the population being served.

C. With respect to *skills,* culturally competent counselors:
  - are able to engage in a variety of verbal and nonverbal helping responses. They are able to send and receive both verbal and nonverbal messages accurately and appropriately. They are not tied to only one method or approach to helping but recognize that helping styles and approaches may be culture bound.
  - acquire skills that are consistent with the life experiences and cultural values of their clients.

- are able to exercise institutional intervention skills on behalf of their clients. They can help clients determine whether a problem stems from racism or bias in others so that clients do not inappropriately personalize problems.
- are not adverse to seeking consultation with traditional healers or religious and spiritual leaders and practitioners in the treatment of culturally different clients when appropriate.
- take responsibility for interacting in the language requested by the client and, if not feasible, make appropriate referrals.
- have training and expertise in the use of traditional assessment and testing instruments.
- attend to and work to eliminate biases, prejudices, and discriminatory contexts in conducting evaluations and providing interventions and develop sensitivity to issues of oppression, sexism, heterosexism, elitism, and racism.
- take responsibility for educating their clients to the processes of psychological intervention, such as goals, expectations, legal rights, and the counselor's orientation.

For a more detailed description of these competencies, see Sue and Sue (2013, chap. 2).

The Case of Talib

Talib, an immigrant from the Middle East, is a graduate student in a counseling program. During many class discussions, his views on gender roles become clear, yet he expresses his beliefs in a respectful and nondogmatic fashion. Talib's attitudes and beliefs about gender roles are that the man should be the provider and head of the home and that the woman is in charge of nurturance, which is a full-time job. Although not directly critical of his female classmates, Talib voices a concern that these students may be neglecting their family obligations by pursuing a graduate education. Talib bases his views not only on his cultural background but also by citing experts in this country who support his position that the absence of women in the home has been a major contributor to the breakdown of the family. There are many lively discussions between Talib and his classmates, many of whom hold very different attitudes regarding gender roles.

Halfway through the semester, his instructor, Dr. Berny, asks Talib to come to her office after class. Dr. Berny tells Talib that she has grave concerns about him pursuing a career in counseling in this country with his present beliefs. She encourages him to consider another career if he is unable to change his "biased convictions" about the role of women. She tells him that unless he can open his thinking to more contemporary viewpoints he will surely encounter serious problems with clients and fellow professionals.

- If you were one of Talib's classmates, what would you want to say to him?
- What assumptions underlie Dr. Berny's advice to Talib?
- If you were a faculty member, what criteria would you use to determine that students are not suited for a program because of their values?
- How would you approach a person whose views seem very different from your own? How would you respond to Talib?

Commentary. Dr. Berny seemed to assume that because Talib expressed strong convictions he was rigid and would impose his values on his clients. She did not communicate a respect for his value system along with her concern that Talib might impose his values on clients. She did not use this situation as a teaching opportunity in the classroom to explore the issue of value imposition.

As a faculty member, Dr. Berny is charged with helping to evaluate whether Talib possess the competence and character to become a mental health professional. Although her concern about his attitudes may be warranted, her supervisory intervention appears to be based on assumptions about how Talib manages his own attitudes when working with clients. Ironically, Dr. Berny conveys the very disrespect for cultural differences that she accuses Talib of demonstrating. We cannot assume that Talib will necessarily impose his value system on his clients.

Students such as Talib who express strong values are often told that they should not work with certain clients. As a result, these students may hesitate to expose their viewpoints if they differ from the "acceptable norm." In our view, a critical feature of multicultural counseling and therapy is the personal development of trainees, which includes helping them clarify a set of values and beliefs concerning culture that increases their chances of functioning effectively in working with culturally diverse client populations. We want to teach students that having strong convictions is not the same as imposing them on others. Students are challenged to become aware of their value systems and to be open to exploring them. However, their role is not to go into this profession to impose these values on others, nor is their role to declare their superiority about their cultural values. If trainees maintain a rigid position regarding the way people should live, regardless of their cultural background, educators must be prepared to address these issues with trainees. •

Our Views on Multicultural Training

We recommend these four dimensions of training in multicultural counseling: (1) self-exploration, (2) didactic coursework, (3) internship, and (4) experiential approaches. The first step in the process of acquiring multicultural counseling skills is for students to become involved in a **self-exploratory journey** to help identify any potential blind spots. Ideally, this would be required of all trainees in the mental health professions and would be supervised by someone with experience in multicultural issues.

In addition to self-exploration, students can take coursework dealing exclusively with multicultural issues and diverse cultural groups. **Coursework** is essential for understanding and applying cultural themes in counseling. It is our position that multicultural topics need to be integrated throughout the curriculum, and not simply limited to a single course.

Bemak, Chung, Talleyrand, Jones, and Daquin (2011) describe how the Counseling and Development Program at George Mason University was revamped to emphasize multicultural social justice work, which entailed redesigning 98% of the course curriculum. To be consistent with their mission statement, which adopted social justice as a core value, this program focused on recruiting faculty of color and attracting students of color. As the authors note, the faculty are committed to supporting their students once admitted to ensure they are successful in the program; thus students are presented with information and materials with which they can identify and that are culturally relevant.

In a training program that holds diversity as a central value, supervised experiences in the field and internships are given special prominence. Trainees should participate in at least one required **internship** in which they have multicultural experiences or reframe their experiences from a multicultural viewpoint. Trainees should be encouraged to select supervised field placements and internships that will challenge them to work on gender and cultural concerns, developmental issues, and other areas of diversity. Through well-selected internship experiences, trainees expand their own consciousness as they increase their knowledge of diverse groups, which provides a basis for acquiring intervention skills.

Experiential Approaches to Training In addition to didactic approaches to acquiring knowledge and skills in multicultural competence, we strongly favor **experiential approaches** as a way to increase self-awareness and to identify and examine attitudes associated with diversity competence. Experiential approaches encourage trainees to pay attention to their thoughts, feelings, and actions in exploring their worldviews.

In conjunction with coursework, experiential learning can assist students in developing self-awareness, knowledge, and the skills that are a part of becoming a culturally competent counselor. It is also essential for counselors who work extensively with a specific cultural group to immerse themselves in knowledge and approaches specific to that group through reading, cultural events, workshops, and supervised practice. Revisiting the model adopted by the faculty of George Mason University, trainees engage in community-driven social justice projects outside of the classroom that involve serving marginalized populations (Bemak et al., 2011).

In *Social Justice Counseling,* Chung and Bemak (2012) devote a chapter to the reflections of their graduate students at George Mason University who enrolled in two classes: Multicultural Counseling and Counseling and Social Justice. The Counseling and Development Program has the core mission of training future multicultural and social justice counselors. The student reflections give examples of students' life changes, the risks they demonstrated in critically evaluating their values and life experiences, and the courage they had in speaking out and acting on social injustices. Rita Chung required that her students participate in a character portrayal, "assuming the identity" of a person of a different gender, class, sexual orientation, race, or ethnic group from their own. Each character described and advocated for a particular issue.

For many students these activities were a life-transforming event. Some students entered the program thinking there was not much more they could learn. The safety created by the professor enabled students to participate in difficult conversations and allowed for significant shifts in students' attitudes. The students were involved in a reading program and wrote about significant turning points for them and how they experienced transformation through activism and social change. One student struggled with the concept of White privilege, and found that Janet Helms's (2008) book, *A Race Is a Nice Thing to Have,* helped her move beyond her anger and continue to develop an identity as a White person. Helms wrote this book to help White people take responsibility for ending racism, understand how racism affects Whites as well as others, analyze racism, and discover positive alternatives for living in a multicultural society. Another White female student said she experienced anger, guilt, embarrassment, and shame when reading Helms's book. She became aware of what it was like for her to grow up with family members who viewed the world through a racist lens.

Get the Most From Your Training To get the most from your training, we suggest that you acknowledge and accept your limitations and be patient with yourself as you expand your vision of how your culture continues to influence the person you are today. Overwhelming yourself by all that you do not know will not help you. You will not become more effective in multicultural counseling by expecting that you must be completely knowledgeable about the cultural backgrounds of all your clients, by thinking that you should have a complete repertoire of skills, or by demanding perfection. Rather than feeling that you must understand all the subtle nuances of cultural differences when you are with a client, we suggest that you develop a sense of interest, curiosity, and respect when faced with client differences and behaviors that are new to you. Take the initiative in educating yourself about the cultural background of clients with whom you work. It is not your client's job to provide information on all aspects of his or her culture; however, you may want to ask your client about the personal significance of certain cultural practices. Recognize and appreciate your efforts toward becoming a more effective person and counselor, and remember that becoming a multiculturally competent counselor is an ongoing process. In this process there are no small steps; every step you take is creating a new and significant direction for you in your work with diverse client populations.

Chapter Summary

Over the past couple of decades mental health professionals have been urged to learn about their own culture and to become aware of how their experiences affect the way they work with those who are culturally different. By being ignorant of the values and attitudes of a diverse range of clients, therapists open themselves to criticism and ineffectiveness. We are all culture bound to some extent, and it takes a concerted effort to monitor our positive and negative biases so that they do not impede the establishment of helping relationships. In our view, imposing one's own vision of the world on clients not only leads to negative therapeutic outcomes but also constitutes unethical practice.

Culture can be interpreted broadly to include racial or ethnic groups, as well as gender, age, religion, economic status, nationality, physical capacity or disability, or sexual orientation. We are all limited by our experiences in these various groups, but we can increase our awareness by direct contact with a variety of groups, by reading, by special coursework, and by in-service professional workshops. Our practices must be accurate, appropriate, respectful, and meaningful for the clients with whom we work. This entails rethinking our theories and modifying our techniques to meet clients' unique needs and not rigidly applying interventions in the same manner to all clients. Ongoing examination of our assumptions, attitudes, and values is basic to understanding how these factors may influence our practice.

Suggested Activities

1. Select two or three cultures or ethnic groups different from your own. What attitudes and beliefs about these cultures did you hold while growing up? In what ways, if any, have your attitudes changed and what has contributed to the changes?

2. Which of your values do you ascribe primarily to your culture? Have any of your values changed over time, and if so, how? How might these values influence the way you work with clients who are culturally different from you?

3. Interview students or faculty members who identify themselves as ethnically or culturally different from you. What might they teach you about differences that you can apply as a counselor to more effectively work with clients?

4. Do you have a good sense of how people from other cultural groups perceive you? What perceptions do you think others have about you? How do you feel these perceptions reflect on how you see yourself? In what ways might this play out in your work with clients who differ from you culturally? Be specific.

5. To what degree have your courses and field experience contributed to your ability to work effectively with people from other cultures? What training experiences would you like to have to better prepare you for multicultural counseling?

6. How often are students in your program encouraged to engage in difficult dialogues around issues of difference? Do you think the faculty models this for students and creates an environment in which you are willing to share your views regarding differences?

7. People from various ethnic groups are often pressured to give up their beliefs and ways in favor of adopting the ideals and customs of the dominant culture. What do you think your approach would be in working with clients who feel such pressure? How might you work with clients who see their own ethnicity or cultural heritage as a burden to be overcome?

8. What was your own "internal dialogue" as you read and reflected on this chapter? Share some of this internal dialogue in small group discussions. Did you find yourself challenged by any of the content in this chapter? What ideas most resonated with you, and what ideas triggered strong reactions from you? How can you continue your self-reflection process around the information presented in this chapter?

9. In small groups, discuss a few of your assumptions that are likely to influence the manner in which you counsel others. From the following list, select one of the assumptions discussed in this chapter that most applies to you. Explore and share your attitudes.

    - What assumptions do you make about the value of self-disclosure on the part of clients?
    - What are your assumptions pertaining to autonomy, independence, and self-determination?
    - To what degree do you assume that it is better to be assertive than to be nonassertive?
    - How would you describe an authentic person?
    - What other assumptions can you think of that might either help or hinder you in counseling diverse client populations?

10. In small groups, explore what you consider to be the main ethical issues in counseling lesbian, gay, bisexual, and transgender clients. Review the discussion of the case

of *Bruff v. North Mississippi Health Services* on pages 127–129. What legal issues are involved in this case? What are the ethical issues in this case? To what degree do you think the counselor imposed her values on her client? Do you think counselors have a right to refuse to provide services to homosexual clients because of the counselors' personal beliefs?

11. Select any one of the many cases described in this chapter, and reflect on how you would deal with this case from an ethical perspective. After you select the case that most interests you, review the steps in the ethical decision-making process described in Chapter 1, and then go through these steps in addressing the issues involved in the case.

12. In small groups review the list of traits of the culturally encapsulated counselor who exhibits cultural tunnel vision. If you recognize any of these traits in yourself, what do you think you might do about them?

13. *The Color of Fear*, produced and directed by Lee Mun Wah, is an emotional and insightful portrayal of racism in America.* Its aim is to illustrate the type of dialogue and relationships needed if we are to have a truly multicultural society based on equality and trust. After viewing the film in class, share what it brought out in you.

14. Check out the Teaching Tolerance website at www.tolerance.org for interesting material on topics explored in this chapter. The website contains information pertaining to a range of issues that can be the topics of discussion in small groups and in class.

15. Are you aware of any prejudices you have held toward others on the basis of cultural differences? Have you been the object of prejudice or discrimination? Engage in an honest, courageous, and respectful dialogue with classmates about prejudice and discrimination and ways to combat the *isms* that continue to be a destructive force in society and in the lives of many clients.

16. Replicate Dr. Rita Chung's character portrayal exercise and assume the identity of a person of a different gender, class, race, or ethnic group from your own. In a small group, discuss some of the challenges you might face as this person in society. Discuss what you imagine it is like to be this person.

Ethics in Action Video Exercises

17. In video role play 3, Challenging the Counselor: Culture Clash, the client (Sally) directly questions the counselor's background. She says that she didn't expect the counselor (Richard) to be so young and seemingly inexperienced. She presses him further about whether he knows much about the Chinese culture. Role-play a situation in which a clash between you and a client might develop (such as difference in age, race, sexual orientation, or culture).

18. In video role play 6, Multicultural Issues: Seeking More From Life, the client (Lucia) is presenting her struggle, which can be understood only to the extent that the counselor (Janice) understands her client's cultural values. In this case, Lucia is struggling with a decision of what she wants to do with her life. Her parents would like her to stay at home and take care of her children. She asks Janice how she might be able to

---

The Color of Fear is available from Stir Fry Productions in Berkeley, California. The Stir Fry Productions Company provides trained facilitators (in some areas) to assist with discussion after the film is shown.

help her. The counselor lets Lucia know that the most important thing is that she is at peace with whatever decision she makes. This situation can be role-played in class or a small group and can then be used as a springboard for discussion of what it takes for a counselor to be able to ethically and effectively counsel diverse clients.

19. Refer to the section titled "Becoming an Effective Multicultural Practitioner" in the *Ethics in Action* video. Complete the self-examination of multicultural counseling competencies. Bring your answers to class and explore in small discussion groups what you need to do to become competent as a counselor of clients whose cultural background differs from your own.

MindTap for Counseling

Go to MindTap® for digital study tools and resources that complement this text and help you be more successful in your course and career. There's an interactive eBook plus videos of client sessions, skill-building activities, quizzes to help you prepare for tests, apps, and more—all in one place. If your instructor *didn't* assign MindTap, you can find out more about it at CengageBrain.com.

5

Client Rights and Counselor Responsibilities

LEARNING OBJECTIVES

1. Explain what is involved in the informed consent process

2. Describe the basic content of an informed consent document

3. Understand a counselor's responsibility in record keeping

4. Explore ethical issues related to online counseling

5. Identify some legal issues and risk management strategies for providing online counseling

6. Discuss ethical issues in working with minors

7. Address issues regarding suspected unethical behavior of colleagues

8. Clarify what is involved in the concept of malpractice

9. Examine the basis for malpractice liability in the therapy profession

10. Delineate practical strategies for risk management

11. Understand an appropriate course of action in dealing with a malpractice complaint

SELF-INVENTORY

Directions: For each statement, indicate the response that most closely identifies your beliefs and attitudes. Use the following code:

5 = I *strongly agree* with this statement.

4 = I *agree* with this statement.

3 = I am *undecided* about this statement.

2 = I *disagree* with this statement.

1 = I *strongly disagree* with this statement.

_____ 1. If there is a conflict between a legal and an ethical standard, a therapist must always adhere to the ethical standard.

_____ 2. Practitioners who do not use written consent forms are unprofessional and unethical.

_____ 3. To practice ethically, therapists must become familiar with the laws related to their profession.

_____ 4. Clients in therapy should *not* have access to their clinical files.

_____ 5. Clients should be made aware of their rights at the outset of a therapeutic relationship.

_____ 6. Therapists have an ethical responsibility to become knowledgeable about community resources.

_____ 7. Before entering therapy, clients should be made aware of the purposes, goals, techniques, policies, and procedures involved.

_____ 8. In certain circumstances, it is *not* necessary or appropriate to inform clients at the initial counseling session of the limits of confidentiality.

_____ 9. Informed consent is an ongoing process.

_____ 10. It is primarily the therapist's responsibility to determine the appropriate time for termination of therapy for most clients.

_____ 11. A therapeutic relationship should be maintained only as long as it is clear that the client is benefiting.

_____ 12. Counselors should keep detailed clinical notes and share these notes with clients when they request them.

_____ 13. When a child is in psychotherapy, the therapist has an ethical and legal obligation to provide the parents with information they request.

_____ 14. Minors should be allowed to seek psychological assistance regarding pregnancy and abortion counseling *without* parental consent or knowledge.

_____ 15. Clinicians have an ethical responsibility to discuss possible termination issues with clients on a periodic basis.

Introduction

To practice in an ethical and legal manner, the rights of clients are paramount. In this chapter we deal with ways of educating clients about their rights and responsibilities as partners in the therapeutic process. Special attention is given to the role of informed consent and to the ethical and legal issues that arise when therapists fail to provide sufficient informed consent. We also deal with some of the ethical and legal issues involved in counseling children and adolescents and in counseling involuntary clients.

Part of ethical practice is talking with clients about their rights. Clients are not always aware of their rights, and they may find the therapeutic process mysterious. Vulnerable and sometimes desperate for help, clients may unquestioningly accept whatever their therapist says or does. Clients may see their therapist much like they see their physician and expect the therapist to have an accurate diagnosis and an immediate solution to their problem. For most people the therapeutic situation is a new one, and they may not realize that the therapist's duty is to help clients find their own solutions. The therapeutic process involves a collaborative endeavor in which a therapist and a client form a partnership to attain goals the client has chosen. For these reasons, the therapist is held responsible for protecting clients' rights and teaching clients about these rights. The ethics codes of most professional organizations require that clients be given adequate information to make informed choices about entering and continuing the client–therapist relationship (see the Ethics Codes box titled "The Rights of Clients and Informed Consent" for examples from several ethics codes). By alerting clients to their rights and responsibilities, the practitioner is encouraging a sense of autonomy and personal power. Therapists also protect themselves from ethics complaints by informing clients of their rights and responsibilities.

ETHICS CODES: The Rights of Clients and Informed Consent

American Psychological Association (2010)
(a) When obtaining informed consent to therapy as required in Standard 3.10, *Informed Consent*, psychologists inform clients/patients as early as is feasible in the therapeutic relationship about the nature and anticipated course of therapy, fees, involvement of third parties, and limits of confidentiality and provide sufficient opportunity for the client/patient to ask questions and receive answers.

(b) When obtaining informed consent for treatment for which generally recognized techniques and procedures have not been established, psychologists inform their clients/patients of the developing nature of the treatment, the potential risks involved, alternative treatments that may be available, and the voluntary nature of their participation. (10.01)

National Association of Social Workers (2008)
Social workers should provide services to clients only in the context of a professional relationship based, when appropriate, on valid informed consent. Social workers should

use clear and understandable language to inform clients of the purpose of the services, risks related to the services, limits to services because of the requirements of a third party payer, relevant costs, reasonable alternatives, clients' right to refuse or withdraw consent, and the time frame covered by the consent. Social workers should provide clients with an opportunity to ask questions. (1.03.a.)

American Counseling Association (2014)

Counselors explicitly address with clients the nature of all services provided. They inform clients about issues such as, but not limited to, the following: the purposes, goals, techniques, procedures, limitations, potential risks, and benefits of services; the counselor's qualifications, credentials, relevant experience, and approach to counseling; continuation of services upon the incapacitation or death of a counselor; the role of technology; and other pertinent information.

Counselors take steps to insure that clients understand the implications of diagnosis, and the intended use of tests and reports. Additionally, counselors inform clients about fees, and billing arrangements, including procedures for nonpayment of fees. Clients have the right to confidentiality and to be provided with an explanation of its limits (including how supervisors and/or treatment or interdisciplinary team professionals are involved), to obtain clear information about their records, to participate in the ongoing counseling plans, and to refuse any services or modality change and to be advised of the consequences of such refusal. (A.2.b.)

Code of Professional Ethics for Rehabilitation Counselors (CRCC, 2010)

Rehabilitation counselors recognize that clients have the freedom to choose whether to enter into or remain in a rehabilitation counseling relationship. Rehabilitation counselors respect the rights of clients to participate in ongoing rehabilitation counseling planning and to make decisions to refuse any services or modality changes, while also ensuring that clients are advised of the consequences of such refusal. Rehabilitation counselors recognize that clients need information to make an informed decision regarding services and that professional disclosure is required in order for informed consent to be an ongoing part of the rehabilitation counseling process. Rehabilitation counselors appropriately document discussions of disclosure and informed consent throughout the rehabilitation counseling relationship. (A.3.b.)

The American Mental Health Counselors Association (2015)

Mental health counselors provide information that allows clients to make an informed choice when selecting a provider. Such information includes but is not limited to: counselor credentials, issues of confidentiality, the use of tests and inventories, diagnosis, reports, billing, and therapeutic process. Restrictions that limit clients' autonomy are fully explained. (I.B.2.a.)

American Association for Marriage and Family Therapy (2015)

Marriage and family therapists obtain appropriate informed consent to therapy or related procedures and use language that is reasonably understandable to clients. When persons, due to age or mental status, are legally incapable of giving informed consent, marriage and family therapists obtain informed permission from a legally authorized person, if such substitute consent is legally permissible. The content of informed consent may vary depending upon the client and treatment plan; however, informed consent generally necessitates that the client: (a) has the capacity to consent; (b) has been adequately informed of significant information concerning treatment processes and procedures; (c) has been adequately informed of potential risks and benefits of treatments for which generally recognized standards do not yet exist; (d) has freely and without undue influence expressed consent; and (e) has provided consent that is appropriately documented. (1.2.)

In addition to the ethical aspects of safeguarding clients' rights, legal parameters also govern professional practice. When we attend continuing education workshops on ethics in clinical practice, the focus is often on legal matters and risk management. Practitioners express their fears of lawsuits and are eager to learn risk management strategies that will protect them from malpractice. These concerns are realistic but need to be kept in perspective. Our emphasis should be on *both* nonmaleficence (avoiding doing harm) and beneficence (doing what is best for the client). Pope (2015) relates this idea specifically to record keeping. He asserts that practicing *defensive record keeping*—that is, making risk management one's primary focus in record keeping and in other areas of practice—may lead clinicians to lose sight of their ethical and clinical responsibilities. When we act in the best interest of the client and can demonstrate this through a process of consultation and documentation, we are less likely to be sanctioned for ethical or legal violations.

Counseling can be a risky venture, and you must be familiar with the laws that govern professional practice. However, we hope you will avoid becoming so involved in legalities that you lose sight of the ethical and clinical implications of what you do with your clients. You will surely want to protect yourself legally, but not to the point that you immobilize yourself and inhibit your professional effectiveness.

The Client's Right to Give Informed Consent

The first step in protecting the rights of clients is the informed consent document. **Informed consent** involves the right of clients to be informed about their therapy and to make autonomous decisions pertaining to it. Informed consent is a shared decision-making process in which a practitioner provides adequate information so that a potential client can make an informed decision about participating in the professional relationship (Barnett, Wise, Johnson-Greene, & Bucky, 2007). Informed consent is both an ethical and a legal obligation of the clinician, and providing information to clients is also a good quality enhancement strategy. Attending to informed consent not only meets legal and ethical standards but represents excellent clinical care as well (Knapp et al., 2015). Informed consent for treatment is a powerful clinical, legal, and ethical tool (Wheeler & Bertram, 2015).

Mental health professionals are required by their ethics codes to disclose to clients the risks, benefits, and alternatives to proposed treatment. The intent of an **informed consent document** is to define boundaries and clarify the nature of the basic counseling relationship between the counselor and the client. One benefit of informed consent is that it increases the chances that clients will become actively involved, educated, and willing participants in the assessment process and in their therapy. When clients understand what is expected of them to get positive results from therapy, the therapeutic alliance is enhanced. It may not be possible or clinically appropriate to discuss informed consent in great detail at the first session due to the emotional state of a client. Dealing with a client's crisis takes precedence over a discussion of informed consent, but informed consent must be addressed as soon as it is clinically appropriate. It is crucial that topics such as the limits of confidentiality be explained at the first session, even in crisis cases. If this is not done and the client discloses a matter that must be reported, the therapist may face both legal and ethical problems.

Most professionals agree that it is crucial to provide clients with information about the therapeutic relationship, but the manner in which this is done in practice varies considerably among therapists. It is a mistake to overwhelm clients with too much detailed information at once, but it is also a mistake to withhold important information that clients need if they are to make wise choices about their therapy. The counselor must strike a balance between providing necessary information to the client and attending to the emotional state of the client.

Professionals have a responsibility to their clients to make reasonable disclosure of all significant facts, the nature of the procedure, and some of the more possible consequences and difficulties. Clients have the right to have treatment explained to them. The process of therapy is not so mysterious that it cannot be explained in a way that clients can comprehend how it works. For instance, most residential addictions treatment programs require that patients accept the existence of a power higher than themselves. This "higher power" is defined by the patient, not by the treatment program. Before individuals agree to entering treatment, they have a right to know this requirement. It is important that clients give their consent *with* understanding. Professionals need to avoid subtly coercing clients to cooperate with a therapy program to which they are not freely consenting. It is the responsibility of professionals to assess the client's level of understanding and to promote the client's free choice. In doing so therapists can model a social justice perspective for clients, many of whom may experience oppression and discrimination. If informed consent procedures are implemented properly, open exchanges between therapists and clients are promoted that may result in empowered collaboration, or shared decision making (Knapp & VandeCreek, 2012). Clients are empowered when they are educated about their rights and responsibilities in the therapeutic process.

Legal Aspects of Informed Consent

Generally, informed consent requires that the client understands the information presented, gives consent voluntarily, and is competent to give consent to treatment (Wheeler & Bertram, 2015). Therapists must give clients information in a clear way and check to see that they understand it. Disclosures should be given in simple language in a culturally sensitive manner and must be understandable to clients. To give valid consent, it is necessary for clients to have adequate information about both the therapy procedures and the possible consequences.

Educating Clients About Informed Consent

A good foundation for a therapeutic alliance is for therapists to employ an educational approach, encouraging clients' questions about assessment or treatment and offering useful feedback as the treatment process progresses. Here are some questions therapists and clients should address at the outset of the therapeutic relationship:

- What are the goals of the therapeutic endeavor?
- What are the potential risks and benefits of counseling?
- What services will the counselor provide?
- What are the techniques, procedures, and potential benefits and risks of the services provided?
- What is expected of the client?
- What is the practitioner's approach to counseling?
- What are the qualifications of the provider of services?
- What professional experience does the counselor have with the client's problem?
- What are the financial arrangements?
- To what extent is the clinician available between sessions?
- How does the clinician handle missed appointments without notification?
- To what extent can the duration of therapy be predicted?
- What are the procedures for managing crises or severe emotional distress after hours?
- What are the limitations of confidentiality?
- In what situations does the practitioner have mandatory reporting requirements?

A basic part of the informed consent process involves giving clients an opportunity to raise questions and to explore their expectations of counseling. We recommend viewing clients as partners with their therapists in the sense that they are involved as fully as possible in each aspect of therapy. Practitioners cannot presume that clients clearly understand what they are told initially about the therapeutic process. Furthermore, informed consent is not easily completed in the initial session by asking clients to sign forms. The *Canadian Code of Ethics for Psychologists* (CPA, 2015) states that informed consent involves a process of reaching an agreement to work collaboratively rather than simply having a consent form signed (Section 1.17).

The more clients know about how therapy works, including the roles of both client and therapist, the more clients will benefit from the therapeutic experience. Most of the codes of ethics make it clear that educating clients about the therapeutic process is an ongoing endeavor. Informed consent is not a single event; rather, it is best viewed as a process that continues for the duration of the professional relationship as issues and questions arise (Barnett & Johnson, 2015; Pope & Vasquez, 2016; Wheeler & Bertram, 2015).

Clients may not feel empowered to challenge their counselor, especially in the beginning stages of treatment, due to cultural beliefs, attitudes about authority, or feelings of intimidation. At the beginning of the informed consent process, therapists have an opportunity to join with their clients and engage with them in forming a working alliance through the process of informed consent. This is the time to explain to clients how they can become the experts on their own lives and the implications of this at all stages of treatment.

Issues of power and control can be central in the therapy process, especially in the case of clients who have been victimized. The informed consent process can help to minimize the power differential. The process of informing clients about therapy is geared toward making the client–therapist relationship a collaborative partnership, which is basic to effective therapy.

Informed Consent and Managed Care

Practitioners are ethically bound to offer the best quality of service available, and clients have a right to know that managed care programs, with their focus on cost containment, may influence the quality of care available. Clinicians are expected to provide prospective clients with clear information about the benefits to which they are entitled and the limits of treatment. Informed consent forms should state that the managed care company may request a client's diagnosis, results of any tests given, a wide range of clinical information, treatment plans, and perhaps even the entire clinical record of a client. Clinicians who work in a managed care system are ethically bound to inform clients about policies that could affect them before they enter into a therapeutic relationship.

Braun and Cox (2005) recommend that clinicians inform clients about the limits of confidentiality and the potential repercussions of disclosing personal information to insurance providers. Clients need to understand that some services may not be covered under their insurance plans and "that the insurance plan and utilization review direct the type and length of treatment received, and that payment for treatment might be terminated before the client and/or the counselor believe(s) the goals of therapy have been achieved" (p. 430). Counselors under any managed care contracts should be aware of their obligations and offer acceptable alternatives to clients during the informed consent process (Nancy Wheeler, personal communication, June 28, 2016). Counselors should include a statement about the client's ultimate responsibility for payment in case the insurance does not cover the services provided (Maureen Kenny, personal communication, September 25, 2016).

Informed Consent in Private Practice and Agency Settings

How do practitioners assist clients in becoming informed partners? Pomerantz and Handelsman (2004) state that clients have a right to know what the therapy process entails because they are buying a service from a professional. Some of the topics they have developed include a series of questions pertaining to what therapy is and how it works, the clinician's approach, alternatives, appointments, confidentiality, fees, procedures for filing for insurance reimbursement, and policies pertaining to managed care. Pomerantz and Handelsman believe that an open discussion of a wide range of questions about the therapy process enhances the therapeutic alliance and lays the groundwork for a relationship based on empowerment through information.

Best practice involves providing information about the therapeutic process to clients both verbally and in writing. A written consent form can augment verbal informed consent discussions. In many agencies, clients read and sign the informed consent form. It is a good practice for clinicians to document that they reviewed the written form with clients and answered client questions. In general, client misunderstanding is reduced through the effective use of informed consent procedures. An adequate informed consent process also tends to reduce the chances a client will file a liability claim. Both the practitioner and the client benefit from this practice.

We have emphasized the importance of the therapist's role in teaching clients about informed consent and encouraging clients' questions about the therapeutic process. With this general concept in mind, put yourself in the counselor's place in the following case. Identify the main ethical issues in this case, and think about what you would do in this situation.

The Case of Kiara

At the initial interview the therapist, Kiara, does not provide an informed consent form and touches only briefly on the process of therapy. In discussing confidentiality, she states that whatever is said in the office will stay in the office, with no mention of the limitations of confidentiality. Three months into the therapy, the client exhibits some suicidal ideation. Kiara has recently attended a conference at which malpractice was one of the topics of discussion, and she worries that she may have been remiss in not providing her client with adequate information about her services, including confidentiality and its limitations. She hastily reproduces an informed consent document that she received at the conference and asks her client to sign the form at the next session. This procedure seems to evoke confusion in the client, and he makes no further mention of suicide. After a few more sessions, he calls in to cancel an appointment and does not schedule another appointment. Kiara does not pursue the case further.

- What are the ethical and legal implications of the therapist's practice? Explain your position.
- If you had been in Kiara's situation, what could you have done?
- Would you have contacted this client after he canceled? Why or why not? What are your thoughts about Kiara not doing that?

Commentary. This case illustrates the absolute importance of making sure the informed consent process is attended to from the outset of therapy. If we only address critical issues when they arise, clients may be justifiably angry and the quality of the therapeutic relationship may be jeopardized. Unfortunately, Kiara focused solely on her own interests in this case, and her actions may have placed her at greater risk of legal action. The belated use of an informed consent form and Kiara's willingness to allow the client to terminate abruptly do not enhance the client's best interests or protect him from harm. When this client canceled the appointment, Kiara had an ethical responsibility to pursue the matter to determine whether he had terminated therapy because of her belated attention to the informed consent process. •

Consider the following case as you think about your personal stance on what you might include in your informed consent document regarding your personal beliefs and values.

The Case of Derik

Derik is a counselor in a community agency setting, and he has strong religious beliefs. He is open about this in his professional disclosure statement, explaining that his religious beliefs play a major part in his personal and professional life. Aida comes to Derik for counseling regarding what she considers to be a disintegrating marriage. Derik has strong convictions about preserving the family unit. After going through an explanation of the informed consent document, Derik asks Aida if she is willing to join him in a prayer for the successful outcome of the therapy and for the preservation of the family. Derik then takes a history and assures Aida that everything can be worked out. He adds that he would like to include Aida's husband in the sessions. Aida leaves and does not return.

- Do you see any potential ethical violations on Derik's part?
- If Derik came to you for consultation, what would you say to him?
- Is it ever appropriate to include your personal values and beliefs in the informed consent process? Do clients have a right to know your personal values? If a client asks you about your personal values or beliefs, how would you respond? How might knowing your values help or hinder your client's work with you?

Commentary. We have some concerns with Derik's approach to Aida. He does not assess the client's state of mind, her religious convictions, if any, the strength of her convictions, or her degree of comfort with his approach. Aida may have felt pressured to agree with him in this first session, or she may not have deemed it appropriate to disagree openly. We question whether Aida is able to give truly informed consent under these circumstances. It is not appropriate for the therapist to introduce prayer into the session, even though he tells clients that this is part of his philosophy. If this is important to Aida, it would be her place to introduce prayer in the session. The ethical issue is captured in this question: "Did Derik take care of the client's needs, or did he take care of his own needs at Aida's expense?" Keep in mind that providing clear informed consent about one's convictions does not relieve counselors of the duty to respect clients' cultural traditions—including religious beliefs—and the prohibition regarding imposing one's values on clients. •

LO2

The Content of Informed Consent

One of the main aims of the first meeting is to establish rapport and create a climate of safety in the therapeutic situation. Realizing that informed consent is an ongoing process, the challenge is to provide clients with the right amount of information at this session for them to make informed choices. The types and amounts of information, the specific content of informed consent, the style of presenting information, and the timing of introducing this information must be considered within the context of state licensure requirements, work setting, agency policies, the specific population being served, and the nature of the client's concerns. Counselors practicing online must pay careful attention to informed consent. The role and place of technology and social media must be discussed at the earliest stage of therapy (Wilcoxon, 2015). There is no assurance that practitioners can avoid legal action, even if they do obtain written informed consent. Rather than focusing on legalistic documents, we suggest that you develop informed consent procedures that stress client understanding and foster client–counselor dialogue within the therapeutic partnership.

Topics selected for discussion during early counseling sessions are best guided by the concerns, interests, and questions of the client. Although it is essential to review informed consent with clients in the initial sessions, doing so only at this time is not adequate. Clients are often anxious during their first sessions and are likely to miss important details. As concerns arise in therapy, clients can be informed about the key aspects of the informed consent process and invited to discuss relevant topics. Let's examine in more detail some of the topics about which clients should be informed.

The Therapeutic Process

It may be difficult to give clients a detailed description of what occurs in their therapy, but some general ideas can be explored. We support the practice of letting clients know that counseling might open up levels of awareness that could cause pain and anxiety. Clients who require long-term therapy need to know that they may experience changes that could produce disruptions and turmoil in their lives. Some clients may choose to settle for a limited knowledge of themselves rather than risk this kind of disruption, and this should be explored but also respected. We believe it is appropriate to use the initial sessions for a frank discussion of how change happens. Clients should understand the procedures and goals of therapy and know that they have the right to refuse to participate in certain therapeutic techniques.

For a further discussion of change processes in therapy, an excellent book from a research perspective is *The Heart & Soul of Change: Delivering What Works in Therapy* by Duncan, Miller, Wampold, and Hubble (2010).

Assessment of a Client's Background

It is a good practice to inform clients about the assessment process. Therapists ask many questions of clients during the intake session and the assessment process, and clients are more likely to cooperate in providing honest information if they know why they are being questioned. This first session is different from others in that the client is being asked more questions than usual to obtain a quality assessment. This assessment often includes areas typically influencing the quality of life, such as family of origin, culture, divorce, substance abuse, immigration status, traumatic events, and religious and spiritual background. Such questioning may reveal areas of a client's life that shed light on the presenting problem, identifying areas for potential exploration during the therapy process.

Background of the Therapist

Therapists can provide clients with a description of their training and education, their credentials, licenses, any specialized skills, their theoretical orientation, and the types of problems that are beyond the scope of their competence. State licensure boards often make giving this information a legal requirement. If the counseling will be done by an intern or a paraprofessional, clients must be made aware of this fact. Likewise, if the provider will be working with a supervisor, this fact should be made known to the client. This description of the practitioner's qualifications, coupled with a willingness to answer any questions clients have about the process, reduces the unrealistic expectations clients may have about therapy; it also reduces the chances of complaints to a licensing board and malpractice actions (Nancy Wheeler, personal communication, June 28, 2016).

Costs Involved in Therapy

All costs involved in counseling or psychological services, including methods of payment, must be provided at the beginning of these services. A therapist's policy on charging for missed appointments or late cancellations should be clearly stated. Clients need to be informed about how insurance reimbursement will be taken care of and any limitations of their health plan with respect to fees. If fees are subject to change, this should be made clear in the beginning, preferably both verbally and in writing.

Most ethics codes have a standard pertaining to establishing fees. Matters of finance are delicate and, if handled poorly, can lead to problems. Clark and Sims (2014) note that the topic of setting and collecting fees tends to be difficult for some practitioners, especially those struggling with their beliefs regarding their self-worth, their sense of competency, and the value of the therapy services they offer. Practitioners new to the profession often experience a sense that they do not deserve the fees they are receiving. Family-of-origin issues also may influence therapists' comfort levels in discussing fees. Clark and Sims point out that therapists who were raised to put others' needs before their own or who were taught that discussing finances was impolite may be hesitant to broach the issue of fees because doing so is embarrassing and uncomfortable.

In establishing fees, practitioners might consider a fee range that is commonly accepted in a given community. It is best practice to come to an agreement on fees at the beginning of a professional relationship. Matters of fees should be documented in the client's record. Mental health practitioners put themselves and the therapeutic relationship at risk if they allow a client to accrue a large debt without discussing a plan for payment. Although therapists can initiate legal action against a client for nonpayment of fees, this is likely to damage the therapeutic relationship. It is generally not legally advisable either because it can result in the client filing a counterclaim against the counselor. The manner in which fees are handled has much to do with the tone of the therapeutic partnership.

Most professional codes of ethics have a *pro bono* guideline that encourages practitioners to share their expertise with those who cannot afford to pay for services. Individual practitioners will aspire to different standards regarding pro bono work, but denying needed services to clients as soon as their insurance has been exhausted raises concerns regarding ethical practice and standards of care. In the spirit of aspirational ethics, therapists would do well to allow for some low fee sessions in their practice. Clinicians should strive to see that clients obtain the services they need.

The Length of Therapy and Termination

Clients should be told that they can choose to terminate therapy at any time, yet it is important for the client to discuss the matter of termination with the therapist.

Part of the informed consent process involves providing clients with information about the length of treatment and the termination of treatment. Regardless of the length of treatment, it is important for clients to be prepared for a termination phase. Termination should be addressed at the outset of the professional relationship and revisited at various stages of therapy, especially when termination is anticipated. An effective termination process is critical in securing trust in the overall therapy process and minimizing the return of symptoms or feelings of exploitation. Termination is a key phase of every client's treatment, and therapists should help clients plan for it, prepare for it, and process it (Younggren, Fisher, Foote, & Hjelt, 2011).

Many agencies have a policy limiting the number of sessions provided to clients. These clients should be informed at the outset that they cannot receive long-term therapy. Under a managed care system, clients are often limited to 6 sessions, or a specified amount for a given year, such as 20 sessions. The limited number of sessions needs to be brought to their attention more than once. Furthermore, clients have the right to expect a referral so that they can continue exploring whatever concerns initially brought them to therapy. If referrals are not possible but the client still needs further treatment, the therapist should describe other alternatives available to the client.

Because practitioners differ with respect to an orientation of long-term versus short-term therapy, it is important that they inform clients of the basic assumptions underlying their orientation. In a managed care setting, practitioners need to have expertise in assessing a client's main psychological issues and matching each client with the most appropriate intervention. They also need to acquire competency in delivering brief interventions.

Part of informing clients about the therapeutic process entails giving them relevant facts about brief interventions that may not always meet their needs. Clients have a right to know how their health care program is likely to influence the course of their therapy as well as the limitations imposed by the program. The managed care dictum appears to be "the shorter, the better." Clients are vulnerable to the judgment of others (the HMO provider) regarding length of treatment, nature of treatment, techniques to be used, and content of treatment sessions. From our perspective, the best length of treatment is the one that generates healing and client growth in the most efficient time.

Clients have a right to expect that their therapy will end when they have realized the maximum benefits from it or have obtained what they were seeking when they entered it. The therapist and the client need to explore the reality of termination early in the therapy process. As a part of the informed consent process, therapists should discuss what they expect from clients and how those expectations relate to termination. Some clinical reasons for termination—clients not making progress, the failure of clients to cooperate with the basic elements of treatment, clients not paying their therapy bills—should be discussed openly early in the therapy process (Knapp et al., 2015). Termination of therapy, with or without managed care involvement, is of critical concern in the therapeutic relationship. It demands the same kind of care and attention that initiated the professional relationship.

Consultation With Colleagues

Student counselors generally meet regularly with their supervisors and fellow students to discuss their progress and any problems they encounter in their work. It is good policy for counselors to inform their clients that they may consult with other professionals on their cases. Experienced clinicians schedule consultation meetings with their peers when they sense the need to do so. Even though it is ethical for clinicians to discuss their cases with other professionals, it is wise to routinely let clients know about this. Clients will then have less reason to feel that the trust they are putting in their counselor is being violated. When consulting with colleagues, the name of the client and other specific identifying information should not be disclosed under most circumstances.

Interruptions in Therapy

Most ethics codes specify that therapists should consider the welfare of their clients when it is necessary to interrupt or terminate the therapy process. It is a good practice to explain early in the course of treatment with clients the possibilities for both expected and unexpected interruptions in therapy and how they might best be handled. A therapist's absence might appear as abandonment to some clients, especially if the absence is poorly handled. As much as possible, therapists should have a plan for any interruptions in therapy, such as vacations or long-term absences. When practitioners plan vacations, ethical practice entails providing clients with another therapist in case of need. Clients need information about the therapist's method of handling emergencies as part of their orientation to treatment. Practitioners will need to obtain a client's written consent to provide information to their substitutes. It is recommended that therapists include in their informed consent document the name of at least one professional colleague who is willing to assume their professional responsibilities in the event of an emergency, such as the therapist becoming incapacitated through injury or death (McGee, 2003). Contact information for the therapist's records custodian or emergency response team also can be included in the informed consent document. For more information on this topic, we recommend *Private Practice Preparedness: The Health Care Professional's Guide to Closing a Practice Due to Retirement, Death or Disability* (Wheeler & Reinhardt, 2014).

Benefits and Risks of Treatment

Clients should have some information about both the benefits and the risks associated with a treatment program. Clients are largely responsible for the outcomes of therapy, so it is a good policy to emphasize the client's responsibility. Clients need to know that no promises can be made about specific outcomes, which means that ethical practitioners avoid promising success. When therapists use nontraditional techniques, clients need to be informed about the potential risks involved. For example, clients who choose online services must be told the advantages and disadvantages of this form of service delivery. Only then can clients decide whether this approach to therapy is right for them.

Informed Consent for the Provision of Psychological Services Using Telecommunication Technology

Clients have a right to know basic information about the provision of psychological services that involve telecommunication technology. Some of the delivery modalities include e-therapy, videoconferencing, and text messaging. Clients need to have information regarding how they can contact the counselor electronically as part of the informed consent process. Clients should be given information about the differences between in-person services and telecommunication technology so they can make an informed decision about participating in some form of e-therapy. Murphy and Pomerantz (2016) provide a framework for facilitating and enhancing the informed consent process for technologies such as interactive videoconferencing, email, telephone, text, and Internet. They note that clients who receive e-therapy are buying a service and have a right to raise questions such as these with the practitioner:

- What are the potential benefits and risks associated with e-therapy compared to in-person therapy?
- How can we know if in-person services are appropriate for my treatment?
- How much do I need to know about technology to participate in e-therapy?
- Are there limits to how and when I can electronically communicate with you?
- If I begin e-therapy, can I switch to in-person treatment?
- What are the fees involved for different forms of telecommunication?
- Will insurance pay for e-therapy?

Drum and Littleton (2014) contend that very little attention has been paid to establishing therapeutic and professional boundaries when delivering services via telecommunication. Practitioners using telecommunication technology are advised to consider how to maintain appropriate boundaries in the relationship as a way of preventing harm and optimizing treatment gains. By being aware of potential boundary crossings in providing services via forms of telecommunication, clinicians can educate clients about the unique role of maintaining professional boundaries. Clinicians are challenged to ensure that services via digital technology be conducted in ways that are both ethical and efficacious.

Alternatives to Traditional Therapy

According to the ethics codes of some professional organizations, clients need to know about alternative helping systems. It is a good practice for therapists to learn about community resources so they can present these alternatives to a client. Some alternatives to psychotherapy include self-help programs, stress management, personal-effectiveness training, peer self-help groups, indigenous healing practices, bibliotherapy, 12-step programs, support groups, and crisis intervention.

This information about therapy and its alternatives can be presented in writing, through an audiotape or videotape, or during an intake session. An open discussion of therapy and its alternatives may, of course, lead some clients to choose sources of help other than therapy. For practitioners who make a living providing therapy services, asking their clients to consider alternative treatments can produce financial anxiety. However, openly discussing therapy and its alternatives may reinforce clients' decisions to continue therapy. Clients have a right to know about alternative therapeutic modalities (such as different theoretical orientations and medication) that are known to be effective with particular clients and conditions.

Recording Therapy Sessions or Live Observations

Many agencies require that interviews be recorded for training or supervision purposes. Clients must consent before a therapist or trainee may audiotape or videotape any session, and this consent must be documented in the clinical record (Nagy, 2011). Therapists sometimes make recordings because they can benefit from listening to them or by having colleagues listen to their interactions with clients and give them feedback. Some agencies allow recordings, but more and more do not support this training method due to HIPPA and confidentiality concerns. In these cases, live observations may be an option for students in education programs as well as those who are participating in supervision. Clients have a right to decline recordings or live observations. It is critical that clients understand why the recordings and live observations are made, how they will be used, who will have access to them, how they will be stored, and how and when recordings will be destroyed.

Clients' Right of Access to Their Files

Clinical records are kept for the benefit of clients. Remley and Herlihy (2016) maintain that clients have a legal right to inspect and obtain copies of records kept on their behalf by professionals. Clients have the ultimate responsibility for decisions about their own health care and, in most circumstances, also have the right of access to complete information with respect to their condition and the care provided. A professional should write about a client in descriptive and nonjudgmental ways with the expectation that the client may see the file someday. A clinician who operates in a professional manner should not have to worry if these notes were to become public information or were read by a client.

Some clinicians question the wisdom of sharing counseling records with a client. They may assume that their clients are not sophisticated enough to understand their diagnosis and the clinical notes, or they may think that more harm than benefit could result from disclosing such information to clients. Rather than automatically providing clients access to what is written in their files, some therapists give clients an explanation of their diagnosis and the general trend of what kind of information they are recording. Other clinicians are willing to grant their clients access to information in the counseling records they keep, especially if clients request specific information. If a decision is made to show the clinical records to a client, Knapp and VandeCreek (2012) recommend that the clinician be present. Clients may misconstrue the language contained in the records unless the therapist is present to interpret the data.

Giving clients access to their files seems to be consistent with the consumer-rights movement, which is having an impact on the fields of mental health, counseling, rehabilitation, and education. One way to reduce malpractice suits and other legal problems is to allow clients to see their medical records, even while hospitalized. In some situations it might not be in the best interests of clients to see the contents of their records. Clients requesting access to their files may be signaling a deeper concern, and the counselor should explore this further before granting a client's request. The clinician needs to make a professional determination of those times when seeing records could be counterproductive. Later in this chapter we discuss procedures for keeping records.

Rights Pertaining to Diagnostic Classifying

One of the major obstacles for some therapists to the open sharing of files with clients is the need to give clients a diagnostic classification as a requirement for receiving third-party reimbursement for psychological services. Some clients are not informed that they will be so classified, what those classifications are, or that the classifications and other confidential material will be given to insurance companies. Clients also do not have control over who receives this information. For example, in a managed care system, office workers will have access to specific information about a client, such as a diagnosis. Ethical practice includes informing clients that a diagnosis can become a permanent part of their file, and that can have ramifications in terms of costs of insurance, long-term insurability, and employment. Remley and Herlihy (2016) recommend that a phrase regarding diagnosis be included in the informed consent document. They believe that counselors should disclose the diagnosis to the client when the diagnosis is placed in the client's clinical record. If an initial diagnosis is later revised as a result of a reassessment of the client's condition, this change should also be discussed with the client.

The well-documented risks of diagnosis, such as the potential of being stigmatized at work or school, should be disclosed to clients (Kress, Hoffman, Adamson, & Eriksen, 2013). "In the short term, it might seem more beneficent to give clients information that will encourage them to receive the services they seem to need, but for some clients the long-term consequences of diagnosis may outweigh the treatment benefits" (p. 18). For example, it is possible that future employers or insurance providers may deny a person a job or insurance coverage, respectively, based on a preexisting condition that is part of the individual's permanent record. Moreover, employers may label some clients as unsuitable employees "because their mental health needs are severe or from fear that they will raise employer insurance premiums" (p. 20). Kress and colleagues advise counselors to provide their clients with the following information about the diagnostic process: (a) whether the client's insurance provider requires a diagnosis; (b) the typical problems associated with a diagnosis; (c) the benefits of receiving a diagnosis; and (d) the options a client can pursue should he or she choose not to receive a diagnosis or not to have an insurance provider involved.

The Nature and Purpose of Confidentiality

Clients must be informed and educated about matters pertaining to confidentiality, privileged communication, and privacy (see Chapter 6). All of the professional codes have a clause stating that clients have a right to know about any limitations of confidentiality from the outset. The *Code of Ethics of the American Mental Health Counselors Association* (AMHCA, 2015) contains the following statement:

> Confidentiality is a right granted to all clients of mental health counseling services. From the onset of the counseling relationship, mental health counselors inform clients of these rights including legal limitations and exceptions. (I.A.2.a.)

Putting this principle into action educates clients and promotes trust. The effectiveness of the client–therapist relationship is built on a foundation of trust. If trust is lacking, it is unlikely that clients will engage in significant self-disclosure and self-exploration.

Part of establishing trust involves making clients aware of how certain information will be used and whether it will be given to third-party payers. Pomerantz and Handelsman (2004) indicate that clients have a right to expect answers from the therapist on questions such as these: "How do governmental regulations, such as federal Health Insurance Portability and Accountability Act (HIPAA) regulations, influence the confidentiality of records?" "How much and what kind of information will you be required to give the insurance company?"

Traditionally, confidentiality is considered an ethical and legal duty imposed on therapists to protect client disclosures. Within a managed care context, however, confidentiality may no longer be presumed in the therapeutic relationship. Clients in a managed care program need to be told that the confidentiality of their communications might well be compromised. Clients should be aware that managed care contracts may require therapists to reveal sensitive client information to a third party who is in a position to authorize initial or additional treatment. Clinicians have no control over confidential information once it leaves their offices, and many managed care contracts require practitioners to submit all progress notes before payment is issued. Practitioners can no longer assure their clients of confidential therapy at any level.

When a practitioner contracts with a third-party payer, a client's records come under the scrutiny and review of the system doing the reimbursing. Pope (2015) contends that it "may be impossible to overstate the importance and complexity of third-party issues in discussions of clinical records' nature, purposes, content, uses and misuses, risks, and unintended effects" (p. 352). Thus some clients may want to safeguard their privacy and confidentiality by seeking treatment that does not involve third-party reimbursement. Clients may choose to opt out of using managed care to finance their therapy when they fully understand its potential impact. This presents an ethical and legal dilemma for therapists bound by managed care contracts.

As you will see in Chapter 6, confidentiality is not an absolute. Certain circumstances demand that a therapist disclose what was said by a client in a private therapy session or disclose counseling records. Fisher (2008, 2016) believes clients have a right to be informed about conditions and limitations of confidentiality *before* they consent to a professional relationship, regardless of the clinical consequences of that conversation. If a conversation about the nature and extent of information that may be disclosed does not take place, clients lose their right to make autonomous decisions regarding entering the relationship and accepting the confidentiality risks. Fisher (2016) stresses the importance of obtaining *truly informed consent*, which involves far more than simply having the client sign a consent form.

The Professional's Responsibilities in Record Keeping

From an ethical, legal, and clinical perspective, an important responsibility of mental health practitioners is to keep adequate records on their clients. The standard of care for all mental health professionals requires keeping current records for all professional contacts. Many state licensing laws and regulations establish minimum guidelines for maintaining client records, but more often it is up to the discretion of the clinician to determine the content of records (Knapp & Vande-Creek, 2012).

"Clinical records hold life-changing power," says Pope (2015, p. 348). He adds that a record's facts, conclusions, inferences, inaccuracies, gaps, wording, and tone can all affect whether a person gets a security clearance, maintains custody of a child, receives life-saving assistance in a crisis, or gets needed accommodations for a disability in the workplace. Record keeping serves multiple purposes. The primary reasons for keeping records are to provide high-quality service for clients and to maintain continuity of care when a client is transferred from one professional to another. Good record keeping also protects counselors because it can demonstrate that adequate care was provided, which could be an issue in a disciplinary hearing. Counselors are expected to document decisions they have made and actions they have taken (Remley & Herlihy, 2016). From a *clinical* perspective, record keeping provides a history that a therapist can use in reviewing the course of treatment. From an *ethical* perspective, records can assist practitioners in providing quality care to their clients. From a *legal* perspective, state or federal law may require keeping a record, and many practitioners believe that accurate and detailed clinical records can provide an excellent defense against certain malpractice claims. From a *risk management* perspective, keeping adequate records is the standard of care (Welfel, 2016; Wheeler & Bertram, 2015). Accurate, relevant, and timely documentation is useful as a risk management strategy.

Record Keeping From a Clinical Perspective

Maintaining clinical notes serves a dual purpose: (a) to provide the best service possible for clients, and (b) to provide evidence of a level of care commensurate with the standards of the profession. Although keeping records is a basic part of a counselor's practice, Remley and Herlihy (2016) believe doing so should not consume too much time and energy. Remley and Herlihy suggest that it is wise for counselors to document actions they take when they are carrying out ethical or legal obligations, yet it is not appropriate for them to neglect serving clients in order to write excessive notes that are basically self-protective. Practitioners need to balance client care with legal and ethical requirements for record keeping.

It is important to distinguish between *progress notes* and *process notes*. **Progress notes** are a means of documenting aspects of a client's treatment and are kept in a client's clinical record. These notes may be used to document significant issues or concerns related to a client's treatment. Writing progress notes can be a simple and straightforward process, and most sessions can be effectively and briefly documented. Progress notes are *behavioral* in nature and address what people say and do. They contain information on diagnosis, functional status, symptoms, treatment plan, prognosis, and client progress. Here is an example of what might be recorded in a client's progress notes:

> Client reports feeling less anxious this week. Client appears fully alert and oriented and no signs of acute distress were observed. Client has been recording levels of anxiety on a daily basis, with "1" *being not at all anxious* and "10" *being unbearably anxious.* At the previous session client reported experiencing a level "7" anxiety most days of the week. This week she reports a level "4-5" anxiety. Client says the following activities have helped her to lower overall anxiety: meditation, talking with friends, taking walks, and cutting back on caffeine. She states that her goal would be to have her anxiety levels at a "3" or below in order to feel good about the outcome of therapy. Therapist and client agreed to do some guided imagery at the next session.

Process notes, or *psychotherapy notes*, are not synonymous with progress notes; process notes deal with client reactions such as transference and the therapist's subjective impressions of a client. Other areas that might be included in the process notes are intimate details about the client; details of dreams or fantasies; sensitive information about a client's personal life; and a therapist's own thoughts, feelings, and reactions to clients. Process notes are not meant to be readily or easily shared with others. They are intended for the use of the practitioners who created them. One way of thinking about process (or psychotherapy) notes is to view them as a form of self-consultation and a way to organize ideas to bring up in supervision. As a general rule, it is best to exclude from process notes matters pertaining to diagnosis, treatment plan, symptoms, prognosis, and progress.

The law requires clinicians to keep a clinical record (progress notes) on all clients, but the law *does not* require clinicians to keep process (psychotherapy) notes. The HIPAA privacy rule allows clinicians to keep two sets of records, but it does not mandate it. When introduced, this HIPAA provision was "heralded as a major benefit for mental health practitioners" (DeLettre & Sobell, 2010, p. 160), and its low utilization has been a surprise to some researchers. DeLettre and Sobell discovered that 79% of the 464 doctoral-level psychologists they surveyed were aware of the HIPAA privacy rule allowing for a separate set of notes, but only 46% reported using such notes. The idea and benefit of keeping two sets of records is that one set (progress notes) is more general, less private, and more readily accessible to insurers and clients. The other set (process or psychotherapy notes) is more private and for the use of the therapist. Psychotherapy notes may contain the therapist's clinical hunches, matters to raise for supervision, personal reactions to the client, or hypotheses for further exploration. If a therapist does keep process notes, they must be kept separately from the individual's clinical record. Legal requests for documentation in the context of litigation may include requests for process notes as well as progress notes, so it is prudent to consider that process notes may also someday become the subject of courtroom scrutiny. Here is an example of what might be included in process notes:

> Client avoided eye contact with counselor and sat silent for much of the session. Upon questioning, client stated that he was angry at the therapist for suggesting that he was not working hard enough in his therapy. Therapist acknowledged client's courage in addressing his feelings and reviewed with client what was triggered in him when the therapist challenged him to be more active in treatment at a previous session. After processing further with the client, he made connections to feeling inadequate as a child and never feeling that he was good enough for his mother. Therapist will follow up with client at next session to see if there are any residual feelings surrounding this encounter.

A client's clinical record is not the place for a therapist's personal opinions or personal reactions to the client, and record keeping should reflect professionalism. The American Psychological Association revised its *Record Keeping Guidelines* (APA, 2007), originally published in 1993, to better assist psychologists in determining appropriate methods for developing, maintaining, disclosing, protecting, and disposing of clinical documentation (Drogin, Connell, Foote, & Sturm, 2010). According to Drogin and colleagues, "records may serve as useful roadmaps for treatment, documenting the need for services, the treatment plan, the course of treatment, and the process of termination" (p. 237).

We offer the following guidelines in record keeping practices:

- If a client misses a session, it is a good practice to document the reasons.
- In writing progress notes, use clear behavioral language. Focus on describing specific and concrete behavior and avoid jargon.
- Consider the possibility that the contents of a clinical record might someday be read in a courtroom with the client present.
- Although professional documentation is expected to be thorough, it is best to keep notes as concise as possible.
- Be mindful of the dictum, "If you did not document it, then it did not happen."
- In the clinical record, address client and therapist behavior that is clinically relevant. Include in clinical records interventions used, client responses to treatment strategies, the evolving treatment plan, and any follow-up measures taken.

Some therapists choose to devote their time to delivering service to clients rather than recording process and progress notes. However, these notes are an important part of practice. At times, therapists may operate on the assumption that keeping clinical records is not an effective use of the limited time they have, which means they would likely adopt a minimalist approach to record keeping. Clinicians may not keep notes because they believe that they can remember what clients tell them, because they are concerned about violating a client's confidentiality and privacy, because they do not want to assume a legalistic stance in their counseling practice, or because they think they do not have time to keep notes on their clients. Regardless of the reason for not keeping records, in today's climate this is inexcusable and violates the common standards of practice. Keeping records is no longer a voluntary task; it is now an ethical, clinical, and legal requirement.

As mentioned earlier, providing clients with access to their files and records seems to be in line with the consumer-rights movement, which is having an impact on the human service professions. Reflect on these questions:

- What are your thoughts on providing your clients with this information?
- What information would you want to share with your clients?
- How would you provide clients with this information?
- What might you do if there were a conflict between your views and the policies of the agency that employed you?

The Case of Maxim

Maxim is a therapist in private practice who primarily sees relatively well-functioning clients. He considers keeping records to be basically irrelevant to the therapeutic process for his clients. As he puts it: "In all that a client says to me in one hour, what do I write down? and for what purpose? If I were seeing high-risk clients, then I certainly would keep notes. Or if I were a psychoanalyst, where everything a client said matters, then I would keep notes." One of his clients, Lucia, assumed that he kept notes and one day after a session asked to see her file. Maxim had to explain his lack of record keeping to Lucia.

- What do you think of Maxim's attitude on record keeping? Do you consider it unethical? Why or why not?
- Taking into consideration the kind of clientele Maxim sees, is his behavior justified? If you disagree, what criteria would you use in determining what material should be recorded?
- What if a legal issue arises during or after Lucia's treatment? How would documenting each session help or not help both the client and the counselor?
- Assuming that some of Maxim's clients will move to other locales and see new therapists, does the absence of notes to be transferred to the new therapist have ethical or clinical implications?
- If keeping notes were not mandated, would you still keep notes? Why or why not?

Commentary. Keeping adequate clinical records is a legal and ethical requirement regardless of the degree of functioning of a client. Keeping notes is a requirement for third-party payments as well. Note taking is a critical component of therapy; it can help the therapist remember relevant information and is useful as a review of clinical procedures used with a client. Few therapists, if any, can remember everything that is covered in a given session over the course of time. Maxim may have to justify in a courtroom how his decision not to keep clinical records affected the standard of care for his clients. Bennett and colleagues (2006) remind us that the legal requirement for maintaining clinical records involves much more than following a set of arbitrary rules: "Good documentation demonstrates that you used a reasonable standard of care in conceptualizing, planning, and implementing treatment" (p. 34). Good documentation is also critical for clinicians who work in agencies. A client may come to the agency in an emergency, and his or her treating clinician may not be available. The clinician who sees this client would benefit from reviewing the treating clinician's documents to appropriately understand and conceptualize what the client needs. ●

Record Keeping From a Legal Perspective

According to Rivas-Vazquez and his colleagues (2001), the adage "if it is not documented, it did not happen" has never been more relevant than in a climate of heightened awareness of potential liability exposure. These authors outline the specific domains required for comprehensive documentation practices. Professional ethics codes also outline the requirements of good record keeping (see the Ethics Codes box titled "Record Keeping"), and as noted earlier, the American Psychological Association has updated its *Record Keeping Guidelines* as well (APA, 2007).

ETHICS CODES: Record Keeping

Code of Professional Ethics for Rehabilitation Counselors (CRCC, 2010)
Rehabilitation counselors include sufficient and timely documentation in the records of their clients to facilitate the delivery and continuity of needed services. Rehabilitation counselors take reasonable steps to ensure that documentation in records accurately reflects progress and services provided to clients. If errors are made in records, rehabilitation counselors take steps to properly note the correction of such errors according to agency or institutional policies. (B.6.a.)

American Mental Health Counselors Association (2015)
Mental health counselors create and maintain adequate clinical and financial records.
 (a) Mental health counselors create, maintain, store, transfer, and dispose of client records in ways that protect confidentiality and are in accordance with applicable regulations or laws.
 (b) Mental health counselors establish a plan for the transfer, storage, and disposal of client records in the event of withdrawal from practice or death of the counselor that maintains confidentiality and protects the welfare of the client. (E.1.)

National Association of Social Workers (2008)
 (a) Social workers should take reasonable steps to ensure that documentation in records is accurate and reflects the services provided.
 (b) Social workers should include sufficient and timely documentation in records to facilitate the delivery of services and to ensure continuity of services provided to clients in the future.
 (c) Social workers' documentation should protect clients' privacy to the extent that is possible and appropriate and should include only information that is directly relevant to the delivery of services.
 (d) Social workers should store records following the termination of services to ensure reasonable future access. Records should be maintained for the number of years required by state statutes or relevant contracts. (3.04.)

American Psychological Association (2010)
Psychologists create, and to the extent the records are under their control, maintain, disseminate, store, retain, and dispose of records and data relating to their professional and scientific work in order to (1) facilitate provision of services later by them or by other professionals, (2) allow for replication of research design and analyses, (3) meet institutional requirements, (4) ensure accuracy of billing and payments, and (5) ensure compliance with law. (6.01)

Guidelines for Records With Violent or Aggressive Clients It is a wise policy for counselors to document their actions in crisis situations such as cases involving potential danger of harm to oneself, others, or physical property. Reeves (2011) offers some useful guidelines for nurses for recording the use of physical restraint with violent or aggressive patients. These guidelines were specifically devised to be used on child and adolescent inpatient units; however, they could be applied more broadly to other clinical settings in which clients become aggressive. Reeves states that a record of an incident should be made available within 24 hours of its occurrence. Some issues that should be documented include the following:

- Events leading up to the incident, including the client's behavior and others' responses to this behavior
- Alternative strategies attempted and any departures from the plan of care
- Rationale for using physical interventions and the risks involved
- Methods and duration of each restraint used
- Difficulties encountered in monitoring the client's physical well-being and actions taken as a result of these difficulties
- How the restraint ended

Guidelines for Maintaining Adequate Clinical Records Wheeler and Bertram (2015) state that practitioners who fail to maintain adequate clinical records are vulnerable to claims of professional malpractice because inadequate records do not conform to the standard of care expected of mental health practitioners. They maintain that competent record keeping is one of the most effective tools counselors have for successfully responding to licensing board complaints or threats of a malpractice suit. Even if a mental health provider acts reasonably and keeps good records, there is no guarantee that he or she will not be sued. Occasionally a competent practitioner will be found liable for damages.

Case notes should *never* be altered or tampered with after they have been entered into the client's record. Tampering with a clinical record after the fact can cast a shadow on the therapist's integrity in court. Enter notes into a client's record as soon as possible after a therapy session, and sign and date the entry. If you keep client notes in a computer, it is essential that your program has a time and date stamp so that if your records are subpoenaed there will be no question of altering material at a later date.

The content and style of a client's records are often determined by agency or institutional policy, state counselor licensing laws, or directives from other regulatory bodies. The particular setting and the therapist's preference may determine how detailed the records will be. The APA (2007) lists the following content areas for inclusion in record keeping:

- Identifying data
- Fees and billing information
- Documentation of informed consent
- Documentation of waivers of confidentiality
- Presenting complaint and diagnosis
- Plan for services

- Client reactions to professional interventions
- Current risk factors pertaining to danger to self or others
- Plans for future interventions
- Assessment or summary information
- Consultations with or referrals to other professionals
- Relevant cultural and sociopolitical factors

Guidelines for Keeping Records With Couples, Families, and Groups The *Record Keeping Guidelines* (APA, 2007) also document procedures for practitioners working with multiple individuals in couples, family, or group therapy. When therapists work with multiple clients, the issues involved in record keeping can become complex (Drogin et al., 2010). Disclosure of information on one client may compromise the confidentiality of other clients. It may be useful to create and maintain a separate record for each person participating in group therapy. Drogin and his colleagues suggest that critical issues relevant to individual group members be documented in their individual files.

When counseling a couple or a family, the identified client may be the system, in which case a practitioner might keep a single record for the couple or the family. In counseling couples, whether records are kept on individuals or a conjoint record is maintained depends on a number of factors. Various jurisdictions have different record keeping requirements. This matter is also determined to some extent by whether the *couple is the client* or *each individual* is a separate client. If the couple is considered the client, there is a basis for a single record (Harway, Kadin, Gottlieb, Nutt, & Celano, 2012). Drogin and his colleagues (2010) note that "experienced psychologists usually develop a philosophy of documentation for couple and family psychotherapy that fits their own treatment model and practice settings" (p. 241). They acknowledge that it may be crucial to document "relational data" in their client records, not simply clinical information specific to individual clients. They believe it is "imperative to inform each party about record maintenance and who will have access to information" when treating multiple clients, whether in a group therapy context or a couples or family therapy context (p. 241). This discussion should take place at the outset of services.

Record Keeping for Managed Care Programs

Practitioners working within a managed care setting are required to maintain adequate documentation of treatment services. A managed care program may audit a practitioner's reports at any time. By law, managed care practitioners are required to keep accurate charts and notes and must provide this information to authorized chart reviewers.

Case law, licensure board statutes and rules, and Medicare/Medicaid reimbursement regulations all contribute to defining the minimum information that mental health records must contain in the managed care context. This information includes the following: client-identifying information; client's chief complaints, including pertinent history; objective findings from the most recent physical examination; intake sheet; documentation of referrals to other providers, when appropriate; findings from consultations and referrals to other health care workers; pertinent reports of diagnostic procedures and tests; signed informed consent for treatment form; diagnosis, when determined; prognosis, including significant continuing problems or conditions; the existence of treatment plans, containing specific target problems and goals; signed and dated progress notes; types of services provided; precise times and dates of appointments made and kept; termination summary; the use and completion of a discharge summary; and release of information obtained. A managed care company may demand a refund for services rendered if the records do not contain a complete description of all the services rendered.

Record Keeping for School Counselors

In some counseling settings, it may be difficult to keep up with record keeping. For example, in school counseling a student-to-counselor ratio of 400:1 (or more) is not uncommon. How realistic is it to expect a school counselor to keep detailed notes on every contact with a student? Birdsall and Hubert (2000) indicate that a well-kept record may be useful to demonstrate that the quality of counseling provided was in line with an acceptable standard of care. Keeping records is particularly important in cases involving moderate to severe social or emotional problems or when students may be at risk of suicide (Remley, 2009). Maintaining records on parent contacts is also essential. School counselors are cautioned about the importance of safeguarding the confidentiality of any records they keep. Many schools maintain a computer-based note system where the school counselor can easily log contacts without much detail (Maureen Kenny, personal communication, September 25, 2016).

The *Ethical Standards for School Counselors* (ASCA, 2016) addresses the issue of student records:

> School counselors abide by the Family Educational Rights and Privacy Act (FERPA), which defines who has access to students' educational records and allows parents the right to review and challenge perceived inaccuracies in their child's records. (A.12.a.)

School counselors need to understand the provisions of the Family Educational Rights and Privacy Act of 1974. This federal law requires that schools receiving federal funds provide access to all school records to parents of students under the age of 18 and to students themselves once they reach 18. This law outlines a method for releasing records to clients. Student records are not to be released to third parties without the written consent of parents of minors, or the written consent of adult students (Remley & Hermann, 2000).

Securing Records Now and in the Future

Clients' records must be handled confidentially. ACA's (2014) *Code of Ethics* provides guidelines for storing, transferring, sharing, and disposing of clinical records (see sections B.6.g. and B.6.h.). Counselors have the responsibility for storing client records in a secure place and exercising care when sending records to others by mail or through electronic means. Due to technological innovations in the production, storage, protection, and retrieval of digital information over the past several years, this seemingly straightforward issue has become increasingly complex. Pope (2015) believes that to "create a sound approach to clinical records, professionals must do a better job of recognizing and responding proactively to threats to confidentiality" (p. 348). He echoes the view shared by others that "these threats may come from the rapidly evolving technologies used to record, store, and communicate clinical information" (p. 348). He adds that threats to confidentiality may come from a number of sources including advertisers, industries, credit companies, government agencies, and thieves looking for access to confidential information to use for their own self-interests. Pope cautions us that threats may result from our failure to adequately safeguard clinical records.

Technological advances such as "cloud" computing have occurred at breakneck speed in recent years. Although counselors may enjoy the benefits of this technology (for example, improved service delivery), helping professionals who utilize the cloud as an off-site storage tool may be exposing themselves and their clients to unforeseen risks. "As records are moved to the cloud, psychologists' [and other practitioners'] ability to exert control over them may diminish to some unknown degree. . . . Furthermore, the aggregation of sensitive data in such large centers may increase the appeal for potential cybercriminals to steal the information" (Devereaux & Gottlieb, 2012, p. 629). Data may be encrypted to reduce this risk, but other technical difficulties are possible such as technical support staff working for the cloud service provider having access to confidential client data. To learn more about record keeping in the cloud and steps that can be taken to reduce the threats associated with cloud computing, refer to Devereaux and Gottlieb (2012).

Be aware that the information in the client's record belongs to the client, and a copy may be requested at any time. It is mandatory to treat clients in an honest and respectful fashion, and it is expected that accurate records will be kept. Mental health practitioners bear the ultimate responsibility for what they write, how they store and access records, what they do with these records, and when and how they destroy them (Nagy, 2005). Clinicians are ethically and legally required to keep records in a secure manner and to protect client confidentiality. They are also responsible for taking reasonable steps to establish and maintain the confidentiality of information based on their own delivery of services, or the services provided by others working under their supervision.

Practitioners need to consider relevant state and federal laws and the policies of their work setting in determining how long to retain a client's records. It is key to determine the specific time period for retention of records that is required by the jurisdiction in which you practice. Whether records are active or inactive, counselors are expected to maintain and store them safely and in a way in which timely retrieval is possible. Extra care should be taken if information is stored electronically.

It is wise to think about what will happen to your clinical records after your death or if you are otherwise incapacitated. Most state laws do not specify how records are to be handled upon a therapist's death, so while you are still able to be involved in the decision making, consider creating a professional will that names another professional who, at least temporarily, will handle your files and clients if you die or become otherwise incapacitated. Here are some questions to consider:

- Who will have access to your clinical records in the event of your death?
- Have you identified a colleague in your area who is willing to take over your practice in the case of your death?

It is important to answer these questions to safeguard your estate. A client can bring suit against your estate after your death if you have failed to consider some of these matters. Even death does not shield us from a malpractice suit! (See Wheeler & Reinhardt, 2014.)

Ethical Issues in Online Counseling

LO4

In this section we consider a few key ethical issues in the use of online counseling and the many forms of service delivery via the Internet. Mental health professionals now have a wide range of digital and electronic options to communicate with and to provide a range of clinical services to their clients, some of which include audio recordings, email chat, videochat, social networking websites, text messaging, self-guided Web-based interventions, and smartphone apps (Reamer, 2017).

Haberstroh, Barney, Foster, and Duffey, (2014) explored the scope of ethical and legal practice for online psychotherapy for the major mental health professions. They observed a trend toward more states and professions endorsing online therapy as a treatment modality. Only a few state regulatory boards address online clinical practice through state laws or ethics codes, but Haberstroh and his colleagues found that no states actually prohibited it. This rapidly developing field involves both benefits and risks, and just as with any new practice area, practitioners have an obligation to consider the best interests of the client, to strive to do no harm, and to adhere to legal requirements. Mental health professionals have the responsibility of evaluating the ethical, legal, and clinical issues related to providing counseling and behavioral services to individuals over a distance (Mallen, Vogel, & Rochlen, 2005). Ethical issues such as informed consent, confidentiality, privacy, self-disclosure, boundaries, and multiple relationships can have special significance when Internet technologies are involved. A significant ethical concern pertains to who is actually on the other end when providing distance counseling. Mental health professionals must make decisions about how they wish to incorporate technology in the delivery of services in their practices, and these decisions should be informed by the standards set forth by the professional associations to which they belong.

Ethics Codes and Technology

The *Code of Ethics of the American Mental Health Counselors Association* (AMHCA, 2015) includes guidelines for online counseling that address issues pertaining to confidentiality, client and counselor identification, client waiver, establishing the online counseling relationship, competence, and legal considerations. The APA (2010) ethics code states that psychologists who offer online services inform clients of the risks to privacy and the limits of confidentiality. The ACA (2014) ethics code states that counselors are expected to inform clients of the benefits and limitations of using technology in the counseling process.

The AAMFT (2015) ethics code has the following guideline for electronic therapy:

> Prior to commencing therapy services through electronic means (including but not limited to phone and Internet), marriage and family therapists ensure that they are compliant with all relevant laws for the delivery of such services. Additionally, marriage and family therapists must: (a) determine that electronic therapy is appropriate for clients, considering professional, intellectual, emotional, and physical needs; (b) inform clients or supervisees of the potential risks and benefits associated with technologically-assisted services; (c) ensure the security of their communication medium; and (d) only commence electronic therapy or services after appropriate education, training, or supervised experience using the relevant technology. (6.1.)

Emerging Issues in Online Counseling

The ethics of online therapy are vigorously debated in the profession, with major cautions centering on its value for clients experiencing significant psychological distress, recurrent psychopathology, and suicidal or homicidal intent. The application of the standard regarding the *duty to protect* when a client discloses threats of harm to self or others via email or another electronic medium is an issue receiving thoughtful attention (Welfel, 2009). From a risk management perspective, Rummell and Joyce (2010) point out that clinicians who conduct online counseling need to know the true identity and location of their clients in the event of an emergency, such as the ones mentioned here. Although acknowledging the benefits of online counseling, they identify many ethical challenges that must be considered when engaging in online counseling. Competence to provide online counseling is a fundamental ethical concern. Practitioners need to develop the skills and competencies necessary to facilitate a meaningful and viable therapeutic relationship online. The "enduring challenge in social work [and other helping professions] is to locate and walk what can be a fine line between valuable innovation that has therapeutic benefits and harmful, possibly exploitative, treatment of vulnerable clients" (Reamer, 2013, p. 171).

Reamer (2013) stresses that ethical mistakes in the delivery of online services can occur by either omission or commission. Examples of *mistakes of omission* include the failure to:

- Obtain clients' fully informed consent before providing online services
- Limit clients' access to personal information on the clinician's social networking site
- Obtain a clinical license to practice in the state in which the client resides
- Comply with HIPAA confidentiality requirements pertaining to electronic communications
- Respond in a timely manner to clients' text or email messages

Examples of *mistakes of commission* include:

- Terminating online services to clients abruptly
- Claiming expertise in providing online services outside the scope of one's education and training
- Providing online services to clients whose clinical needs are so severe that they require in-person services

Advantages and Disadvantages of Online Counseling

Most experts agree that Internet counseling cannot be considered traditional psychotherapy, but some believe this form of service delivery may benefit consumers who are reluctant to seek more traditional treatment. The benefits of online interventions are vast because of the potential for greater numbers of people to receive services. Reamer (2017) reports that research is demonstrating the effectiveness of distance counseling with a variety of populations and conditions. Proponents make a case for the capacity of digital technology to reach and enhance the delivery of services to vulnerable people. For example, Web-based treatment interventions offer an opportunity for practitioners to provide specific behavioral treatments tailored to individuals who may need to seek professional assistance from their own homes. Clients with certain disabilities or chronic illnesses that render them immobile could find online counseling beneficial. Kolmes (2017) claims that "the explosion of social media culture is opening up new opportunities for connection for psychotherapists and their clients" (p. 193). Rummell and Joyce (2010) state that "one of the most commonly described benefits of online counseling is that it allows the clinician to access hard to reach populations, such as those in a rural or otherwise remote environment where a trip to a psychological clinic is difficult, unrealistic, or impossible" (p. 484). One study on Australian adolescents' preferred modes of delivery for mental health services found that only 16% favored online treatment; those who expressed a preference for this modality emphasized benefits such as remaining anonymous, finding information easily accessible online, and finding others in chat rooms who had similar experiences (Bradford & Rickwood, 2014). Glasheen, Shochet, and Campbell's (2016) study of Australian secondary school students found that more than 80% claimed they would definitely use or might use online services offered by the school counselor, especially to deal with concerns of a sensitive or personal nature such as sexuality. One possible benefit of discussing personal issues online is that students with concerns about their sexuality can control their visibility.

Ravis (2007) contends that the benefits of distance counseling outweigh the risks. With adequate preparation, support, and resourcefulness, counselors may find that the challenges involved in distance counseling are less daunting than might be imagined. Ravis offers some suggestions for counselors considering online counseling:

- Before offering distance counseling, acquire the appropriate competencies related to this evolving specialty.
- Learn how to adapt traditional methods for effective application to distance counseling.

- Screen clients for suitability with respect to the specific distance services you are considering using.
- As a part of informed consent, educate your clients about the difficult situations that may occur during distance counseling.
- Familiarize yourself with the ethical guidelines that have been developed to inform your specific scope of practice.
- Be aware of the legal issues and state licensure board regulatory policies that govern your specific practices when delivering online counseling.

Simply having a technology available does not mean that it is appropriate for every client, or perhaps for any client. The potential benefits need to be greater than the potential risks for clients to ethically justify any form of technology that is used for counseling purposes. Here are some of the *disadvantages* in the use of online and distance counseling:

- Inaccurate diagnosis or ineffective treatment may be provided due to lack of behavioral clues and the lack of nonverbal information.
- Confidentiality and privacy cannot be guaranteed; digital technology expands the ways clients' privacy and confidentiality can be breached (Reamer, 2017).
- Therapists' duty to warn or protect others is limited.
- Clients who are suicidal, suffering extreme anxiety or depression, or who are in crisis may not receive adequate immediate attention.
- Some online service providers may not be qualified to provide competent services and may misrepresent themselves and their qualifications.
- Clinicians' use of digital technology introduces some complex challenges to therapeutic boundaries, especially multiple relationships (Reamer, 2017).
- Anonymity enables minors to masquerade as adults seeking treatment and enables other clients to misrepresent themselves as well.
- It is possible for individuals other than the client to log on and engage in a session, as if they were the client.
- Transference and countertransference issues are difficult to address.
- It is difficult to develop an effective therapeutic alliance with an individual who has never been seen in the traditional face-to-face counseling context.
- Distance counseling services may not be appropriate for clients with very complex or long-term psychological problems (Reamer, 2017).

Shaw and Shaw (2006) point out that the debate on the usefulness of online counseling will continue until there are adequate data on outcome effectiveness for this medium. They suggest that informed consent documents state that online counseling is not a replacement for traditional face-to-face counseling, but it may be a useful supplement to traditional ways of delivering counseling services.

Legal Issues and Regulation of Online Counseling

Because providing counseling services over the Internet (also known as remote services or distance counseling) is relatively new and controversial, a host of legal questions will not be addressed until lawsuits are filed pertaining to its use, or misuse, in counseling practice. One of the most pressing issues regarding the use of remote services or Internet counseling is whether it is legal for a mental health practitioner who is licensed in one state to treat a client in another state by telephone or over the Internet.

A clinician's license is intended for practice in the state where he or she is licensed to practice. Some states have ruled that licensed mental health professionals cannot practice online counseling in states in which they are not licensed. However, this is a complex matter, and some state licensing laws are archaic and do not recognize contemporary digital realities (Zur, 2016). Counselors need to stay current regarding the changing laws pertaining to counseling across states. Counselors are advised to check the laws both in the state where they practice and in the state where their client is located. Check with legal counsel or one's licensure board before engaging in online counseling or telephone counseling with out-of-state clients. It is a good idea for counselors also to check with their malpractice insurance carrier if they plan to engage in these activities. According to Zur, the state in which the client resides is more likely to be concerned about whether its laws were violated by a therapist who is not licensed in that state. Licensing boards have a legal mandate to protect consumers who live in their state; they do not have an obligation to consumers who do not reside in their state.

Can clients who cross state lines receive professional services via a telephone or video session when they have a matter they want to discuss with their therapist without jeopardy to the practitioner? According to Leslie (2016), clients have a right to expect that their therapist will continue to be available during the course of the professional relationship, especially during a crisis situation or in times of need, even when temporarily out of state. Leslie criticized a licensing board that published a notice to California consumers that if they are traveling to another state and want to participate in counseling via the telephone (or online) with their California-licensed therapist, the therapist needs to check with the state where clients are temporarily located to see if this is permitted. Leslie contends that this notice is contrary to decades of safe and ethical practice nationwide in which clients' best interests are given priority and continuity of care with their therapist of choice is expected.

To address barriers to providing psychological services across geographical boundaries, a movement has been initiated to make clinical licensure for psychologists transferable and valid in all 50 states. Some progress is being made on this front. In July 2012 the Association of State and Provincial Psychology Boards (ASPPB) announced that it had received a licensure portability grant from the federal government to fund development and implementation of the ASPPB Psychology Licensure Universal System (PLUS). Once jurisdictional issues are ironed out by the state licensing boards, therapists who choose to offer professional services online will have to give careful thought to ways of limiting their legal liability and to reducing potential harm to their clients.

Harris and Younggren (2011) note that an abundance of literature addresses how the electronic age has created new and improved ways to deliver health care services. They cite studies that challenge the assumption that in-person psychotherapy is superior to remote treatment. However, if the psychological community is to make full use of the services of the electronic world, they believe mental health practitioners must address a host of ethical and legal issues and assess the risks associated with delivering services via electronic means. Harris and Younggren believe practitioners interested in risk management will choose in-person delivery, unless a case can be made for relying on remote services. They identify the following situations that justify the use of remote services consistent with ethical practice and in keeping with regulatory standards:

- When service is provided in the context of an existing therapy relationship
- When in-person treatment is either difficult or impossible to access due to client's remote location
- When remote services offer practical advantages over in-person treatment (such as clients' busy schedule make remote sessions more efficient)
- When the client desires remote sessions and the therapist has sufficient information about the client to determine that this is a rational and informed decision

Harris and Younggren (2011) maintain that if the client does not have a past relationship with the therapist and lives in an area in which many therapists have similar skills, referral to local resources is the prudent approach to take from a professional and risk management perspective. "A proper analysis of risk should lead to a delivery model that is ethically sound, consistent with standards of professional practice, and respectful of the law" (p. 416).

Use of Smartphones

The smartphone has been used more and more over the past few years by mental health providers. Increasingly, clinical programs are encouraging or even requiring clients to download apps on their smartphones to record information about their clinical symptoms, moods, and behaviors; to obtain psychoeducation information or automated messages from clinicians (e.g., supportive messages); and to obtain links to local resources, such as the locations of nearby 12-step meetings (Reamer, 2015).

From an ethical perspective, smartphone use may have unintended consequences, so psychotherapists must assess whether smartphones are a useful and appropriate adjunct to treatment on a client-by-client basis. Some clients may become overly dependent on their smartphones, which could result in increased anxiety when they are without these devices.

Eonta and colleagues (2011) build a case for ways that technology can lead to better and more accessible client care. The smartphone is just one example of a widely available technology that can individualize the nature of client care and can tailor assessment and treatment strategies to the needs and preferences of each client. They issue the caution that "it is crucial to remain flexible and creative as psychotherapists in order to ensure that our interventions and assessments are best suited to the clients we treat, and that we are not using a 'one size fits all' approach to client care. Technology is one way of individualizing treatment and increasing efficiency of the treatment approaches we use" (p. 519).

Competent Counseling Online

Competence is a basic ethical issue when practitioners provide remote services. If complaints are filed, professionals who provide remote services will have to demonstrate competence in both the services they offer and the technology they are using to render services. Practitioners need to determine what kinds of services they can and cannot appropriately offer, and they need to assess the benefits and risks of delivery of services remotely. Therapists who choose to counsel clients online should acquire special training to become competent. In addition to acquiring technical competence, Kolmes (2012) contends that clinicians must gain a deeper understanding of how clients use and experience social networking sites. She notes:

> The cultural divide between digital natives and digital immigrants may make it more difficult for some clinicians to understand individuals who are dealing with challenges related to the merging of social, professional, and support networks in online spaces. (p. 610)

Therapists who are involved in online counseling must anticipate problems with technologically unsophisticated clients. For example, therapists should address the limitations of confidentiality and discuss what actions might be taken in the event that confidentiality is compromised. Therapists can also discuss with the client, in advance, what to do during service disruptions, such as a technological failure. A discussion of issues such as these is a basic part of the informed consent process, especially when the therapist and client are evaluating whether remote therapy is the right choice (Harris & Younggren, 2011).

Our Perspective on Online Counseling

Therapists do not have to choose between online counseling and traditional face-to-face counseling. Technology can be used in the service of clients and can address some unique needs, especially if therapists combine remote therapy and in-person sessions. For example, therapists might require one to three face-to-face sessions, if at all possible, to determine the client's suitability for online counseling and to establish a working therapeutic relationship. We think this will increase the likelihood that online services will be effective. During these face-to-face sessions, time could be allocated for orienting the client to the counseling process and securing informed consent, taking the client's history, conducting an assessment and formulating a diagnostic impression, collaboratively identifying counseling goals, developing a general treatment plan, and formulating a specific plan of action. As the action plan is carried out following these initial sessions, online sessions could be used to monitor specific homework assignments. Depending on the client's needs and situation, there might be face-to-face sessions scheduled at regular intervals along with online counseling. Integrating traditional in-person therapy with remote therapy in this way can accommodate consumers who would not take advantage of counseling delivered exclusively by face-to-face sessions due to financial considerations or restrictions imposed by traveling long distances.

Some fields of counseling seem better suited for remote services, such as career counseling and educational counseling, which involve gathering and processing information. In this endeavor, technology may have some useful applications. However, we have reservations about the effectiveness of online counseling for clients with deeply personal or interpersonal concerns. Many clinical problems involve complex variables that require human-to-human interaction. At the present time, we do not think online counseling should be used as an exclusive or primary means of delivering services, but in some cases it could be an important adjunct to face-to-face counseling. If you were to make online counseling part of your practice, what ethical considerations would you consider? What difficulties most need to be addressed in this area?

Working With Children and Adolescents

The definition of a minor varies from state to state (Barnett & Johnson, 2015). The upper range is 18 to 21 years of age, although some states authorize 16-year-olds to consent to their own health care in some circumstances. Consistent with the increasing concern over the rights of children in general, more attention is being paid to issues such as the minor's right of informed consent. Barnett and Johnson maintain that therapists should clearly discuss the limits of confidentiality with minors as part of the informed consent process, even in those cases when a parent or guardian consents to treatment.

Legal and ethical questions faced by human-service providers who work with children and adolescents include the following:

- To what degree should minors be allowed to participate in setting the goals of therapy and in providing consent to undergo it?
- What are the limits of confidentiality in counseling minors? Would you discuss these limits with minor clients even though a parent or guardian consents to treatment of the minor?
- What does informed consent consist of in working with minors?

We consider some of these questions next and focus on the rights of children when they are clients.

Parental Right to Information About a Minor's Treatment

Each state has specific statutes and regulations that offer guidance to clinicians working with children and adolescents, and practitioners should become familiar with the laws in their state pertaining to minors. In most states, for a minor to enter into a counseling relationship, it is necessary to have informed parental or guardian consent or for counseling to be court ordered, although there are exceptions to this general rule. Parents or guardians generally have the legal right to know the contents of counseling sessions with their children (Remley & Herlihy, 2016).

Informed consent of parents or guardians may not be legally required when a minor is seeking counseling for addictions to dangerous drugs or narcotics, for sexually transmitted diseases, for pregnancy and birth control, or for an examination following alleged sexual assault of a minor over 12 years of age (Lawrence & Kurpius, 2000). The justification for allowing children and adolescents to have access to treatment without parental consent is that some minors might not otherwise seek needed treatment. Some children and adolescents who seek help when given independent access might not do so without the guarantee of privacy. It is important that you check with your state regarding the current laws if you are a school counselor or school psychologist. Marriage and family therapists, clinical social workers, licensed clinical mental health counselors, and psychologists may operate under different laws. For example, a recent California law allows mental health practitioners to provide counseling services to a consenting minor age 12 or older if the practitioner determines the minor is mature enough to participate intelligently in the treatment (California Board of Behavioral Sciences, 2017).

School Counseling and Parental Consent

Counselors working with minors must know the laws in their state or jurisdiction and understand the policies of the settings in which they work. School counselors do not have a legal obligation to obtain parental consent for counseling unless a state statute requires this. Many schools have a student handbook, a part of which typically describes information about counseling services available to students. This handbook is often sent to parents at the beginning of a school year to provide them with school rules and policies, as well as general information about various services offered by the school. At the end of the handbook, there is typically a page that asks for parents' signatures indicating their consent for their children to use the services provided by the school. Such a procedure is a means of securing required consent. If parents do not want their children to receive any kind of counseling, this could be indicated at the end of the handbook on the signature page.

In the section on counseling, some handbooks give examples of individual and group counseling activities. For example, counseling sessions may focus on themes such as improving study habits, time management, making good choices, substance abuse prevention, anger management, career development, and other personal or social concerns. At times, specific approval may be required if children want to participate in special counseling (such as a children of divorce group). If parents have questions about any counseling activities, they are given the name of a person to contact at the school. Parents who object to their child's participation in counseling generally have a legal right to do so. If you are not required by law to get parental consent for treatment, but you decide to ask for their permission and they decline, you cannot counsel their children. Florida and some other states allow counselors to see children in crisis without parental consent for a period of time.

Seeing Minors Without Parental Consent

Counselors faced with the issue of when to counsel minors without parental consent must consider various factors. What is the competence level of the minor? What are the potential risks and consequences if treatment is denied? What are the chances that the minor will not seek help or will not be able to secure parental permission for needed help? How serious is the problem? What are the laws pertaining to providing therapy for minors without parental consent? If practitioners need to make decisions about accepting minors without parental consent, they should know the relevant statutes in their state. They would also be wise to consult with other professionals or with their professional organizations in assessing the ethical issues involved in each case.

California enacted a law in 2011 allowing mental health practitioners to treat minors (12 years or older) if the practitioner determines the minors are mature enough to participate intelligently in outpatient treatment or mental health counseling. However, the statute does require parental (or guardian) involvement in the treatment unless the therapist finds, after consulting with the minor, that this involvement would be inappropriate under the circumstances. Therapists have the responsibility for noting in the client's records whether they attempted to contact the minor's parent or guardian, whether this attempt was successful or unsuccessful, or why it was deemed inappropriate to make this contact. This law protects the right to seek treatment of certain populations of youth, such as young people from immigrant families, homeless youth, people who are gay, and young people from cultural backgrounds that do not condone receiving mental health services (Leslie, 2010).

Informed Consent Process With Minors

Minors are not always able to give informed consent. The APA (2010) code provides guidance on this matter:

> For persons who are legally incapable of giving informed consent, psychologists nevertheless (1) provide an appropriate explanation, (2) seek the individual's assent, (3) consider such persons' preferences and best interests, and (4) obtain appropriate permission from a legally authorized person, if such substitute consent is permitted or required by law. When consent by a legally authorized person is not permitted or required by law, psychologists take reasonable steps to protect the individual's rights and welfare. (3.10.b.)

The ACA (2014) *Code of Ethics* also addresses this topic:

> When counseling minors, incapacitated adults, or other persons unable to give voluntary consent, counselors seek the assent of clients to services, and include them in decision-making as appropriate. Counselors recognize the need to balance the ethical rights of clients to make choices, their capacity to give consent or assent to receive services, and parental or familial legal rights and responsibilities to protect these clients and make decisions on their behalf. (A.2.d.)

Therapists working with children and adolescents have the ethical responsibility of providing information that will help minor clients become active participants in their treatment. If children lack the background to weigh risks and benefits and if they cannot give complete informed consent, therapists should still attempt to explain the therapy process and general procedures of therapy to them. Even though minors usually cannot give informed consent for treatment, they can give their *assent* to counseling. Assent to treatment implies that counselors involve minors in decisions about their own care, and that to the greatest extent possible they agree to participate in the counseling process (Welfel, 2016).

There are both ethical and therapeutic reasons for involving minors in their treatment. By giving them the maximum degree of autonomy within the therapeutic relationship, the therapist demonstrates respect for them. Also, it is likely that therapeutic change is promoted by informing minors about the process and enlisting their involvement in it. In general, the older and more mature a child is, the more he or she can be included in the process of ongoing informed consent. Factors to consider are what the child can and cannot understand, as well as the degree to which the child is able to understand, participate in, and benefit from informed consent.

Involving Parents in the Counseling Process With Minors

To work effectively with a minor it is often necessary to involve the parents or guardians in the treatment process. To the extent that it is possible, it is a good practice for counselors to involve the parents or guardians in the initial meeting with their child to arrive at a clear, mutual agreement regarding the nature and extent of information that will be provided to them. This also gives the therapist an opportunity to see how the child behaves in the presence of the parents and also how the parents react to their child. This policy makes it possible to create clear boundaries for sharing information and establishes a three-way bond of trust (Lawrence & Kurpius, 2000). The American Psychiatric Association (2013b) offers this guideline:

> Careful judgment must be exercised by the psychiatrist in order to include, when appropriate, the parents or guardian in the treatment of a minor. At the same time, the psychiatrist must assure the minor proper confidentiality." (4.7.)

The *Ethical Standards for School Counselors* (ASCA, 2016) addresses the matter of the school counselor's responsibilities to parents:

> School counselors recognize that providing services to minors in a school setting requires school counselors to collaborate with students' parents/guardians as appropriate. (B.1.a.)

Ethical and Legal Challenges Pertaining to Confidentiality With Minors

Mental health professionals must take special care to protect the rights of minors, but clinicians often experience difficulty when applying ethics codes guidelines in their work with children and adolescents. A study of Australian psychologists found a high level of variation in their opinions regarding when to breach confidentiality to inform parents in cases involving adolescents engaging in risky behaviors (Duncan, Williams, & Knowles, 2013). According to Benitez (2004), counselors who work with minors are frequently challenged to balance the minor's need for confidentiality and the parents' requests for information about the minor's counseling. Benitez claims that it is a wise policy for practitioners to make it clear to parents of minors that effective counseling requires a sense of trust in the therapist. Information that will or will not be disclosed to parents or guardians must be discussed at the outset of therapy with both the child or adolescent and the parent or guardian. If the matter of confidentiality is not clearly explored with all parties involved, problems can be expected to emerge in the course of therapy.

Therapists cannot guarantee blanket confidentiality to minors. If the parents or guardians of minors request information about the progress of the counseling, the therapist may be expected to provide some feedback. Remley and Herlihy (2016) contend that counselors have legal duties to parents or guardians of minors and that in some circumstances counselors will determine that parents or guardians must be given information that a minor client has disclosed in a counseling session. For example, if a counselor makes the judgment that a minor client is at risk of harm (to self or others), the counselor usually is required to inform the minor's parents or guardians. However, if the minor client has threatened harm against a third party, merely notifying the client's parents or guardians may not be sufficient to insulate the counselor from liability. There also may be a duty to notify the potential victim, the potential victim's parents or guardians, or the police, depending on state law (Nancy Wheeler, personal communication, June 28, 2016). If a counselor had relevant information and did not take appropriate action to prevent a minor client from injuring him- or herself, or if the minor client harmed another person, the counselor may be held legally accountable.

Minors who engage in self-injurious behaviors raise complex issues regarding the limits of confidentiality. Wester (2009) points out that there is little in the ethics codes of the ACA or the APA to assist counselors in determining when to breach confidentiality for minors who engage in self-injurious behavior. It is crucial to set limitations to confidentiality specifically related to self-injurious behavior at the outset of a professional relationship. Wester adds that counselors should seek supervision and consultation when necessary so that they are working within the boundaries of their competence.

Because of the high correlation between self-injury and suicide (Whitlock et al., 2013), counselors need to understand the distinction between self-injury and suicidal behavior. Furthermore, counselors need to have the expertise to identify self-injury when it is presented in counseling by a client. Assessment instruments can be used to screen for self-injury and suicide and to address the functions self-injury serves for clients. A number of researchers have devoted time and attention to this complex topic in recent years (Evans & Hurrell, 2016; Hawton et al., 2016; Kress, Newgent, Whitlock, & Mease, 2015; Lewis, Heath, Michal, & Duggan, 2012; Nock, 2014; Plener, Schumacher, Munz, & Groschwitz, 2015; Victor, Styer, & Washburn, 2015; Walsh & Muehlenkamp, 2013; Wester, Ivers, Villalba, Trepal, & Henson, 2016; Whitlock, Prussien, & Pietrusza, 2015), but additional research is needed to fully understand this phenomenon. We encourage mental health practitioners and school counselors to remain abreast of the literature on self-injury and suicidal behavior.

Although minor clients have an *ethical* right to privacy and confidentiality in the counseling relationship, the law still favors the rights of parents over their children. However, some sensitive information, if revealed or disclosed, may be detrimental to the therapy process. Disclosure of a minor's personal information can result in the child no longer trusting the therapist due to fears that this personal information will be disclosed to parents. This should be explained to parents or guardians during the informed consent process.

Parents and guardians usually have a *legal* right to information pertaining to counseling sessions with their children, although a court may hold otherwise due to specific state statutes (Remley & Herlihy, 2016). When parents or legal guardians become involved in the counseling process, counselors must acknowledge that these adults have authority over minors. Marion's case is an example of the challenges a counselor must address in determining how to handle personal information to parents.

The Case of Marion

Marion is a 15-year-old honors student. She discovered that she is pregnant and feels she would be better off dead than being a teenage mom. Marion was born to teenage parents, so she knows they will never allow her to have an abortion. Marion went to see the school counselor to talk about her situation. The counselor educated Marion on the different options she had with regard to her pregnancy. Marion stated that she wanted to abort her pregnancy. If her parents would not allow her to have an abortion, Marion said she would kill herself. The school counselor persuaded Marion to agree to see a family therapist with her parents, and during the family session Marion's father stated he would not hear of Marion's having an abortion. Marion then stated with conviction that she would kill herself. The family therapist has reason to believe that Marion will act on her threat of suicide.

- If your state had a law requiring parental consent for abortion, how would this influence the interventions you would make in this case?
- Might you encounter a conflict between ethics and the law if you were counseling Marion? How would you deal with her suicidal threat?
- Knowing what Marion told you about her parents' values, would you have involved them in this case? Why or why not?
- Would you use Marion's threat of suicide to influence her parents, or would you ignore this threat? Explain.
- What other options would you consider?

Commentary. The family therapist can act on the suicidal threat, which could result in a 72-hour hospitalization. This takes care of the therapist's legal responsibility, yet this does not solve the problem of Marion's suicidal threats. This case reminds us of the importance of knowing about available resources when there is a suicidal threat, and the need for consultation and documentation. After Marion is released, the therapist will need to continue working with the family.

Marion's case illustrates the importance of ensuring one's own competence to counsel various types of clients. In this case, the counselor must be competent to work with minors and their families in crisis. ●

At this point we suggest that you think about these legal and ethical considerations in providing counseling for minors:

- Many parents argue that they have a right to know about matters that pertain to their adolescent daughters and sons. They assert, for example, that parents have a right to be involved in decisions about abortion. What is your position?
- If the state in which you practice has a law requiring parental consent for abortion, how would this influence your interventions with minors who were considering an abortion?
- Some people argue for the right of minors to seek therapy without parental knowledge or consent because needed treatment might not be given to them otherwise. When, if at all, would you counsel a minor without parental knowledge and consent?

- What kinds of information should be provided to children and adolescents before they enter a therapeutic relationship?
- If therapists do not provide minors with the information necessary to make informed choices, are they acting unethically? Why or why not?

Counseling Reluctant Children and Adolescents

Some young people resent not having a choice about entering a therapeutic relationship. Adolescents often resist therapy because they become the "identified patient" and the focus is on changing them. These adolescents are frequently aware that they are only *part* of the problem in the family unit. Although many minors indicate a desire to participate in treatment decisions, few are given the opportunity to become involved in a systematic way. Unwillingness to participate in therapy can be minimized if therapists take time to explore the reasons for adolescents' unwillingness.

The Case of Kody

Kody was expelled from high school for getting explosively angry at a teacher who, according to Kody, had humiliated him in front of his class. Kody was told that he would not be readmitted to school unless he sought professional help. His mother called a therapist and explained the situation to her, and the therapist agreed to see him. Although Kody was uncomfortable and embarrassed over having to see a therapist, he was nevertheless willing to talk. He told the therapist that he knew he had done wrong by lashing out angrily at the teacher but that the teacher had provoked him. He said that although he was usually good about keeping his feelings inside, this time he had "just lost it."

After a few sessions, the therapist determined that there were many problems in Kody's family. He lived with an extreme amount of stress, and to work effectively with Kody it would be essential to see the entire family. Indeed, he did have a problem, but he was not the problem. He was covering up many family secrets, including a verbally abusive stepfather and an alcoholic mother. Hesitantly, he agreed that it would be a good idea to have the entire family come in for therapy. When the therapist contacted the parents, they totally rejected the idea of family therapy. The mother asserted that the problem was with Kody and that the therapist should concentrate her efforts on him. A few days before his next scheduled appointment his mother called to cancel, saying that they had placed Kody in homebound study and that he therefore no longer required counseling.

- What are the ethical responsibilities of the therapist in this situation?
- Should Kody be seen as a condition of returning to school?
- What other strategies might the therapist have used?
- What would you do differently, and why?
- Should the therapist have seen Kody and the teacher?
- Should the therapist have encouraged Kody to continue his therapy even if his family refused to undergo treatment?
- Would it be ethical for the therapist to refuse to continue with Kody once the family refused to join the therapy sessions?

Commentary. One ethical problem in this case was the treatment of the individual as opposed to the treatment of the family. This case highlights the importance of providing thorough informed consent. If a therapist routinely transitions from individual to marital or family therapy, clients need to understand the circumstances that might prompt the therapist to recommend this role shift.

In this case, there was an alcoholic parent in the family. Kody's expulsion from school could have been more a symptom of the family dysfunction than of his own disturbance. Indeed, he did need to learn anger management, as both the school and the mother contended, yet more was going on within this family that needed attention. In this case it might have been best for the therapist to stick to her initial convictions of family therapy as the treatment of choice. If the parents would not agree to this, she could have made a referral to another therapist who would be willing to see Kody in individual counseling. In many states the therapist would be required to make a child abuse report to Child Protective Services because of the alleged verbal and emotional abuse. •

Specialized Training for Counseling Children and Adolescents

The ethics codes of the major professional organizations specify that it is unethical to practice in areas for which one has not been trained. It is important not to begin counseling with minors without requisite coursework and supervision by a specialist in this area. Many human-service professionals have been trained and supervised in "verbal therapies," but there are distinct limitations in applying these therapeutic interventions to children. Practitioners who want to counsel children may have to acquire supervised clinical experience in play therapy, art and music therapy, and recreational therapy. These practitioners also must understand the developmental issues pertaining to the population with which they intend to work. They need to become familiar with laws relating to minors, to be aware of the limits of their competence, and to know when and how to make appropriate referrals. It is essential to know about community referral resources, such as Child Protective Services.

LO7

Dealing With Suspected Unethical Behavior of Colleagues

Throughout this book our focus has been on your own professional behavior and the importance of practicing in an ethical manner. In this section we take up the difficult question of what to do should you become aware of unethical behavior on the part of a colleague. You may wonder whether it is your place to judge the practices of other practitioners. Even if you are convinced that the situation involves clear ethical violations, you may be in doubt about the best way to deal with it. Should you first discuss the matter with the person? Assuming that you do and that the person becomes defensive, what other actions should you consider? When would a violation be serious enough that you would feel obligated to bring it to the attention of an appropriate local, state, or national committee on professional ethics?

Although the ethics codes of most professional organizations clearly place the responsibility for addressing problems of competence or unethical behavior of colleagues on the members of their profession, Johnson and colleagues (2012) state that mental health professionals are reluctant to address such problems. Professionals admit they might not directly approach a colleague they believe is functioning below thresholds for competence or behaving unethically, even though they have an ethical duty to address the situation. Ignoring evidence of peer misconduct is an ethical violation in itself (see the Ethics Code box titled "Unethical Behavior of Colleagues").

Professionals have an obligation to deal with colleagues when they suspect unethical conduct. Koocher and Keith-Spiegel (2016) recommend informal peer monitoring as one way to assume responsibility for watching out for each other. Informal peer monitoring provides an opportunity for corrective interventions to ethically questionable acts. Actions can be taken directly by confronting a colleague, or indirectly by advising clients how to proceed when they have concerns about another professional's actions. If unethical behavior by a colleague cannot be satisfactorily resolved informally, you have an ethical obligation to file a formal complaint.

Generally, the best way to proceed when you have concerns about the behavior of a colleague is to deal directly with the colleague, unless doing so would compromise a client's confidentiality. In cases of egregious offenses, such as sexual exploitation of clients or general incompetence, informal measures are not enough. Depending on the nature of the complaint and the outcome of the discussion, reporting a colleague to a professional board is one of several options open to you.

The Case of Melanee

Melanee's lunch at the university's cafeteria was interrupted when she became distracted by a conversation in the booth directly behind her. A male—his voice only vaguely familiar at first—was regaling a female lunch companion with a story about someone's extreme social anxiety and fear of women. As Melanee looked around the cafeteria, she noticed a few other patrons glancing at the therapist who was talking loudly, undoubtedly overhearing the discussion just as she was. As Melanee listened, it became clear the man was referring to a mental health client. The man recounted specific experiences his client had shared and some of the exposure therapy assignments the man had given his client earlier that day. Melanee realized the client information and some of the specific stories were familiar to her because she had heard some of this material earlier in the week during group supervision. The voice belonged to Lonny, one of her fellow counseling interns at the university's student counseling center.

Upset over Lonny's poor judgment, concerned at the prospect that the client or one of his friends might be overhearing Lonny's conversation, yet equally determined not to overreact, Melanee did her best to collect her thoughts. Melanee decided to tell Lonny what she had overheard and asked him if he understood how his behavior may have compromised his client's confidentiality. Rather than accusing or threatening, Melanee's tone and demeanor were concerned and caring, but nonetheless firm.

Sensing that Melanee had both his own and his client's best interests at heart, Lonny was quick to admit his blunder and instantly embarrassed and remorseful. He admitted having "completely blown it" and thanked Melanee for her candor. Several times during the remainder of the internship year, Lonny thanked Melanee again and described the experience as a turning point in his understanding of his obligations to clients—both in and outside of the counseling session.

- What are your thoughts about how Melanee dealt with this situation?
- Should Melanee have gone straight to the program dean and reported Lonny's behavior?
- Should Melanee file an ethics complaint with the university or the state counseling board?
- If you were in Melanee's place, what do you imagine you would have done?
- What would you think of Melanee if she had decided she had no right to confront Lonny with his behavior?

Commentary. Ethical guidelines and standards in the mental health professions require professionals to remain both aware of and responsive to the functioning of colleagues. Whenever possible, make your best effort to informally communicate any concerns about a colleague's diminished competence or unethical behavior directly to that colleague. Do your best to be respectful and nonthreatening, but clearly state both your concerns and the ethical requirement at issue. Melanee effectively confronted Lonny and helped him to understand how he had gotten off track and why it was a serious concern. She refrained from putting Lonny on the defensive or needlessly escalating the matter. •

Johnson and his colleagues (2012) suggest that the current APA *Ethics Code* (APA, 2010) lacks care and compassion as general guiding principles. They believe a clearer focus on care and compassion for both individual psychologists and for members of the professional community is required. They contend that a humanistic concern for others is a foundational component of professionalism and, thus, concern for colleagues warrants increased attention in the ethics code.

Malpractice Liability in the Helping Professions

How vulnerable are mental health professionals to malpractice actions? What are some practical safeguards against being involved in a lawsuit? In this section we examine these questions and encourage you to develop a prudent approach to risk management in your practice.

What Is Malpractice?

The word **malpractice** means "bad practice." Malpractice is the failure to render professional services or to exercise the degree of skill that is ordinarily expected of other professionals in a similar situation. Malpractice is a legal concept involving alleged negligence that results in injury or loss to the client. **Professional negligence** can result from unjustified departure from usual practice or from failing to exercise proper care in fulfilling one's responsibilities.

Practitioners are expected to abide by legal standards and adhere to the ethics code of their profession in providing care to their clients. Unless practitioners take due care and act in good faith, they may be liable in a civil lawsuit for failing to do their duty as provided by law. A malpractice lawsuit alleges negligence in meeting one's professional responsibilities or duties. The plaintiff may claim that a practitioner's actions (or lack of actions) deviated from the acceptable standard of care and directly caused harm to the client (Knapp & VandeCreek, 2012). The primary focus of a negligence suit lies in determining what **standard of care** to apply in deciding whether a breach of duty to a client has taken place. Clinicians are judged according to the standards that are commonly accepted by the profession; that is, whether a reasonably prudent counselor in a similar circumstance would have acted in the same manner (Wheeler & Bertram, 2015).

Remley and Herlihy (2016) remind us: "Although malpractice lawsuits against mental health professionals have increased dramatically over the past decade, the total number of these lawsuits is relatively small" (p. 189). However, students taking an ethics class seem particularly anxious about making mistakes and becoming involved in a malpractice suit. Practitioners are not infallible, but they are expected to possess and exercise the knowledge, skill, and judgment common to other members of their profession. It is a good policy for practitioners to maintain a reasonable view of the realities involved in dealing with high-risk clients. No matter how ethical and careful you try to be, you can still be accused of malpractice. However, the more careful and ethical you try to be, the less likely you are to be successfully sued. The best defense against becoming embroiled in a malpractice suit or having a complaint filed with the licensing board is to practice quality client care and establish and maintain effective relationships with your clients. Younggren, Harris, and Martin (2016) recommend that clinicians "develop and nurture relationships with clients. Not only is this good psychotherapy, but it is also good risk management" (pp. 405–406).

To succeed in a malpractice claim, these four elements of malpractice must be present: (1) a professional relationship between the therapist and the client must have existed; (2) the legal duty based on this relationship must have been breached: the therapist must have acted in a negligent or improper manner, or have deviated from the "standard of care" by not providing services that are considered "standard practice in the community"; (3) the client must have suffered harm or injury, such as emotional distress or physical harm, which must be verified; and (4) there must be a legally demonstrated causal relationship between the practitioner's negligence or breach of duty and the damage or injury claimed by the client.

It should be noted that anyone, at any time, can file a suit against you. Even if the suit does not succeed, it can take a toll on you in terms of time, money, and emotional stress. You may have to spend many hours preparing and supplying documents and responding to requests for information. However, the burden of proof that harm actually took place is the client's, and the plaintiff must demonstrate that all four elements applied in his or her situation.

In the case of suicide, for example, two factors determine a practitioner's liability: foreseeability and reasonable care. Most important is *foreseeability*, which involves assessing the level of risk. Failing to conduct a comprehensive risk assessment and to document this assessment would be a major error on the therapist's part. If you are not competent to make such an assessment, then a referral is mandatory so that an assessment can be made. Practitioners need to demonstrate that their judgments were based on data observed and that these judgments were reasonable. The second factor in liability is whether *reasonable care* was provided. Once an assessment of risk is made, it is important to document that appropriate precautions were taken to prevent a client's suicide.

Reasons for Malpractice Suits

Malpractice is typically found in the following kinds of situations: (1) the procedure used by the practitioner was not within the realm of accepted professional practice; (2) the practitioner employed a technique that he or she was not trained to use; (3) the professional did not follow standard counseling procedures, which resulted in harm to the client; (4) the therapist failed to warn others about and protect them from a violent client; (5) informed consent to treatment was not obtained or not documented; or (6) the professional did not explain the possible consequences of the treatment (Wheeler & Bertram, 2015). In the social work field, malpractice typically results from a practitioner's active violation of a client's rights (Reamer, 2015).

Many areas of a therapist's practice could lead to a legal claim, but we focus on the types of professional negligence that most often put therapists at legal risk. Wheeler and Bertram (2015, p. 69) report that common complaints lodged against counselors and other mental health providers by the state licensure board involve sexual/romantic interaction with current clients, client's partners, or client's family members; failure to practice within the boundaries of competence; improper sharing of confidential material without client consent or legal justification; failing to make fees and charges clear to clients; misrepresenting credentials; altering records; using false advertising; and practicing while impaired.

Knapp and VandeCreek (2012) report that no standardized set of data exists of the most common ethical infractions of psychologists. However, a general analysis of common sources of complaints lodged against psychologists are in these areas: multiple relationships (both sexual and nonsexual); incompetence in diagnosis and treatment; disputes arising out of child custody evaluations; premature termination; and fee disputes. Other complaints include inadequate supervision; inadequate record keeping; impairment; and breach of confidentiality. Professional journals reveal an increase in citations for the abuse of alcohol and drugs because of its impairment possibility.

In a survey of ethical questions of both psychologists and clients, Wierzbicki, Siderits, and Kuchan (2012) noted that the Wisconsin Psychological Association has a mechanism for assisting psychologists and their clients who have questions about ethical psychological practice. Questions most often raised by psychologists about their own practice involved matters such as self-disclosure, multiple relationships, and maintaining confidentiality. Questions raised by their clients concerned sexual intimacies, maintaining confidentiality, and reporting ethical violations. Among concerns most frequently raised by clients were fees, financial arrangements, and the termination process. Wierzbicki and colleagues recommend consulting regularly with colleagues through meetings in a peer consultation group. They also suggest asking for regular feedback from clients about the degree to which they are satisfied with the psychological services rendered to them.

The following discussion of these risk categories is an adaptation of malpractice liability and lawsuit prevention strategies suggested by various writers (Bennett et al., 2006; Calfee, 1997; Kennedy, Vandehey, Norman, & Diekhoff, 2003; Kirkland, Kirkland, & Reaves, 2004; Knapp & VandeCreek, 2012; VandeCreek & Knapp, 2001; Wheeler & Bertram, 2015; Younggren et al., 2016).

Failure to Obtain or Document Informed Consent Therapists need to recognize that they can be liable for failure to obtain appropriate informed consent even if their subsequent treatment of the client is excellent from a clinical perspective. Although written informed consent may not be needed legally, it is wise to have clients sign a form to acknowledge their agreement with the terms of the proposed therapy. Without a written document, it may be very difficult to ascertain whether counselors communicated clearly and effectively to clients about the therapeutic process and whether clients understood the information.

Refusal to Counsel Clients Due to Value Differences As the *Bruff* case demonstrates (see Chapter 4), therapists who refuse to work with clients due to value conflicts may be liable for legal action and malpractice suits. The codes of ethics of most professional organizations state that clinicians may not discriminate against specific categories of people. If a counselor refuses to work with a client because of value conflicts, or if the counselor attempts to impose his or her values on a client, the client may have legal and ethical grounds to file a complaint.

Client Abandonment and Premature Termination Younggren and Gottlieb (2008) define **termination** as "the ethically and clinically appropriate process by which a professional relationship is ended" (p. 500). They define **abandonment** as "the failure of the psychologist to take the clinically indicated and ethically appropriate steps to terminate a professional relationship" (p. 500). A central concern associated with termination is avoiding abandonment of a client. Clinical records should give evidence that they were not terminated inappropriately. It is useful to document the nature of a client's termination, including who initiated the termination, how this was handled, the degree to which initial goals were met, and referrals provided when appropriate.

The codes of ethics of professional organizations state that mental health practitioners do not abandon clients. When a psychologist unilaterally terminates a professional relationship with a client, even after careful reflection, the client may experience this as abandonment (Wierzbicki et al., 2012). Ideally, termination of therapy is a collaborative effort involving both client and therapist. Clients need to be informed about termination and, as much as possible, should be involved in making decisions about when to end their treatment. When both client and therapist agree that the goals of therapy have been achieved and that therapy is no longer required, there is a very low risk that the client will file a malpractice complaint. Under managed care programs, termination typically is not the result of a collaborative process but of company policy. Under managed care plans, therapists may be accused of abandonment when they terminate a client based on the allocated number of sessions rather than on the therapeutic needs of the client. It is the responsibility of therapists to inform clients that the request for additional sessions may or may not be granted by their managed care provider and to work with clients to explore alternatives.

Practitioners who work on a fee-for-service basis can usually terminate treatment when they are not receiving payment for their services because the original remuneration contract is not being honored. Therapists have no *legal* duty to provide free psychological services and can stop treatment when the client stops paying for the services (Younggren et al., 2011). How termination is handled is critical, and at the very least the client should be given referral options. Premature termination from therapy is a significant problem and has negative effects on clients who do not complete treatment as well as on providers and the agencies that work with them. Approximately 20% of all clients drop out of therapy prematurely, with higher rates among some types of clients and in some settings (Swift, Greenberg, Whipple, & Kominiak, 2012).

Courts have determined that the following acts may constitute abandonment: failure to follow up on the outcomes with a client who has been hospitalized; consistently not being able to be reached between appointments; failure to respond to a request for emergency treatment; or failure to provide for a substitute therapist during vacation times. Terminating a client who clearly needs continuing care may be sufficient grounds for a malpractice suit (Knapp & VandeCreek, 2012). Clients have a case for abandonment when the facts indicate that a therapist unilaterally terminated a professional relationship and that this termination resulted in some form of harm. However, as Younggren (Younggren et al., 2011) notes, there are legitimate grounds for terminating a professional relationship, such as when no progress is taking place in the therapy or when clients are not cooperating with the treatment. In these situations, termination is likely to be the appropriate course of action and to do otherwise could put the practitioner at risk.

Sexual Misconduct With a Client Related to the topic of unhealthy transference relationships is the area of sexual boundary violations, one of the most common grounds for malpractice suits. It is *never* appropriate for therapists to engage in sexual contact with clients. (This topic is explored in detail in Chapter 7.) Court cases suggest that no act is more likely to create legal problems for therapists than engaging in a sexual relationship with a client. Furthermore, initial consent of the client will not be a defense against malpractice actions. Even in the case of sex between a therapist and a former client, courts do not easily accept the view that therapy has ended.

Marked Departures From Established Therapeutic Practices If counselors employ unusual therapy procedures, they put themselves at risk. They bear the burden of demonstrating a rationale for their techniques. If it can be shown that their procedures are beyond the usual methods employed by most professionals, they are vulnerable to a malpractice action. Appropriate use of evidence-based practices are a general safeguard against claims of departure from the standard of care.

Practicing Beyond the Scope of Competency Mental health practitioners have been held liable for damages for providing treatment below a standard of care. If the client follows the treatment suggested by a professional and suffers damages as a result, the client can initiate a civil action. Professional health care providers should work only with those clients and deliver only those services that are within the realm of their competence. Accepting a case beyond the scope of a counselor's education and training is not only a breach of ethics but also can result in a malpractice suit.

Mental health professionals have an obligation to work closely with physicians to ensure that a medical condition or side effects from a medication are not causing the psychological symptoms. A client may need to be referred to a physician for a medication evaluation in some instances, and collaboration as well as a referral may become necessary.

If counselors have any doubts about their level of competency to work with certain cases, they should receive peer input or consultation. If a counselor is accused of unethical practice, the counselor must prove that he or she was properly prepared in that area of practice (Chauvin & Remley, 1996). Clinicians can refine their skills by participating in continuing education, taking graduate coursework, or seeking direct supervision from a colleague who has relevant clinical experience.

Negligent Assessment and Misdiagnosis Negligent assessment can be the basis for complaints to a state licensing board, an ethics committee, and for malpractice action. Areas of high risk involve assessment in child custody cases and in employment evaluations (Knapp & VandeCreek, 2012). Lacking the ability to demonstrate diagnostic competence can result in making a misdiagnosis or missed diagnosis, which could leave the practitioner vulnerable to an allegation of malpractice (Wheeler & Bertram, 2015). It is generally not the court's role to question the therapist's diagnosis. However, in cases where it can be shown through the therapist's records that a diagnosis was clearly unfounded and below the standard of care, a case of malpractice might be successful. In court, an expert witness is often questioned to determine whether the therapist used appropriate assessment procedures and arrived at an appropriate diagnosis. It is wise for mental health practitioners to require a prospective client to undergo a complete physical examination, as the results of this examination might have a bearing on the client's diagnosis and affect his or her treatment (Calfee, 1997).

Repressed or False Memory A memory is considered false if it is arrived at through an untested intervention by the therapist rather than being the client's actual memory. Therapists have been sued and found guilty of such induced memories. A jury in Minnesota awarded more than $2.6 million to a woman who claimed she was injured by false memories of abuse induced after her psychiatrist suggested that she suffered from a multiple personality disorder, which most likely was the result of repeated sexual abuse by relatives (Wheeler & Bertram, 2015). Certainly, the style in which a therapist questions a client can influence memories, particularly for young children. Repeated questioning can lead a person to believe in a "memory" of an event that did not occur. A trusted therapist who suggests past abuse as a possible cause of problems or symptoms can greatly influence the client.

What is the best course for you to follow when you suspect that past sexual abuse is related to a client's present problem? How can you best protect the client, the alleged abuser, and other family members, without becoming needlessly vulnerable to a malpractice suit? Wheeler and Bertram (2015) recommend following these basic clinical and ethical principles:

- Be attentive to the kinds of questions you ask clients.
- Remain nonjudgmental and demonstrate empathy as you talk to a client about possible memories of abuse.
- Avoid prejudging the truth of the client's reports.
- If a client reports a memory, explore it with the person.
- Make use of established assessment and treatment techniques.
- Avoid pressuring the client to believe events that may not have actually occurred.
- Do not minimize a client's reported memories.
- Do not suggest to clients that they terminate the relationship precipitously.
- If you are not specifically trained in child abuse assessment and treatment, consult with a supervisor or a professional with expertise in this area, or refer the client for a clinical assessment. (p. 81)

Wheeler and Bertram (2015) suggest carefully documenting in the client's clinical record the allegations, the circumstances under which the memory was revealed, the techniques used to assess the veracity of the memory, and the treatment options considered, including consultation or referral to other professional colleagues.

Unhealthy Transference Relationships The importance of understanding how transference and countertransference play out in the therapy relationship is considered in Chapter 2. The mere existence of countertransference feelings is not an ethical or legal issue. However, if a therapist's personal reactions to a client cannot be managed effectively, an abuse of power is likely, and this can have both ethical and legal consequences. In cases involving mishandling of a client's transference or a counselor's countertransference, allegations have included sexual involvement with clients, inappropriate socialization with clients, getting involved with clients in a business situation, and burdening clients with a counselor's personal problems. When a therapist gets involved in multiple relationships with a client, it is always the client who is most vulnerable to abuse because of the power differential.

It is a good practice for the counselor who is considering a referral to explore this matter in supervision or in consultation with a colleague before deciding whether making the referral is warranted and in the best interest of the client. In our work with counselors in training, we teach them that the client who most triggers them can be a valuable teacher. Although we do not want the counselor's development to be at the expense of the client, it is important to push ourselves to work with clients who may make us personally uncomfortable.

Failure to Assess and Manage a Dangerous Client Therapists may have a duty to intervene when clients pose a grave danger to themselves or to others. However, it is difficult to determine when a given client actually poses a danger to self or others. We discuss this topic in greater detail in Chapter 6.

A number of states have duty-to-warn or duty-to-protect statutes that instruct practitioners regarding what they must do, must not do, or may do in treating clients who pose a potential threat to others (Knapp & VandeCreek, 2012). These statutes are intended to protect mental health professionals who breach confidentiality to report danger to others as well as to protect the public. Reporting dangerousness is required by California statute, and there is no privilege in cases involving dangerous patients (Leslie, 2010). Even in states where such a warning is not legally mandated, ethical practice demands a proper course of action on the therapist's part.

Risk Management Strategies

Risk management is the practice of focusing on the identification, evaluation, and treatment of problems that may injure clients and lead to filing an ethics complaint to a licensing board or a malpractice action. One of the best precautions against malpractice is personal and professional honesty and openness with clients. Providing quality professional services to clients is the best preventive step you can take. Although you may not make the "right choice" in every situation, it is crucial that you know your limitations and remain open to seeking consultation in difficult cases. Misunderstandings between therapist and client can result in a stronger therapist–client working relationship if the client and the therapist talk through the misunderstanding. Minor errors can become significant, however, and can lead to malpractice actions when they are repeated and are not recognized by the therapist. It is critical that clinicians remain alert for possible misunderstandings that, if not recognized or poorly handled, could lead to a therapeutic rupture or premature termination of therapy.

Some recommendations for improving risk management include the following:

- Become aware of local and state laws that pertain to your practice, as well as the policies of any agency for whom you work. Stay current with legal and ethical changes by becoming actively involved in professional organizations and attending risk management workshops.
- Make use of treatment contracts that present clients with written information on confidentiality issues, reasons for contacting clients at home, fee structures and payment plans, a policy on termination, and suicide provisions (Kennedy et al., 2003). Review this information with the client and document informed consent with a signature. Recognize that the disclosure statement establishes a contract between you and your client (Chauvin & Remley, 1996).
- Present information to your clients in clear language and be sure they understand the information.

- Contemporaneously engage in assessment and document your decisions (Werth, Welfel, Benjamin, & Sales, 2009).
- Explain your diagnosis, the treatment plan, and its risks and benefits in sufficient detail to be sure the client understands it, and document this as well. Documentation is one of the cornerstones of good risk management, and also of quality care (Werth et al., 2009). Carefully document your clients' treatment process.
- Inform clients that they have the right to terminate treatment any time they choose. Exceptions may include clients who are court-ordered for treatment. Although mandated clients may terminate early, they will face consequences. The reasons for a client's termination should be documented.
- Restrict your practice to clients for whom you are qualified by virtue of your education, training, and experience. Refer clients whose conditions are obviously not within the scope of your competence.
- Document not only what you do and why, but what you decided not to do in certain cases (Werth et al., 2009).
- Maintain good financial and clinical records, and recognize your ethical, professional, and legal responsibility to preserve the confidentiality of client records.
- Be aware that not enough information in a client's record may be problematic when your professional conduct is being evaluated (Younggren et al., 2016).
- Develop clear and consistent policies and procedures for creating, maintaining, transferring, and destroying client records (Remley & Herlihy, 2016).
- Report any case of suspected child abuse, elder, or dependent abuse as required by law.
- Evaluate how well you keep boundaries in your personal life. If you have clarity and responsibility in your personal life, then you are more likely to have the same in your professional life.
- Before engaging in any multiple relationship, seek consultation and talk with your client about the possible repercussions of such a relationship. Realize that such relationships can lead to problems for both you and your client.
- Be thorough about informed consent, documentation, and consultation when crossing boundaries or engaging in multiple relationships with high-risk clients.
- In deciding whether or not to accept a gift or to engage in bartering, consider the relevant cultural and clinical issues.
- Do not engage in sexual relationships with current or former clients or with current supervisees or students.
- Not keeping your appointments may feel like abandonment to a client. If you have to miss a session, be sure to call the client. Provide coverage for emergencies when you are not available.
- When in doubt, consult with colleagues and document the discussions. Before consulting with others about a specific client, obtain consent from the client for the release of information. Consultation shows that you have a commitment to sound practice and that you are willing to learn from other professionals to further the best interests of your clients.
- Develop a network of consultants who can assist you with considering options without necessarily telling you what to do (Werth et al., 2009).

- Get training in the assessment of clients who pose a danger to themselves or others, or have an experienced and competent therapist to whom you can refer.
- If you are working with a suicidal client, consult and document the nature of the consultation.
- If you make a professional determination that a client is dangerous, take the necessary steps to protect the client or others from harm.
- Recognize that a mental health professional is a potential target for a client's anger or transference feelings. Be attentive to how you react to your clients and monitor your countertransference.
- Treat your clients with respect by attending carefully to your language and your behavior.
- Foster the therapeutic alliance and assess and discuss treatment progress and satisfaction throughout the course of therapy (Swift et al., 2012).
- The best protection against malpractice liability is to be concerned first and foremost with providing quality care and secondly to strive for ways to reduce risk (Werth et al., 2009).
- Have a theoretical orientation that justifies the techniques you employ.
- Support your practice, whenever possible, with evidence-based procedures.

This list of risk management strategies may appear overwhelming. It contains many of the points that have been discussed in this chapter or that will be addressed in other chapters. Our intention is to remind you of appropriate actions and also to provide a checklist to expand your awareness of ethical and professional behavior. Most ethical practitioners are already taking these steps. Increased use of the legal system may lead to excessive caution on the part of therapists because of their concern about being sued. The best way to reduce the chance of being sued is to know the ethical and legal standards and to follow them.

Laws often take center stage when what is most needed is a language for placing laws into an ethical context (Fisher, 2008). Fisher points out that taking a risk management perspective can raise practitioners' anxiety, which may lead them to focus on avoiding risks to *themselves* rather than considering their ethical obligations and the potential risks to *clients*. Zur (2010) contends that current risk management policies pose several serious risks to clinical effectiveness. Risk management policies can erode the foundation of healing, damage the therapeutic alliance, and inhibit creativity. When following risk management advice, Zur believes therapists may be attempting to protect themselves at the expense of their clients. He maintains that the recent wave of risk management practices has propelled the profession in the direction of fear-based interventions that often compromise clinical integrity.

Course of Action in a Malpractice Suit

LO11

Even though you practice prudently and follow the guidelines previously outlined, you still may be sued. Malpractice claims are not reserved exclusively for the irresponsible practitioner. Clients may make allegations of unethical conduct or file a legal claim due to negligence, even though the counselor may have acted ethically and appropriately. In the event that you are sued, consider these recommendations by Bennett and his associates (1990):

- Treat the lawsuit seriously, even if it represents a client's attempt to punish or control you.
- Do not attempt to resolve the matter with the client directly because anything you do might be used against you in the litigation.
- Contact the ethics and risk management services of your professional associations, if applicable. If you consult with an attorney, prepare summaries of any pertinent events about the case that you can use.
- Become familiar with your liability policy, including the limits of coverage, and contact your insurance company immediately.
- Never destroy or alter files or reports pertinent to the client's case.
- Do not discuss the case with anyone other than your attorney. Avoid making self-incriminating statements to the client, to his or her attorney, or to the press.
- Determine the nature of support available to you from professional associations to which you belong.
- Do not continue a professional relationship with a client who is bringing a suit against you.

Legal assistance is a must if the licensing board has opened an investigation. This usually occurs before the filing of a malpractice claim and can be just as devastating as a lawsuit. If you face going to court, you would do well to consult with an attorney and take steps to prepare yourself for your appearance. Ideally, you should consult with your professional association prior to any legal action. If you have concerns that any of your actions or omissions could lead to a lawsuit, it is wise to seek legal consultation as soon as possible.

Legal Liability in an Ethical Perspective

Legal liability and ethical practice are not identical, but they do overlap in many cases. Legal issues give substance and direction to the evolution of ethical issues. If you are involved in a malpractice action, an expert case reviewer will probably evaluate your clinical records to determine whether your practice reflected the appropriate standard of care. Records are vital to review the course of treatment. How you document treatment may determine the outcome of the case. The case reviewer will probably look for deviations from your process of reasoning and application of knowledge in trying to determine whether there has been a gross deviation from the standards. As a practitioner, you cannot guarantee the outcome, but you are expected to demonstrate that you applied a reasonable approach to the presenting problem of your client. Although you are not expected to be perfect, it is beneficial to evaluate what you are doing and why you are practicing as you are. Engaging in self-reflection and dialogue with colleagues can go a long way toward reducing your legal liability and increasing your efforts to be an ethical practitioner.

This discussion of malpractice and risk management strategies is not meant to scare you or make you overly cautious. It is easy to be anxious over the possibility of being sued, but this is not likely to bring out the best in you as a practitioner. We hope our discussion of malpractice increases your awareness of the range of professional responsibilities and suggests ways you can meet these responsibilities in an ethical fashion.

Chapter Summary

The ethics codes of all mental health organizations specify the centrality of informed consent. Clients' rights can best be protected if therapists develop procedures that aid their clients in making informed choices. Legally, informed consent entails the client's ability to act freely in making rational decisions. The process of informed consent includes providing information about the nature of therapy as well as the rights and responsibilities of both therapist and client. A basic challenge therapists face is to provide accurate and sufficient information to clients yet at the same time not to overwhelm them with too much information too soon. Informed consent can best be viewed as an ongoing process aimed at increasing the range of choices and the responsibility of the client as an active therapeutic partner.

In addition to a discussion of the rights of clients, this chapter has considered the scope of professional responsibility. Therapists have responsibilities to their clients, their agency, their profession, the community, the members of their clients' families, and themselves. Ethical dilemmas arise when there are conflicts among these responsibilities, for instance, when the agency's expectations conflict with the concerns or wishes of clients. Members of the helping professions need to know and to observe the ethics codes of their professional organizations, and they must make sound judgments within the parameters of acceptable practice. We have encouraged you to think about specific ethical issues and to develop a sense of professional ethics and knowledge of state laws so that your judgment will be based on more than what "feels right."

Associated with professional responsibilities are professional liabilities. Risks cannot be eliminated when professionals are delivering services to consumers. However, risks can be assessed, controlled, minimized, and managed through proper risk management practices (Younggren et al., 2016). If practitioners ignore legal and ethical standards or if their conduct is below the expected standard of care, they may be sued. Practitioners who fail to keep adequate records of their procedures are opening themselves to liability. Good record-keeping practices will help practitioners avoid legal trouble and will enhance the quality of their service to clients. Certainly, it is realistic to be concerned about malpractice actions and ethics complaints to a licensing board; following the professional practices described here can reduce these risks. It is our hope that practitioners do not become so preoccupied with making mistakes and self-protective strategies that they render themselves ineffective as clinicians. Being committed to doing what is best for the client is a very powerful risk management strategy.

Suggested Activities

1. In small groups, create an informed consent document. What does your group think clients must be told either before therapy begins or during the first few sessions? How can therapists provide informed consent without overwhelming clients? After discussing this, role-play the informed consent process with a partner who adopts the role of the client, and include an observer. Switch roles so that each person in the triad has an opportunity to play each role.

2. Select some of the open-ended cases presented in this chapter to role-play with a classmate. One of you chooses a client you feel you can identify with, and the other becomes the counselor. Conduct a counseling interview. Afterward, talk about how each of you felt during the interview and discuss alternative courses of action that could have been taken. You might include a third person to observe the role play.

3. Research your state's laws regarding providing mental health services to minors. What are you able to find on topics such as informed consent with minors? treatment of minors with and without parental/guardian consent? confidentiality issues with minors? legal issues to consider in working with minors?

4. Consider inviting an attorney who is familiar with the legal aspects of counseling practice to address your class. Some possible questions for discussion are: What are the legal rights of clients in therapy? What are the main legal responsibilities of therapists? What are the best ways to become familiar with laws pertaining to counselors? What are the grounds for lawsuits, and how can counselors best protect themselves from being sued?

5. Interview practicing counselors about some of their most pressing ethical concerns in carrying out their responsibilities. How have they dealt with these ethical issues? Have technological innovations such as cloud computing and online counseling raised new ethical concerns? What are some of their legal considerations? What are their concerns, if any, about malpractice suits?

6. Debate the pros and cons of online counseling. Be sure to include ethical considerations that arise when using electronic technology in the counseling process.

7. Explore this question in small groups: In reviewing the common reasons for malpractice suits against counselors, which of the behaviors were most surprising to you?

8. Discuss your concerns about professional liability. What can you do to lessen the probability of being accused of not having practiced according to acceptable standards?

Ethics in Action Video Exercises

9. In video role play 1, Counseling Adolescents: Teen Pregnancy, the client is a 13-year-old who just found out she is pregnant. She begs the counselor not to tell her parents. In this situation, what are the rights of the minor client? What rights do the parents have for access to certain information? What ethical and legal issues are involved in this case? What role would parental consent laws play in this case? What kind of informed consent process would you implement if you were counseling minors?

MindTap for Counseling

Go to MindTap® for digital study tools and resources that complement this text and help you be more successful in your course and career. There's an interactive eBook plus videos of client sessions, skill-building activities, quizzes to help you prepare for tests, apps, and more—all in one place. If your instructor *didn't* assign MindTap, you can find out more about it at CengageBrain.com.

6

Confidentiality: Ethical and Legal Issues

LEARNING OBJECTIVES

1. Differentiate between confidentiality, privacy, and privileged communication

2. Clarify the purpose and limitations of confidentiality

3. Identify privacy issues with telecommunications devices

4. Understand the implications of HIPAA for mental health providers

5. Explain the distinction between duty to warn and duty to protect

6. Recognize landmark court cases and implications for practice

7. Describe guidelines for dealing with dangerous clients

8. Explain the implications of duty to warn and to protect for school counselors

9. Evaluate ethical and legal duties pertaining to suicide

10. Delineate guidelines for assessing suicidal behavior

11. Understand the duty to protect children, dependent adults, and the elderly from harm, abuse, and maltreatment

12. Discuss several confidentiality issues in HIV/AIDS counseling

SELF-INVENTORY

Directions: For each statement, indicate the response that most closely identifies your beliefs and attitudes. Use the following code:

5 = I *strongly agree* with this statement.

4 = I *agree* with this statement.

3 = I am *undecided* in my opinion about this statement.

2 = I *disagree* with this statement.

1 = I *strongly disagree* with this statement.

_____ 1. I am not clear about how much to tell my clients about confidentiality.

_____ 2. There are no situations in which I would disclose what a client had told me without the client's permission.

_____ 3. Absolute confidentiality is necessary if effective psychotherapy is to occur.

_____ 4. If I were working with a client whom I had assessed as potentially dangerous to another person, it would be my duty to protect the potential victim(s).

_____ 5. Once I make an assessment that a client is suicidal, it is my ethical and legal obligation to take appropriate action.

_____ 6. As a helping professional, it is my responsibility to report suspected child abuse, regardless of when it occurred.

_____ 7. I think reporting elder abuse and dependent adult abuse is not the therapist's responsibility.

_____ 8. The abuse of older people and other vulnerable adults deserves the same kind of attention that is paid to abuse of children.

_____ 9. Balancing client confidentiality with protecting the public is a major ethical challenge for mental health professionals.

_____ 10. Self-injury can be a predictor of suicide, but it is a mistake to assume that most people who self-injure are suicidal.

_____ 11. I am concerned that I won't know what actions to take in situations involving the duty to protect.

_____ 12. A written safety plan can be effective in working with high-risk individuals.

_____ 13. Counselors should discuss with their clients both the challenges and safeguards when using email as a mode of communication.

_____ 14. If it became necessary to break a client's confidentiality, I would inform my client of my intended action.

_____ 15. I believe that it is easy to invade a client's privacy unintentionally.

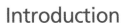

Introduction

Perhaps the central right of the client is knowing that disclosures in therapy sessions will be protected. However, you cannot promise your clients that *everything* they talk about will *always* remain confidential. In this chapter we consider the ethical and legal ramifications of confidentiality and explore the process, importance, and impact of informing your clients from the outset of therapy of those circumstances that limit confidentiality.

The more you consider the legal ramifications of confidentiality, the clearer it becomes that most situations cannot be neatly defined. Even if therapists have become familiar with local and state laws that govern their profession, this legal knowledge alone is not enough to enable them to make sound decisions. Each case is unique. There are many subtle points in the law and at various times conflicting ways to interpret the law. Professional judgment plays a significant role in resolving cases, from both an ethical and a legal perspective.

Confidentiality, Privileged Communication, and Privacy

Confidentiality is a complex responsibility, with both legal and ethical implications. See the Ethics Codes box titled "Confidentiality in Clinical Practice" for some specific guidelines on the obligations mental health practitioners have to maintain the confidentiality of their relationships with clients. Therapists must become familiar with concepts of confidentiality, privileged communication, and privacy, as well as the legal protection afforded to the privileged communications of clients and the limits of this protection.

ETHICS CODES: Confidentiality in Clinical Practice

American Counseling Association (2014)
At initiation and throughout the counseling process, counselors inform clients of the limitations of confidentiality and identify foreseeable situations in which confidentiality must be breached. (B.1.d.)

American Psychiatric Association (2013b)
Psychiatric records, including even the identification of a person as a patient, must be protected with extreme care. Confidentiality is essential to psychiatric treatment. This is based in part on the special nature of psychiatric therapy as well as on the traditional ethical relationship between physician and patient. Growing concern regarding the civil rights of patients and the possible adverse effects of computerization, duplication equipment, and data banks makes the dissemination of confidential information an increasing hazard. Because of the sensitive and private nature of the information with which the psychiatrist deals, he or she must be circumspect in the information that he or she chooses to disclose to others about a patient. The welfare of the patient must be a continuing consideration. (4.1.)

American Psychological Association (2010)
Psychologists have a primary obligation and take reasonable precautions to protect confidential information obtained through or stored in any medium, recognizing that the extent and limits of confidentiality may be regulated by law or established by institutional rules or professional or scientific relationship. (4.01.)

American School Counselor Association (2016)
Inform students of the purposes, goals, techniques and rules of procedure under which they may receive counseling. Disclosure includes informed consent and clarification of the limits of confidentiality. Informed consent requires competence, voluntariness and knowledge on the part of students to understand the limits of confidentiality and, therefore, can be difficult to obtain from students of certain developmental levels, English-language learners and special-needs populations. If the student is able to give assent/consent before school counselors share confidential information, school counselors attempt to gain the student's assent/consent. (A.2.b.)

Canadian Counselling Association (2007)
Counselling relationships and information resulting therefrom are kept confidential. However, there are the following exceptions to confidentiality:

- when disclosure is required to prevent clear and imminent danger to the client or others;
- when legal requirements demand that confidential material be revealed;
- when a child is in need of protection. (B.2.)

American Association for Marriage and Family Therapy (2015)
Marriage and family therapists disclose to clients and other interested parties at the outset of services the nature of confidentiality and possible limitations of the clients' right to confidentiality. Therapists review with clients the circumstances where confidential information may be requested and where disclosure of confidential information may be legally required. Circumstances may necessitate repeated disclosures. (2.1.)

National Association of Social Workers (2008)
Social workers should protect the confidentiality of all information obtained in the course of professional service, except for compelling professional reasons. The general expectation that social workers will keep information confidential does not apply when disclosure is necessary to prevent serious, foreseeable, and imminent harm to a client or other identifiable person. In all instances, social workers should disclose the least amount of confidential information necessary to achieve the desired purpose; only information that is directly relevant to the purpose for which the disclosure is made should be revealed. (1.07.c.)

American Mental Health Counselors Association (2015)
Mental health counselors have a primary obligation to safeguard information about individuals obtained in the course of practice, teaching, or research. Personal information is communicated to others only with the person's consent, preferably written, or in those circumstances, as dictated by state laws. Disclosure of counseling information is restricted to what is necessary, relevant and verifiable. (Principle 2.)

Confidentiality

Confidentiality, privileged communication, and privacy are related concepts, but there are important distinctions among them. **Confidentiality**, which is rooted in a client's right to privacy, is at the core of effective therapy; it "is the counselor's ethical duty to protect private client communication" (Wheeler & Bertram, 2015, p. 104). Mental health professionals have an ethical responsibility, as well as a legal and professional duty, to safeguard clients from unauthorized disclosures of information given in the therapeutic relationship. Professionals must not disclose this information except when authorized by law or by the client to do so. Hence, there are limitations to the promise of confidentiality. Court decisions have underscored that there are circumstances in which a therapist has a duty to warn and to protect the client or others, even if it means breaking confidentiality. Also, because confidentiality is a client's right, psychotherapists may legally and ethically reveal a client's confidences if a client waives this right. Confidentiality belongs to the client, and counselors generally do not find it problematic to release information when the client requests that they do so.

Fisher (2008, 2016) has designed a six-step ethical practice model for protecting confidentiality rights that places legal mandates in an ethical context. The six steps include the following:

Preparation. To inform your clients about the limits of confidentiality, you must understand the limits yourself. This involves doing your legal homework and engaging in personal soul searching regarding your own moral principles. Clarify your ethical position about confidentiality and its limits, and devise an informed consent document that reflects your policies and intentions. Discuss confidentiality and its limits with your clients in clear language, and document this discussion. Provide clients with an opportunity to address any questions they have about confidentiality at the outset of therapy, and continue to share the limits of confidentiality when necessary. Just as informed consent is an ongoing process, clients must also understand the limits of confidentiality throughout the counseling relationship.

Tell clients the truth. Inform your clients about the limits you intend to impose on confidentiality, and obtain your client's consent to accept these limits as a condition of entering into a professional relationship with you. Explain any roles that might affect confidentiality.

Obtain "truly informed consent" before disclosing voluntarily. Make disclosures only if legally unavoidable. Obtain and document your client's signed consent before disclosing this information.

Respond ethically to legal demands for information. Notify your client of a pending legal demand for disclosure without his or her consent. Limit disclosure of confidential information to the extent that is legally possible.

Avoid preventable breaches of confidentiality. Avoid making unethical exceptions to the confidentiality rule; establish and maintain policies aimed at protecting confidentiality; monitor your note taking and record keeping practices; avoid dual roles that create conflicts of interest in the courtroom; anticipate legal demands and your response to such requirements; empower clients to act protectively on their own behalf; and do not confuse laws that *permit* disclosure with laws that *require* disclosure.

Talk about confidentiality. Model ethical behavior and practice; invite a dialogue with clients about confidentiality as needed; teach ethical practices to students and supervisees; and educate attorneys, judges, and consumers.

Fisher's (2008) model can assist mental health professionals to frame ethical questions more clearly and to help identify questions to explore in the process of consultation. "In short, psychologists can use this practice model to reclaim their status as experts about the confidentiality ethics of their profession" (p. 12).

Privileged Communication

Privileged communication is a legal concept that generally bars the disclosure of confidential communications made to a psychotherapist from any judicial proceedings or court of law (Knapp & VandeCreek, 2012). All states have enacted into law some form of psychotherapist–client privilege, but the specifics of this privilege vary from state to state. Clinicians need to understand the privilege laws in the states in which they practice. Some privileged communication statutes protect client–counselor relationships to the fullest extent that the law allows; statutes in other jurisdictions are quite weak (Remley & Herlihy, 2016). When a client–therapist relationship is covered as privileged communication by statute, clinicians may not disclose confidential information. Therapists can refuse to answer questions in court or refuse to produce a client's records in court. These laws ensure that personal and sensitive client information will be protected from exposure by therapists in legal proceedings.

Again, this privilege belongs to the client and is designed for the client's protection rather than for the protection of the counseling professional. If a client knowingly and rationally waives this privilege, the professional has no legal grounds for withholding the information. Professionals are obligated to disclose information that is *necessary and sufficient* when the client requests it, but only the information that is specifically requested and only to the individuals or agencies that are specified by the client. In some circumstances, the therapist can make a clinical decision to withhold all or some information if the client waves his or her privilege. For example, if the therapist believes the client is not mentally competent to make such a decision, the therapist may not abide by the client's request to waive privilege.

Privileged Communication in Group Counseling, Couples and Family Therapy, and Child and Adolescent Therapy

The legal concept of privileged communication generally does *not* apply to group counseling, couples counseling, family therapy, or child and adolescent therapy. However, the therapist is still bound by confidentiality with respect to circumstances not involving a court proceeding. Statements made in the presence of a third party may not be protected in a court proceeding. Members of a counseling group can assume that they could be asked to testify in court concerning certain information revealed in the course of a group session, unless there is a statutory exception. In states where no law exists to cover confidentiality in group therapy, courts may use the ethics codes of the professions regarding confidentiality. If a situation arises, therapists may need to demonstrate the means they used to create safety for the group members. A written group contract defining members' responsibility for maintaining confidentiality of whatever takes place in a group can be used for this purpose.

Similarly, couples therapy and family therapy are not subject to privileged communication statutes in many states. In the case of child and adolescent clients, there are restrictions on the confidential character of disclosures in the counseling relationship. No clear judicial trend has emerged for communications that are made in the presence of third persons. Clients have a right to be informed about any limitations on confidentiality in group work, child and adolescent therapy, and couples and family therapy. Ambiguity may exist regarding who the client is and the specific nature of the therapy goals when counseling couples or families. When more than one client is in the consulting room at a time, the confidentiality mandate can become complex. Confidentiality and its exceptions must be addressed at the outset of treatment and at any time during treatment when confidentiality issues become salient. Furthermore, therapists working with couples or families should clearly communicate their policy about keeping, or not keeping, secrets disclosed by one of the partners or family members in advance of starting counseling (Barnett & Johnson, 2015). Some therapists may choose to provide their clients with this policy in writing to be sure that clients are fully informed. We discuss this topic in more detail in Chapter 11.

The *Jaffee* Case and Privileged Communication The basic principles of privileged communication have been reaffirmed by case law. On June 13, 1996, the United States Supreme Court ruled that communications between licensed psychotherapists and their clients in the course of diagnosis or treatment are privileged and therefore protected from forced disclosure in cases arising under federal law. The Supreme Court ruling in *Jaffee v. Redmond* (1996), written by Justice John Paul Stevens, states that "effective psychotherapy depends upon an atmosphere of confidence and trust in which the patient is willing to make frank and complete disclosure of facts, emotions, memories, and fears." The 7–2 decision in this case represented a victory for mental health organizations because it extended the confidentiality privilege.

In the *Jaffee* case, an on-duty police officer, Mary Lu Redmond, shot and killed a suspect while attempting an arrest. The victim's family sued in federal court, alleging that the victim's constitutional rights had been violated. The court ordered Karen Beyer, a licensed clinical social worker, to turn over notes she made during counseling sessions with Redmond after the shooting. The social worker refused, asserting that the contents of her conversations with the police officer were protected against involuntary disclosure by psychotherapist–client privilege. The court rejected her claim of psychotherapist–client privilege, and the jury awarded the family $545,000.

The Court of Appeals for the Seventh Circuit reversed this decision and concluded that the trial court had erred by refusing to afford protection to the confidential communications between Redmond and Beyer. Jaffee, an administrator of the victim's estate, appealed this decision to the Supreme Court.

The Supreme Court upheld the appellate court's decision, clarifying for all federal court cases, both civil and criminal, the existence of the privilege. The Court recognized a broadly defined psychotherapist–client privilege and further clarified that this privilege is not subject to the decision of a judge on a case-by-case basis. The Court's decision to extend federal privilege (which already applied to psychologists and psychiatrists) to licensed social workers leaves the door open for inclusion of other licensed psychotherapists, such as licensed marriage and family therapists, licensed professional counselors, and mental health counselors.

In discussing the impact on the law of the *Jaffee v. Redmond* case, Shuman and Foote (1999) indicate that the case is not constitutionally based. Instead, *Jaffee* is an interpretation of the Federal Rules of Evidence that apply in actions tried in federal courts. Thus, *Jaffee* applies only in federal cases, both civil and criminal, governed by the Federal Rules of Evidence.

Privacy

Privacy, as a matter of law, refers to the constitutional right of individuals to be left alone and to control their personal information (Wheeler & Bertram, 2015). Privacy is the right to be protected from visibility, access, or intrusion by others (Fisher, 2016). Practitioners should exercise caution with regard to the privacy of their clients. It is easy to invade a client's privacy unintentionally. Examples of some of the most pressing situations in which privacy is an issue include an employer's access to an applicant's or an employee's psychological tests, parents' access to their child's school and health records, and a third-party payer's access to information about a client's diagnosis and prognosis.

If counselors have occasion to meet clients outside of the professional setting, it is essential that they do not violate their privacy. This is especially true in small towns, where such meetings can be expected. In the course of treatment, you may realize that you and the client belong to the same house of worship, that your children attend the same school, or that your children play on the same soccer team. It is a good practice to let your client know that encounters may occur and to talk with your client about how you might interact when you meet. Consider what you might do in the following case.

The Case of Erica

Helena is a counselor in the student services department at a community college. She has been counseling Erica for several months for a variety of problems having to do with her body image and eating behaviors. One evening Helena and a friend go out to a local cafe for a light meal and a coffee. Helena is surprised when the waitress comes up to her cheerily and says hello. She looks up and realizes it is Erica. She chats briefly with Erica who then takes her order and goes off to serve other customers. Helena's friend then asks who Erica is and how she knows her?

- If you were the counselor, would you introduce Erica to your friend? If so how?
- If you were the counselor, how would you answer your friend's question?
- If Erica acknowledged that you were her counselor in front of your friend, how would you respond to her?
- If Erica began to discuss her sessions with you, what would you do?

Commentary. These chance meetings are often unavoidable. If Helena had ignored Erica, not only could this be seen as being rude, but Erica might feel offended. It is inappropriate for Helena to acknowledge to her friend that Erica is her client. If Erica began discussing matters pertaining to her counseling sessions, Helena should find a way to steer the interaction to a general conversation. Helena's dilemma reminds us that during the informed consent process it is a good idea to discuss how clients would like you to handle chance encounters outside of therapy; this is especially important if you live and practice in a small community or at a college or university campus. •

Most professional codes of ethics contain guidelines to safeguard a client's right to privacy. An example of the privacy standard, designed to minimize intrusions on privacy, is found in the APA (2010) ethics code:

> Psychologists disclose confidential information without the consent of the individual only as mandated by law, or where permitted by law for a valid purpose such as to (1) provide needed professional services; (2) obtain appropriate professional consultations; (3) protect the client/patient, psychologist, or others from harm; or (4) obtain payment for services from a client/patient, in which instance disclosure is limited to the minimum that is necessary to achieve the purpose. (4.05.b.)

Practitioners who also teach courses, offer workshops, write books and journal articles, and give lectures must ensure that client privacy is protected. It is of the utmost importance that practitioners take measures to adequately disguise their clients' identities when using examples from clinical practice, and it is prudent not to use current clients as examples. Sperry and Pies (2010) discuss the ethical considerations in writing about clients. They identify three options for presenting case material: (1) seek the client's permission to publish, which some consider ethically questionable because it entails inserting the clinician's professional agenda into the client's treatment; (2) disguise case material for publication, which may or may not release the therapist from needing to secure the client's permission; or (3) develop composite case material from two or more clients. Most of the case examples and commentaries we include in this book are fictional cases we have created. In the few actual clinical examples, we have taken care to disguise any identifying details.

Students should be advised to adequately disguise identities of their clients in any reports they give in class. Of course, students' personal comments in class are also to be kept confidential.

Confidentiality and Privacy in a School Setting

Managing confidentiality is a challenge most school counselors face. School counselors need to balance their ethical and legal responsibilities with three groups: the students they serve, the parents or guardians of those students, and the school system. When minors are unable to give informed consent, parents or guardians provide this informed consent, and they may need to be included in the counseling process. Counselors have an ethical obligation to safeguard the confidentiality of minors to the extent that it is possible, but in most states their discussions with students are not privileged communication (Stone & Dahir, 2016).

School counselors are ethically obliged to respect the privacy of minor clients and maintain confidentiality, yet this obligation may be in conflict with laws regarding parental rights to be informed about the progress of treatment and to decide what is in the best interests of their children. The ASCA (2016) ethics code states that school counselors "recognize their primary ethical obligation for confidentiality is to the student but balance that obligation with an understanding of the parents'/guardians' legal and inherent rights to be the guiding voice in their children's lives" (A.2.f.).

School counselors have an ethical responsibility to ask for client permission to release information, and they should clearly inform students of the limitations of confidentiality and how and when confidential information may be shared. The ASCA (2016) guideline regarding parents is that the school counselor "informs parents/guardians of the counselor's role to include the confidential nature of the school counseling relationship between the school counselor and student" (B.1.f.). Although school counselors may be required to provide certain information to parents and school personnel, they need to do so in a manner that will minimize intrusion of the child's or adolescent's privacy and in a way that demonstrates respect for the counselee. To the degree possible, school counselors aim to establish collaborative relationships with parents and school personnel.

Laws regarding confidentiality in school counseling differ. In some states, therapists in private practice are required to demonstrate that attempts have been made to contact the parents of children who are younger than 16, whereas school counselors are not required to do so. Schools that receive federal funding are generally bound by the provisions of the Family Educational Rights and Privacy Act of 1994 (FERPA). It is necessary that school counselors exercise discretion in the kind and extent of information they reveal to parents or guardians about their children.

School personnel and administrators may operate under different guidelines regarding confidentiality, and they may not understand the mental health professions' requirements. When a school counselor withholds information from school personnel and administrators about students in counseling, especially with regard to risk-taking behaviors, the counselor "may be seen as something other than a team player (i.e., school administrators may view school counselors' protecting the confidentiality of students as insubordination)" (Moyer, Sullivan, & Growcock, 2012, p. 99). This is a complex area that requires careful thought and consideration, as the following case examples illustrate.

The Case of Serena

Serena, a school counselor, shifted her career from private practice to counseling in an elementary school. She was particularly surprised by the differences between private practice and school counseling with respect to confidentiality issues. She remarked that she was constantly fielding questions from teachers such as "Whom do you have in that counseling group?" "How is Alex doing?" "It's no wonder this girl has problems. Have you met her parents?"

Although Serena talked to the principal and teachers about the importance of maintaining a safe, confidential environment for students in counseling situations, she would still receive questions from them about students, some of whom were not in their classes. In addition to the questions from teachers, Serena found that she had to deal with inquiries from school secretaries and other staff members, some of whom seemed to know everything that was going on in the school. They would ask her probing questions about students, which she, of course, was not willing to answer. For example, although she would not tell a secretary whom she was counseling, a teacher might have told the secretary that she was seeing one of his students.

Serena observed that the principal and parents also asked for specific information about the students she was seeing. She learned the importance of talking to everyone about the need to respect privacy. If she had not exercised care, it would have been easy for her to say more than would have been ethical to teachers, staff members, and parents. She also learned how critical it was to talk about matters of confidentiality and privacy in simple language with the schoolchildren she counseled.

- If you were asked some of the questions posed to Serena, how would you respond?
- How would you protect the privacy of the students and at the same time avoid alienating the teachers and staff members?
- How would you explain the meaning of confidentiality and privacy to teachers? staff members? parents? administrators? the children?
- Would you consider listening to some school personnel to gather information pertaining to your client(s)? Why or why not?
- Might you consider collaborating with school personnel to provide some type of treatment for the client? Why or why not?

Commentary. This case illustrates the importance of a school counselor taking the initiative to educate parents, administrators, and staff members about the need to respect privacy and protect confidentiality of minor clients. Serena took steps to protect the privacy of the children by educating all concerned about the importance of confidentiality in counseling. A further step Serena might take is to offer in-service training for all school staff regarding the importance of confidentiality and the process of counseling. Serena might consider inviting a local health care attorney to offer training at her school. Because school counselors are part of an educational community, they often consult with parents, teachers, and administrators and may be asked to reveal student confidences. Moyer, Sullivan, and Growcock (2012) point out that school counselors must be able to determine when administrators have the ethical right to gain access to confidential information about students, especially in cases of risk-taking behavior by students. In addition, "the issue is confounding because the administrator on campus is often the school counselor's direct supervisor" (p. 99). •

The Case of Jeremy

Jeremy, a third grade boy in an elementary school, reports to his school counselor that he was with his mother when she stole a dress from a store. Jeremy also reports that after he and his mother left the store, she told him that she at times stole food because she couldn't afford it. Jeremy requests that the counselor not say anything to his mother because she has been very depressed about not having a job and he worries about what she might do if she learns that he is talking to a counselor about her. After the session, the counselor initiates a conversation with Jeremy's fourth grade sister, who is a student in the same school, to further explore the allegation of the mother's stealing.

- Was this school counselor behaving inappropriately by initiating a conversation with a client's sibling to further explore an alleged crime?
- As a counselor, do you have a legal obligation in this case?
- Would you consider calling Jeremy's mother to schedule a meeting with her? Why or why not?
- If the mother's actions are indicative of financial desperation and a lack of resources, what community referrals or resources might you find to help the family?

- Do you have any ethical, legal, or clinical concerns about the counselor acting as a "detective"?
- What would you have done if you were counseling Jeremy?

Commentary. Whether or not the therapist is trying to confirm Jeremy's story or gain additional information, talking to Jeremy's sister is a violation of his confidentiality. If the mother is indeed stealing from stores, she may be arrested, which could be traumatic for the children. However, the school counselor's primary duty is to address Jeremy's fear and his well-being. The therapist may suggest that Jeremy ask his mother to attend a session with him so Jeremy has an opportunity to express his fears in a conjoint session. A school counselor may have an ethical and legal responsibility to report a parent for an alleged crime, especially when there is risk of harm to the minor such as dealing drugs from the home, driving drunk with children in the car, or leaving the children alone for long periods of time. However, crimes that do not threaten the safety of a child do not have to be reported. Even when such a report is necessary, it is important to simultaneously work to keep the minor client engaged. The role of the counselor is not to be a detective or to investigate details of an alleged crime but to focus on the clinical needs and safety of the minor client.

An important clinical issue in this case is to understand the meaning of the mother's behaviors. Stealing is not an ideal choice, but if Jeremy's mother is doing so to provide for her children, she needs additional support. One way the therapist could intervene is to locate resources available to help with the family's financial needs and provide this information to the mother.

A Case of Academic Dishonesty

Miles, a high school counselor, is told by Tess, a student, that she and some friends have stolen a chemistry final exam. Tess requests that Miles not say a word about it to anyone because she is presently failing chemistry and needs to do well on the final exam to pass the course and graduate from high school. Miles decides not to divulge any information, respecting the student's request to maintain confidentiality.

- What are your thoughts about Miles's decision?
- How might this dilemma for the counselor raise questions concerning the limits to confidentiality?
- What interventions can Miles make with Tess without breaking confidentiality? Can he encourage her to make different choices, and what might those be?
- What would you have done if you were the counselor in this situation?
- Can school policies be included as you explain the limits to confidentiality to students in your role as a school counselor? Why or why not?

Commentary. The counselor has no obligation to breach confidentiality because there is no danger to life. If it is school policy that such matters must be reported, this information should be clearly stated in an informed consent document. One clinical issue that could be explored is why this student told Simon about the theft.

Ethical and Legal Ramifications of Confidentiality and Privileged Communication

Clients in counseling are involved in a deeply personal relationship and have a right to expect that what they discuss will be kept private. The compelling justification for confidentiality is that it is necessary in order to encourage clients to develop the trust needed for full disclosure and for the other work involved in therapy. For example, the school counselor has the task of providing a safe and trusting environment for counseling relationships to take root. If students do not believe their communications with a counselor will be kept confidential, they may not participate in counseling services (Stone & Dahir, 2016). Clients must feel free to explore all aspects of their lives without fear that these disclosures will be released outside the therapy room. Counselors are ethically obligated to help clients appreciate the meaning of confidentiality by presenting it in language the client can understand and that respects the cultural experiences of the client (Barnett & Johnson, 2015). The meaning of confidentiality may be interpreted in different ways depending on the client's culture. By encouraging an ongoing dialogue about how, when, and with whom information will be shared, counselors establish a collaborative spirit in their relationships with clients (Wheeler & Bertram, 2015).

When it does become necessary to break confidentiality, it is good practice to inform the client of the intention to take this action and also to invite the client to participate in the process. For example, all states now have statutes that require professionals who suspect any form of child abuse to report it to the appropriate agencies, even when the knowledge was gained through confidential communication with clients. A professional who reports suspected child abuse, in good faith, is immune from civil liability and criminal prosecution as a mandated reporter (Jensen, 2006).

Exceptions to Confidentiality and Privileged Communication Counselors must help clients understand the limits of confidentiality and address any exceptions to confidentiality clients may encounter. Although ethical standards provide guidelines regarding the circumstances under which confidentiality cannot be maintained, therapists must exercise their own professional judgment in specific situations. When assuring their clients that what they reveal will ordinarily be kept confidential, therapists should point out that they also have obligations to others. Therapists are legally and ethically bound to protect others from harm. Most major professional organizations have taken the position that practitioners may need to reveal certain information when there is *serious and foreseeable danger* to an individual or to society. The ASCA's (2016) ethical standard states this clearly:

> School counselors keep information confidential unless legal requirements demand that confidential information be revealed or a breach is required to prevent serious and foreseeable harm to the student. Serious and foreseeable harm is different for each minor in schools and is determined by students' developmental and chronological age, the setting, parental rights and the nature of the harm. School counselors consult with appropriate professionals when in doubt as to the validity of an exception. (A.2.e.)

It is the responsibility of counselors to clarify the ethical and legal restrictions on confidentiality. Practitioners cannot provide absolute confidentiality and must inform clients about conditions under which confidentiality cannot be protected (Fisher, 2016). It is best to include these exceptions in the informed consent document as well as discussing them verbally with the client. Consider these exceptional circumstances in which it is permissible to share information with others in the interest of providing competent services to clients:

- When the client requests a release of information
- When reimbursement or other legal rules require disclosure
- When clerical assistants handle confidential information, as in managed care
- When the counselor consults with experts or peers
- When the counselor is working under supervision
- When other mental health professionals request information and the client has given consent to share
- When other professionals are involved in a treatment team and coordinate care of a client

Remley and Herlihy (2016) identify 15 exceptions to confidentiality and privileged communication and underscore the importance of consultation (and documentation) whenever practitioners are in doubt about their obligations regarding confidentiality or privileged communication. Among the conditions that warrant disclosure of information shared in the counseling relationship are these legally mandated exceptions to confidentiality and privileged communication:

- Disclosure of confidential information is ordered by a court
- Client waiver of the privilege
- Clients file complaints and litigation against their counselors
- Clients claim psychological damage in a lawsuit
- Civil commitment proceedings are initiated
- Statutes involving child abuse or elder abuse mandate disclosure
- Clients pose a danger to others or to themselves

The limitations of confidentiality may be greater in some settings and agencies than in others. In addition, exceptions to confidentiality vary by jurisdiction, and counselors are required to know the laws that govern their area of practice. If clients are informed about the conditions under which confidentiality may be compromised, they are in a better position to decide whether or not to enter counseling. If clients are involved in involuntary counseling, they can decide what they will disclose in their sessions. It is generally accepted that clients have a right to understand in advance the circumstances under which therapists are required or allowed to communicate information about them to third parties. Unless clients understand the exceptions to confidentiality, their consent to treatment is questionable.

In an addiction treatment center, the policy may be "what is said to one staff member is said to all." One reason for this practice may be to avoid triangulation of the staff, which would be detrimental to patients. This frees the entire treatment staff to share information about patients as a part of the treatment process, and it eliminates concerns about breaching confidentiality. When a crisis occurs and the therapist is not available, other staff members can step in to handle the situation. Of course, the patients should be made aware of this policy. When patients suffer a relapse during addiction treatment and public safety is jeopardized, counselors have a duty to report. If being intoxicated on the job can seriously threaten the lives of others, such as clients who are airline pilots or bus drivers, counselors have a duty to disclose this.

If you breach confidentiality in an unprofessional manner (in the absence of a recognized exception), you open yourself to both ethical and legal sanctions, including expulsion from a professional association, loss of certification, license revocation, and a malpractice suit. To protect yourself against such liability, it is essential to become familiar with all applicable ethical and legal guidelines pertaining to confidentiality, including state privilege laws and their exceptions, child and elder abuse reporting requirements, and the parameters of the duty-to-protect exceptions in your state.

The Case of Lorenzo

Lorenzo, 16 years old, is sent to a family therapy clinic by his parents. During the first session the counselor sees Lorenzo and his parents together. She tells the parents in his presence that what she and Lorenzo discuss will be confidential and that she will not disclose information acquired through the sessions without his permission. The parents seem to understand that confidentiality is necessary for trust to develop between their son and his counselor.

At first Lorenzo is reluctant to come in for counseling. Eventually, as the sessions go on, he discloses that he has a serious drug problem. Lorenzo's parents know he used drugs at one time, but he has told them he is no longer using them. The counselor listens to anecdote after anecdote about Lorenzo's use of illegal drugs, about how "I am loaded at school every day," and about a few brushes with death when he was under the influence of illegal substances. Finally, she tells Lorenzo that she does not want the responsibility of knowing he is experimenting with illegal drugs and that she will not agree to continue the counseling relationship unless he stops using them. At this stage she agrees not to inform his parents, on the condition that he quits using drugs, but she does tell him that she will be talking with one of her colleagues about the situation.

Lorenzo apparently stops using drugs for several weeks. However, one night while he is under the influence of methamphetamine he has a serious car accident. As a result of the accident, Lorenzo is paralyzed for life. Lorenzo's parents angrily assert that they had a legal right to be informed that he was seriously involved in drug use, and they file suit against both the counselor and the agency.

- What is your general impression of the way Lorenzo's counselor handled the case?
- Do you think the counselor acted in a responsible way toward the client? the parents? the agency?
- If you were convinced that Lorenzo was likely to hurt himself or others because of his drug use and his emotional instability, would you have informed his parents, even at the risk of losing Lorenzo as a client? Why or why not?
- Which of the following courses of action could you have taken if you had been Lorenzo's counselor? Check as many as you think are appropriate:

    _____ State the legal limits on you as a therapist during the initial session.

    _____ Consult with the supervisor of the agency as well as with other colleagues.

    _____ Refer Lorenzo for psychological testing to determine the degree of his emotional disturbance.

    _____ Refer Lorenzo to a psychiatrist for treatment.

    _____ Continue to see Lorenzo without any stipulations.

    _____ Insist on a session with Lorenzo's parents as a condition of continuing counseling.

_____ Inform the police or other authorities.

_____ Document your decision-making process with a survey of pertinent research.

- What potential ethical violations do you see in this case?

Commentary. This case emphasizes the importance of doing a thorough assessment of a client. When Lorenzo spoke of "a few brushes with death," it was clear that he was a danger to himself, which was cause for the counselor to take immediate action. This therapist wanted to believe Lorenzo's story and failed to take the necessary steps to prevent harmful consequences to her client. This case demonstrates how important it is to set limits to confidentiality based on the counselor's assessment (danger to self or others) and highlights the issue of informed consent. Although the counselor promised confidentiality at the outset, many circumstances and jurisdictional requirements may necessitate disclosure of confidential information to both an official agency and to the parents or legal guardians. When explaining informed consent, counselors who routinely work with minors need to clarify the various exceptions to confidentiality in language minor clients can understand.

Additional Cases for Your Reflection We have provided commentaries on many cases involving ethical dilemmas. Based on what you have learned and from your own deliberations, select the most ethical course of action in each of the following cases.

1. You are a student counselor. For your internship you are working with college students on campus. Your intern group meets with a supervisor each week to discuss your cases. One day, while you are having lunch in the campus cafeteria with three other interns, they begin to discuss their cases in detail, even mentioning names of clients. They joke about some of the clients they are seeing, while nearby there are other students who may be able to overhear this conversation. What would you do in this situation?

_____ I would tell the other interns to stop talking about their clients where other students could overhear them and to continue their conversation in a private place.

_____ I would bring the matter up in our next practicum meeting with the supervisor.

_____ I would take no action.

2. You are leading a counseling group on a high school campus. The members have voluntarily joined the group. In one of the sessions several of the students discuss the drug use on their campus, and two of them reveal that they sell illegal substances to their friends. You discuss this matter with them, and they claim that there is nothing wrong with using these drugs and emphasize that many people support the legalization of marijuana. They think you are making a much bigger deal out of the matter than it deserves. They argue that most of the students on campus use drugs, that no one has been harmed, and that there isn't any difference between using drugs (which they know is illegal) and using alcohol. What would you do in this situation?

_____ Because their actions are illegal, I would report them to the police or campus authorities.

_____ I would do nothing because I would not want to jeopardize their trust in me.

_____ I would report the situation to the school authorities but keep the identities of the students confidential.

_____ I would let the students know that I planned to inform the school authorities of their actions and their names.

_____ I would explore with the students their reasons for making this disclosure.

_____ I would start an education program pertaining to drug abuse.

3. You are counseling children in an elementary school. Miriana is referred to you by her teacher because she is becoming increasingly withdrawn. After several sessions Miriana tells you that she is afraid that her father might kill her and that he frequently beats her. Until now she has lied about obvious bruises on her body, claiming that she fell off her bicycle and hurt herself. She shows you welts on her arms and back but tells you not to say anything to anyone because her father has threatened a worse beating if she tells anyone. What would you do in this situation?

_____ I would respect Miriana's wishes and not tell anyone what I knew.

_____ I would report the situation to the principal and the school nurse.

_____ I would immediately go with Miriana to her home and talk to her parents.

_____ I would report the matter to the police and to Child Protective Services.

_____ I would tell Miriana that I had a legal obligation to make this situation known to the authorities but that I would work with her and not leave her alone with her fears.

Privacy Issues With Telecommunication Devices

Digital technology in the helping professions is wide ranging. Computers (including email and online chat), smartphones, tablets, and other electronic instruments are being used to deliver services to and communicate with clients, manage confidential case records, and access information about clients (Reamer, 2015). Telephone, answering machine, voice mail, fax, cellular phone, text messaging, and email all pose a number of potential ethical problems with regard to protecting client privacy. Counselors in private practice may find text messaging with their clients to be an inexpensive and convenient tool; however, they must be mindful of the ethical issues that can arise from the use of this technology. Potential concerns related to privacy, confidentiality, documentation, appropriateness of use, counselor competence, boundary issues, and misinterpretation must be considered (Sude, 2013).

Barros-Bailey and Saunders (2010) point out that "when communication can be easily captured, copied, transferred, disseminated, and stored in written text (e.g., email, text messaging), through picture or video means (e.g., smart phone cameras, VoIP technology such as Skype), or verbally (e.g., recording devices in all sorts of portable media from cell phones to MP3 players or recorders), the danger for a breach of confidentiality substantially increases" (p. 256). Rummell and Joyce (2010) recommend "password protection, data encryption, use of secure socket layer encryption for Internet traffic between psychotherapist and client computers, and use of a firewall" to promote confidentiality of client information (p. 488). Yet they admit that even these measures cannot guarantee confidentiality. Accidental interception, unauthorized email access, and email snooping are potential mishaps that can occur. Reamer (2015) advises practitioners not to assume that Internet sites and electronic tools they use are necessarily encrypted; the ethical burden is on clinicians to ensure trustworthy encryption by cautiously examining statements and guarantees made by software vendors.

Compared to other forms of electronic technology, Brenes, Ingram, and Danhauer (2011) suggest the telephone may be the preferred method for providing psychological services. Neither therapists nor clients need instructions on how to use the telephone, which reduces the barriers to service. A few phone sessions may be appropriate when a client is seriously ill and cannot come to an office. However, more research is needed to determine who might benefit most from telephone-delivered therapy, and in what situations it is appropriate. Brenes and colleagues point out a number of challenges of telephone-delivered therapy. Mental health practitioners must exercise caution in discussing confidential or privileged information with anyone over the telephone and especially when employing digital and mobile technologies. Therapists must set firm boundaries with clients from the beginning and address matters such as avoiding interruptions and privacy. It is critical to disclose the limits of confidentiality with clients if wireless telephones are used; Brenes and colleagues recommend land lines to ensure greater privacy and confidentiality for clients.

Therapists should discuss the use of technology and the method for securing, protecting, and handling data with clients in the informed consent process and as needed throughout the therapeutic sessions. It is important that the informed consent document clearly explain, justify, and present accurate risks to data storage and communication (Lustgarten, 2015).

Using fax machines and email to send confidential material is another source of potential invasion of a client's privacy. It is the counselor's responsibility to make sure fax and email transmissions arrive in a secured environment in such a way as to protect confidential information. Tran-Lien (2012) recommends that therapists who plan to exchange emails with their clients provide clients with a statement (as part of the informed consent process) that details the therapist's guidelines and limitations on the use of email, the potential risks to confidentiality, and the expected turnaround time. She notes that "communicating with your clients via e-mail can be done, but careful consideration should be given to the guidelines and relevant legal and ethical issues" (p. 22). Both the challenges and the safeguards in using email as a mode of communication should be clearly explained.

Therapists and their clients should carefully consider privacy issues before agreeing to send email messages to clients' workplaces or homes. If emails are sent directly to your smartphone, the risks to privacy and confidentiality increase. A good policy is to limit email and text message exchanges to basic information such as an appointment time. Courts have ruled that email sent or received on computers used by employees is considered to be the property of the company;

therefore, privacy and confidentiality do not exist. It is important to take appropriate measures to safeguard privacy and security when using email. Tran-Lien (2012) offers several tips for therapists regarding email:

- Remember that anything sent via email to clients ultimately ends up in their possession and may be shared with third parties at their discretion.
- Consider including a confidentiality disclaimer notice stating that the information in the email is confidential and should not be shared with others without authorization from the sender.
- Do not email clients on a public computer for privacy and security reasons.

This discussion of privacy may seem to be just a matter of common sense, but we have become so accustomed to relying on technology that careful thought is not always given to the subtle ways privacy can be violated. Exercise caution and pay attention to ways you could unintentionally breach the privacy of your clients when using various forms of communication. Apprise your clients of potential problems of privacy regarding a wide range of technology and discuss how they might best contact you between office visits and how you might leave messages for them. Take preventive measures so that both you and your clients understand and have a signed agreement detailing these important concerns. You may face legal problems due to violations of privacy and confidentiality in this era of electronic communication, so it is important to determine whether your liability insurance covers email and other electronic communications with clients (Bradley, Hendricks, Lock, Whiting, & Parr, 2011).

Implications of HIPAA for Mental Health Providers

The **Health Insurance Portability and Accountability Act of 1996** (HIPAA) was passed by Congress to promote standardization and efficiency in the health care industry and to give patients more rights and control over their health information. HIPAA is a federal law that contains detailed provisions regarding client privacy, informed consent, and transfer of records. HIPAA regulations require practitioners who are covered entities under HIPAA to provide prospective clients with a clear written explanation of how health information is used, disclosed, and kept (Fisher, 2016). HIPAA includes provisions designed to encourage electronic transactions and requires certain new safeguards to protect the security and confidentiality of health information. The **HIPAA Privacy Rule** was designed to provide a uniform level of privacy and security on the federal level. This Privacy Rule, which applies to both paper and electronic transmissions of protected health information by covered entities, developed out of the concern that transmission of health care information through electronic means could lead to widespread gaps in the protection of client confidentiality. The Privacy Rule requires health plans and other covered entities to establish policies and procedures to protect the confidentiality of health information about their patients. It requires technical, administrative, and physical safeguards to protect security of protected health information in electronic form (Wheeler & Bertram, 2015). The Privacy Rule provides patients with rights concerning how their health information is used and disclosed by health care providers who fall within the domain of HIPAA.

Health care providers need to determine whether they are covered entities under HIPAA. If providers transmit any protected health information in electronic form (such as health care claims, health plan enrollment, or coordination of benefits), or if they hire someone to electronically transmit protected health care information, they must comply with all applicable HIPAA regulations (Wheeler & Bertram, 2015). If you submit a claim electronically, even once, you are likely to be considered a covered entity for HIPAA purposes.

Jensen (2003b) explains that there are three types of **covered entities**: health plans, health care clearinghouses, and health care providers who transmit health information by electronic means. To determine that you are a "covered entity," you need to answer affirmatively to all three of these questions:

1. Are you a health care provider?
2. Do you transmit information electronically?
3. Do you conduct covered transactions?

According to Jensen, if you do not answer "yes" to all of these questions, or if you do not employ someone to conduct the covered transactions for you, then you are not a covered entity and HIPAA does not apply to you.

If you want to avoid becoming a covered entity, Jensen (2003e) offers these suggestions:

- Do not use your computer to conduct one of the standard/covered transactions.
- Use only your telephone, the mail, or your fax machine.
- Avoid hiring a person to do your billing services to clients if he or she conducts one of the standard/covered transactions electronically.
- Do not allow health plans to communicate with you electronically.
- Make certain that health plans communicate with you about clients only by phone, mail, or fax machine.

In his article, "HIPAA Overview," Jensen (2003b) describes the four standards of HIPAA: (1) privacy requirements, (2) electronic transactions, (3) security requirements, and (4) national identifier requirements. Let's examine each in more detail.

Privacy requirements. The Privacy Rule requires practitioners to take reasonable precautions in safeguarding patient information. Licensed health care providers are expected to have a working knowledge of and guard patients' rights to privacy in disclosure of information, health care operations, limiting the disclosure of protected information, payment matters, protected health information, psychotherapy notes and a patient's medical record, and treatment activities.

Electronic transactions. HIPAA aims at creating one national form of communication, or "language," so that health care providers can communicate with one another electronically in this common language.

Security requirements. Minimum requirements are outlined in HIPAA that are designed to safeguard confidential information and prevent unauthorized access to health information of patients. Technological advances, including electronic record keeping, challenge practitioners' abilities to maintain security (Lustgarten, 2015).

National identifier requirements. It is essential that covered entities be able to communicate with one another efficiently. Health care providers and health plans are required to have national identification numbers that identify them when they are conducting standard transactions.

Only mental health providers who fall within the definition of *covered entity* are subject to HIPAA requirements. Those providers who do not fall within this scope of practice are not required to comply with HIPAA requirements, unless they choose to do so (Jensen, 2003e). Wheeler and Bertram (2015) suggest that some HIPAA requirements could be good practices from a risk management perspective even if the practitioner is not technically a covered entity.

Handerscheid, Henderson, and Chalk (2002) state that HIPAA privacy requirements are meant to protect confidential patient information irrespective of the form in which the information is stored. To comply, covered entities first need to review their routine business practices to assess how well patient information is protected against inappropriate disclosures. Policies and procedures need to be in place. The second step involves modifying business policies or practices once any problems are detected. The third step involves working with consumers to inform them of their rights, advise them about providing written authorization for release of information, and describe grievance procedures clients can use if they believe their privacy has been violated.

The Duty to Warn and to Protect

LO5

Mental health professionals, spurred by the courts, have come to realize that they have a dual professional responsibility: to protect other people from potentially dangerous clients and to protect clients from themselves. Balancing client confidentiality and protecting the public is a major ethical challenge that mental health professionals must assess in considering these competing interests. The American Psychiatric Association (2013b) provides this standard: "When, in the clinical judgment of the treating psychiatrist, the risk of danger is deemed to be significant, the psychiatrist may reveal confidential information disclosed by the patient." (4.8.). In this section we look first at therapists' responsibilities to protect potential victims from violence and then at the problems posed by clients who are suicidal.

The Duty to Protect Potential Victims

One of the most difficult tasks therapists grapple with is deciding whether a particular client is dangerous. It is extremely difficult to decide when it is justified to breach confidentiality and notify and protect potential victims. Although practitioners are not generally legally liable for their failure to render perfect predictions of violent behavior of a client, an inadequate assessment of client dangerousness can result in liability for the therapist, harm to third parties, and inappropriate breaches of client confidentiality. Therapists faced with potentially dangerous clients should take specific steps to protect the public and to minimize their own liability. They should take careful histories, advise clients of the limits of confidentiality, keep accurate notes of threats and other client statements, seek several consultations, and record steps they have taken to protect others. Practitioners should consult with a supervisor or an attorney because they may be subject to liability for failing to notify those who are in danger. If a determination is made that an individual poses a high risk for harming an identifiable third party, mental health practitioners must develop and implement an intervention plan.

Mossman (2009) suggests that "violence prediction alone may be a futile approach to reducing violence" (p. 137). Referencing rampage shootings in the United States, Mossman points out that in hindsight we often perceive tragedies as being more easily foreseeable than they really were. Mossman points out that the risk factors we have are imperfect indicators of actual future violent acts. He believes clinical attention should be paid to risk prevention (rather than risk prediction) and that society should seek broad measures aimed at addressing known risks for violent behaviors among people who have and who do not have mental health problems.

Nearly every jurisdiction has a different interpretation of the duty to warn and the duty to protect, with some having no statute or case law related to the issues and others with very specific legal guidelines (Welfel, Werth, & Benjamin, 2009). Most states permit (if not require) therapists to breach confidentiality to warn or protect victims. Some states specify how that duty is to be discharged. Some states grant mental health practitioners immunity or protection from being sued for breaching confidentiality if they can demonstrate that they acted in good faith to notify or protect third parties. A few states have no mandatory duty to warn and to protect third parties, and therapists have no specific grant of immunity from civil suits for breaching confidentiality in those states. Some practitioners are concerned that laws requiring, rather than permitting, a warning may dissuade potentially violent individuals from seeking treatment or fully revealing their intentions, or that potential liability may discourage therapists from treating such clients because their ability to predict violent behavior is limited (Widgery & Winterfeld, 2013). Despite these concerns, counselors must be prepared to handle such disclosures.

In 1999 in the case of *Thapar v. Zezulka,* the Texas Supreme Court ruled that mental health workers do not have a duty to warn and protect their clients' known and intended victims. Basing its decision on the Texas statute governing the legal duty of mental health professionals to protect clients' confidentiality, the court found that it was unwise to impose a duty to warn on mental health practitioners. This decision reflected the justices' reluctance to violate existing state confidentiality statutes. Given the fact that various states have different interpretations of the duty to warn and protect, the most important message is to know the law in your state.

Welfel, Werth, and Benjamin (2009) differentiate between the duty to warn and the duty to protect. The **duty to warn** applies to those circumstances where case law or statute requires the mental health professional to make a reasonable effort to contact the identified victim of a client's serious threats of harm, or to notify law enforcement of the threat. The **duty to protect** applies to situations in which the mental health professional has a legal obligation to protect an identified third party who is being threatened; in these cases the therapist generally has other options in addition to warning the person of harm. The duty to protect provides ways of maintaining the client's confidentiality; the duty to warn requires a disclosure of confidential information to the person who is being threatened with harm.

Exercising a duty to warn can result in inappropriate breaches of confidentiality that damage the therapeutic relationship, which can end treatment. Furthermore, this course of action cannot guarantee another person's safety. Most mental health practitioners assume that they are mandated to take reasonable steps to warn an identified person of a foreseeable and imminent danger of serious harm when a client communicates an intention to harm a victim. However, in many situations, warning is not the only option or the best course to follow. Other appropriate actions include hospitalizing the client, increasing the frequency of therapy sessions, notifying the police, or referring a client for a psychiatric consult or for prescribing medication (DeMers & Siegel, 2016). Absent specific state laws mandating the duty to warn and to protect, Wheeler and Bertram (2015) believe mental health professionals may have an ethical duty to disclose information when it is necessary "to prevent clear and imminent danger to the client or others" (p. 145). They suggest the real question for counselors to ponder is: "How can I fulfill my legal and ethical duties to protect human life, act in the best interest of the client, and remain protected from potential liability?" (p. 145).

Implications of Landmark Court Cases

The responsibility to protect the public from dangerous acts of violent clients entails liability for civil damages when practitioners neglect this duty by (1) failing to diagnose or predict dangerousness, (2) failing to warn potential victims of violent behavior, (3) failing to commit dangerous individuals, or (4) prematurely discharging dangerous clients from a hospital (APA, 1985). The first two of these legally prescribed duties are illustrated in the case of *Tarasoff v. Board of Regents of the University of California* (1976), which has been the subject of extensive analysis in the psychological literature. As noted by Bersoff (2014), due to "the proliferation of mass shootings in the recent past, the ongoing push for legislation to control access to firearms, and the alleged connection between mental illness and violence, it may be particularly timely to revisit *Tarasoff v. Regents of the University of California*" (p. 461). The other two duties are set forth in additional landmark court cases. These cases provide case law governing the duty to warn only for the states in which the judgments were made. There is no overarching federal framework regarding these issues.

The *Tarasoff* Case In August 1969 Prosenjit Poddar was a voluntary outpatient at the student health service at the University of California, Berkeley and was in counseling with a psychologist named Moore. Poddar had confided to Moore his intention to kill an unnamed woman (who was readily identifiable as Tatiana Tarasoff) when she returned from an extended trip in Brazil. In consultation with other university counselors, Moore made the assessment that Poddar was dangerous and should be committed to a mental hospital for observation. Moore later called the campus police and told them of the death threat and of his conclusion that Poddar was dangerous. The campus officers did take Poddar into custody for questioning, but they later released him when he gave evidence of being "rational" and promised to stay away from Tarasoff. He was never confined to a treatment facility. Moore followed up his call with a formal letter requesting the assistance of the chief of the campus police. Later, Moore's supervisor asked that the letter be returned, ordered that the letter and Moore's case notes be destroyed, and asked that no further action be taken in the case. Tarasoff and her family were never made aware of this potential threat.

Shortly after Tarasoff's return from Brazil, Poddar killed her. Her parents filed suit against the Board of Regents and the employees of the university for having failed to notify the intended victim of the threat. When a lower court dismissed the suit in 1974, the parents appealed, and the California Supreme Court ruled in favor of the parents in 1976, holding that a failure to warn an intended victim was professionally irresponsible. The court's ruling requires that therapists breach confidentiality in cases where the general welfare and safety of others is involved. This was a California case, and courts in other states are not bound to decide a similar case in the same way.

Under the *Tarasoff* decision, the therapist must first accurately diagnose the client's tendency to behave in dangerous ways toward others. This first duty is judged by the standards of professional negligence. In this case the therapist did not fail in this duty. He even took the additional step of requesting that the dangerous person be detained by the campus police. However, the court held that merely notifying the police was not sufficient to protect the identifiable victim.

In the first ruling, in 1974, the lower court cited a **duty to warn**, but this duty was expanded by the 1976 California Supreme Court ruling, which said: "When a therapist determines . . . that his patient presents a serious danger of violence to another, he incurs an obligation to use reasonable care to protect the intended victim against such danger." Richard Leslie (2008) states that the "duty" created by the California Supreme Court in the *Tarasoff* decision was *not* a "duty to warn." According to Leslie, the court described the duty simply as a "duty to exercise reasonable care to protect the foreseeable victim" from the serious danger of violence against him or her.

According to Jensen (2012), the *duty to protect* can be discharged in a variety of ways, one of which involves hospitalization, whether voluntary or involuntary. Therapists can protect others through traditional clinical interventions such as reassessment, medication changes, and referral. Other steps therapists may take include warning potential victims, calling the police, or informing the state child protection agency. Negligence lies in the practitioner's failure to conduct an assessment for potential violence, failure to warn a third party of imminent danger, not in failing to predict any violence that may be committed. The goal of doing an assessment of dangerousness is to arrive at a reasoned and informed judgment about a client's capacity for seriously harming or killing another person: "In other words, you do not have to be perfect in predicting what will happen; you just have to be reasonably competent in assessing for what *could* happen" (p. 46).

The *Tarasoff* decision made it clear that client confidentiality can be readily compromised; indeed, "the protective privilege ends where the public peril begins" (as cited in Perlin, 1997). Mental health professionals have ethical and legal responsibilities to their clients, and they also have legal obligations to society. These dual responsibilities sometimes conflict, and they can create ambiguity in the therapeutic relationship. Welfel (2016) points out that courts interpret the duty to warn and protect to include situations in which therapists *should have known* about the danger. If ignorance about a dangerous situation is the result of incompetent or negligent practice, then professionals have neglected this duty. State courts and legislatures vary in their interpretations of *Tarasoff,* and practitioners remain uncertain about the nature of their duty to protect or to warn. However, the codes of ethics of most mental health professions incorporate this concept, and it is generally assumed that the duty to warn and to protect is a federal legal requirement. Although state laws differ on the specifics of notifying intended victims, for the most part, psychotherapists are required to take proactive steps when a client reveals a serious intention of harming another person (Knapp & VandeCreek, 2012). "A lawsuit alleging breach of this duty has been filed against the psychiatrist whose patient allegedly killed 12 people and injured dozens more in a movie theater in Aurora, Colorado" (Widgery & Winterfeld, 2013, p. 7).

Mandatory reporting laws only apply to threats regarding *future* violence. Reports by clients of *past* violence may not be reported and are protected as confidential information (Barnett & Johnson, 2015). A study conducted by Walfish, Barnett, Marlyere, and Zielke (2010) examined the incidence of client disclosures to their therapists of violent crimes they had committed for which they had not been prosecuted. Crimes such as murder, sexual assault, and physical assault were revealed. Based on their findings, Walfish et al. commented, "during the course of clinicians' careers there is a very high likelihood (69%) that a client will tell them he or she has physically assaulted someone, a moderate likelihood (33%) that a client will tell them that he or she has sexually assaulted someone, and a small (13%) but not infinitesimal chance that he or she has even murdered someone, outside of killing a person in the line of duty in the military or as a public peace officer, without being reported to the proper authority and/or prosecuted" (p. 319).

Mental health professionals should be familiar with the warning signs and risk factors for violence and the potential for acting out. Therapists should conduct a formal risk assessment with all clients who show any warning signs for violence. They should also be familiar with the treatment options and resources for managing high-risk clients in their local area (Barnett & Johnson, 2015). The first critical step in applying *Tarasoff* is to assess for dangerousness. This assessment may lead you to the conclusion that your client poses a serious risk of killing or physically injuring another person. If this judgment is made, your records need to reflect why you believe your client is reasonably likely to commit violence. According to Bersoff (2014):

> *Tarasoff* and the cases that adopt its holding present the therapist with complex problems requiring nuanced decisions. The therapist must tread a thin line between protecting confidentiality and protecting the potential victim. An error on either side of this line can lead to liability—either for malpractice in unreasonably breaching

confidentiality or for wrongful death for failure to warn in the face of a real threat. But beyond the private interests at stake, these cases raise a more fundamental issue, the dilution of privacy" (p. 466).

Therapists are often concerned about legal responsibility when the identity of the intended victim is unknown. VandeCreek and Knapp (2001) recommend seeking consultation with other professionals who have expertise in dealing with potentially violent people and documenting the steps taken. They add that therapists do well to adhere to risk management strategies in dealing with dangerous clients. In particular, therapists need to be especially careful about grounds for liability including abandonment; failure to consult, refer, or coordinate treatment with a physician; maintaining adequate records; and responding appropriately if a suit is filed.

In *Ewing v. Goldstein* (2004) the California courts broadened the practitioner's duty to warn by declaring that therapists must break confidentiality if they receive information from a family member about a client's intention to seriously harm another person (Nagy, 2011). This court decision means that licensed therapists in California could be held liable for failure to issue a *Tarasoff* warning when the information regarding the dangerousness of a client comes from a client's family member rather than from the client. "Ultimately *Tarasoff* comes down to two responsibilities: assessing for violence, and if the assessment reveals the likelihood of violence, discharging the duty to protect" (Jensen, 2012, p. 50).

The *Bradley* Case A second case illustrates the duty not to negligently release a dangerous client. In *Bradley Center v. Wessner* (1982) the patient, Wessner, had been voluntarily admitted to a Georgia facility for psychiatric care. Wessner was upset over his wife's extramarital affair. He had repeatedly threatened to kill her and her lover and had even admitted to a therapist that he was carrying a weapon in his car for that purpose. He was given an unrestricted weekend pass to visit his children, who were living with his wife. He met his wife and her lover in the home and shot and killed them. The children filed a wrongful death suit, alleging that the psychiatric center had breached a duty to exercise control over Wessner. The Georgia Supreme Court ruled that a physician has a duty to take reasonable care to prevent a potentially dangerous patient from inflicting harm (Laughran & Bakken, 1984).

The *Jablonski* Case A third legal ruling underscores the duty to commit a dangerous individual. The intended victim's knowledge of a threat does not relieve therapists of the duty to protect, as can be seen by the decision in *Jablonski v. United States* (1983). Meghan Jablonski filed suit for the wrongful death of her mother, Melinda Kimball, who was murdered by Philip Jablonski, the man with whom she had been living. Earlier, Philip Jablonski had agreed to a psychiatric examination at a hospital. The physicians determined that there was no emergency and thus no basis for involuntary commitment. Kimball later again accompanied Jablonski to the hospital and expressed fears for her own safety. She was told by a doctor that "you should consider staying away from him." Again, the doctors concluded that there was no basis for involuntary hospitalization and released him. Shortly thereafter Jablonski killed Kimball. The Ninth U.S. Circuit Court of Appeals found that failure to obtain Jablonski's prior medical history constituted malpractice. The essence of *Jablonski* is a negligent failure to commit (Laughran & Bakken, 1984).

The *Hedlund* Case A fourth legal ruling, *Hedlund v. Superior Court* (1983), extends the duty to warn in California to a foreseeable, identifiable person who might be near the intended victim when the threat is carried out and thus might also be in danger. LaNita Wilson and Stephen Wilson had received psychotherapy from a psychological assistant, Bonnie Hedlund. During treatment Stephen Wilson told the therapist that he intended to harm LaNita Wilson. Later he did assault her, in the presence of her child. The allegation was that the child had sustained "serious emotional injury and psychological trauma."

In keeping with the *Tarasoff* decision, the California Supreme Court held (1) that a therapist has a duty first to exercise a "reasonable degree of skill, knowledge, and care ordinarily possessed and exercised by members [of that professional specialty] under similar circumstances" in making a prediction about the chances of a client's acting dangerously to others; and (2) that therapists must "exercise reasonable care to protect the foreseeable victim of that danger." One way to protect the victim is by giving a warning of peril. The court held that breach of such a duty with respect to third persons constitutes "professional negligence" (Laughran & Bakken, 1984).

In the *Hedlund* case the duty to warn of potentially dangerous conduct applied to the mother, not to her child, against whom no threats had been made. However, the court found that a therapist could be held liable for injuries sustained by the intended victim's child if the violent act was carried out. The court held that a therapist must consider the welfare of the intended victim as well as the welfare of persons in close relationship to the victim when determining how to best protect the potential victim.

Guidelines for Dealing With Dangerous Clients

Most counseling centers and community mental health agencies now have guidelines regarding the duty to warn and protect when the welfare of others is at stake. These guidelines generally specify how to deal with emotionally disturbed individuals, violent behavior, threats, suicidal possibilities, and other circumstances in which counselors may be legally and ethically required to breach confidentiality. In response to the April 16, 2007, school shooting on the Virginia Tech campus in which 33 people were killed, task forces were formed in several states to create significant changes to the policies and procedures at college counseling centers and campus security offices (Davenport, 2009). According to Davenport, "what constitutes 'risk' on our college campuses is continually changing and intensifying" (p. 181), leading college counselors to increasingly adopt the role of risk managers. Despite measures taken by secondary schools and postsecondary institutions to prepare for such crisis situations, devastating acts of violence and mass shootings continue to plague the United States. There have been 215 school shootings in the United States since the massacre of 20 children and six adults at Sandy Hook

Elementary School in Newtown, Connecticut, on December 14, 2012 (Everytown for Gun Safety, 2015).

As clinicians, we believe one of the problems with being able to piece together a true picture of potential for violence is a lack of communication between all parties working with, or on behalf of, a potentially violent client. Counselors working with potentially high-risk clients should have a release of information in place so a more complete picture of the client's level of functioning can be determined. The dangerous behaviors or warning signs may be witnessed in one or more arenas, but key health care workers often do not have permission to speak to one another.

Understandably, many counselors find it difficult to predict when clients pose a serious threat to others. Clients are encouraged to engage in open dialogue in therapeutic relationships. Although clients at times may express feelings or thoughts about doing physical harm to others, this does not mean that these threats will be carried out. Thus, it is not realistic to expect counselors to routinely reveal all verbal threats. Notifying a third party of a threat is a relatively rare event. Breaking confidentiality can seriously harm the client–therapist relationship as well as the relationship between the client and the person "threatened." Such disclosures should be carefully evaluated. In making decisions about when to warn, counselors should seek consultation, exercise reasonable professional judgment, and apply practices that are commonly accepted by professionals in the specialty. In most cases therapists will not have advanced warning that a client is dangerous. Therefore, therapists must be prepared for such an eventuality. We offer the following suggestions:

- Examine your informed consent document. Is it clear in terms of the forfeiture of confidentiality because of a threat of violence to self or others?
- Know how to contact your professional organization for assistance. For example, the American Counseling Association's Ethics and Risk Management Services are available to members. You also may want to consider consulting with your own local health care attorney.
- Review the code of ethics of your professional organization on matters applicable to your practice.
- Familiarize yourself with professionals who are experienced in dealing with violence and know how to reach them.
- In the initial interview, if there is any hint of violence in the client's history, request clinical records from previous therapists, if they exist.
- Take at least one workshop in the assessment and management of dangerous clients.
- Determine that the limits of your professional liability insurance are adequate.

Wheeler and Bertram (2015) suggest some practical risk management guidelines in dealing with duty to warn and protect situations:

- Consult with colleagues or a supervisor.
- Consult with an attorney if you are not clear about your legal duty.
- Know the law in your state and whether it requires a communicated threat against a specifically identifiable victim or if it encompasses a broader duty.
- Obtain prior medical and behavioral history.

- Inquire about a client's access to weapons, homicidal ideation, and intentions, which would include whether a specific victim is involved.
- In cases of immediate threat by a client, do not hesitate to take steps to prevent harm to yourself even if it means potentially fracturing your relationship with the client.
- Make referrals where appropriate.
- Consider all appropriate steps to take and the consequences of each.
- Know and follow the policy of your institution.
- Document the people you consulted, all the actions you take, those you reject, and the rationale behind each of your decisions.

If you have prepared yourself for the eventuality of a dangerous client, you will have a better sense of what to do in these circumstances. In addition, your liability will be reduced if you have followed a prudent course of action and can demonstrate that you acted within the standard of care expected of a competent mental health professional.

As you think about the following case, ask yourself how you would assess the degree to which Isaac is potentially dangerous. What would you do if you were the therapist in this case?

The Case of Isaac

Isaac has been seeing Dr. Schultz, his therapist, for several months. One day he comes to the therapy session inebriated and very angry. He has just found out that a close friend is having an affair with his girlfriend. He is deeply wounded over this incident. He is also highly agitated and even talks about killing the friend who betrayed him. As he puts it, "I am so damn mad I feel like getting my gun and shooting him." Isaac experiences intense emotions in this session. Dr. Schultz does everything she can to defuse his rage and to stabilize him before the session ends. The session continues for about 2 hours (instead of the usual hour), and she asks him to call her a couple of times each day to check in. Before he leaves, she develops a safety plan with him that includes an agreement that he will not go over to this man's house and that he will not act out his urges. Because of the strength of the therapeutic relationship, she assessed Isaac as not being a violent person and decided not to follow through with the duty to warn. He follows through and calls her every day. When he comes to the session the following week, he admits to still being in a great deal of pain over his discovery, but he no longer feels so angry. As he puts it, "I am not going to land in jail because of this jerk!" He tells Dr. Schultz how helpful the last session was in allowing him to get a lot off his chest.

- Do you think Dr. Schultz followed the proper ethical and legal course of action in this case?
- Did she fulfill her responsibilities by making sure that Isaac called her twice a day and by developing a safety plan with him? Why or why not?
- Some would say that she should have broken confidentiality and warned the intended victim. What do you think? Explain your reasoning.
- What criteria could you use to determine whether the situation is dangerous enough to warn a potential victim? What is the fine line between overreacting and failing to respond appropriately in this kind of case?
- If Dr. Schultz had sought you out for consultation in this case immediately after the session at which Isaac talked about wanting to kill his friend, how would you have advised her?
- Is there any evidence that Dr. Schultz acted negligently in any way?

Commentary. Dr. Schultz did an assessment of dangerousness and received several commitments from Isaac to restrain his behavior. Although a verbal threat of the intent to harm another person is a key factor, other factors to consider include the context in which the threat is made, the intent, Isaac's history of violence, use of drugs and alcohol, and the availability of opportunity. Dr. Schultz's assessment that Isaac was not dangerous was based on her 5-month relationship with him and her trust in him to honor their agreements. To her credit, she implemented a safety plan with Isaac, which could identify alternative behaviors in a stepwise fashion to reduce risk and deescalate dangerous behavior. From both an ethical and legal perspective, it is critical that Dr. Schultz seek consultation in the process of making her decision on how to deal with Isaac's threat. Dr. Schultz may be less inclined to see Isaac as violent, even if he is, because of her therapeutic relationship with him. By not consulting with colleagues, Dr. Schultz potentially put herself, her client, and others at risk. •

Implications of Duty to Warn and to Protect for School Counselors

The basic standard of care for school counselors is clear; courts have uniformly held that school personnel have a duty to protect students from foreseeable harm (Hermann & Remley, 2000). The duty to protect vulnerable children is also a well-articulated standard in the field of psychology. School personnel may need to act on student reports of their peers' plans related to intended violence. Furthermore, school officials may be held accountable if a student's writing assignments contain evidence of premeditated violence.

Hermann and Finn (2002) contend that school counselors are legally and ethically obligated to work toward preventing school violence. They state that school counselors may find themselves legally vulnerable because of their role in determining whether students pose a risk of harm to others and deciding on appropriate interventions with these students. Current case law reveals that all indicators of potential violence should be taken seriously.

Moyer and coauthors (2012) suggest that ethics codes "provide no explanation as to what constitutes a potentially disruptive or damaging behavior, and individual school counselors are likely to interpret this differently" (p. 98). Despite the lack of guidance in the codes, preventing students from harming other students seems to be implicit in the duty of school personnel. Courts have consistently found that school counselors have a duty to exercise reasonable care to protect students from foreseeable harm, but they are only exposed to legal liability if they fail to exercise reasonable care (Hermann & Remley, 2000).

School counselors try to provide a safe place for students to disclose their personal problems, but these counselors also have a reporting duty in many instances. School counselors need to assess a student's dangerousness by evaluating the student's plans for implementing the violent act and his or her ability to carry out the act. Moyer and colleagues (2012) surveyed school counselors to get their impressions of when it is ethical to inform administrators about risky student behaviors. In their study, counselors deemed it more ethical to break confidentiality when the behaviors were directly observed rather than when reported by students and when the risk-taking behaviors occurred during school hours on the school campus. These counselors also showed a greater willingness to breach confidentiality when they were supported by written school policies guiding their interventions. Given the context of emerging case law and the violent climate of today's schools, school counselors would do well to take threats of violence seriously. The central ethical concern surrounding this issue involves the commitment of mental health professionals to develop organized prevention efforts in response to school violence.

School counselors and mental health professionals must be prepared to respond to crises when they do occur. Given the high level of visibility of school violence today, Fein, Carlisle, and Isaacson (2008) suggest that school counselors be prepared to lead and to assume responsibilities that may be beyond the scope of their formal training. They may have to respond to the needs and demands of students, staff, and administrators and adopt multiple roles, which may create inherent role conflicts.

The following case illustrates a challenge school counselors might face in dealing with students who pose a danger to others.

The Case of Blaise

Blaise is a high school student who seems to have the potential for violence. During his sessions with you, he talks about his impulses to hurt others and himself, and he describes times when he has seriously beaten his girlfriend, Lucy. He tells you that she is afraid to leave him because she thinks he will beat her even more savagely. He later tells you that sometimes he gets so angry that he feels like killing her. You believe Blaise could seriously harm and possibly even kill Lucy. Which of the following would you do? Check all that apply.

_____ 1. I would notify Lucy that she might be in grave danger, if I knew of her identity.

_____ 2. I would notify the police or other authorities.

_____ 3. I would keep Blaise's threats to myself because I could not be sure that he would act on them.

_____ 4. I would seek a second opinion from a colleague.

_____ 5. I would inform my director or supervisor.

_____ 6. I would refer Blaise to another therapist.

_____ 7. I would arrange to have Blaise hospitalized.

Would you answer differently if Blaise showed real promise in therapy and seemed to really want to change his behavior?

Commentary. Because Blaise is voluntarily seeing a therapist and is disclosing his impulses and behavior, he may want to change. However, you must consider specific actions, comments, and threats that Blaise has made in determining the appropriate course of action to take. He has seriously beaten Lucy and she is afraid to leave him. He also tells you that sometimes he gets so angry that he feels like killing her, and you believe he is capable of this violence. The seriousness of Blaise's actions poses a clear danger to others, which you cannot ethically or legally ignore. Notifying the police is in order because Lucy cannot be relied upon to inform the police. You may be able to continue therapy after notifying the police if Blaise agrees to this, or you can help him find other appropriate resources, such as an anger management program. ●

The Duty to Protect Suicidal Clients

In the preceding discussion we emphasized the therapist's obligation to protect others from dangerous individuals. The guidelines and principles outlined in that discussion often apply to the client who poses a danger to self. As part of the informed consent process, therapists must inform clients that they have an ethical and legal obligation to break confidentiality when they have good reason to suspect suicidal behavior. Even if clients argue that they can do what they want with their own lives, including taking them, therapists have a legal **duty to protect suicidal clients.** The crux of the issue is knowing when to take a client's hints seriously enough to report the condition. Certainly not every mention of suicidal thoughts or feelings justifies extraordinary measures.

The evaluation and management of suicidal risk can be a source of great stress for therapists. Clinical practitioners must face many troublesome issues, including their degree of influence, competence, level of involvement with a client, responsibility, legal obligations, and ability to make life-or-death decisions. If a client dies by suicide, the risk of a malpractice action is greatly reduced if the therapist can demonstrate that a reasonable assessment and intervention process took place; professional consultation was sought; clinical referrals were made when appropriate; and thorough and current documentation was done (Jobes & O'Connor, 2009). Counselors can be accused of malpractice for neglecting to take action to prevent harm when a client is likely to take the step of suicide, yet they are also liable if they overreact by taking actions that violate a client's privacy when there is not a justifiable basis for doing so (Remley & Herlihy, 2016).

The law does not require practitioners to always make correct assessments of suicide risk, but therapists do have a legal duty to make assessments from an informed position and to carry out their professional obligations in a manner comparable to what other reasonable professionals would do in similar situations. If a counselor makes a determination that a client is at risk for suicide, the counselor should take the least intrusive steps necessary to prevent the harm (Remley & Herlihy, 2016). Consult with experienced colleagues when you are faced with clients who are at risk for self-harm, and be sure to document the nature of your discussions with colleagues.

Ethical Issues in Assessing and Treating Nonsuicidal Self-Injury

Although self-injury is a predictor of suicide, it is a mistake to assume that most people who self-injure are suicidal. However, counselors who work with clients who self-injure will most likely deal with ethical dilemmas regarding safety and duty to warn/protect. Whisenhunt, Stargell, and Perjessy (2016) state that "nonsuicidal self-injury is a complex and often misunderstood issue that may require counselors to reevaluate their assumptions and biases before providing safe and effective treatment" (p. 40). They suggest that counselors need education and training in effective ways of intervening with clients who self-injure. Whisenhunt and colleagues believe practitioners need to understand the futility of focusing mainly on stopping the behavior and instead address the underlying dynamics of self-injurious behavior if they hope to facilitate behavioral change with individuals who self-injure. Self-injury can be a way to transform emotional pain into physical pain, which is often easier to cope with for many people. Lecturing such individuals will not lead to a readiness for change, whereas supporting clients in sharing their stories can be therapeutic.

It is important to monitor and continually assess for the risk of serious harm and the potential for suicide, especially when counseling minors. Confidentiality and privacy need to be explained during the informed consent process, including how self-injury might result in mandatory reporting.

School Counselor Liability for Student Suicide

Suicide by a student is perhaps the greatest tragedy on a campus, and one that shocks the entire school community. Recognizing signs of potential suicide and preventing suicide certainly have to be among the major challenges school counselors face. School counselors are expected to be aware of the warning signs of suicidal behavior and need to have the skills necessary to assess a student's risk for suicide (Capuzzi & Gross, 2008). To manage the legal risks associated with their jobs, school counselors must be prepared to determine whether a student may be at risk for suicide (Capuzzi, 2009). Evans and Hurrell's (2016) systematic review of qualitative research on the role schools play in children's self-harm and suicide found that only the most severe forms of self-harm are defined as such by school personnel. Thus many problematic behaviors are rendered invisible. This issue is compounded by structural barriers, such as the limited time staff have to spend with individual students, which reduce opportunities for detection and disclosure.

School counselors who do not possess competency in identifying and managing students who may be suicidal need supervision, consultation, and direction from counselors who possess such expertise (Remley, 2009). Although school counselors are not expected to predict all suicide gestures or attempts, they are expected to use sound judgment in making clinical decisions, and their reasoning should be documented in their notes. In cases where school counselors make an assessment that a student is at risk for suicide, it is imperative that the student's parents or guardians be notified that such an assessment took place. Parents or guardians have a legal right to know when their child may be in danger.

Court Cases In school settings, some courts have found a special relationship between school personnel and students. Hermann (2001) has documented this, and our discussion is based on her work. One of the first cases that addressed school counselor liability for student suicide was *Eisel v. Board of Education* (1991). In this case, 13-year-old Nicole was involved in Satanism. Nicole made a suicide pact with another student, who subsequently shot Nicole and then shot herself. Fellow students had told their school counselor that Nicole wanted to take her own life. When the school counselor confronted Nicole about her suicidal intentions, she denied making any such statements. The counselor did not attempt to contact Nicole's parents. In *Eisel* the court found that school counselors have a duty to use reasonable means to attempt to prevent a suicide when they know about a student's suicidal intentions. The reasoning of the court was that an adolescent is more likely to share thoughts of suicide with friends than with a school counselor, teacher, or parent. The court found that reasonable care would have included notifying Nicole's parents that their daughter was at risk for suicide. Although the suicide occurred off the school premises, the court held that legally the school could be held liable for failure to exercise reasonable care to prevent a foreseeable injury.

Even if the risk of the student actually committing suicide is remote, the possibility may be enough to establish a duty to contact the parents or the guardians and to inform them of the potential for suicidal behavior. Courts have found that the burden involved in making a telephone call is minor considering the risk of harm to a student who is suicidal. In short, school personnel are advised to take every suicide threat seriously and to take every precaution to protect the student.

The courts have addressed the need for training school employees in suicide prevention. The *Wyke v. Polk County School Board* (1997) case involved a 13-year-old named Shawn, who attempted suicide two times at school before finally killing himself at home. School officials were aware of the suicide attempts, yet they failed to notify Shawn's mother. During the trial, several experts in the field of suicide prevention testified about the need for suicide prevention training in schools, including mandatory written policies requiring parental notification, holding students in protective custody, and arranging for counseling services. The experts who testified at the trial believed the school board failed to provide adequate training for school personnel. Without training, school personnel will most likely underestimate the lethality of suicidal thoughts, statements, and attempts. The conclusion of this expert testimony was that Shawn would not have committed suicide if the employees had been adequately trained. Persuaded by this input, the court held that the school could be found negligent for failing to notify the decedent's mother.

If you are aiming for a career as a school counselor, you will need more than this basic knowledge regarding your ethical and legal obligations to respond in a professional manner in situations where students may pose a danger to themselves or others. It is important that you know the school district's policy on dealing with suicidal clients. Continuing education is of the utmost importance, as is your willingness to seek appropriate consultation when you become aware of students who are at risk.

The Case of Vijay

Vijay, a 16-year-old high school student, is being seen by the school psychologist, Dr. Roshawn, at the request of his parents. Vijay's school work has dropped off, he has become withdrawn socially, and he has expressed to his parents that he has thought of suicide, even though he has not made a specific plan. After the psychologist has seen Vijay for several weeks of individual counseling, his concerned parents call and ask how he is doing. They wonder whether they should be alert to possible suicide attempts. Vijay's parents tell Dr. Roshawn that they want to respect confidentiality and are not interested in detailed disclosures but that they want to find out if they have cause for worry. Without going into detail, Dr. Roshawn reassures them that they really do not need to worry.

- Is Dr. Roshawn's behavior ethical? Would it make a difference if Vijay were 25 years old?
- Does Dr. Roshawn have an ethical obligation to inform Vijay of the conversation with his parents?

- If the parents were to insist on having more information, does Dr. Roshawn have an obligation to say more?

- Did Dr. Roshawn have sufficient information to justify telling the parents that they have no need to worry?

- If Dr. Roshawn provides details to the parents, does he have an obligation to inform Vijay before talking with his parents?

- Would Dr. Roshawn be remiss if he had not informed Vijay about the limits of confidentiality?

- Other than doing what this school psychologist did, do you see other courses of action?

- If Vijay were indeed suicidal, what ethical and legal obligations would Dr. Roshawn have toward the parents? Would he have to inform the school principal?

Commentary. This case shows the importance of knowing the law in your state or jurisdiction pertaining to confidentiality in counseling minors. What are the rights of the parents/guardians? What are the minor client's rights? To prevent later misunderstandings, it is good practice initially to have a dialogue with both the minor client and the parents/guardians regarding what details may be shared regarding the progress of therapy. A discussion of the limits of confidentiality is also in order. Good practice also involves informing the minor client of any times when there is a discussion between the parents and the therapist. When Vijay's parents asked the therapist for information, they could have been invited to a session with their son (with his permission) to express their concerns with him being present. This would enable Vijay to be part of the discussion and, with the counselor's help, to choose what to disclose directly to his parents. ●

Guidelines for Assessing Suicidal Behavior

Mental health professionals cannot predict or prevent all client suicides, but they can learn to recognize common crises that may precipitate a suicide attempt and reach out to people who are experiencing these crises. Counselors must take the "cry for help" seriously. Mental health professionals are expected to complete a comprehensive assessment of clients, especially with clients who pose a threat to themselves. Suicide risk assessment requires clinicians to identify client risk factors, warning signs, and protective factors that can work to mitigate the risk. Learning about these warning signs and risk factors is a key component of assessing for suicidal behavior (Granello, 2010).

Wheeler and Bertram (2015) assert that therapists who fail to conduct an adequate assessment of a client are vulnerable to a malpractice claim. If a client denies suicidal intent, yet shows evidence of serious depression, the therapist should inquire further and possibly make a referral to a psychiatrist for further evaluation. In an assessment interview, it is important to focus on evaluating depression, suicide ideation, suicide intention, suicide plans, and the presence of any risk factors associated with suicide. Granello (2010) notes that it is critical to uncover a client's underlying message because there are as many reasons for a suicide as there are suicidal individuals. Understanding the underlying message will determine, to a great extent, the interventions to use. In the assessment, it is useful to obtain information about a client's past treatment. In crisis counseling, assess your clients for suicidal risk during the early phase of therapy, and keep alert to this issue during the course of therapy. Danger signs, such as the following, should be evaluated:

- Take direct verbal warnings seriously, as they are one of the most useful single predictors of a suicide. Be sure to document your actions.
- Find out if there were previous suicide attempts, as these are the best single predictor of lethality.
- Identify clients suffering from depression, a characteristic common to all suicide victims. Sleep disruption, which can intensify depression, is a key sign. For people with clinical depression the suicide rate is about 20 times greater than that of the general population.
- Be alert for feelings of hopelessness and helplessness, which seem to be closely associated with suicidal intentions. Explore the client's ideational and mood states. Individuals may feel desperate, guilt-ridden, and worthless.
- Consider the client's level of impulsivity, which can increase risk for both planned and unplanned suicide. This may be especially true for adolescents and young adults.
- Consider the client's ability to problem solve. Limited problem-solving abilities can exacerbate risk, whereas complex problem-solving abilities can help to insulate against suicide risk (e.g., the client's ability to see alternate solutions to difficult life events).
- Explore carefully the interpersonal stressor of loss and separation, such as a relationship breakup or the death of a loved one.
- Monitor severe anxiety and panic attacks.
- Ascertain whether there has been a recent diagnosis of a serious or terminal health condition.
- Determine whether the individual has a plan. The more definite the plan, the more serious is the situation. Suicidal individuals should be asked to talk about their plans and be encouraged to explore their suicidal fantasies.
- Identify clients who have a history of severe alcohol or drug abuse, as they are at greater risk than the general population. Alcohol is a contributing factor in one fourth to one third of all suicides.
- Be alert to client behaviors such as giving away prized possessions, finalizing business affairs, or revising wills.
- Determine whether clients have a history of previous psychiatric treatment or hospitalization. Clients who have been hospitalized for emotional disorders are more likely to be inclined to suicide.
- Determine whether the individual has access to lethal means, especially firearms, and take steps to limit this access. This may involve working with family members or loved ones to remove lethal means from the home.
- Assess the client's support system. If there is no support system, the client is at greater risk.
- Ascertain whether there has been any suicide in the family; risk is particularly elevated when a parent was lost to suicide.
- If the client verbalizes suicidal ideation, talk with the person about whether he or she wants to die or wants the pain to end. The latter is likely more amendable to therapeutic intervention.

Therapists have the responsibility to prevent suicide if they can reasonably anticipate it. Once it is determined that a client is at risk for serious harm to self, the professional is legally and ethically required to take appropriate action aimed at protecting the person. Liability generally arises when a counselor fails to act in such a way as to prevent the suicide or when a counselor does something that might contribute to it. Obtain consultation from knowledgeable colleagues or from clinical supervisors (Wheeler & Bertram, 2015). Counselors with limited experience in suicide assessment should not rely on their own clinical judgment; rather, they should seek consultation and supervision from professionals with experience in this area. Mental health professionals are expected to make their assessments from an informed position and to fulfill their obligations to a client by acting in a professional manner (Remley & Herlihy, 2016). Even clinicians with years of experience can benefit from consultation on their assessment and decisions when dealing with potentially suicidal individuals. Therapists' clinical decisions and their reasoning should be recorded in their notes.

The final decision about the degree of suicidal risk is a subjective one that demands professional judgment. In evaluating liability the courts assess the reasonableness of professional judgment in treating a suicidal person. If a client demonstrates suicidal intent, and the therapist does not exercise reasonable precautions, there are grounds for liability. If a client makes a serious declaration of ending his or her life, the therapist is justified in intervening rapidly by voluntary hospitalization or other measures to protect the client (Knapp & VandeCreek, 2012).

Steps in Suicide Prevention Suicidal individuals often hope that somebody will listen to their cry. Many are struggling with short-term crises, and if they can be given help in learning to cope with the immediate problem, their potential for suicide can be greatly reduced.

Expectations for action by mental health professionals dealing with suicidal clients differ depending on the setting. In school settings, the law imposes a duty to take precautions to protect students who may be suicidal. A similar standard exists in hospital settings. However, legal opinions are not consistent when addressing suicidal clients in outpatient settings. It should be noted that successful lawsuits have been brought against therapists who did not follow standard procedures to protect a client's life (Austin, Moline, & Williams, 1990).

Safety Plans Written safety plans have become a common intervention in suicide prevention with high-risk clients. Templates for a safety plan are available in a variety of formats. The therapist and client collaborate in developing a personalized safety plan, which is designed to assist the client in weathering the storm of suicidal thoughts and impulses. The safety plan usually has an introductory paragraph designed to instill hope in clients, reminding them that most suicidal thoughts are transitory and decrease when individuals engage in alternative behaviors. Clients are then asked to list their reasons for living. If they cannot think of any reason to live, this may be diagnostic and indicative for the need of a higher level of care. Subsequently, clients are asked to identify a few self-soothing behaviors in which they can engage (e.g., listening to music, taking a bath, going for a walk). They are then asked to list the names and phone numbers of two people they can call for assistance or just to have a conversation as a distraction from suicidal thoughts. Again, if clients are unable to identify a single person to call, this may be indicative of the need for a higher level of care. Clients are provided with the phone numbers of emergency suicide prevention resources (suicide hotlines, mobile crisis intervention teams) and are advised to go to the nearest emergency room if they try everything on the safety plan and are still feeling suicidal. The safety plan is an intervention used outside of the consulting room, and it is provided in writing because clients who are in suicidal crisis often are unable to remember everything that was recommended in the therapy session.

Safety plans can be usefully applied in cases involving client self-injury as well. Even if suicidal ideation is not present, clients can use safety plans when they are experiencing distress and emotional pain. A no-harm contract has many limitations, but safety plans are an effective way to enhance the therapeutic relationship and minimize risk of serious harm. Whisenhunt and colleagues (2016) stress the importance of conducting suicide risk assessments at intake and periodically with clients who self-injure. It is essential to create a safe and nonjudgmental climate that encourages clients to talk about their emotional pain and to explore alternative coping strategies to stress beside self-injury. Safety plans can provide a context for exploring healthy ways of coping with stress. "At a minimum, safety plans include identification of warning signs, internal coping strategies, positive distractions, people to ask for help, professionals/agencies to ask for help and ways to make the environment safer" (p. 44).

Managing Suicidal Clients The following recommendations for managing suicidal behavior have been collected from a variety of sources (see Austin et al., 1990; Barnett & Johnson, 2008, 2015; Bednar, Bednar, Lambert, & Waite, 1991; Bennett et al., 1990, 2006; Bonger, 2013; Granello, 2010; Peruzzi & Bongar, 1999; Pope & Vasquez, 2016; Remley, 2004, 2009; Remley & Herlihy, 2016; Rosenberg, 1999; Sommers-Flanagan & Sommers-Flanagan, 1995; Wheeler & Bertram, 2015):

- Know how to determine whether a client may be at risk for attempting suicide.
- Assess each new client for suicidal thoughts, regardless of the reason the client is seeking counseling.
- Deal candidly with matters of confidentiality, privilege, and privacy.
- Be knowledgeable about the legal requirements bearing on mandatory reporting of suicidal clients and limits of confidentiality in your jurisdiction.
- Clearly outline the limits of confidentiality and the steps you will need to take if your client poses a risk of self harm.
- Obtain education, training, and supervision in suicide risk assessment, suicide prevention, and crisis intervention methods.
- Keep up to date with current research, theory, and practice regarding suicide prevention.
- Work with the suicidal client to create a supportive environment.
- Periodically collaborate with colleagues and ask for their views regarding the client's condition. Consult with as many colleagues as possible when making

difficult decisions and document these discussions. This collaboration can be critical in understanding the level of risk.

- Consult with and involve family members and significant others, when appropriate.
- Collaborate with clients in developing a written safety plan that addresses steps they can take to reduce suicidal risk. Remind these clients of their personal strengths and reasons for living; provide contact information for emergency suicide prevention services (hotlines, mobile crisis teams) and explain how to access the nearest emergency room should all other strategies fail.
- Specify your availability to your clients; let them know how they can contact you during your absences.
- Realize that you may have the responsibility to prevent suicide if the act can be reasonably foreseen.
- Recognize the limits of your competence and know when and how to refer.
- Use sensitivity and caution in terminating or referring a client who has been or is currently suicidal. Be careful to ensure that this transition goes smoothly and that the client does not feel abandoned in the process.
- Consider hospitalization, weighing the benefits and the drawbacks.
- For services that take place within a clinic or agency setting, ensure that clear and appropriate lines of responsibility are explicit and are fully understood by everyone.
- Work with clients so that dangerous instruments are not within easy access. If the client possesses any weapons, put them in the hands of a third party.
- Consider increasing the frequency of the counseling sessions.
- Work with clients' strengths and desires to remain alive.
- Attempt to communicate a realistic sense of hope.
- Be willing to communicate your caring.
- As much as possible, involve the client in the decisions and actions being taken. It is important for clients to share in the responsibility for their ultimate decisions.
- Document the client's mental status, your ongoing risk assessments, and your treatment plan decisions in the client's record. Document options you considered, options you ruled out, actions taken, results of your interventions, and follow-up. "According to the law, a suicide risk assessment that is not documented did not happen" (Granello, 2010, p. 368).
- Know your personal limits and your own reactions to working with suicidal clients. Recognize the stresses involved and the toll this work takes on you personally and professionally. Seek appropriate consultation, practice self-care, and try to limit the number of suicidal clients with whom you work.
- Attempt to develop a supportive network of family and friends to help clients face their struggles. Discuss this with clients and enlist their help in building this resource of caring people.

Remember that clients are ultimately responsible for their own actions and that there is only so much that you can reasonably do to prevent self-destructive actions. Even though you take specific steps to lessen the chances of a client's suicide, the client may still take this ultimate step. The courts recognize that not all suicides are preventable, and they tend to support mental health practitioners who make consistent and systematic efforts to protect their clients (Granello, 2010).

What is your position with respect to your ethical obligations to recognize, evaluate, and intervene with potentially suicidal clients? To what degree do you agree with the guidelines discussed in this chapter? Which guidelines make the most sense to you? After clarifying your own thoughts underlying the professional's role in assessing and preventing suicide, reflect on the following case of a client who is contemplating suicide.

The Case of Emmanuel

Emmanuel is a middle-aged widower who complains of emptiness in life, loneliness, depression, and a loss of the will to live. He has been in individual therapy for 7 months with a psychologist. Using psychodiagnostic procedures, she has determined that Emmanuel has serious depressive tendencies and is potentially self-destructive. In their sessions he talks about the history of his failures, the isolation he feels, the meaninglessness of his life, and his feelings of worthlessness and depression. With her encouragement he experiments with new ways of behaving in the hope that he will find reasons to go on living. Finally, after 7 months of searching, he decides that he wants to take his own life. He tells his therapist that he is convinced he has been deluding himself in thinking that anything in his life will change for the better and that he feels good about deciding to end his life. He informs her that he will not be seeing her again.

The therapist expresses her concern that Emmanuel is very capable of taking his life. She acknowledges that the decision to end his life by suicide is not a sudden one, but she lets him know that she wants him to give therapy more of a chance. He says that he is truly grateful to her for helping him. He says firmly that he does not want her to attempt to obstruct his plans in any way. She asks that he postpone his decision for a week and return to discuss the matter more fully. He tells her he isn't certain whether he will keep this appointment, but he agrees to consider it.

The therapist does nothing further. During the following week she hears from a friend that Emmanuel has ended his own life.

- What do you think of the way the therapist dealt with her client?
- What would you have done differently if you had been Emmanuel's therapist?
- How would your viewpoint regarding suicide influence your approach with Emmanuel?
- What personal values or issues of your own would be triggered by this case?
- What steps might you take to help resolve any issues that you might have following the suicide of a client?
- Which of the following actions might you have pursued?

  _____ Committed him to a psychiatric hospital for observation, even against his will, for 72 hours

  _____ Consulted with another professional as soon as he began to discuss suicide as an option

  _____ Respected his choice of suicide, even if you did not agree with it

  _____ Informed the police and reported the seriousness of his threat

  _____ Informed members of his family of his intentions, even though he did not want you to

  _____ Bargained with him in every way possible in an effort to persuade him to keep on trying to find some meaning in life

Discuss in class any other steps you could have taken in this case.

Commentary. Although prediction of both danger to others and to self is difficult, courts may impose liability on therapists who predict incorrectly. Suicidal clients, like dangerous clients, pose a high risk for therapists. In Emmanuel's case, we would report the client's suicidal intent to the most appropriate authority in his jurisdiction (a mental health evaluation team or the police department). In light of the fact that Emmanuel is not terminally ill and is suffering from depression, this course of action is required both ethically and legally. In this instance, we may break confidentiality and contact a close friend or family member to increase Emmanuel's support system. ●

Protecting Children, the Elderly, and Dependent Adults From Harm

Mental health providers have an ethical and legal obligation to protect children, older adults, and dependent adults from abuse and neglect. Whether you work with children or adults in your practice, you are expected to know how to assess potential abuse and to report it in a timely fashion. Confidentiality does not apply in cases of child abuse and neglect, nor does it apply in cases of elder and dependent adult abuse. Such matters constitute a situation of **reportable abuse**. If children, the elderly, or other dependent adults disclose that they are being abused or neglected, the professional is required to report the situation under penalty of fines and imprisonment. If adults reveal in a therapy session that they are abusing or have abused their children, the matter must be reported. If the therapist has reason to believe that abuse is taking place, most states require a report. The practice of **mandatory reporting** is designed to encourage reporting of any suspected cases of child, elder, or dependent adult abuse; and therapists are advised to err on the side of reporting in uncertain circumstances (Benitez, 2004). The goal of reporting is to protect the child or older person who is being abused. The professional has an obligation to protect those who cannot advocate for themselves.

In 1974 Congress enacted the National Child Abuse Prevention and Treatment Act (PL 93-247), which defines child abuse and neglect as follows:

> Physical or mental injury, sexual abuse or exploitation, negligent treatment, or maltreatment of a child under the age of eighteen or the age specified by the child protection law of the state in question, by a person who is responsible for the child's welfare, under circumstances which indicate that the child's health or welfare is harmed or threatened thereby.

All states now require mental health professionals and school personnel to report incidents of child abuse, or suspected child abuse. Most states have enacted laws that impose liability on professionals who fail to report abuse or neglect of children, the elderly, and other dependent adults. States also provide immunity by law from civil or criminal suits that may arise from reporting suspected child abuse and neglect, or of abuse of the elderly or other dependent adults, if the reports are made in good faith. Some states require that professionals complete continuing education workshops on assessment of abuse and proper reporting as a condition of the granting of a license or of renewing a license.

Know the laws of your state because the threshold for reporting, penalties, and who is mandated to report vary from state to state. There is no substitute for knowing the specific law in your state (Bennett et al., 2006; Welfel, 2016). In Pennsylvania, for example, therapists are required to file a report if the client appears to be the victim of abuse. In New York, therapists must report abuse whether they learn about the situation from the child in therapy, the abuser who is in therapy, or a relative. The laws of some states now require therapists to report disclosures by adult clients about child sexual abuse that occurred years before treatment. It is recommended that you report even if you think it has already been reported (Maureen Kenny, personal communication, September 25, 2016).

The abuse of older people and other vulnerable adults deserves the same kind of attention that is paid to abuse of children. However, Zeranski and Halgin (2011) state that elder abuse has received scant attention in the research literature. Dramatic cases of battery and abandonment can be easily recognized and reported, but many instances of elder abuse occur within the home at the hands of a spouse or an adult child. Knapp and VandeCreek (2012) note that states vary in reporting requirements for elder abuse. Some states permit therapists to break confidentiality and file a report; some states require that therapists do so. In general, the duty to protect elders from harm is stronger than a practitioner's obligation to maintain client confidentiality.

All 50 states have statutes related to elder abuse; in 45 states mental health professionals are mandated to report neglect or abuse of dependent elders (Welfel, 2016). Zeranski and Halgin (2011) state that mental health providers should report when they have reasonable grounds to believe that an elder is suffering from abuse or neglect. In addressing future directions of elder abuse reporting, Zeranski and Halgin contend that "elder abuse will remain a concerning issue for professional psychologists who have legal and ethical obligations to protect people who cannot protect themselves" (p. 299).

The major types of elder abuse are physical abuse, sexual abuse, psychological abuse, neglect, abandonment, and financial or material exploitation (see the box titled "Types of Elder Abuse").

Types of Elder Abuse

Physical abuse involves the use of physical force that often results in bodily injury, physical pain, or impairment.

Sexual abuse consists of nonconsensual sexual contact of any kind with an older adult.

Psychological or emotional abuse involves inflicting anguish, pain, or distress through verbal or nonverbal acts. This kind of abuse might include verbal assaults, insults, threats, intimidation, humiliation, and harassment.

Neglect is the failure of caregivers to fulfill their responsibilities to provide an elderly person with basic necessities. Neglect can be either intentional or unintentional, and can be either self-inflicted or inflicted by others.

Abandonment involves the desertion of an elderly person by a person who has assumed responsibility for being a caregiver.

Financial or material exploitation is the illegal or improper use of an elder's funds, property, or assets.

The National Center on Elder Abuse (NCEA) is dedicated to educating the public about elder abuse, neglect, and exploitation and its tragic consequences. NCEA is an internationally recognized resource for policy leaders, practitioners, prevention specialists, researchers, advocates, families, and concerned citizens. Abusers of older people can be anyone they depend on or come into contact with.

From both an ethical and legal perspective, mental health practitioners are expected to inform clients about the limits of confidentiality pertaining to the duty to report cases of abuse. Although therapists are likely to accept their professional responsibility to protect innocent children, older adults, and dependent adults from physical and emotional mistreatment, they may have difficulty determining how far to go in making a report. It is often difficult to reconcile ethical responsibilities with legal obligations. Therapists may think they have been placed in the predicament of behaving either unethically (by reporting and thus damaging the therapy relationship) or illegally (by ignoring the mandate to report all cases of suspected child or elder abuse). Clinicians must develop a clear position regarding the assessment and reporting of child, elder, and dependent adult abuse. Sometimes reporting is mandatory; sometimes it is discretionary. Some states require permission from the elderly client; other states do not. Review the laws regarding reporting abuse in the state in which you practice.

Many therapists wonder whether they have sufficient information or suspicion to report abuse. Mental health professionals who fail to file a mandated report because of the concern that nothing will be done about it, or who fear that a report could make matters worse, or because they are not certain that their suspicions are valid are likely to be in violation of the law and the ethics codes of most professional organizations (Barnett & Johnson, 2015). Fortunately, professional associations in some states provide legal assistance to help therapists make a determination about when and whether to report abuse. Child Protective Services is also useful in helping to determine when to report a situation. Consult with a colleague when you have a reasonable suspicion that abuse occurred. Reporting the matter best protects the client and also protects you as a mandated reporter.

To what degree are you prepared to carry out your duty to protect children, the elderly, and other dependent adults from abuse or neglect? Evaluate your preparedness by answering the following questions:

- How well prepared do you think you are in determining when to report suspected abuse of a child, an older person, or a dependent adult?
- How would you account for cultural differences in assessing abuse?
- Can you think of ways in which you could file a report on an adult abuser and continue working with the client therapeutically?
- What struggles, if any, have you encountered with respect to following the laws regarding reporting child, dependent adult, or abuse of older adults?
- If you follow the law in all cases, are you also following an ethical course? What potential conflicts are there between doing what is legal and what is ethical?
- If an adult admits having abused a child, what are your thoughts about a therapist who argues that keeping the client in therapy is the best way to help him or her work through this problem, even if it means failing to report the abuse to authorities?

- Do you think therapists should have some flexibility in deciding when it would be best to make a report? Why or why not?
- What personal experiences, if any, have you had in your own life that might be triggered by working with child abuse and reporting issues?
- How might you handle a parent who comes to you enraged because you called Child Protective Services on him or her or on a spouse?

To help you clarify your position with respect to situations involving child, elder, or dependent adult abuse, consider the following three case examples. In the first case, ask yourself how far you should go in reporting suspected abuse. Does the fact that you have reported a matter to the officials end your ethical and legal responsibilities? In the second case, look for ways to differentiate between what is ethical and what is legal practice. Ask yourself what you would be inclined to do if you saw a conflict between ethics and the law. In the third case, ask yourself whether it is better to error on the side of caution rather than assuming there is no reality base to the allegations. What steps could you take to separate fact from fantasy?

The Case of Martina

Martina, a high school counselor, has reason to believe that one of her students is being physically abused. As part of the abuse, critical medication is being withheld from the student. Martina reports the incident to Child Protective Services and gives all the information she has to the caseworker. She follows up the phone conversation with the caseworker with a written report. A week later, the student tells her that nothing has been done.

- Has Martina adequately fulfilled her responsibility by making the report? Does she have a responsibility to report the agency for not having taken action?
- If the agency does not take appropriate action, does Martina have a responsibility to take other measures?
- Would it be ethical for Martina to take matters into her own hands and to call for a family session or make a house call, especially if the student requests it?
- Does Martina have an obligation to inform the administration? Does the school have a responsibility to see that action is taken?

Commentary. Suspected physical abuse and denying the child critical medication are immediate reportable matters. Although the therapist complied with her legal duty to protect the child by reporting the matter to Child Protective Services, she has an ethical obligation to follow up on the report until the matter has been officially investigated and actions have been taken. Martina might want to begin with another phone call to the original caseworker. Should this course of action prove unsatisfactory, she might contact the caseworker's supervisor to emphasize the urgent medical issues at hand. Martina should document these efforts as well as any consultations she makes while handling the case. •

A Case of Protecting an Older Client

Rose, an older adult, takes great pride in her independence, her ability to take care of herself, and in not being a burden to her family. Her therapist, Arman, is impressed with her independent spirit. Rose eventually divulges to Arman several episodes of forgetting to turn off the gas flame in the kitchen. She laughs it off by saying, "I guess I'm not perfect." Every so often,

Rose discloses similar episodes of forgetfulness that have potential lethal consequences. Arman becomes increasingly concerned and suggests that she notify her family of her problem. Rose lets Arman know that this is not an option because her family has wanted her to move to a nursing home. Rose is adamant in her refusal to go along with their plan. She tells Arman, "If you make me leave my home, there is no point in living."

- If you were Rose's counselor, what course of action would you take?
- What ethical, legal, and medical issues can you identify in this case?
- Is there a duty to protect in this situation?

Commentary. The therapist cannot afford to become sidetracked by Rose's insistence that there is no reason to worry or by ignoring Rose's hint of suicide. It is more important for the therapist to take action to help the client than it is to have her like the therapist. As Arman suggests, a meeting with the family can be of great benefit to all concerned. In our view, Arman does have a duty to protect Rose from accidentally harming herself, and possibly others, as a result of her cognitive impairment. By working closely with Rose, her family, and appropriate authorities, he may be able to help Rose transition to an arrangement that is both safe and acceptable to her. The counselor might also help Rose see some of the potential positive elements in leaving her home, such as fewer things to worry about and being given useful assistance. •

A Case of Protecting a Dependent Adult

You are working with individuals with mental disabilities, many of whom are institutionalized. One of your clients, Carlos, who has a severe mental disability and lives in a residential home, leads you to believe that he is being sexually abused by at least one member of the staff. You are not really sure about this because it is difficult to separate fact from fantasy when talking with him about other things.

- Are you required to make a report to Adult Protective Services so that they can determine the validity of the allegation?
- Could you be legally liable for not making a report to protective services?

Commentary. In a case such as this it is better to error on the side of caution rather than assuming there is no reality base to the allegations. When there is a reasonable suspicion of any abuse or neglect, a report must be made to the appropriate agency within the time frame specified in local laws (Barnett & Johnson, 2015). Valuable information can be gleaned from a meeting with the multidisciplinary treatment team to make a more accurate assessment and to determine the course of action to take with Carlos. •

Confidentiality and HIV/AIDS-Related Issues

AIDS affects a large population with diverse demographics and continues to gain prominence as a public health and social issue. Most mental health practitioners will inevitably come in contact with people who have AIDS, with people who have tested positive as carriers of the virus, or with people who are close to these people.

People who receive an HIV-positive test are usually in need of immediate short-term help. They need to establish a support system to help them through the troubled times they will endure. Those who are HIV-positive often live with the anxiety of not knowing when or whether they may be diagnosed with AIDS.

Many also struggle with the stigma attached to AIDS. They live in fear not only of developing a life-threatening disease but also of being discovered and rejected by society and by friends and loved ones. In addition to feeling different and stigmatized, anger, which is likely to be directed toward others, especially those who have infected them, can be extreme. These clients have often been discriminated against, so it is important that professionals respect their situation, obtain informed consent, and educate them about their rights and responsibilities.

Therapists need to inform themselves about the limits of confidentiality, matters of reporting, and their duty to protect third parties, and they need to communicate their professional responsibilities to their clients from the outset. If therapists decide that they cannot provide competent services to HIV-infected people, it is ethically appropriate that they refer these clients to professionals who can provide assistance. We recommend that you review the earlier discussion in this chapter regarding the therapist's duty to protect and think about how that duty applies to people who have AIDS or are HIV-positive.

As a counselor you may indeed work with clients who are HIV-positive. You might accept a client and establish a therapeutic relationship only to find out months later that this person had recently tested positive. If this were the case, how would you answer the following questions:

- Can you think of any reason that it would be ethical to terminate the professional relationship and make a referral?
- Who might you consult with regarding this case?
- Do you have an ethical responsibility to warn or otherwise protect third parties in cases of those who are HIV-positive and who are putting others at risk by engaging in unprotected sex or needle sharing?
- If you do your best to convince your client to disclose his or her HIV status to a partner, and if your client refuses to share this information, what course of action might you take?
- What values or life experiences have you had that may influence the way you work with clients who are HIV-positive?

Consider your ethical responsibilities to respond to this population *before* you encounter possible difficult situations. The case described here is designed to help you clarify your position on the ethical dimensions of counseling clients who have AIDS or are HIV-positive.

The Case of Levi and Makena

Levi and Makena are seeing Sarina for couples counseling. After a number of sessions Makena requests an individual session, in which she discloses that she has tested HIV-positive. Sarina finds herself in a real dilemma: She has concerns for the welfare of the couple, but she is also concerned about Makena's painful predicament.

- Does Sarina have a duty to warn and protect Levi? Why or why not?
- What alternatives does she have to warning that would serve to protect Levi?
- Would such a duty supersede any implied confidentiality of the private session?
- Would it be more therapeutic for Sarina to persuade Makena to disclose her condition to Levi rather than taking the responsibility for this disclosure herself?

- If Makena refused to inform her husband, should Sarina discontinue therapy with the couple? If she were to discontinue working with them, how might she ethically explain her decision to the couple?

- If Sarina felt obligated to continue therapy with the couple, how would she handle the secret, and what ethical issues arise from keeping such a secret?

- Are there factors in this situation that would compel Sarina to treat Makena's secret differently from other major secrets in couples therapy?

Commentary. The law is not clear pertaining to the duty to protect in cases pertaining to HIV status. It is extremely important to know the specific law in your jurisdiction and to seek consultation from a colleague experienced with reporting requirements. In some states therapists could lose their license to practice if they breached confidentiality by warning in cases involving HIV status. A number of our colleagues who have faced this kind of dilemma claim that they are generally successful in convincing the person who is HIV-positive to disclose his or her health status. This is especially true if the therapist is willing to continue to provide support to both of the partners once the disclosure has been made. It is hard to imagine that couples counseling could be successful if this secret is not addressed. It is crucial for clinicians to maintain a focus on the individual who is infected and to help that person navigate the multitude of issues that will arise. Because of our own fears and biases around HIV and AIDS, as counselors we can too quickly become concerned with protecting "others" and miss helping the person who is sitting in front of us. •

Ethical and Legal Considerations in AIDS-Related Cases

Much has been written about the conditions under which confidentiality might be breached in AIDS-related therapy situations. Courts have not applied the duty to protect to mental health professionals in cases involving HIV infection. Thus, therapists' legal responsibilities for protecting sexual partners of HIV-positive clients remain unclear.

From a legal perspective, breaching confidentiality because of a client's HIV status is not one of the exceptions to confidentiality. Until a landmark court case determines a precedent, mental health professionals will continue to struggle with doing what they think is morally and ethically right without any guarantee of legal protection. Legal consultation could be critical in providing a safeguard against legal action.

Duty to Protect Versus Confidentiality Earlier in this chapter we discussed the principles involved in situations in which therapists may have a duty to protect innocent victims. The duty to protect *may* arise when a therapist is convinced that a client who is HIV-positive intends to continue to have unprotected sex, or to share needles, with unsuspecting but reasonably identifiable third parties.

Determining whether a duty to protect applies in the case of a client who is HIV-positive is one of the more controversial and emotion-laden issues practitioners might encounter. For practitioners who work with people who are HIV-positive, the choice is often between protecting the client–therapist relationship and breaching confidentiality to protect people at risk of infection. This situation can put practitioners in a moral, ethical, legal, and professional bind.

Knowing your state's law is crucial when dealing with clients who have contagious and life-threatening diseases. Earlier versions of the ACA code required counselors to confirm that a client had HIV or another contagious life-threatening disease prior to disclosing this information to a person at risk. The 2014 ACA *Code of Ethics* has replaced this requirement with reliance on relevant laws (Kaplan et al., 2017). State laws differ regarding HIV and the limits of confidentiality, and the law is often different for medical professionals than for licensed psychotherapists. All states now have statutes governing reporting of HIV and AIDS cases to public health authorities and corresponding confidentiality duties, but many of the laws that either permit or require reporting are limited to reporting by physicians (Wheeler & Bertram, 2015). Some state laws forbid any disclosure of HIV status to third parties, and others allow some disclosure to at-risk third parties by physicians and psychiatrists, but not by other mental health professionals. Some states prohibit psychotherapists from warning identifiable victims of people who are HIV-positive. In some states, therapists who disclose a client's disease status without first attempting to confirm the diagnosis or striving to reach an agreement with the client to protect others are vulnerable to an ethical or legal violation (Barnett & Johnson, 2015). Other states have yet to address this issue by statute. Thus, therapists are advised to know what statutes, if any, define the actions they should take regarding reporting of HIV or AIDS cases; they should then follow the statutory mandate. If you are uncertain about how to proceed in reporting HIV or AIDS cases, your state public health department can provide information regarding your obligations. You can also seek advice from an attorney, your professional organizations, and colleagues who are well-versed in ethical decision making (Wheeler & Bertram, 2015).

Careful consideration should be given to breaching confidentiality due to the danger to others posed by HIV-positive clients. The following recommendations for therapists can help in making this decision:

- All limits to confidentiality should be discussed with the client at the onset of treatment. When this is done early in the therapeutic relationship, it is less likely that therapists will encounter dilemmas over breaching confidentiality. The implications of disclosing confidentiality, as well as other alternatives, can be explored with HIV-positive clients within the counseling context at this time.
- Therapists need to keep current with regard to relevant medical information related to the transmission of HIV, know which sexual practices are safer and which are not, and encourage their clients to practice safer sex.
- Therapists should speak directly and openly with their clients about their concerns regarding the danger of certain behaviors and the risk to third parties. They can use the therapeutic process to educate their clients about the effects their behavior can have on others, teach safer sex practices, obtain commitments from the client to notify partners, and offer help in communicating information to partners.
- If the client continues to resist using safer sex practices or refuses to inform partners, then the therapist needs to determine what course of action to follow. Practitioners should consult with the public health agency, knowledgeable peers, or attorneys to determine whether their intended course of action is ethically and legally sound.
- In disclosing HIV information, therapists need to follow the statutory guidelines and safeguard the client's privacy as much as possible.

Bennett and colleagues (2006) recommend thinking about these situations from a clinical perspective. Attempt to understand the reasons a client is not willing to disclose his or her HIV status. Is it because of fear of domestic abuse? fear of being abandoned? social rejection? Or is the nondisclosure due to some other relationship issue? If you explore the clinical aspects of your client's situation, it may not be necessary to take steps to warn or protect others.

VandeCreek and Knapp (2001) assert that warning an identifiable victim should be considered as a last resort. Many courses of action are open to practitioners besides warning a third party and breaking confidentiality. If psychotherapy is given a chance to work, there is a good chance that the client will voluntarily disclose this information to his or her partner.

In summary, dealing responsibly with the dilemmas posed in this section demands an awareness of the ethical, legal, and clinical issues involved in working with clients with HIV/AIDS. There are no simple solutions to the complex issues practitioners face, and this topic is surely one of the more challenging ones.

Chapter Summary

Along with their duties to clients, therapists have responsibilities to their agency, to their profession, to the community, to the members of their clients' families, and to themselves. Ethical dilemmas involving confidentiality arise when there are conflicts between responsibilities. Members of the helping professions should know and observe the ethics codes of their professional organizations and make sound judgments that are within the parameters of acceptable practice. We have encouraged you to think about specific ethical issues and to develop a sense of professional ethics and knowledge of state laws so that your judgment will be well-founded.

The roles of school counselors are increasingly complex. Emerging case law and the violent climate in schools today require that school counselors take all threats of violence seriously. Developing prevention strategies to make the school community a safer place for all students is challenging. School counselors also have a legal duty to protect students who may pose a danger to themselves, and school counselors would do well to take the initiative in obtaining continuing education on developments in the field of student suicide to help save lives and limit their legal liability.

Court decisions have provided an expanded perspective on the therapist's duty to protect the public. As a result of the *Tarasoff* case, and subsequent legislation and case law, therapists are now becoming aware of their responsibility to the potential victims of a client's violent behavior. All 50 states now have laws regarding the duty to warn. This duty spans interventions from warning threatened individuals to involuntary commitment of clients. Therapists also have an ethical and legal duty to protect clients who are likely to injure or kill themselves.

States have enacted laws that require professionals to report child, elder, and dependent adult abuse whenever they suspect or discover it in the course of their professional activities. Clients have a right to know that therapists are legally and ethically bound to breach confidentiality in situations involving child, elder, or dependent adult abuse. Therefore, this should be included in your informed consent document.

Because state laws vary on breaching confidentiality of a client's HIV status to warn or protect potential victims, practitioners are advised to know their state laws and to consult professional colleagues, and perhaps an attorney, before taking any action regarding disclosing a client's HIV status to a person at risk. Breaching confidentiality should be the last resort, implemented only after less obtrusive measures have failed, and only if the disclosure does not conflict with state law.

Suggested Activities

1. In small groups discuss the cases and guidelines presented in this chapter on the duty to protect victims from violent clients or students. If you found yourself faced with a potentially dangerous client or student, what specific steps might you take to carry out this duty?

2. Structure a class debate around the arguments for and against suicide prevention. Consider debating a specific case of a client who is terminally ill and decides that he wants to end his life because of his suffering and because there is no hope of getting better.

3. Ask several students to investigate the laws of your state pertaining to confidentiality and privileged communication and present their findings to the class. What kinds of mental health providers in your state can offer their clients privileged communication? What are the exceptions to this privilege? Under what circumstances are you legally required to breach confidentiality? Regarding confidentiality in counseling minors, what state laws should you know?

4. In small groups discuss specific circumstances in which you would break confidentiality, and see whether you can agree on some general guidelines.

5. Discuss some ways in which you can prepare clients for issues pertaining to confidentiality. What could you do to educate clients about the purposes of confidentiality and the legal restrictions on it? Examine how you would do this in various situations, such as school counseling, group work, couples and family counseling, and counseling with minors.

6. In a class debate, have one side take the position that absolute confidentiality is necessary to promote full client disclosure. The other side can argue for a limited confidentiality that still promotes effective therapy.

7. Do an Internet search on one another in class and see what types of information your clients would be able to find out about you. Are you posting information on social networking sites that you would not want a client to see?

Ethics in Action Video Exercises

8. Refer to video role play 8, Sexuality: Promiscuity, and think of ways to reenact a role play with different students demonstrating a variety of ways to deal with this woman who is having unprotected casual sexual encounters. If she told you that she just found out that she is HIV-positive—and that she absolutely does not intend to reveal this news to her partner—what would your stance be? Would you protect the client's confidentiality? Or would you see this as a duty to warn and protect case? Devise alternative role plays showing a variety of approaches for dealing with the ethical and legal dimensions in this case.

MindTap for Counseling

Go to MindTap® for an eBook, videos of client sessions, activities, practice quizzes, apps, and more—all in one place. If your instructor didn't assign MindTap, you can find out more information at CengageBrain.com.

7

Managing Boundaries and Multiple Relationships

LEARNING OBJECTIVES

1. State the ethical guidelines regarding dual or multiple relationships

2. Appreciate various perspectives on multiple relationships

3. Identify factors to consider before entering into a multiple relationship

4. Differentiate between boundary crossings and boundary violations

5. Critically evaluate the controversies on boundary issues

6. Understand ethical challenges in managing multiple relationships in small communities

7. Explore the pros and cons of bartering for professional services

8. Formulate guidelines on receiving gifts from clients

9. Describe ethical issues regarding forming social relationships with current or former clients

10. Articulate guidelines for dealing with sexual attractions in the therapy relationship

11. Recognize the ethical and legal aspects of sexual misconduct

12. Clarify guidelines for the use of touch in the therapy relationship

SELF-INVENTORY

Directions: For each statement, indicate the response that most closely identifies your beliefs and attitudes. Use the following code:

5 = I *strongly agree* with this statement.

4 = I *agree* with this statement.

3 = I am *undecided* about this statement.

2 = I *disagree* with this statement.

1 = I *strongly disagree* with this statement.

_____ 1. A good therapist gets involved in the client's case without getting involved with the client emotionally.

_____ 2. Nonerotic touching is best avoided in counseling because it can easily be misunderstood by the client.

_____ 3. Nonerotic touching can be beneficial to a client.

_____ 4. Social relationships with clients while they are in counseling may be unwise, but such relationships are permissible after counseling ends.

_____ 5. If I were a truly ethical professional, I would never be sexually attracted to a client.

_____ 6. If I were counseling a client who was sexually attracted to me, I would refer this client to another counselor.

_____ 7. I might be inclined to barter my therapeutic services for goods if a client could not afford my fees.

_____ 8. If a client initiated the possibility of exchanging services in lieu of payment, I would consider bartering as an option.

_____ 9. The topic of dealing with sexual attractions in therapy should be addressed throughout the counselor's training program.

_____ 10. It is essential to consider the cultural context in deciding on the appropriateness of bartering, accepting gifts, and the counselor assuming multiple roles with a client.

_____ 11. Dual and multiple relationships should not be considered inappropriate or unethical in all circumstances, but should be decided on a case-by-case basis.

_____ 12. I would have no trouble accepting a close friend as a client if it were clear that our personal relationship is separate from our professional one.

_____ 13. It will be relatively easy for me to establish clear and firm boundaries with my clients.

_____ 14. Before I would engage in a dual relationship, I would discuss the potential problems with the client and actively involve the client in the decision-making process.

_____ 15. Multiple relationships can be potentially beneficial to clients.

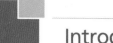

Introduction

The terms *dual relationships* and *multiple relationships* are used interchangeably in various professional codes of ethics, and the ACA (2014) uses the term *nonprofessional relationships*. In this chapter we use the broader term of *multiple relationships* to encompass both dual relationships and nonprofessional relationships.

The APA (2010) ethics code defines a **multiple relationship** as one in which a practitioner is in a professional role with a person in addition to another role with that same individual, or with another person who is close to that individual. When clinicians blend their professional relationship with a nonprofessional relationship with a client, ethical concerns must be considered. In these situations, it is often difficult to determine what is in the best interests of the client.

Multiple relationships occur when professionals assume two or more roles at the same time or sequentially with a client. This may involve assuming more than one professional role (such as instructor and therapist) or blending a professional and a nonprofessional relationship (such as counselor and friend or counselor and business partner). Multiple relationships also include providing therapy to a relative or a friend's relative, socializing with clients, becoming emotionally or sexually involved with a client or former client, combining the roles of supervisor and therapist, having a business relationship with a client, borrowing money from a client, or loaning money to a client. Boundary crossings or multiple relationships increase the *possibility* that therapists may misuse their power to influence and exploit clients for their own benefit and to the clients' detriment (Zur, 2007). Although some suggest that it is good practice to abstain from crossing boundaries or engaging in multiple relationships, this is not always possible.

Mental health professionals must learn how to effectively and ethically manage multiple relationships, including dealing with the power differential that is a part of most professional relationships, managing boundary issues, and striving to avoid the misuse of power (Herlihy & Corey, 2015b). Although codes can provide some general guidelines, good judgment, the willingness to reflect on one's practices, and being aware of one's motivations are critical dimensions of an ethical practitioner. Mental health professionals can fail to heed warning signs in their relationships with clients. They may not pay sufficient attention to the potential problems involved in establishing and maintaining professional boundaries. Practitioners may be unaware of the implications of their actions and may not recognize when they are engaged in unprofessional or problematic conduct.

The underlying theme of this chapter is the need for counselors to be honest and self-searching in determining the impact of their behavior on clients. In cases that are not clear-cut, it is especially important to make an honest appraisal of your behavior and its effect on clients and to consult with trusted colleagues. To us, behavior is unethical when it reflects a lack of awareness or concern about the impact of the behavior on clients. Some counselors may place their personal needs above the needs of their clients by engaging in more than one role with clients to meet their own financial, social, or emotional needs.

This chapter focuses on boundary issues in professional practice, establishing appropriate boundaries, the difference between boundary crossings and boundary violations, multiple relationships, role blending, a variety of nonsexual multiple relationships, and sexual issues in therapy. We also examine the more subtle aspects of sexuality in therapy, including sexual attractions and the misuse of power. Multiple relationship issues cannot be resolved with ethics codes alone; therapists must think through all of the ethical and clinical dimensions involved in a wide range of boundary concerns.

LO1

The Ethics of Multiple Relationships

The codes of ethics of most professional organizations warn of the potential problems of multiple relationships (see the Ethics Codes box titled "Standards on Multiple Relationships"). These codes caution professionals against any involvement with clients that might impair their judgment and objectivity, affect their ability to render effective services, or result in harm or exploitation of clients. Nonsexual multiple relationships are not inherently unethical, and most ethics codes acknowledge that some multiple relationships are unavoidable. However, when multiple relationships exploit clients, or have significant potential to harm clients, they are unethical.

ETHICS CODES: Standards on Multiple Relationships

American Association for Marriage and Family Therapy (2015)
Marriage and family therapists are aware of their influential position with respect to clients, and they avoid exploiting the trust and dependency of such persons. Therapists, therefore, make every effort to avoid conditions and multiple relationships with clients that could impair professional judgment or increase the risk of exploitation. Such relationships include, but are not limited to, business or close personal relationships with a client or the client's immediate family. When the risk of impairment or exploitation exists due to conditions or multiple roles, therapists document the appropriate precautions taken. (1.3.)

American Mental Health Counselors Association (2015)
Mental health counselors are aware of their influential position with respect to their clients and avoid exploiting the trust and dependency of the client. (Principle 3.)

National Association of Social Workers (2008)
Social workers should not engage in dual or multiple relationships with clients or former clients in which there is a risk of exploitation or potential harm to the client. In instances when dual or multiple relationships are unavoidable, social workers should take steps to protect clients and are responsible for setting clear, appropriate, and culturally sensitive boundaries. (Dual or multiple relationships occur when social workers relate to clients in more than one relationship, whether professional, social, or business. Dual or multiple relationships can occur simultaneously or consecutively.) (1.06.c.)

continued

Canadian Psychological Association (2015)

Manage dual or multiple relationships or any other conflict-of-interest situation entered into in such a way that bias, lack of objectivity, and risk of exploitation or harm are minimized. This might include involving the affected party(ies) in clarification of boundaries and expectations, limiting the duration of the relationship, obtaining ongoing supervision or consultation for the duration of the dual or multiple relationship, or involving a third party in obtaining consent (e.g., approaching a primary client or employee about becoming a research participant). (3.34.)

American School Counselor Association (2016)

School counselors establish and maintain appropriate professional relationships with students at all times. School counselors consider the risks and benefits of extending current school counseling relationships beyond conventional parameters, such as attending a student's distant athletic competition. In extending these boundaries, school counselors take appropriate professional precautions such as informed consent, consultation and supervision. School counselors document the nature of interactions that extend beyond conventional parameters, including the rationale for the interaction, the potential benefit and the possible positive and negative consequences for the student and school counselor. (A.5.b.)

American Counseling Association (2014)

Counselors are prohibited from engaging in counseling relationships with friends or family members with whom they have an inability to remain objective. (A.5.d.)

Counselors are prohibited from engaging in a personal virtual relationship with individuals with whom they have a current counseling relationship (e.g., through social and other media). (A.5.e.)

Counselors consider the risks and benefits of accepting as clients those with whom they have had a previous relationship. These potential clients include individuals with whom the counselor has had a casual, distant, or past relationship. Examples include mutual or past membership in a professional association, organization, or community. When counselors accept these clients, they take appropriate professional cautions such as informed consent, consultation, supervision, and documentation to ensure that judgment is not impaired and no exploitation occurs. (A.6.a.)

American Psychological Association (2010)

(a) A multiple relationship occurs when a psychologist is in a professional role with a person and (1) at the same time is in another role with the same person, (2) at the same time is in a relationship with a person closely associated with or related to the person with whom the psychologist has the professional relationship, or (3) promises to enter into another relationship in the future with the person or a person closely associated with or related to the person.

A psychologist refrains from entering into a multiple relationship if the multiple relationship could reasonably be expected to impair the psychologist's objectivity, competence, or effectiveness in performing his or her functions as a psychologist, or otherwise risks exploitation or harm to the person with whom the professional relationship exists.

Multiple relationships that would not reasonably be expected to cause impairment or risk exploitation or harm are not unethical.

(b) If a psychologist finds that, due to unforeseen factors, a potentially harmful multiple relationship has arisen, the psychologist takes reasonable steps to resolve it with due regard for the best interests of the affected person and maximal compliance with the Ethics Code.

(c) When psychologists are required by law, institutional policy, or extraordinary circumstances to serve in more than one role in judicial or administrative proceedings, at the outset they clarify role expectations and the extent of confidentiality and thereafter as changes occur. (3.05.)

Differing Perspectives on Multiple Relationships

There is a wide range of viewpoints on multiple relationships. As you work to clarify your position on this issue, you will encounter conflicting advice. Some writers focus on the problems inherent in multiple relationships, especially the legal implications of entering into multiple relationships. If a client suffers harm or is exploited due to a multiple relationship, the client could file a malpractice lawsuit against the mental health provider. Others see the entire discussion of multiple relationships as subtle and complex, defying simplistic solutions or absolute answers. Despite certain clinical, ethical, and legal risks, in many situations some blending of roles is unavoidable For example, in military settings multiple relationships are common and can be a healthy part of communal life. These relationships can improve morale, decrease the stigma attached to seeking psychological assistance, and improve access to care (Johnson & Johnson, 2017).

Although the codes of ethics of most professions caution against engaging in nonsexual multiple relationships, they are not necessarily problematic, and some are beneficial (Herlihy & Corey, 2015b). For example, "mentoring" involves blending roles, yet both mentors and learners can certainly benefit from this relationship. Casto, Caldwell, and Salazar (2005) point out that mentors often balance a multiplicity of roles, some of which include teacher, counselor, role model, guide, and friend. They add that the mentoring relationship is a personal one, in which both mentor and mentee may benefit from knowing the other personally and professionally. Casto and colleagues emphasize the importance of maintaining boundaries between mentorship and friendship, which requires vigilance of the power differential and how it affects the mentee. They contend that the focus of mentoring is always on the mentee's personal and professional development.

After reviewing the literature on the topic of multiple relationships, Herlihy and Corey (2015b) conclude that there is no clear consensus regarding nonsexual multiple relationships in counseling. When considering such a relationship, practitioners must examine their motivations and consult with other professionals to determine the appropriateness of the relationship. Practitioners should be cautious about entering into more than one role with a client unless there is sound clinical justification for doing so, and they must take measures to minimize the likelihood of harm coming to the client. It is good practice to document precautions practitioners take to protect clients when such relationships are unavoidable.

Factors to Consider Before Entering Into a Multiple Relationship

Moleski and Kiselica (2005) believe multiple relationships range from the destructive to the therapeutic. Although some multiple relationships are harmful, other secondary relationships complement, enable, and enhance the counseling relationship. Moleski and Kiselica encourage counselors to examine the potential positive and negative consequences that a secondary relationship might have on the primary counseling relationship. They suggest that counselors consider forming multiple relationships only when it is clear that such relationships are in the best interests of the client.

Younggren and Gottlieb (2004) suggest applying an ethical, risk-managed, decision-making model when practitioners are analyzing a situation involving the pros and cons of a multiple relationship. They "acknowledge that these types of relationships are not necessarily violations of the standards of professional conduct, and/or the law, but we know enough to recommend that they have to be actively and thoroughly analyzed and addressed, although not necessarily avoided" (p. 260). Younggren and Gottlieb recommend that practitioners address these questions to make sound decisions about multiple relationships:

- Is entering into a relationship in addition to the professional one necessary, or should I avoid it?
- Can the multiple relationship potentially cause harm to the client?
- If harm seems unlikely, would the additional relationship prove beneficial? If it is beneficial, is the benefit focused more on the client, the counselor, or both?
- Is there a risk that the multiple relationship could disrupt the therapeutic relationship?
- Can I evaluate this matter objectively? (pp. 256–257)

In answering these questions, practitioners must carefully assess the risk for conflict of interests, loss of objectivity, and implications for the therapeutic relationship. It is good practice to discuss the potential problems involved in a multiple relationship with the client and to actively involve the client in the decision-making process.

If the multiple relationship is judged to be appropriate and acceptable, the therapist should document the entire process, including having the client sign an informed consent form. In addition, therapists would do well to adopt a risk management approach to the problem. This involves a careful review of various issues such as diagnosis, level of functioning, therapeutic orientation, community standards and practices, and consultations with professionals who could support the decision. Younggren and Gottlieb conclude with this advice: "Only after having taken all these steps can the professional consider entering into the relationship, and he or she should then do so with the greatest of caution" (p. 260).

Barnett (Barnett, Lazarus, et al., 2007) suggests some guidelines to increase the likelihood that a client's best interests are being served:

- The therapist is motivated by what the client needs rather than by his or her own needs.
- The boundary crossing is consistent with a client's treatment plan.
- The client's history, culture, values, and diagnosis have been considered.
- The rationale for the boundary crossing is documented in the client's record.
- The boundary crossing is discussed with the client in advance to prevent misunderstandings.
- Full recognition is given to the power differential, and the client's trust is safeguarded.
- Consultation with colleagues guides the therapist's decisions.

Boundary Crossings Versus Boundary Violations

Certain behaviors of professionals have the potential for creating a multiple relationship, but they are not inherently considered to be multiple relationships. Examples of these behaviors include accepting a client's invitation to a special event such as a graduation; bartering goods or services for professional services; accepting a small gift from a client; attending the same social, cultural, or religious activities as a client; or giving a supportive hug after a difficult session. Gutheil and Gabbard (1993) caution that engaging in boundary crossings paves the way to boundary violations and to becoming entangled in complex multiple relationships. They distinguish between boundary crossings (changes in role) and boundary violations (exploitation of the client at some level). A **boundary crossing** is a departure from commonly accepted practices that could potentially benefit clients; a **boundary violation** is a serious breach that results in harm to clients and is therefore unethical. Gutheil and Gabbard note that not all boundary crossings should be considered boundary violations. Interpersonal boundaries are fluid; they may change over time and may be redefined as therapists and clients continue to work together. Yet behaviors that stretch boundaries can become problematic, and boundary crossings can lead to a pattern of blurring of professional roles. The key is to take measures to prevent boundary crossings from becoming boundary violations.

Johnson and Johnson (2017) contend that military mental health providers must increase their tolerance for routine boundary crossings and contacts with clients outside the consulting room. If military therapists demonstrate calm acceptance of their multiple roles and relationships, clients are likely to become calmer about these unavoidable multiple relationships. Military therapists need to be mindful of client confidentiality in interactions with clients outside of therapy and remain vigilant to possible adverse effects of multiple roles on clients or on the therapeutic relationship.

A common type of boundary crossing is therapist self-disclosure. If a counselor engages in lengthy self-disclosure, a client might well wonder whether he or she is being heard in the therapy session. Many theoretical models encourage appropriate and timely disclosure on the therapist's part, but such self-disclosure must be in the service of the client. Therapist self-disclosure should never burden the client or result in the client feeling a need to take care of the therapist. Counselors must consider a range of factors such as the client's history, his or her presenting problem, cultural factors, the client's comfort with disclosures on the part of the therapist, and a therapist's comfort with disclosing. It is critical that therapists understand their motivations for sharing personal experiences or reactions to what is going on in a session.

In examining ethical complaints and violations received by the Commission on Rehabilitation Counselor Certification from 2006 to 2013, Hartley and Cartwright (2015) found that boundary violations were the most pervasive themes. Barnett (Barnett, Lazarus, et al., 2007) states that even for well-intentioned clinicians, thoughtful reflection is required to determine when crossing a boundary results in a boundary violation. If a therapist's actions result in harm to a client, it is a boundary violation. Failing to practice in accordance with prevailing community standards, as well as other variables such as the role of the client's diagnosis, history, values, and culture, can result in a well-intentioned action being perceived as a boundary violation. Pope and Vasquez (2016) caution that crossing a boundary entails risks: "Done in the wrong situation, or at the wrong time, or with the wrong person it can knock the therapy off track, sabotage the treatment plan, and offend, exploit, or even harm the patient" (p. 253). Barnett (2017a) states that "one client's boundary crossing may be another client's boundary violation" (p. 27) and recommends that therapists openly discuss concerns regarding multiple relationships with clients as part of the informed consent process. Barnett adds that crossing boundaries may be clinically relevant and appropriate in some cases, and that avoiding crossing some boundaries could work against the goals of the therapeutic relationship. Pope and Vasquez (2016) point out that refusing to engage in a boundary crossing may be a lost opportunity that can damage the therapeutic alliance. If a client gives her therapist a small painting she created as a token of gratitude and her therapist declines the gift, the client may feel rejected because she personally created the gift. She also may be offended if giving gifts is considered to be an important part of her cultural tradition.

Consistent yet flexible boundaries are often therapeutic and can help clients develop trust in the therapy relationship. Smith (2011) recommends finding a balanced framework for the therapeutic relationship that is neither too tight nor too loose. Smith states that appropriate boundaries provide "both patient and therapist freedom to explore past and present, conscious and unconscious, fact and fantasy. Boundaries offer safety from the possibility of rule by impulse and desire" (p. 63).

Setting Appropriate Boundaries in Home-Based Therapy Changes in mental health care laws and practice have increased the need for outreach psychotherapists in recent years (Rogers, 2014). Some clients may have difficulty getting to an office due to a lack of transportation or physical limitations. Others may be struggling with poverty and a host of problems that limit their access to office services. Offering therapy in a client's home can aid in building a therapeutic relationship and provides the clinician with the opportunity to observe the client's experience firsthand. Despite the benefits of outreach psychotherapy, graduate programs continue to emphasize in-clinic training and are not adequately preparing students for the challenges encountered when meeting clients in their homes or working in the community. Some training programs would like to provide outreach therapy experiences for students but cannot due to the limits of malpractice insurance at their university. Rogers (2014) lists some concerns that may be encountered when serving clients at home: challenging mental health issues, safety concerns, distracting environment issues, a lack of collegial support and supervision in the field, role confusion, feelings of isolation, countertransference, and blurred boundaries. These concerns are unlike those experienced in an office setting, and it is likely that boundary crossing issues will need to be addressed in the home environment.

Hartley and Cartwright (2015) describe an increasing trend toward providing rehabilitation counseling services in clients' homes and natural environments.

One of the challenges that accompany this trend is that the practitioner may be asked to take on tasks outside of the counseling role such as running errands or attending to visitors coming to client's home. Hartley and Cartwright believe "there is a need for continued discussion toward how to sustain appropriate roles and relationships with clients when providing services to reduce the potential of nonsexual boundary violations" (p. 161).

Zur (2008) also makes a case for taking professional relationships beyond the office walls. He writes about the advantages of out-of-office experiences, such as home visits, attending celebrations of a client, adventure or outdoor therapy, and other encounters with clients. For example, he describes how he accompanied a client to the gravesite of a child for whom she had not grieved. This intervention proved to be therapeutic for the woman who had been depressed for years prior to beginning her therapy with Zur.

In some situations, out-of-office contact is required on a regular basis. Psychologists who work with athletes and coaches may travel with teams, attend practice sessions and competitions, eat meals with their clients (the athletes), and share hotel rooms with coaches (Moles, Petrie, & Watkins, 2016). Sport psychology consultants often engage in behaviors that cross boundaries typically associated with mental health settings. Developing trusting and credible relationships requires sport psychologists to meet athletes where they practice their sport; these relationships are considered appropriate because of the context of the sport environment and the culture of sport (Haberl & Peterson, 2006; Moles et al., 2016).

We recommend that therapists who make it a practice to venture outside of the office or engage in nontraditional activities with clients make this clear at the outset of therapy during the informed consent process. Furthermore, therapists might do well to consult with their insurance carrier about such practices as these activities may have implications for their liability exposure.

A Cultural Perspective on Boundaries Speight (2012) argues for the need to reconsider boundaries in the therapeutic relationship and calls for a reexamination of the traditional perspective on understanding boundaries, boundary crossings, the counselor's role, and the counseling relationship. She discovered that many African American clients expect a warm, reciprocal, and understanding relationship and perceive therapists' objective detachment as uncaring and uninvolved. Speight proposes the concept of *solidarity*, rooted in the ties within a society that bind people together, as a culturally congruent way of understanding, defining, and managing boundaries. "Solidarity between myself and my clients both allowed and required me to be myself, to give primacy to the real relationship, to establish close boundaries, and to act in clients' best interests" (p. 147). By embracing a broader understanding of boundaries, Speight was able to be genuine and close in her therapeutic relationships without being inappropriate and exploitative. "I was flexible with my boundaries, in a way that felt entirely consistent culturally but was inconsistent with my prior training and education. No longer was I a distant, detached professional, but I was an engaged and involved counseling psychologist, and this was just 'the type of psychologist' I wanted to be" (p. 141).

Speight advocates for learning how to tolerate complexity and for developing role flexibility in therapeutic situations. She encourages clinicians to be mindful of the fine line between boundaries that are too close and those that are too distant.

Role Blending Some roles that professionals play involve an inherent multiplicity of roles. **Role blending**, or combining roles and responsibilities, is quite common in some professions. For example, counselor educators serve as instructors, but they sometimes act as therapeutic agents for their students' personal development. At different times, counselor educators may function in the role of teacher, therapeutic agent, mentor, evaluator, or supervisor. School counselors must often function in multiple roles such as counselor, teacher, and chaperon.

Role blending is not necessarily unethical, but it does call for vigilance on the part of the professional to ensure that exploitation does not occur. Herlihy and Corey (2015b) assert that role blending is inevitable in the process of educating and supervising counselor trainees and that it can present ethical dilemmas when there is a loss of objectivity or a conflict of interests. Functioning in more than one role involves thinking through potential problems *before* they occur and building safeguards into practice. Whenever a potential for negative outcomes exists, professionals have a responsibility to design safeguards to reduce the potential for harm.

Avoiding the Slippery Slope Professionals get into trouble when their boundaries are poorly defined and when they attempt to blend roles that do not mix (such as professional and social roles). A gradual erosion of boundaries can lead to very problematic multiple relationships that harm clients. Gutheil and Gabbard (1993) and Gabbard (1994) cite the **slippery slope phenomenon** as one of the strongest arguments for carefully monitoring boundaries in psychotherapy. Once a practitioner crosses a boundary, the tendency to engage in a series of increasingly serious boundary violations can lead to a progressive deterioration of ethical behavior. Furthermore, if professionals do not adhere to uncompromising standards, their behavior may foster relationships that are harmful to clients.

Many practitioners are critical of the slippery slope argument, stating that it tends to result in therapists practicing in an overly cautious manner that may harm clients (Lazarus & Zur, 2002; Pope & Vasquez, 2016; Speight, 2012; Zur, 2007). Gottlieb and Younggren (2009) believe the slippery slope does exist but that it is not as steep or as slippery as many fear. They state that most boundary crossings are done in a thoughtful manner that is appropriate to the therapeutic context and that entail minimal risks to clients. Gottlieb and Younggren conclude that the increased flexibility in maintaining boundaries is a healthy sign but that as relationships with clients become more complex, more careful management and thoughtful decision making are required.

Managing multiple roles and relationships can be extremely complex, and seasoned professionals are often challenged to follow the most ethical course when it comes to crossing boundaries. Managing multiple relationships can be even more challenging to students, trainees, and beginning professionals. Those with relatively little clinical experience might be well advised to avoid engaging in multiple relationships whenever possible. On the other hand, as Dallesasse (2010) points out, graduate students often serve in a number of positions during their course of study, for example, as student, instructor, counselor, researcher, and adviser. These advanced students may encounter dilemmas regarding nonsexual multiple relationships, and they need to have a framework for sorting through different courses of action.

Consider these slippery slope scenarios and reflect on whether you could see yourself saying "yes" to some of these boundary crossings:

- A client asks to "friend" you on Facebook or follow you on Instagram or Twitter
- A client invites you to his or her graduation
- A client asks if he or she can bring you lunch when you meet at noon
- A client texts you photos of her children from time to time
- A client asks what general practice doctor you use because he or she is looking for a good referral

What reactions do you have to these scenarios? Do you find yourself leaning toward saying "yes" or "no" more often? How do your responses to these situations reflect your counseling theory?

Issues to Consider in Addressing Multiple Relationships In *Boundary Issues in Counseling: Multiple Roles and Responsibilities,* Herlihy and Corey (2015b) identify a number of key themes surrounding multiple roles in counseling, some of which follow:

1. Multiple relationship issues affect most mental health practitioners, regardless of their work setting or clientele.
2. Most professional codes of ethics caution practitioners about the potential exploitation in multiple relationships, and more recent codes acknowledge the complex nature of these relationships.
3. Not all multiple relationships (and boundary crossings) can be avoided, nor are they necessarily always harmful; they can be beneficial.
4. Multiple role relationships challenge us to monitor ourselves and to examine our motivations for our practices.
5. Whenever you consider becoming involved in a multiple relationship, seek consultation from trusted colleagues, a supervisor, or your professional organization. It is a good idea to document the nature of this consultation.
6. Few absolute answers exist to neatly resolve multiple relationship dilemmas.
7. Being cautious about entering into multiple relationships should be for the benefit of our clients rather than to protect ourselves from censure.
8. In determining whether to proceed with a multiple relationship, consider whether the potential benefit outweighs the potential for harm. To the extent possible, include the client in making this decision.

The Changing Perspectives on Nonsexual Multiple Relationships

In his thoughtful book, *Boundaries in Psychotherapy,* Zur (2007) addresses the changing perspectives on professional boundaries. Concerns about therapeutic boundaries came to the forefront during the 1960s and 1970s, largely due to a widespread lack of any sense of boundaries on the part of many mental health professionals and the resulting exploitation of clients. There was pressure within the culture at large as well as in the mental health professions to provide specific guidelines for appropriate and ethical conduct in the practice of psychotherapy. The 1980s saw increased injunctions against boundary crossing and an increased emphasis on risk management practices. Most boundary crossings and dual relationships were viewed from a risk management perspective as hazards that should be avoided.

In the 1990s, a shift in thinking about psychotherapeutic boundaries began to emerge. There was increased recognition that some boundary crossings, such as therapist self-disclosure and nonsexual touch, can be clinically valuable. Topics such as appropriate therapeutic boundaries, potential conflicts of interest, and ethical and effective ways of managing multiple relationships were addressed in some ethics codes.

The absolute ban on multiple relationships has been replaced with cautions against taking advantage of the power differential in the therapeutic relationship and exploiting the client, while acknowledging that some boundary crossings can be beneficial. Many professionals now agree that flexible boundaries can be clinically helpful when applied ethically and that boundary crossings need to be evaluated on a case-by-case basis (Herlihy & Corey, 2015b).

Consider the circumstances in which you may decide upon flexible boundaries. What multiple relationships might be unavoidable, and what can you do in these situations? What kinds of relationships place you in professional jeopardy? Consider, for example, how refusing to attend a social event of a client could complicate the therapeutic relationship. In struggling to determine what constitutes appropriate boundaries, you are likely to find that occasional role blending is inevitable. Therefore, it is crucial to learn how to manage boundaries, how to prevent boundary crossings from turning into boundary violations, and how to develop safeguards that will prevent the exploitation of clients.

Perspectives on Boundary Issues

Arnold Lazarus (1998, 2001) has taken the position that a general proscription against dual and multiple relationships has led to unfair and inconsistent decisions by state licensing boards, brought sanctions against practitioners who have done no harm, and sometimes impeded a therapist's ability to perform optimum work with a client. Lazarus contends that professionals who hide behind rigid boundaries often fail to be of genuine help to their clients. He argues for a non-dogmatic evaluation of boundary questions when deciding whether to enter into a secondary relationship. Lazarus sums up his perspective on ethics and boundaries in this way:

> To my way of thinking, here is what I regard as really important: develop rapport; earn your client's trust; respect and honor confidentiality; display genuine warmth and caring; stringently avoid any form of disparagement, exploitation, abuse, harassment, inconsiderateness, and sexual contact. Above all, do no harm and always keep the best interests of the client in mind. (personal communication, April 6, 2013)

Advantages of Boundary Crossings

A rigid risk-avoidance application of boundaries can be harmful to clients by creating a sterile relationship that works against establishing a positive therapeutic alliance (Barnett, 2017a). Examples of such rigidity include never touching a client under any circumstances, refusing every small gift, or refusing to extend a session for any reason. In many situations, it may be difficult for clinicians to readily discern the difference between a positive boundary crossing and a boundary violation.

There are advantages to crossing boundaries in certain circumstances. The counselor can do a lot to build a relationship with a student by attending a student's school play, musical recital, or sports event. However, we recommend that school counselors ask these questions: "How will I respond if this client continues to ask me to participate in other activities?" "How will I respond to other students who make similar requests?" "How will I deal with these extra demands on my time?"

Consider the client population with whom you are dealing. Not all clients are alike. Age, diagnosis, life experiences such as abuse, and culture are key elements to consider when establishing boundaries. Another important element is the character of the therapist. In our opinion, the therapist's character and values have more influence than training and orientation. Consider how boundaries were respected in your family of origin and how you manage boundaries in your own personal life. How sensitive are you to the boundaries of others in your personal life? If we establish and maintain appropriate boundaries in our personal lives, it is unlikely that we will be indifferent to boundaries in our professional lives, or unwittingly ignore them.

Your Thinking on Crossing Boundaries Before you read about the various forms of multiple relationships therapists may encounter, clarify your thinking on these issues:

- What are your reactions to the position that some multiple relationships and boundary crossings can enhance treatment outcomes?
- Do you think nonsexual multiple relationships necessarily lead to exploitation, sex, or harm? What are your thoughts regarding the slippery slope argument?
- Do you think the ethics codes of the various professional organizations are reasonable as they pertain to boundary issues, nonprofessional relationships, and multiple relationships?
- What challenges, if any, do you face in establishing and maintaining boundaries in your personal life?
- Might certain multiple relationships alter the power differential between you and your client in such a manner as to facilitate better health and healing?
- Would your fears of a malpractice suit alter the way you deal with boundaries with clients? If so, what are you doing now that could be viewed as being unethical?
- What topics pertaining to managing boundaries, multiple roles, and multiple relationships would you want to address with your clients from the initial session?

As you read the rest of this chapter, think of some challenges you might encounter in managing multiple relationships.

Managing Multiple Relationships in a Small Community

Learning to manage multiple relationships is essential for practitioners in small communities. Practitioners in rural settings often find themselves involved in multiple relationships (Barnett, 2017b) as they balance the roles of being a clinician, a neighbor, a friend, and perhaps even a spiritual leader. Other challenges include professional isolation, high visibility in the community, spending a great deal of time traveling between professional engagements, and coping with the inevitability of multiple relationships (Bray, 2016). Practitioners who work in small communities often have to blend their professional role with a variety of community-oriented roles, such as being a member of a religious group, a member on various boards, an educational consultant, or a sports coach (Bradley, Werth, & Hastings, 2012). Clinicians may attend the same church or community activities as the clients they serve. A therapist who is a recovering alcoholic and attends Alcoholics Anonymous meetings may meet a client at one of these meetings. In an isolated area, a clergy person may seek counseling for a personal crisis from the only counselor in the town—someone who also happens to be a parishioner. Managing boundaries and multiple relationships are realities faced by all therapists who live and practice in small communities.

Coping With Challenges of Practice in Rural Communities

Counselors who practice in a rural area clearly experience challenges, but Bray (2016) believes these challenges can best be met by being creative and willing to collaborate with clients and others in the community. "Rural counseling is anything but the neat-and-tidy model in which a practitioner sees each individual client one hour per week in a single office" (pp. 33–34). To protect client confidentiality in small, closely knit communities where therapists commonly need to balance multiple roles, potential concerns about boundary issues and how best to safeguard client privacy should be discussed at the beginning of the counseling relationship. Barnett (2017b) believes that the goal for rural therapists is not to avoid all multiple roles and relationships but to manage these relationships in an ethical and thoughtful manner.

A counselor who worked in a community agency in a rural area described how he addressed confidentiality matters with one of his clients:

> One of my clients disclosed to me in our first session together that he was gay, but he did not want the director of the agency to know that about him because they attended the same church. My client was in the process of coming out to significant others in his life, and it was important to him to feel a sense of control over the disclosure of this information. Earlier in that session, as I was discussing informed consent with him, I had revealed that the director of the agency was my clinical supervisor and that it was customary for me to discuss all of my cases with him. After my client shared his concerns, we brainstormed how we could work together so that he would feel comfortable

and I would have access to supervision. The client granted me permission to share with the director the basic dilemma without sharing the specific issue that he didn't want me to reveal. The director was understanding and wanted to respect the client's boundaries and confidentiality. He allowed me to seek supervision for this one case from another therapist on staff. The client was satisfied with this solution, and we had a productive therapeutic relationship.

Another challenge in practicing therapy in a small community is illustrated by Henry's case. Henry owned a farm supply store in a midwestern town. He was given an ultimatum by his wife to seek therapy or face a divorce, and Henry reluctantly agreed to meet with a local therapist to address his anger management issues. A major factor contributing to his stress and anger was that another farm supply store had recently opened in the community, which put a strain on his business. The therapist was familiar with the new farm supply store because her son had recently been hired at this store. The therapist decided to disclose that her son was working there. If she withheld this information from Henry and he later discovered it on his own, he would likely feel betrayed.

Henry was worried about people knowing he was going to therapy, and the therapist and Henry spent time during the first session discussing how they could take precautions to protect his confidentiality. In addition to addressing the source of his anger and ways to manage it constructively, the therapist assisted Henry in identifying resources that support small businesses. She encouraged him to join a regional small business advocacy group that met monthly, and Henry found this group to be helpful.

Practicing counseling in rural communities comes with both advantages and challenges. Advantages related to a rural lifestyle such as less traffic and crime and a slower pace draws practitioners to these communities, and Fifield and Oliver (2016) state that the "challenges of rural practice are well documented and tend to cluster around ethical issues regarding professional competence, ensuring confidentiality, and avoiding/managing multiple relationships" (p. 77). If practitioners isolate themselves from the surrounding community, they are likely to alienate potential clients and reduce their effectiveness. Practitioners must be prepared to face the ethical dilemmas unique to rural practice. For example, if a therapist shops for a new snow plow he risks violating the letter of the ethics code if the only person in town who sells snow plows happens to be a client. However, if the therapist were to buy a snow plow elsewhere, this could strain relationships within the community because of the value rural communities place on loyalty to local merchants. Or consider clients who wish to barter goods or services for counseling services. Some communities operate substantially on swaps rather than on a cash economy. This does not necessarily have to become problematic, yet the potential for conflict exists in the therapeutic relationship if the bartering agreements do not work well.

Minimizing Risks of Practicing in Small Communities

Practitioners in rural communities experience greater visibility than those in urban settings, which has a bearing on the way therapists take care of themselves and how they balance their personal and professional life. Schank (Schank, Helbok,

Haldeman, & Gallardo, 2010) states that practitioners in small communities can minimize risk and practice ethically and professionally by following these steps:

- Obtain informed consent
- Document thoroughly
- Set clear boundaries and expectations, both for yourself and with your clients
- Pay attention to matters of confidentiality
- Get involved in ongoing consultation or a peer supervision group

Fifield and Oliver (2016) conducted a needs assessment to identify ways to increase the perceived competency of rural practitioners. Those who responded to the survey reported that training specific to rural counseling would be helpful in strengthening their perceived competence. In addition to workshops and conferences, survey participants cited online communities, online interest networks, and regional resource guides hosted on the websites of professional organizations as potential resources.

A Case of a Multiple Relationship in a Small Community

Millie, a therapist in a small community, experienced heart pain one day. The fire department was called, and the medic on the team turned out to be her client, Andres. To administer proper medical care, Andres had to remove Millie's upper clothing. During subsequent sessions, neither Andres nor Millie discussed the incident, but both exhibited a degree of discomfort with each other. After a few more sessions, Andres discontinued his therapy with Millie.

- Can this case be considered an unavoidable dual relationship? Why or why not?
- What might Millie have done to prevent this outcome?
- Should Millie have discussed her discomfort in the therapy session following the incident? Why or why not?
- If you were in Millie's situation, what would you have done?

Commentary. This case illustrates how some roles can shift and how some multiple relationships are unavoidable, especially in small communities where therapists need to anticipate frequent boundary crossings with clients. In our view, Millie should have discussed with Andres how he would like to handle chance encounters in the community during the informed consent process. Even so, we doubt that Millie could have predicted this awkward boundary crossing with Andres. Clinically, Millie might have salvaged the therapy relationship by processing her own discomfort with a colleague, and then processing the event with Andres. By allowing the discomfort to remain hidden, Millie failed to practice with the best interests of her client in mind. In this instance, neither Millie's nor Andres's needs were being met in the therapeutic relationship. •

Practicing Ethically in a Small Community

I (Marianne Schneider Corey) practiced for many years as a marriage and family therapist in a small town. This situation presented a number of ethical considerations involving safeguarding the privacy of clients. Even in urban areas, therapists will occasionally encounter their clients in other situations. However, in a rural area such meetings are more likely to occur.

I discussed with my clients the unique variables pertaining to confidentiality in a small community. I informed them that I would not discuss professional concerns with them should we meet at the grocery store or the post office, and I respected their preferences regarding interactions away from the office. Knowing that they were aware that I saw many people from the town, I reassured them that I would not talk with anyone about who my clients were, even when I might be directly asked. Another example of protecting my clients' privacy pertained to the manner of depositing checks at the local bank. Because the bank employees knew my profession, it would have been easy for them to identify my clients. Again, I talked with my clients about their preferences. If they had any discomfort about my depositing their checks in the local bank, I arranged to have them deposited elsewhere.

Practicing in a small town inevitably meant that I would meet clients in many places. For example, the checker at the grocery store might be my client; the person standing in line before me at the store could be a client who wants to talk about his or her week; at church there may be clients or former clients in the same Bible study group; in restaurants a client's family may be seated next to the table where my family is dining, or the food server could be a client; and on a hiking event I may discover that in the group is a client and his or her partner. As I was leaving the hairstyling salon in town one day, I encountered a former client of many years ago who enthusiastically greeted me. I stopped and acknowledged her, and she then went on in detail telling the hairstylist about her therapy with me. I did not ask her any pointed questions nor did I engage her in any counseling issues. Instead, I kept the conversation general. Had I not acknowledged her, this most likely would have offended her. All of these examples present possible problems for the therapist. Neither my clients nor I experienced problems in such situations because we had talked about the possibility of such meetings in advance. Being a practitioner in a small community demands flexibility, honesty, and sensitivity. In managing multiple roles and relationships, it is not very useful to rely on rigid rules and policies; you must be ready to creatively adapt to situations as they unfold.

The examples I have given demonstrate that what might clearly not be advisable in an urban area might just as clearly be unavoidable or perhaps mandatory in a rural area. This does not mean that rural mental health professionals are free do whatever they please. The task of managing boundaries is more challenging in rural areas, and practitioners often are called upon to examine what is in the best interests of their client.

Now consider these questions:

- What ethical dilemmas do you think you would encounter if you were to practice in a rural area?
- Are you comfortable discussing possible outside contacts with clients up front, and are you able to set guidelines with your clients?
- What are some of the advantages and disadvantages of practicing in a small community?
- Is there more room for flexibility in setting guidelines regarding social relationships and outside business contacts with clients in a small community?

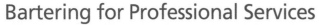

Bartering for Professional Services

When a client is unable to afford therapy, it is possible that he or she may offer a **bartering** arrangement, exchanging goods or services in lieu of a fee. For example, a mechanic might exchange work on a therapist's car for counseling sessions. However, if the client was expected to provide several hours of work on the therapist's car in exchange for one therapy session, this client might become resentful over the perceived imbalance of the exchange. If the therapist's car was not repaired properly, the therapist might resent that client. This would damage the therapeutic relationship. In addition, problems of another sort can occur with dual relationships should clients clean houses, perform secretarial services, or do other personal work for the therapist. Clients can easily be put in a bind when they are in a position to learn personal material about their therapists. The client might feel taken advantage of by the therapist, which could damage his or her therapy. Certainly, many problems can arise from these kinds of exchanges for both therapists and clients.

Ethical Standards on Bartering

Most ethics codes address the complexities of bartering (see the Ethics Codes box titled "Bartering"). We agree with the general tone of these standards, although we would add that bartering should be evaluated within a cultural context. In some cultures, and especially in rural communities, bartering is an accepted practice and frequently conforms to prevailing community standards (Barnett, 2017b). The ethics codes of APA, NASW, AAMFT, AMHCA, and ACA currently take a realistic stance on bartering, and most professional organizations now provide guidelines for the ethical practice of bartering.

ETHICS CODES: Bartering

American Psychological Association (2010)
Barter is the acceptance of goods, services, or other nonmonetary remuneration from clients/patients in return for psychological services. Psychologists may barter only if (1) it is not clinically contraindicated, and (2) the resulting arrangement is not exploitative. (6.05.)

American Counseling Association (2014)
Counselors may barter only if the bartering does not result in exploitation or harm, if the client requests it, and if such arrangements are an accepted practice among professionals in the community. Counselors consider the cultural implications of bartering and discuss relevant concerns with clients and document such agreements in a clear written contract. (A.10.e.)

American Association for Marriage and Family Therapy (2015)
Marriage and family therapists ordinarily refrain from accepting goods and services from clients in return for services rendered. Bartering for professional services may be conducted only if: (a) the supervisee or client requests it, (b) the relationship is not exploitative, (c) the professional relationship is not distorted, and (d) a clear written contract is established. (8.5.)

American Mental Health Counselors Association (2015)

Mental health counselors usually refrain from accepting goods or services from clients in return for counseling services because such arrangements may create the potential for conflicts, exploitation and distortion of the professional relationship. However, bartering may occur if the client requests it, there is no exploitation, and the cultural implications and other concerns of such practice are discussed with the client and agreed upon in writing. (E.2.b.)

National Association of Social Workers (2008)

Social workers should avoid accepting goods or services from clients as payment for professional services. Bartering arrangements, particularly involving services, create the potential for conflicts of interest, exploitation, and inappropriate boundaries in social workers' relationships with clients. Social workers should explore and may participate in bartering only in very limited circumstances when it can be demonstrated that such arrangements are an accepted practice among professionals in the local community, considered to be essential for the provision of services, negotiated without coercion, and entered into at the client's initiative and with the client's informed consent. Social workers who accept goods or services from clients as payment for professional services assume the full burden of demonstrating that this arrangement will not be detrimental to the client or the professional relationship. (1.13.b.)

Before bartering is entered into, both parties need to talk about the arrangement, gain a clear understanding of the exchange, and come to an agreement. It is important that problems that might develop be discussed and that alternatives be examined. Using a sliding scale to determine fees or making a referral are two possible alternatives that might have merit. Bartering is an example of a practice that we think allows some room for therapists, in collaboration with their clients, to use good judgment and consider the cultural context in the situation. Zur (2011a) maintains that bartering can be a dignified and honorable form of payment for those who are cash poor but talented in other ways. He adds that bartering is a healthy norm in many cultures. Bartering can be part of a clearly articulated treatment plan, and like other interventions, bartering must be considered in light of the client's needs, desires, situation, and cultural background. If bartering is done thoughtfully and in a collaborative way, it can be beneficial for many clients and can enhance therapeutic outcomes.

Barnett and Johnson (2008) and Koocher and Keith-Spiegel (2016) acknowledge that bartering arrangements with clients can be both a reasonable and a humanitarian practice when people require psychological services but do not have insurance coverage and are in financial difficulty. Barnett and Johnson (2008) suggest that bartering arrangements can be a culturally sensitive and clinically indicated decision that may prove satisfactory to both parties. However, bartering entails risks, and they emphasize the importance of carefully assessing such arrangements prior to taking them on. Clinicians should seek consultation from a trusted colleague who can provide an objective evaluation of the proposed arrangement in terms of equity, clinical appropriateness, and the danger of potentially harmful multiple relationships.

Both Holly Forester-Miller (2015) and Lawrence Thomas (2002) provide views on the benefits of bartering when clients cannot afford to pay for psychological services. Forester-Miller (2015) addresses the difficulties involved in avoiding overlapping relationships in rural communities and reminds counselors that values and beliefs may vary significantly between urban dwellers and their rural counterparts. She suggests that counselors need to ensure that they are not imposing values that come from a cultural perspective different from that of their clients. Bartering is one way of providing counseling services in some regions to individuals who could not otherwise afford counseling. Forester-Miller recounts her experience providing therapy in the Appalachian culture, where individuals pride themselves on being able to provide for themselves and their loved ones. Forester-Miller once provided counseling for an adolescent girl whose single-parent mother could not afford her usual fee, nor could she afford to pay a reduced fee, as even a small amount would be a drain on this family's resources. When Forester-Miller informed the mother that she would be willing to see her daughter for free, the mother stated that this would not be acceptable to her. However, she asked the counselor if she would accept a quilt she had made as payment for counseling the daughter. The mother and the counselor discussed the monetary value of the quilt and decided to use this as payment for a specified number of counseling sessions. Forester-Miller reports that this was a good solution because it enabled the adolescent girl to receive needed counseling services and gave the mother an opportunity to maintain her dignity in that she could pay her own way.

Thomas (2002) believes bartering is a legitimate means of making psychological services available to people of limited economic means. He maintains that bartering should not be ruled out simply because of the slight chance that a client might initiate a lawsuit against the therapist. His view is that if we are not willing to take some risks as psychotherapy professionals, then we are not worthy of our position. Thomas believes that venturing into a multiple relationship requires careful thought and judgment. In making decisions about bartering, the most salient issue is the "higher standard" of considering the welfare of the client. Thomas recommends a written contract that spells out in detail the nature of the agreement between therapist and client, which should be reviewed regularly. Documenting the arrangement can clarify agreements and can help professionals defend themselves if this becomes necessary. Thomas admits that bartering is a troublesome topic, yet he emphasizes that the role of our professional character is to focus on the higher standard—the best interests of the client.

Making a Decision About Bartering

Barnett and Johnson (2008) maintain that, as a general rule, it is unwise to engage in bartering practices with therapy clients. They add that accepting goods or services for professional services can open the door to misunderstandings, perceived or actual exploitation, boundary violations, and reduced effectiveness as a clinician. Although bartering is not prohibited by ethics or law, most legal experts frown on the practice. Woody (1998), both a psychologist and an attorney, argues against the use of bartering for psychological services. He suggests that it could be argued that bartering is below the minimum standard of practice. If you enter into a bartering agreement with your client, Woody states that you will have the burden of proof to demonstrate that (a) the bartering arrangement is in the best interests of your client; (b) is reasonable, equitable, and undertaken without undue influence; and (c) does not get in the way of providing quality psychological services to your client. Because bartering is so fraught with risks for both client and therapist, Woody believes prudence dictates that it should be the option of last resort.

Zur (2011a) notes that many who are opposed to bartering view this practice as the first step on the slippery slope toward harming clients. Zur believes what is missing in the literature is a discussion of bartering that is done intentionally and deliberately for the benefit of the client. Rather than focusing on the "do no harm" approach, Zur focuses on "doing good," or doing what is most likely to improve the client's mental health.

During an economic crisis therapists may be presented with more frequent requests for bartering. Here are a few guidelines for bartering arrangements:

- Determine the value of the goods or services in a collaborative fashion with the client at the outset of the bartering arrangement.
- Estimate the length of time for the barter arrangement.
- Document the bartering arrangement, including the value of the goods or services and a date on which the arrangement will end.

To these recommendations we add the importance of consulting with experienced colleagues, a supervisor, and especially your professional organization if you are considering some form of bartering in lieu of payment for therapy services.

The client may not realize the potential conflicts and problems involved in bartering. It is the counselor's responsibility to enumerate the potential problems and risks in bartering. We highly recommend a straightforward discussion with your client about the pros and cons of bartering in your particular situation, especially as it may apply to the standards of your community. It may be wise to consult with a third party regarding the value of a fair market exchange. We concur with Thomas (2002), who recommends creating a written contract that specifies hours spent by each party and all particulars of the agreement. If you still have doubts about the agreement, consult with a contract lawyer. Once potential problems have been identified, consult with colleagues about alternatives you and your client may not have considered. Ongoing consultation and discussion of cases, especially in matters pertaining to boundaries and dual roles, provide a context for understanding the implications of certain practices. Needless to say, these consultations should be documented.

Your Stance on Bartering Consider a situation in which you have a client who cannot afford to pay even a reduced fee. Would you be inclined to engage in bartering goods for your services? What kind of understanding would you need to work out with your client before you agreed to a bartering arrangement? Would your decision be dependent on whether you were practicing in a large urban area or a rural area? How would you take the cultural context into consideration when making your decision?

Which services might you be willing to barter for with a client? Think about why you would or would not be comfortable in each situation. Answer "yes," "no," or "uncertain" regarding each of the following services:

- Have my client clean my house or office
- Have my client take care of my pets while I'm on vacation
- Accept my client's art work
- Accept my client cutting my hair or providing manicures
- Accept yoga lessons from my client
- Have my client tutor my child

What do your responses say about your personal and professional boundaries? Are there any cultural factors or contextual factors that might cause you to change your answers?

Consider the following cases and apply the ethical standards we have summarized to your analysis. What ethical issues are involved in each case? What potential problems do you see emerging from these cases? What alternatives to bartering can you think of?

The Case of Macy

Macy is 20 years old and has been in therapy with Sidney for over a year. She has developed respect and fondness for her therapist, whom she sees as a father figure. She tells him that she is thinking of discontinuing therapy because she has lost her job and simply has no way of paying for the sessions. She is obviously upset over the prospect of ending the relationship, but she sees no alternative. Sidney informs her that he is willing to continue her therapy even if she is unable to pay. He suggests that as an exchange of services she can become the babysitter for his three children. She gratefully accepts this offer. After a few months, however, Macy finds that the situation is becoming difficult for her. Eventually she writes a note to Sidney telling him that she cannot handle her reactions to his wife and their children. It makes her think of all the things she missed in her own family. She writes that she has found this subject difficult to bring up in her sessions, so she is planning to quit both her services and her therapy.

- What questions does this case raise for you?
- How would you have dealt with this situation?
- What are your thoughts concerning the therapist's suggestion that Macy babysit for him?
- Do you think Sidney adequately considered the nature of the transference relationship with this client?

Commentary. This case illustrates how a well-meaning therapist created a multiple relationship with his client that became problematic for her. In addition, Sidney suggested a bartering arrangement that involved Macy performing personal services in exchange for therapy; it generally is not a good idea for a therapist to involve his significant others in barter exchanges with the client. Sidney did not explore with Macy her transference feelings for him, nor did he predict potential difficulties with her taking care of his children. Indeed, countertransference on Sidney's part may have led to the blurring of boundaries. The ethics codes of the ACA (2014), APA (2010), NASW (2008), AMHCA (2015), and AAMFT (2015) all specify that bartering may be ethical under certain conditions: if the client requests it; if it is not clinically contraindicated; if it is not exploitative; and if the arrangement is entered into with full informed consent. None of these standards was met in this case. Sidney should have explored other options such as working pro bono, reducing his fees, or a referral to another agency. •

The Case of Thai

Thai is a massage therapist in her community. Her services are sought by many professionals, including Giovani, a local psychologist. In the course of a massage session, she confides in him that she is experiencing difficulties in her long-term relationship. She would like to discuss with him the possibility of exchanging professional services. She proposes that in return for couples therapy she will give both him and his partner massage treatments. An equitable arrangement based on their fee structures can be worked out. Giovani might make any one of the following responses:

Response A: That's fine with me, Thai. It sounds like a good proposal. Neither one of us will suffer financially because of it, and we can each benefit from our expertise.

Response B: Well, Thai, I feel okay about the exchange, except I have concerns about the dual relationship.

Response C: Even though our relationship is professional, Thai, I do feel uncomfortable about seeing you as a client in couples therapy. I certainly could refer you to a competent relationship therapist.

Consider your thoughts about these response options.

- Which do you consider to be ethical? unethical?
- Do you think Thai's proposal is practical?
- What are the ethical implications in this case?
- Do you think Thai's suggestion for an exchange of services reflects her own culturally appropriate standards? If so, how would that affect your response?
- If you were in this situation, how would you respond to Thai?

Commentary. Because of the physically intimate nature of massage work, we would discourage any therapist from entering into this kind of exchange. We do not see any signs that Thai and Giovani adequately assessed the potential risks involved in exchanging these personal services. In addition, no indication of an inability to pay for counseling has been stated by Thai. As with the previous case, other options besides bartering could have been considered. •

The Case of Exchanging Services for Therapy

Vidar is a counselor in private practice who has been seeing a client for a few months. Jana is hard working, dedicated to personal growth, and is making progress in treatment. At her last session she expressed concern about her ability to continue funding her sessions. Jana suggested that Vidar consider allowing her husband's pool company to provide summer pool cleaning service for the months of May through August for Vidar's home pool in return for her continued sessions. The fees would be basically equitable, and Vidar is seriously considering this agreement to assist Jana in her ability to continue counseling.

- Does this arrangement seem like a reasonable request to you?
- What ethical issues related to this situation might cause you concern, if any?
- Which ethical standards apply to this situation?

Commentary. The case of Vidar and Jana is less clear-cut. It is important that the arrangement was suggested by Jana and not by Vidar. It would be beneficial for Vidar to consider some consultation in reviewing the pros and cons of this proposal prior to making a decision. Vidar should also consider whether bartering is a commonly accepted practice in his geographical area. If he decides to participate in this bartering arrangement, he will need to have an explicit written contract of the agreed-upon terms of exchange. Exchanging services for therapy, because of its complexity, is fraught with more inherent problems than is accepting goods from clients. Vidar might suggest an alternative form of bartering, asking Jana to perform some kind of community service for a mutually agreed-upon cause or a nonprofit organization rather than a more direct exchange (Zur, 2007). •

Giving or Receiving Gifts

The codes of ethics of the AAMFT, the AMHCA, and the ACA specifically address the topic of giving or receiving gifts in the therapeutic relationship. See the Ethics Codes box titled "Giving and Receiving Gifts" for specific standards of these organizations.

Lavish gifts certainly present an ethical problem, yet we can go too far in the direction of trying to be ethical and, in so doing, actually damage the therapeutic relationship. Some therapists include a statement regarding gifts from clients in their informed consent document to make their policy clear. Rather than establishing a hard and fast rule, our preference is to evaluate each situation on a case-by-case basis. Let's examine a few of these areas in more detail.

- *What is the monetary value of the gift?* Most mental health professionals would agree that accepting a very expensive gift is problematic and potentially unethical. It would also be problematic if a client offered tickets to the theater or a sporting event and wanted you to accompany him or her to this event. In the novel *Lying on the Couch* (Yalom, 1997), a therapist is offered a $1,600 bonus by a wealthy client to show his appreciation for how a few therapy sessions changed his life. The therapist struggles as he declines this gift, stating that it is considered unethical to accept a monetary gift from a client. The client angrily protests, claiming that rejecting his gift could cancel some of the gains made during their work, and he *insists* that the score be evened. The therapist steadfastly responds that he cannot accept the gift and acknowledges that one topic they did not discuss in therapy was the client's discomfort in accepting help.

- *What are the clinical implications of accepting or rejecting the gift?* It is important to recognize when accepting a gift from a client is clinically contraindicated and that you be willing to explore this with your client. Certainly, knowing the motivation for a client's overture is critical to making a decision. For example, a client may be seeking your approval, in which case the main motivation for giving you a gift is to please you. Accepting the gift without adequate discussion would not be helping your client in the long run. Practitioners may want to inquire what meaning even small gifts have to the client. Zur (2011b) suggests that any gift must be understood and evaluated within the context in which it is given. He mentions that inappropriately expensive gifts or any gifts that create indebtedness, whether of the client or the therapist, are boundary violations. However, Zur (2011b) claims that appropriate gift-giving can be a healthy aspect of a therapist–client relationship and can enhance therapeutic effectiveness.

• *When in the therapy process is the offering of a gift occurring?* Is it at the beginning of the therapy process? Is it at the termination of the professional relationship? It could be more problematic to accept a gift at an early stage of a counseling relationship because doing so may be a forerunner to creating lax boundaries. A gift at the end of therapy may have cultural and symbolic value for clients. Therapists should assess whether accepting a gift from a client is appropriate.

• *What are your own motivations for accepting or rejecting a client's gift?* The giving or receiving of gifts has layers of meaning that should be explored. You must be aware of whose needs are being served by receiving a gift. Some counselors will accept a gift simply because they do not want to hurt a client's feelings, even though they are not personally comfortable doing so. Counselors may accept a gift because they are unable to establish firm and clear boundaries. Other counselors may accept a gift because they actually want what a client is offering. In appropriate circumstances, a gift may be helpful to therapy, but it is the therapist's responsibility to consider the meaning of the gift.

• *What are the cultural implications of offering a gift?* The cultural context plays a role in evaluating the appropriateness of accepting a gift from a client. Sue and Capodilupo (2015) point out that in Asian cultures gift-giving is a common practice to show respect, gratitude, and to seal a relationship. Although such actions are culturally appropriate, Western-trained professionals may believe that accepting a gift would distort boundaries, change the relationship, and create a conflict of interest. However, if a practitioner were to refuse a client's gift, it is likely that this person would feel insulted or humiliated, and the refusal could damage both the therapeutic relationship and the client. Zur (2011b) notes that most practitioners agree that rejecting appropriate gifts of small monetary value but of high relational value can be offensive to clients and negatively affect the therapeutic alliance. Neukrug and Milliken (2011) found that the value of the gift was important in counselors' decisions. Of the counselors they surveyed, 88.3% thought it was unethical to accept a gift from a client worth more than $25, and 94.7% believed it was unethical to give a gift to a client worth more than $25. If you are opposed to receiving gifts and view this as a boundary crossing, you may need to address this issue in your informed consent document.

One of the reviewers of this book stated that students sometimes give school counselors gifts. Such gifts are usually inexpensive, if purchased, or are items made in an art or shop class. He indicates that he could accept the gift and display the gift in his office. If you were a school counselor, would you be inclined to accept inexpensive gifts? Would you display a gift in your office? How would you respond if other students (your clients) or teachers asked you who made the gift that is on display? Under what circumstances, if any, might you be inclined to give a student a gift? To what degree would you be comfortable documenting and having your colleagues learn about a gift you have accepted?

American Association for Marriage and Family Therapy (2015)
Marriage and family therapists attend to cultural norms when considering whether to accept gifts from or give gifts to clients. Marriage and family therapists consider the potential effects that receiving or giving gifts may have on clients and on the integrity and efficacy of the therapeutic relationship. (3.9)

American Counseling Association (2014)
Receiving Gifts. Counselors understand the challenges of accepting gifts from clients and recognize that in some cultures, small gifts are a token of respect and gratitude. When determining whether to accept a gift from clients, counselors take into account the therapeutic relationship, the monetary value of the gift, the client's motivation for giving the gift, and the counselor's motivation for wanting to accept or decline the gift. (A.10.f.)

American Mental Health Counselors Association (2015)
When accepting gifts, mental health counselors take into consideration the therapeutic relationship, motivation of giving, the counselor's motivation for receiving or declining, cultural norms, and the value of the gift. (E.2.d.)

The Case of Suki

Toward the end of her therapy, Suki, a Japanese client, presents an expensive piece of jewelry to her counselor, Joaquin. Suki says she is grateful for all that her counselor has done for her and that she really wants him to accept her gift, which has been in her family for many years. In a discussion with the counselor, Suki claims that giving gifts is a part of the Japanese culture. Joaquin discusses his dilemma, telling Suki that he would like to accept the gift but that he has a policy of not accepting gifts from clients. He reminds her of this policy, which was part of the informed consent document she signed at the beginning of the therapeutic relationship. Suki is persistent and lets Joaquin know that if he does not accept her gift she will feel rejected. She is extremely grateful for all Joaquin has done for her, and this is her way of expressing her appreciation. Joaquin recalls that Suki had told him that in her culture gifts are given with the expectation of reciprocity. A few days after this session, Joaquin received an invitation from Suki to attend her daughter's birthday party where her family would be present.

Put yourself in this situation with Suki. What aspects would you want to explore with your client before accepting or not accepting her gift?

- Do you see a difference between accepting a gift during therapy or toward the end of therapy?

- Would it be important to consider your client's cultural background in accepting or not accepting the gift?

- How would you deal with Suki if she insisted that you recognize her token of appreciation and accept her invitation to her daughter's birthday party?

- If you find that clients frequently want to give you gifts, would you need to reflect on what you might be doing to promote this pattern? Explain.

Commentary. Joaquin was clear about his policy on accepting gifts, which was included in his informed consent document, and he understood that Suki accepted this guideline. To help Joaquin assess the meaning of this gesture and avoid potentially misunderstanding Suki's desire that he accept her gift, Joaquin could discuss with her what importance and meaning the gift has for her. He could also explore with her the cultural implications of her offering him this gift. Counselors must weigh cultural influences and implications in professional relationships, but it is important not to yield to a culture-based request that might ultimately harm the client or the counseling relationship. Joaquin must deal with the pressure to accept the gift if it does not seem right for him to do so. With respect to the invitation to the daughter's birthday party, Joaquin would do well to reflect on how he will deal with possible future requests from this client as well as requests from other clients. •

Social Relationships With Clients

Do social relationships with clients necessarily interfere with therapeutic relationships? Some would say no, contending that counselors and clients are able to handle such relationships as long as the priorities are clear. They see social contacts as particularly appropriate with clients who are not deeply disturbed and who are seeking personal growth. Some peer counselors, for example, maintain that friendships before or during counseling are actually positive factors in establishing trust.

Other practitioners take the position that counseling and friendship should not be mixed. They claim that attempting to manage a social and professional relationship simultaneously can have a negative effect on the therapeutic process, the friendship, or both. Here are some reasons for discouraging the practice of accepting friends as clients or of becoming socially involved with clients: (1) therapists may not be as challenging as they need to be with clients they know socially because of a need to be liked and accepted by the client; (2) counselors' own needs may be enmeshed with those of their clients to the point that objectivity is lost; and (3) counselors are at greater risk of exploiting clients because of the power differential in the therapeutic relationship.

Cultural Considerations

The cultural context can play a role in evaluating the appropriateness of dual relationships that involve friendships in the therapy context. Parham and Caldwell (2015) question Western ethical standards that discourage dual and multiple relationships and claim that such standards can prove to be an obstacle or hindrance in counseling African American clients. In an African context, therapy is not confined to a practitioner's office for 50-minute sessions. Instead, therapy involves multiple activities that might include conversation, playful activities, laughter, shared meals and cooking experiences, travel, rituals and ceremony, singing or drumming, storytelling, writing, and touching. Parham and Caldwell view each of these activities as having the potential to bring a "healing focus" to the therapeutic experience.

In a similar spirit, Sue and Capodilupo (2015) point out that some cultural groups may value multiple relationships with helping professionals. Consider these cultural differences in determining when multiple relationships might be acceptable:

- In some Asian cultures it is believed that personal matters are best discussed with a relative or a friend. Self-disclosing to a stranger (the counselor) is considered taboo and a violation of familial and cultural values. Some Asian clients may prefer to have the traditional counseling role evolve into a more personal one.

- Clients from many cultural groups prefer to receive advice and suggestions from an expert. They perceive the counselor to be an expert, having higher status and possessing superior knowledge. To work effectively with these clients, the counselor may have to play a number of different roles, such as advocate, adviser, change agent, and facilitator of indigenous support systems. Yet counselors may view playing more than one of these roles as engaging in dual or multiple relationships.

Forming Social Relationships With Former Clients

Mental health professionals are not legally or ethically prohibited from entering into a nonsexual relationship with a client after the termination of therapy. However, forming friendships with former clients may pose difficulties for both the client and the therapist. For example, a former client might feel taken advantage of, which could result in a complaint against the therapist. Therapists need to know that it is their responsibility to evaluate the impact of entering into such relationships.

Although forming friendships with former clients may not be unethical or illegal, the practice can lead to problems. The safest policy is probably to avoid developing social relationships with former clients. In the long run, former clients may need you more as a therapist at some future time than as a friend. If you develop a friendship with a former client, then he or she is not eligible to use your professional services in the future. Even in the social relationship, the imbalance of power may not change and you may still be seen as a therapist or you may behave as a therapist. Mental health practitioners should be aware of their own motivations, as well as the motivations of their clients, when allowing a professional relationship to evolve into a personal one, even after the termination of therapy. We question the motivation of helpers who rely on their professional position as a way to meet their social needs. Furthermore, therapists who are in the habit of developing relationships with former clients may find themselves overextended and come to resent the relationships they sought out or to which they consented. Perhaps the crux of the situation involves the therapist being able to establish clear boundaries regarding what he or she is willing to do.

Your Position on Socializing With Current or Former Clients There are many types of socializing, ranging from going to a social event with a client to having a cup of tea or coffee with a client. Social involvements initiated by a client are different from those initiated by a therapist. Another factor to consider is whether the social contact is ongoing or occasional. The degree of intimacy is also a factor; there is a difference between meeting a client for coffee or for a candlelight dinner. In thinking through your own position on establishing a dual relationship with a current client, consider the nature of the social function, the nature of your client's problem, the client population, the setting where you work, the kind of therapy being employed, and your theoretical approach. For example, if you are psychoanalytically oriented, you might adopt stricter boundaries and would be concerned about infecting the transference relationship should you blend any form of socializing with therapy. Weigh the various factors and consider this matter from both the client's and the therapist's perspective.

When professional and social relationships are blended, a great deal of honesty and self-awareness is required by the therapist. Ask yourself why you are considering a social relationship with a client or former client. No matter how clear the therapist is on boundaries, if the client cannot understand or cannot handle the social relationship, such a relationship should not be formed—with either current or former clients. When clear boundaries are not maintained, both the professional and the social relationship can sour. Clients may well become inhibited during therapy out of fear of alienating their therapist. They may fear losing the respect of a therapist with whom they have a friendship. They may censor their disclosures so that they do not threaten this social relationship.

What are your thoughts on this topic? What are the therapist's obligations to former clients? Under what circumstances might such relationships be inappropriate or even unethical? When do you think these relationships might be considered ethical? When you are uncertain about how to proceed, consultation is a priority.

Sexual Attractions in the Client–Therapist Relationship

Are sexual attractions to be expected in therapy? In a classic and pioneering study, Pope, Keith-Spiegel, and Tabachnick (1986) addressed the lack of systematic research into the sexual attraction of therapists to their clients. Pope and his colleagues studied 585 respondents, and only 77 reported never having been attracted to any client. The vast majority (82%) reported that they had never seriously considered actual sexual involvement with a client. An even larger majority (93.5%) reported never having had sexual relations with their clients. Therapists gave a number of reasons for having refrained from acting out their attractions to clients, including a need to uphold professional values, a concern about the welfare of the client, and a desire to follow personal values. Fears of negative consequences were mentioned, but they were less frequently cited than values pertaining to client welfare. Those who had some graduate training in this area were more likely to have sought consultation (66%) than those with no such training.

The tendency to treat sexual feelings as if they are taboo has made it difficult for therapists to acknowledge and accept attractions to clients (Pope, Sonne, &

Holroyd, 1993). Simply experiencing sexual attraction to a client, without acting on it, makes the majority of therapists feel guilty, anxious, and confused. Given these reactions, it is not surprising that many therapists want to hide these feelings rather than acknowledge and deal with sexual feelings by consulting a colleague or by bringing this to their own therapy. Although a majority of therapists report feeling sexually attracted to some clients, and most report discomfort with their feelings, adequate training in this area is relatively rare (Pope & Wedding, 2014). In a survey conducted by Neukrug and Milliken (2011), 10.3% of counselors thought it was ethical to reveal a sexual attraction to a client; 89.7% thought this was unethical.

In the specialty area of sport psychology consulting, little is known about the extent to which practitioners are aware of, manage, or act on their sexual attractions. This lack of knowledge inspired a group of researchers to examine this phenomenon. Moles and colleagues (2016) reported that the vast majority (78.3%) of sport psychology consultants (SPC) in their study received ethics training on this issue while in graduate school, and some also received training after earning their graduate degrees. Of the 275 SPCs surveyed, 112 (40.7%) claimed to have been sexually attracted to *at least* one client-athlete. The majority were attracted to 1–2 client-athletes, 28.6% were attracted to 3–5 client-athletes, 8.9% were attracted to 6–10 client-athletes, and 6.3% were attracted to 11 or more client-athletes. Of the 112 respondents who acknowledged experiencing sexual attractions, only 88 reported on whether they had engaged in sexual behaviors: 13.6% admitted to crossing sexual boundaries "primarily by discussing sexual matters unrelated to their work; no SPC reported kissing, dating, or having sexual intercourse with a client-athlete" (p. 93).

There is a distinction between finding a client sexually attractive and being preoccupied with this attraction. The SPCs who sought supervision to discuss their sexual attraction issues found supervision to be embarrassing and slightly uncomfortable, but also helpful, enlightening, reassuring, supportive, engaging, therapeutic, empowering, and normalizing (Moles et al., 2016). If you find yourself sexually attracted to your clients, it is important to monitor your feelings. If you are frequently attracted, examine this issue in your own therapy and supervision. We recommend Irvin Yalom's (1997) book, *Lying on the Couch: A Novel*, for an interesting case and discourse on the slippery slope of sexual attraction between therapist and client.

Educating Counselor Trainees

Training programs have an ethical responsibility to help students identify and openly discuss their concerns pertaining to sexual dilemmas in counseling practice. Prevention of sexual misconduct is a better path than remediation. Ignoring this subject in training sends a message to students that the subject should not be talked about, which will inhibit their willingness to seek consultation when they encounter sexual dilemmas in their practice. The findings from Harris and Harriger's (2009) study on sexual attraction in conjoint therapy suggest that new marriage and family therapists are not confident about the course of action to take when faced with the issue of sexual attraction. These researchers claim that there is an urgent need to address this topic during a training program and equip therapists in training with the skills to manage sexual attraction in a range of settings.

Pope, Sonne, and Holroyd (1993) believe that exploration of sexual feelings about clients is best done with the help, support, and encouragement of others. They maintain that practice, internships, and peer supervision groups are ideal places to talk about this issue but that this topic is rarely raised. It is a disservice to therapists and clients if training involving sexual ethics is limited to the injunction to "never engage in sex with clients." Young (2010) broadens this topic to include a host of delicate and complicated sexual matters such as sexual attraction, sexual fantasy, sexual advances of clients, romantic relationships with former clients, and sexual discussions in therapy. These topics should be included in training programs.

Suggestions for Dealing With Sexual Attractions

Trainees as well as experienced counselors need to ask themselves how they set boundaries when sexual attraction occurs. Practitioners who have difficulty establishing clear boundaries in their personal life are more likely to encounter problems defining appropriate boundaries with their clients. To prevent sexual feelings of therapists from interfering with therapy, it is important for therapists to recognize their countertransference reactions and deal with and manage them. Burwell-Pender and Halinski (2008) point out that "the potential for sexual impropriety and sexual misconduct is increased with unmanaged countertransference" (p. 43). The vulnerability the client shows when revealing painful material is very powerful and appealing. The attention a caring therapist shows in response is also powerful and appealing. This environment creates the possibility of mutual attraction. When these feelings are acknowledged in a safe setting with a supervisor or a trusted colleague, therapists are more likely to manage their feelings productively.

Perhaps out of a fear of experiencing sexual attraction to clients, or even worse, the temptation to engage in sexual misconduct, some clinicians address the issue proactively by broaching the topic during the informed consent discussion at the initial session. Knapp, Handelsman, Gottlieb, and Vandecreek (2013) point out that harm can be done by disproportionately emphasizing certain rules such as this statement in one clinician's informed consent document: "I recognize that I am here to see Dr. X for professional purposes and that I have no sexual interest in him and will not attempt to involve him in a sexual relationship or even fantasize about him" (p. 375). This practitioner's manner "appeared to place the responsibility for sexual misconduct on the patient and to raise it to a level of importance that most patients would never have considered. Such statements could also cause some patients to wonder if this psychologist had issues with personal control over his own impulses" (p. 375). Behaving in the most honorable and ethical manner possible is important, but this quest should not lead us to make matters worse and detract from our effectiveness as professionals.

A Case of Sexual Attraction Toward a Client

You find yourself sexually attracted to one of your clients. You believe your client may have similar feelings toward you and might be willing to become involved with you. You often have difficulty paying attention during sessions because of your attraction. Which of the following options do you think is most ethical? Which of the following courses of action would you consider to be unethical?

- I can ignore my feelings for the client and my client's feelings toward me and focus on other aspects of the relationship.

- I will tell my client of my feelings of attraction, discontinue the professional relationship, and then begin a personal relationship.

- I will openly express my feelings toward my client by saying: "I'm flattered you find me an attractive person, and I'm attracted to you as well. But this relationship is not about our attraction for each other, and I'm sure that's not why you came here."

- If there was no change in the intensity of my feelings toward my client, I would arrange for a referral to another therapist.

- I would consult with a colleague or seek professional supervision.

Can you think of another direction in which you could proceed? What would you do and why?

Commentary. Some may argue that if you are sexually attracted to a client, he or she will be aware of this and it could easily impede the therapy process. As therapists, we need to control our emotional energy without getting frozen. It is a good practice to monitor ourselves by reflecting on the messages we are sending to a client. It is our responsibility to recognize and deal with our feelings toward a client in a way that does not burden the client. As Fisher (2004) states, therapists have the responsibility to make sure that they take appropriate steps to manage their feelings professionally and ethically.

Koocher and Keith-Spiegel (2016) advise therapists to discuss feelings of sexual attraction toward a client with another therapist, an experienced and trusted colleague, or an approachable supervisor. Doing so can help therapists clarify the risk, become aware of their vulnerabilities when it comes to sexual attraction, provide suggestions on how to proceed, and offer a fresh perspective on these situations. Therapists are always responsible for managing their feelings toward clients; shifting blame or responsibility to the client is never an excuse for unprofessional or unethical conduct. We caution against sharing your feelings of attraction with your client directly; such disclosures often detract from the work of therapy and may be a confusing burden for the client. •

The Case of Adriana

Adriana's husband, a police officer, was killed in the line of duty, leaving her with three school-age boys. She seeks professional help from Clint, the school social worker, and explores her grief and other issues pertaining to one son who is acting out at school. She seems to rely on the social worker as her partner in supporting her son. After 2 years the son is ready to move on to high school. She confesses to Clint that she is finding it increasingly difficult to think of not seeing him anymore. She has grown to love him. She wonders if they could continue to see each other socially and romantically.

At first Clint is taken aback. But he also realizes that throughout the relationship he has come to admire and respect Adriana, and he discloses his fondness for her. He explains to her that because of their professional relationship he is bound by ethical guidelines not to become involved with parents socially or romantically. He suggests to her that they not see each other for a year. If their feelings persist, he will then consider initiating a personal relationship.

- What do you think of Clint's way of handling the situation?
- What possible negative implications might there be for Adriana and her son?
- Is Clint making himself vulnerable to professional misconduct in any way?
- If you were in a similar situation and did not want to pursue the relationship, how might you deal with your client's disclosure?
- What personal values or life experiences have you had that might influence the way you respond in this case?

Commentary. We agree with Clint's decision to refuse to initiate a romantic relationship with Adriana at this time. Clint should carefully consider his ethical obligations bearing on romantic and sexual relationships with former clients or their family members. The ACA (2014) code explicitly prohibits such relationships for a period of 5 years following the termination of services. The APA (2010) code specifies a moratorium of 2 years, and the AAMFT (2015) code prohibits sexual intimacy with former clients regardless of time elapsed. If Clint does commence a romantic relationship with Adriana in the future, he will bear the burden of showing that this change in roles was not harmful to her. If their relationship were to end, Clint would not be protected should Adriana report him for professional misconduct.

If the boundaries involved in the therapeutic relationship are identified in our informed consent document, situations such as this are likely to be less complicated. Growing fond of each other is not an ethical violation, but how we act on our feelings toward our clients determines our degree of ethical and professional behavior. •

Sexual Relationships in Therapy: Ethical and Legal Issues

It is important to realize that the relationship between therapist and client can involve varying degrees of sexuality. Therapists may have sexual fantasies, they may behave seductively with their clients, they may influence clients to focus on sexual feelings toward them, or they may engage in physical contact that is primarily intended to satisfy their own needs. Sexual contact in therapy is not a simple matter limited to having sex with a client. Practitioners need to differentiate between a sexual attraction and acting on this attraction. Sexual overtones can distort the therapeutic relationship and become the primary focus of the sessions. We need to be aware of the effects of our sex-related socialization patterns and how they may influence possible countertransference reactions.

A number of studies have documented the harm that sexual relationships with clients can cause. Other research highlights the damage done to students and supervisees when educators and supervisors enter into sexual relationships with them (see Chapter 9). Later in this section we discuss the negative effects that typically occur when the client–therapist relationship becomes sexualized.

Ethical Standards on Sexual Contact With Clients

Sexual relationships between therapists and clients continue to receive considerable attention in the professional literature. Sexual relationships with clients are clearly unethical, and all of the major professional ethics codes have specific prohibitions against them (see the Ethics Codes box titled "Sexual Contact and the Therapeutic Relationship"). In addition, most states have declared such relationships to be a violation of the law. If therapists have had a prior sexual relationship with a person, many of the ethics codes also specify that they are prohibited from accepting this person as a client. It is clear from the statements of the major mental health organizations that these principles go beyond merely condemning sexual relationships with clients. The existing codes are explicit with respect to sexual harassment and sexual relationships with clients, students, and supervisees. However, they do not, and maybe they cannot, define some of the more subtle ways that sexuality can enter the professional relationship.

ETHICS CODES: Sexual Contact and the Therapeutic Relationship

American Association for Marriage and Family Therapy (2015)
Sexual intimacy with current clients or with known members of the client's family system is prohibited. (1.4.)

American Counseling Association (2014)
Sexual and/or romantic counselor–client interactions or relationships with current clients, their romantic partners, or their family members are prohibited. This prohibition applies to both in-person and electronic interactions or relationships. (A.5.a.)

American Mental Health Counselors Association (2015)
Romantic or sexual relationships with clients are strictly prohibited. Mental health counselors do not counsel persons with whom they have had a previous sexual relationship. (A.4.a.)

American Psychological Association (2010)
Psychologists do not engage in sexual intimacies with current clients/patients. (10.05.)

Psychologists do not engage in sexual intimacies with individuals they know to be close relatives, guardians, or significant others of current clients/patients. Psychologists do not terminate therapy to circumvent this standard. (10.06.) Psychologists do not accept as therapy clients/patients persons with whom they have engaged in sexual intimacies. (10.07.)

National Association of Social Workers (2008)
Social workers should under no circumstances engage in sexual activities or sexual contact with current clients, whether such contact is consensual or forced. (1.09.a.)

Social workers should not provide clinical services to individuals with whom they have had a prior sexual relationship. Providing clinical services to a former sexual partner has the potential to be harmful to the individual and is likely to make it difficult for the social worker and individual to maintain appropriate professional boundaries. (1.09.d.)

American Psychiatric Association (2013b)
The requirement that the physician conduct himself/herself with propriety in his or her profession and in all the actions of his or her life is especially important in the case of the psychiatrist because the patient tends to model his or her behavior after that of his or her psychiatrist by identification. Further, the necessary intensity of the treatment relationship may tend to activate sexual and other needs and fantasies on the part of both patient and psychiatrist, while weakening the objectivity necessary for control. Additionally, the inherent inequality in the doctor-patient relationship may lead to exploitation of the patient. Sexual activity with a current or former patient is unethical. (2.1.)

Sexual misconduct is considered to be one of the more serious of all ethical violations for a therapist, and it is also one of the most common allegations in malpractice suits (APA, 2003b). Grenyer and Lewis (2012) examined the prevalence of all forms of psychologist misconduct reported to the New South Wales Psychologists Registration Board over a period of 4 years. Of the 9,489 registered psychologists, complaints had been filed against 224 of them, resulting in 248 independent notifications of misconduct (some were recipients of more than one complaint). Of these complaints, 24 were related to boundary violations: 10 of the boundary violation complaints involved sexual relationships, and 4 involved sexual behavior without a relationship.

The Scope of the Problem

Many professional journals review disciplinary actions taken against therapists who violate ethical and legal standards, and most of these cases involve sexual misconduct. Brief summaries of a few of these cases provide a picture of how therapists can manipulate clients to meet their own sexual or emotional needs.

• A clinical social worker engaged in unprofessional conduct when he exchanged a romantic kiss with a client. The clinician used his relationship with another client to further his own personal, religious, political, or business interests. He engaged in a sexual relationship with a former client, less than 3 years after termination of the professional relationship (California Association of Marriage and Family Therapists [CAMFT], 2004b, p. 49).

• A licensed marriage and family therapist engaged in inappropriate discussions and sexual relationships with a client. The therapist discussed intimate aspects of his personal life with his client, engaged in multiple relationships with the client, watched a sexually explicit movie with her, and accepted a nude photograph of the client. He failed to schedule appointments with the client at appropriate times, scheduling them instead for the evening hours. He failed to refer her to another therapist (CAMFT, 2004c, p. 50).

• A licensed marriage and family therapist was charged with committing sexual misconduct and gross negligence. When his client, a woman with a history of alcohol dependency and psychologically abusive relationships with men, revealed her sexual attraction to him, this therapist disclosed his mutual attraction to her and did not attempt to redirect her feelings or discuss the transference issue. He talked about his sexual fantasies in their sessions and expressed disappointment that they were prevented from having sex. He revealed personal details about himself and talked to her on the phone at night and on weekends, sometimes in a flirtatious fashion. After talking with her Alcoholics Anonymous sponsor, the client began to understand that her therapist was harming her. The client shared her confusion about their relationship directly with her therapist, but he did not respond well, which left the client feeling distraught. The therapist made no attempts to counsel her or to refer her to a different therapist (CAMFT, 2010, pp. 55–57).

• A licensed clinical social worker was accused of unprofessional conduct in the form of gross negligence. She moved in with a patient who had been under her direct care only 2 months earlier in a hospital setting. She reported feeling a spiritual connection with him and, upon further investigation, was found to be intimately dating him. Her former patient dropped out of two recovery programs, and the social worker moved out of his residence after a few months. Her employment at the hospital was terminated, and she was subject to further disciplinary action for recklessly causing emotional harm to a client (CAMFT, 2011b, pp. 40–41).

Harmful Effects of Sexual Contact With Clients

Studies continue to demonstrate that clients who are the victims of sexual misconduct suffer dire consequences. Erotic contact is totally inappropriate, is always unethical, and is an exploitation of the relationship by the therapist. Therapist–client sexual contact is the most potentially damaging boundary violation. Mental health professionals cannot argue that their clients seduced them. Even if clients behave in seductive ways, it is clearly the professional's responsibility to establish and maintain appropriate boundaries. To blame the client in these cases is as inappropriate as blaming a victim in a rape case.

Bouhoutsos and colleagues (1983), in a pioneering study of sexual contact in psychotherapy, assert that when sexual intercourse begins, therapy as a helping process ends. When sex is involved in a therapeutic relationship, the therapist loses control of the course of therapy. Of the 559 clients in their study who became sexually involved with their therapists, 90% were adversely affected. This harm ranged from mistrust of opposite-gender relationships to hospitalization and, in some cases, suicide. Other effects of sexual intimacies on clients' emotional, social, and sexual adjustment included negative feelings about the experience, a negative impact on their personality, and a deterioration of their sexual relationship with their primary partner. Bouhoutsos and her colleagues conclude that the harmfulness of sexual contact in therapy validates the ethics codes barring such conduct and provides a rationale for enacting legislation prohibiting it.

Decades have passed since that pioneering research was conducted, but their findings remain relevant today. Eichenberg, Becker-Fischer, and Fischer (2010) state that the consequences of sexual misconduct with therapy patients "are consistent in all international literature: all empirical studies that are available to date show very negative consequences for the victims" (p. 1019). These researchers reported that 86.5% of their study participants experienced consequences as a result of the sexual contact they had with their therapists. Of these, 93.3% experienced problematic consequences such as isolation, stronger distrust, fear, depression, feelings of shame and guilt, suicidal tendencies, anger, and posttraumatic stress disorder.

Legal Sanctions Against Sexual Violators

A number of states have enacted legal sanctions in cases of sexual misconduct in the therapeutic relationship, making it a criminal offense. Among the negative consequences for therapists include being the target of a lawsuit, being convicted of a felony, having their license revoked or suspended by the state, being expelled from professional organizations, losing their insurance coverage, and losing their jobs. Therapists may also be placed on probation, be required to undergo their own psychotherapy, be closely monitored if they are allowed to resume their practice, and be required to obtain supervised practice. In addition, their reputation is likely to suffer among their colleagues and other practitioners.

Criminal liability is rarely associated with the practices of mental health professionals. However, some activities can result in arrest and incarceration, and the number of criminal prosecutions of mental health professionals is increasing. The two major causes of criminal liability are sex with clients (and former clients) and fraudulent billing practices (Reaves, 2003).

In California, the law prohibiting sexual activity in therapy applies to two situations: (1) the therapist has sexual contact with a client during therapy, or (2) the therapist ends the professional relationship primarily to begin a sexual relationship with a client. Therapists who have sex with clients are subject to both a prison sentence and fines. For a first offense with one victim, an offending therapist would probably be charged with a misdemeanor, with a penalty of a sentence up to 1 year in county jail and a fine up to $1,000. For second and following offenses, therapists may be charged with misdemeanors or felonies. For a felony charge, offenders face up to 3 years in prison, or up to $10,000 in fines, or both. In addition to criminal action, civil action can be taken against therapists who are guilty of sexual misconduct. Clients may file civil lawsuits to seek money for damages or injuries suffered and for the cost of future therapy sessions (California Department of Consumer Affairs, 2011).

Assisting Victims in the Complaint Process

Each of the mental health professional associations has specific policies and procedures for reporting and processing ethical and professional misconduct. (Chapter 1 lists these organizations and provides contact information.) Mental health professionals have an obligation to help increase public awareness about the nature and extent of sexual misconduct and to educate the public about possible courses of action. The California Department of Consumer Affairs (2011) booklet, "Professional Therapy Never Includes Sex," describes ethical, legal, and administrative options for individuals who have been victims of professional misconduct.

Although the number of complaints of sexual misconduct against therapists has increased, individuals are still reluctant to file complaints for disciplinary action against their therapists, educators, or supervisors. Eichenberg and colleagues (2010) report that two thirds of study respondents said they never thought about taking legal steps, and among those who did, many decided not to follow through and initiate legal action. Clients are often unaware that they can file a complaint, and they frequently do not know the avenues available to them to address sexual misconduct. Each of the following options has both advantages and disadvantages, and it is ultimately up to the client to decide the best course of action.

Clients can file an ethics complaint with the therapist's licensing board. The board reviews the case, and if the allegation is supported, the board has the power to discipline a therapist using the administrative law process. Depending on the violation, the board may revoke or suspend a license. When a license is revoked, the therapist cannot legally practice. When sexual misconduct is admitted or proven, most licensing boards will revoke the therapist's license. The board's action is often published in the journal of the therapist's professional organization.

Legal alternatives include civil suits or criminal actions. A malpractice suit on civil grounds seeks compensatory damages for the client for the cost of treatment and for the suffering involved. Criminal complaints are processed based on state and federal statutes.

Sexual Relationships With Former Clients

Most professional organizations prohibit their members from engaging in sexual relationships with former clients because of the potential for harm. Some organizations specify a time period, and others do not. Most of the organizations state that in the exceptional circumstance of sexual relationships with former clients—even after a 2- to 5-year interval—the burden of demonstrating that there has been no exploitation clearly rests with the therapist. (For guidelines for particular professional associations, refer to the Ethics Codes box titled "Sexual Relationships With Former Clients.")

ETHICS CODES: Sexual Relationships With Former Clients

American Psychological Association (2010)
(a) Psychologists do not engage in sexual intimacies with former clients/patients for at least two years after cessation or termination of therapy.

(b) Psychologists do not engage in sexual intimacies with former clients/patients even after a two-year interval except in the most unusual circumstances. Psychologists who engage in such activity after the two years following cessation or termination of therapy and of having no sexual contact with the former client/patient bear the burden of demonstrating that there has been no exploitation, in light of all relevant factors, including (1) the amount of time that has passed since therapy terminated; (2) the nature, duration, and intensity of the therapy; (3) the circumstances of termination; (4) the client's/patient's personal history; (5) the client's/patient's current mental status; (6) the likelihood of adverse impact on the client/patient; and (7) any statements or actions made by the therapist during the course of therapy suggesting or inviting the possibility of a posttermination sexual or romantic relationship with the client/patient. (10.08.)

American Counseling Association (2014)
Sexual or romantic counselor–client interactions or relationships with former clients or their family members are prohibited for a period of five years following the last professional contact. This prohibition applies to both in-person and electronic interactions or relationships. Counselors, before engaging in sexual and/or romantic interactions or relationships with former clients, their romantic partners, or their family members demonstrate forethought and document (in written form) whether the interaction or relationship can be viewed as exploitive in any way and/or whether there is still potential to harm the former client; in cases of potential exploitation and/or harm, the counselor avoids entering such an interaction or relationship. (A.5.c.)

American Mental Health Counseling Association (2015)
Mental health counselors are strongly discouraged from engaging in romantic or sexual relationships with former clients. Counselors may not enter into an intimate relationship until five years post termination or longer as specified by state regulations. Documentation of supervision or consultation for exploring the risk of exploitation is strongly encouraged. (A.4.b.)

Commission on Rehabilitation Counselor Certification (2010)
Sexual or romantic rehabilitation counselor–client interactions or relationships with former clients, their romantic partners, or their immediate family members are prohibited for a period of five years following the last professional contact. Even after five years, rehabilitation counselors give careful consideration to the potential for sexual or romantic relationships to cause harm to former clients. In cases of potential exploitation and/or harm, rehabilitation counselors avoid entering such interactions or relationships. (A.5.b.)

National Association of Social Workers (2008)
Social workers should not engage in sexual activities or sexual contact with former clients because of the potential for harm to the client. If social workers engage in conduct contrary to this prohibition or claim that an exception to this prohibition is warranted because of extraordinary circumstances, it is social workers—not their clients—who assume the full burden of demonstrating that the former client has not been exploited, coerced, or manipulated, intentionally or unintentionally. (1.09.c.)

American Association for Marriage and Family Therapy (2015)
Sexual intimacy with former clients or with known members of the client's family system is prohibited. (1.5.)

Transforming a Professional Relationship Into a Personal Relationship

A therapist should seek consultation or personal therapy to explore his or her motivations and the possible ramifications of transforming a professional relationship into a personal one. When considering initiating such a relationship, many factors must be evaluated. These include the amount of time that has passed since termination of therapy, the nature and duration of therapy, the circumstances surrounding termination of the professional–client relationship, the client's personal history, the client's competence and mental status, the foreseeable likelihood of harm to the client or others, and any statements or actions by the therapist suggesting a plan to initiate a sexual relationship with the client after termination. Koocher and Keith-Spiegel (2016) state that sexual relationships with former clients involve such a high potential for a number of risks that they strongly discourage them, regardless of the lapse of time stipulated in ethics codes.

Some counselors maintain, "Once a client, always a client." Although a blanket prohibition on sexual intimacies, regardless of the time that has elapsed since termination, might clarify the issue, some contend that this measure is too extreme (Shavit & Bucky, 2004). Others point out the significant differences between an intense, long-term therapy relationship and a less intimate, brief-term one. A blanket prohibition ignores these distinctions. Reflecting the lack of consensus on this issue, 42.9% of the ACA members surveyed by Neukrug and Milliken (2011) thought it was ethical to become sexually involved with a former client at least 5 years after the counseling relationship ended; the other 57.1% viewed this as unethical behavior.

Examine Your Position At this point, reflect on your own stance on the controversial issue of forming sexual relationships once therapy has ended. Consider these questions in clarifying your position:

- Should counselors be free to formulate their own practices about developing sexual relationships with former clients? Give your reasons.
- Does the length and quality of the therapy relationship have a bearing on the ethics involved in such a personal relationship? Would you apply the same standard to a long-term client and a brief therapy client who worked on personal growth issues for 6 weeks?
- Would you favor changing the ethics codes to include an absolute ban on post-termination sexual relationships regardless of the length of time elapsed? Why or why not?
- What ethical guidelines would you suggest regarding intimate relationships with former clients?
- Although it might not be illegal in your state, what are the potential consequences of engaging in sex with former clients? Explain.
- React to the statement, "Once a client, always a client."

A Special Case: Nonerotic Touching With Clients

We include the discussion of nonerotic touching in this chapter because it is perhaps one of the more controversial boundary crossings. Although some are concerned that nonsexual touching can eventually lead to sexual exploitation, nonerotic touching can be appropriate and can have significant therapeutic value. A therapist's touch can be a genuine expression of caring and compassion; touch can be reassuring and a part of the healing process. Such touching also might be done primarily to gratify the therapist's own needs, so therapists must carefully assess the appropriateness of touching clients (Koocher & Keith-Speigel, 2016). It is inappropriate to touch *some* clients under any circumstances. Zur (2007) and Zur and Nordmarken (2009) write that touch needs to be evaluated in the context of client factors, the professional setting, the therapist's theoretical orientation, and the quality of the therapeutic relationship. Client factors include gender, age, culture, class, personal history with touch, presenting problem, diagnosis, and personality. For some clients touching may be appropriate and therapeutic, whereas the same kind of touch may be inappropriate and harmful for other clients. According to Zur and Nordmarken, a growing body of research indicates the potential clinical value of nonerotic touch as an adjunct to verbal therapy. Clinically appropriate touch can increase a client's trust and ease with the therapist and can be effective in enhancing the therapeutic alliance.

There is another side to the issue of nonerotic touching. Some clinicians warn of the dangers of physical contact; others oppose any form of physical contact between counselors and clients on the grounds that it can promote dependency, can interfere with the transference relationship, can be misread by clients, and can become sexualized. Pope and Wedding (2014) remark on other dangers: "When discordant with clinical needs, context, competence, or consent, even the most well-intentioned nonsexual physical contact may be experienced as aggressive, frightening, intimidating, demeaning, arrogant, unwanted, insensitive, threatening, or intrusive" (p. 585). Gutheil and Brodsky (2008) contend that the question of touch in therapy must be approached with caution and clinical understanding. Stating that "there are virtually no circumstances in which it is appropriate for a therapist to initiate a hug with a patient," Gutheil and Brodsky believe a therapist may accept a hug from a client in rare cases, such as from a client in profound grief who reaches out to a therapist or from a client at the conclusion of an extended course of therapy (p. 167).

In our view, it is critical to determine whose needs are being met when it comes to touching. If it comes from the therapist alone, and not from the context of the therapeutic relationship, it should be avoided. If touching occurs, it should be a spontaneous, nonsexual, and honest expression of the therapist's feelings and always done for the client's benefit. It should not be done as a technique. It is unwise for therapists to touch clients if this behavior is not congruent with what they feel. A touch that is not genuine will most likely be detected by clients and could erode trust in the relationship.

Touching is counterproductive when it distracts clients from experiencing what they are feeling, or when clients do not want to be touched. Some clients may interpret any physical contact based on their experience in other dysfunctional past relationships. The therapist must approach any contact with caution as the therapist cannot know how clients will interpret or react to touch. Clients from abusive backgrounds may confuse a therapeutic physical contact with an expression of dominance or as a way of inflicting harm. With these clients, any kind of touch may have sexual connotations (Gutheil & Brodsky, 2008).

Physical contact with clients must be carefully considered in context because a touch given at the right moment can convey far more empathy than words can. Therapists need to be aware of their own motives and to be honest with themselves about the meaning of physical contact. They also need to be sensitive to factors such as the client's readiness for physical closeness, the client's cultural understanding of touching, the client's reaction, the impact such contact is likely to have on the client, and the level of trust that they have built with the client.

Ethical and Clinical Considerations of Nonsexual Touch in Therapy

Practitioners need to formulate clear guidelines and consider appropriate boundaries when it comes to touching. In Neukrug and Milliken's study (2011), 83.9% of the counselors surveyed endorsed the idea that it was ethical to console clients using nonerotic touch, such as touching their shoulder, and 66.7% believed it was ethical to hug clients. Think about your position on the ethical implications of the practice of touching as part of the client–therapist relationship by answering these questions:

- What criteria could you use to determine whether touching your clients is therapeutic or countertherapeutic?
- Do you give hugs routinely in your personal life? If not, what motivates you to give hugs as a professional?
- To what degree do you think your professional training has prepared you to determine when touching is appropriate and therapeutic?
- What factors should you consider in determining the appropriateness of touching clients? (Examples are age, gender, the type of client, the nature of the client's problem, and the setting in which the therapy occurs.)
- What would you do if your client wanted a hug but you were hesitant to do so? How would you explain your reservation to the client?

Zur and Nordmarken (2009) note that touch in therapy is not inherently unethical and that none of the codes of ethics of professional organizations view touch as unethical. They also suggest that practicing risk management by rigidly avoiding touch may be unethical. They do suggest that therapists seek consultation in using touch in complex and sensitive cases. Documentation of the type and frequency of touch, along with the clinical rationale for using touch, is an important aspect of ethical practice. Zur and Nordmarken identify the following ethical and clinical guidelines for nonsexual touch in therapy:

- Touch should be employed only when it is likely to have a positive therapeutic effect.
- Touch should be used in accordance with the therapist's training and competence.
- It is essential that therapists create a foundation of client safety and empowerment before using touch.
- In deciding to touch, it is important to thoughtfully consider the client's potential perception and interpretation of touch.
- Special care is important in using touch with people who have experienced assault, neglect, attachment difficulties, rape, molestation, sexual addictions, or intimacy issues.
- It is the responsibility of therapists to explore their personal issues regarding touch and to seek education and consultation regarding the appropriate use of touch in therapy.
- Therapists should not avoid touch out of fear of licensing boards or the dread of litigation.
- Clinically appropriate touch must be used with sensitivity to clients' variables such as gender, culture, problems, situation, history, and diagnosis.

Zur and Nordmarken emphasize that it is critical for therapists to be mindful of not abusing the trust and power they have in the therapeutic relationship. They remind us that power by itself does not corrupt; rather, it is the lack of personal integrity on the therapist's part that corrupts.

The Case of Sienna

Austin is a warm and kindly counselor who routinely embraces his clients, both male and female. One of his clients, Sienna, has had a hard life, has had no success in maintaining relationships with men, is now approaching her 40th birthday, and has come to him because she is afraid that she will be alone forever. She misreads his friendly manner of greeting and assumes that he is giving her a personal message. At the end of one session when he gives his usual embrace, she holds onto him and does not let go right away. Looking at him, she says: "This is special, and I look forward to your hugs." He is surprised and embarrassed. He explains to her that she has misunderstood his gesture, that this is the way he is with all of his clients, and that he is truly sorry if he has misled her. She is crestfallen and abruptly leaves the office. She cancels her next appointment.

- What are your thoughts on this counselor's manner of touching his clients?
- If Austin had asked for Sienna's permission to hug her at the end of a session, would that have been more acceptable?
- Would you feel differently if Sienna had been the one to initiate the hugs?
- Was the manner in which he dealt with Sienna's embrace ethically sound?
- Would you follow up with Sienna about canceling her appointment?

Commentary. In our opinion, this case is a good example of a situation in which the counselor was more concerned with the bind he was in than the bind his client was in. The nature of a therapist's work is to take care of the client's difficulty first. Austin assumed that he correctly understood Sienna's message, and his response served his emotional needs rather than Sienna's. Had Austin put his client's needs first, he would have encouraged Sienna to discuss the meaning for her of the embrace. Austin also must be mindful of his own possible counter-transference and how this could be affecting the manner in which he interpreted Sienna's comments. Counselors need to be cautious in applying "routine" practices without considering their unique relationship with the client as well as the client's particular concerns being addressed in counseling. Touching should be approached with caution and with respect for the client's boundaries. •

Chapter Summary

In this chapter we have tried to put ethical issues pertaining to multiple relationships into perspective. We have emphasized that dual and multiple relationships are neither inherently unethical nor always problematic. Multiple relationships are unethical, however, when they result in exploitation or harm to clients. We have attempted to avoid being prescriptive and have summarized a range of recommendations offered by others to reduce the risk of boundary crossings and boundary violations—recommendations we expect will increase the chances of protecting both the client and the therapist.

Although ethics codes provide general guidance, you will need to weigh many specific variables in making decisions about what boundaries you need to establish in

your professional relationships. The emphasis in this chapter has been on guidelines for making ethical decisions about nonsexual multiple relationships, which often tend to be complex and defy simplistic solutions. To promote the well-being of their clients, clinicians are challenged with balancing their own values and life experiences with ethics codes as they make choices regarding how to best help their clients (Moleski & Kiselica, 2005).

Sexual relationships with clients are clearly unethical and detrimental to clients' welfare. It is unwise, unprofessional, unethical, and in many states illegal to become sexually involved with clients. However, it is important not to overlook some of the more subtle and perhaps insidious behaviors of the therapist that may in the long run cause serious damage to clients. It is unrealistic for therapists to believe they will never be attracted to certain clients. You are imposing an unnecessary burden on yourself if you believe that you should not have such feelings for clients or if you try to convince yourself that you should not have more feeling toward one client than toward another. It is important to decide how you will deal with these feelings as they affect the therapeutic relationship. Referral to another therapist is not necessarily the best solution, unless it becomes clear that you can no longer be effective with a certain client. Instead, you may recognize a need for consultation or, at the very least, for an honest dialogue with your colleagues. If for some reason your feelings of attraction become known to the client, it is essential that the client be assured that they will not be acted upon. If this creates a problem for the client, a referral should be discussed.

We want to stress the importance of reflecting on what you are doing and on whose needs are primary. A willingness to be honest in your self-examination is your greatest asset in becoming an ethical practitioner. As was mentioned earlier, it is always good to keep in mind whether you would act differently if your colleagues were observing you.

Suggested Activities

1. Investigate the ethical and legal aspects of multiple relationships as they apply to your professional interests. Look for any trends, special problems, or alternatives. Once you have gathered materials and ideas, present your findings in class.

2. Some say that multiple relationships are inevitable, pervasive, and unavoidable and have the potential to be either beneficial or harmful. Form two teams and debate the core issues. Have one team focus on the potential benefits of multiple relationships and argue that they cannot be dealt with by simple legislative or ethical mandates. Have the other team argue the case that multiple relationships are unethical and provide reasons.

3. Write a brief paper on your position on multiple relationships in counseling. Take some small aspect of the problem, develop a definite position on the issue, and present your own views.

4. What are your views about bartering with clients? Discuss the circumstances under which you might agree to barter with a client as well as those under which you would not agree. What guidelines would you need to establish? What are the ethical issues involved?

5. Discuss in a small group the issue of a sexual attraction in counseling. Explore how you might react if you found yourself attracted to a client. How might you respond to a client who reveals an attraction to you?

6. What are your views about forming social relationships with clients during the time they are in counseling with you? after they complete counseling? Consider the topic through several cultural frameworks.

7. What guidelines would you employ to determine whether nonerotic touching was therapeutic or countertherapeutic? Would the population you work with make a difference? Would the work setting make a difference? How comfortable are you as both the recipient and giver of nonerotic touch? What are your ethical concerns about touching?

8. Take some time to review the ethics codes of the various professional associations as they apply to two areas: (a) multiple relationships in general and (b) sexual intimacies with present or former clients. Have several students team up to analyze different ethics codes, make a brief presentation to the class, and then lead a discussion on the code's value.

9. Form small groups to explore the core issues involved in some of the cases in this chapter. Role-play the cases, and then discuss the implications. Role playing the therapist and the client is bound to enliven the discussion and give you a different perspective on the case.

Ethics in Action Video Exercises

10. Using Part III of the DVD/Workbook or online program (boundary issues), bring your completed responses to the self-inventory to class for discussion.

11. In video role play 14, Therapy Outside of the Office: The Picnic, the client (Lucia) would like to meet with the counselor (John) at the park down the street for their counseling sessions so she can get to know him better and feel closer to him. She could bring a lunch for a picnic. John is concerned about creating an environment that would help Lucia the most, and she says "That [meeting in the park] would really help me." Through role playing, demonstrate how you would establish and maintain boundaries with Lucia if she were your client. Under what conditions would you consider counseling a client outside the office?

12. In video role play 15, Beyond the Office Contact: The Wedding, the client (Richard) wants his counselor (Suzanne) to come to his wedding and reception. He stresses that her attendance would mean a lot to him. Suzanne is uncomfortable about going to the reception, but she agrees to attend the marriage ceremony. Through role playing, demonstrate how you might deal with your client's request to attend his wedding and reception.

13. In video role play 16, Social Relationships with Clients: The Friendship, at the last therapy session the client (Charlae) says she would like to continue their relationship because they have so much in common and she has shared things with the counselor (Natalie) that she has not discussed with anyone else. Natalie informs Charlae that this puts her in a difficult situation and she feels awkward. Charlae says, "What if we just go jogging together a couple of mornings a week?" Assume your client would like to meet with you socially and this is the final therapy session. Through role playing, demonstrate how you would handle a client's request to develop a social relationship with you once the professional relationship is terminated.

14. In video role play 17, Counselor Sexual Attraction to Client: Crossing the Line, the counselor (Conrad) shares with the client (Suzanne) that he has been thinking about her a lot and that he is attracted to her. Suzanne responds with, "You are

kidding, right?" She says she came to him because she was having problems with men taking advantage of her and not respecting her. She has bared her soul to him, and now she feels devalued. Suzanne suggests possibly seeing another counselor, but Conrad thinks they can work it out. What are your thoughts about the way the counselor (Conrad) shared his feelings with the client? If you were sexually attracted to a client, what course of action would you follow?

15. In video role play 18, Client Sexual Attraction to Counselor: The Disclosure, the client (Gary) discloses his attraction to his counselor (LeAnne). The counselor attempts to deal with his attraction therapeutically by focusing on how his attraction might be a theme in his life and how it is related to issues he has pursued in counseling, especially his relationships with women. Role-play this situation by showing how you would deal with a client who admits to being sexually attracted to you.

16. In video role play 19, Bartering: Manicuring for Therapy, the client states she can no longer afford to pay for therapy but that she does not like to think about terminating. The counselor (Natalie) takes the initiative of suggesting a bartering arrangement, indicating she would be open to trading manicures and haircuts for therapy services. Discuss the ethical issues involved in this case. What is your stance on bartering for counseling?

17. In video role play 20, Bartering: The Architect, the client (Janice) lost her job and can no longer pay for counseling sessions. She suggests providing architecture services for work on his house. The counselor (Jerry) suggests they discuss the pros and cons and that he wants to be sure that this is in her best interests. He mentions the code of ethics that discourages bartering. Jerry talks about issues of value and timeliness of services. Put yourself into this scene. Assume your client lost her job and could no longer pay for therapy. She suggests a bartering arrangement for some goods or services you value. Role-play how you would deal with her. What issues would you want to explore with your client?

18. In video role play 21, Gift Giving: The Vase, the client (Sally) is grateful for her counselor's (Charlae) help and wants to give her a vase. The client informs the therapist that giving gifts is a part of the Chinese culture. Charlae discusses her dilemma with wanting to accept the gift, but also the fact that the codes discourage her from accepting gifts from clients. Sally lets her counselor know that she would feel rejected if her gift to Charlae is not accepted. Role-play this situation and demonstrate ways of either accepting or not accepting the gift. Discuss guidelines you would use to determine your decision.

19. In video role play 22, Gift Giving: Tickets for Therapy, the client (John) shows his appreciation for his counselor (Marianne) by giving her tickets to the theater. John says, "I got tickets for you so you can go and enjoy it and have a good time." Marianne talks about why she cannot accept the tickets, in spite of the fact that she is very appreciative of his gesture. Put yourself in the counselor's place. What issues would you explore with John? Might you accept the tickets, under any circumstances? Why or why not? Demonstrate, through role playing, what you would say to the client.

MindTap for Counseling

Go to MindTap® for an eBook, videos of client sessions, activities, practice quizzes, apps, and more—all in one place. If your instructor didn't assign MindTap, you can find out more information at CengageBrain.com.

CHAPTER

8

Professional Competence and Training

LEARNING OBJECTIVES

1. Clarify how therapist competence is an ethical issue

2. Describe what is involved in the assessment of competence

3. Ascertain when and how to make referrals

4. Examine ethical issues in training therapists

5. Understand the basis of screening candidates in training programs

6. Recognize how to evaluate knowledge, skills, and personal functioning of trainees

7. Describe the gatekeeping role of faculty in promoting competence

8. Explore issues involved in dismissing students for nonacademic reasons

9. Articulate the purpose of licensing and credentialing

10. Gain a greater appreciation of the role continuing education plays in maintaining competence

Directions: For each statement, indicate the response that most closely identifies your beliefs and attitudes. Use the following code:

5 = I *strongly agree* with this statement.

4 = I *agree* with this statement.

3 = I am *undecided* about this statement.

2 = I *disagree* with this statement.

1 = I *strongly disagree* with this statement.

_____ 1. Counselors are ethically bound to refer clients to other therapists when working with them is beyond their professional training.

_____ 2. It is inappropriate and unethical to refer a client on the basis of a client's sexual orientation.

_____ 3. Possession of a license or certificate from a state board of examiners shows that a person has therapeutic skills and is competent to practice psychotherapy.

_____ 4. Professional licensing protects the public by setting minimum standards of preparation for those who are licensed.

_____ 5. None of us is competent in all settings, with all client populations, with all therapeutic modalities, and with all skills and techniques.

_____ 6. Continuing education coursework should be a requirement for renewal of a license to practice psychotherapy.

_____ 7. To apply our knowledge and skills competently, we must attend to our physical, emotional, mental, social, and spiritual well-being.

_____ 8. Institutions that train counselors should select trainees on the basis of both their academic record and the degree to which they possess the personal characteristics of effective therapists.

_____ 9. The arguments for licensing psychotherapists outweigh the arguments against licensing.

_____ 10. Candidates applying for a training program have a right to know the criteria for selecting trainees.

_____ 11. Once students are admitted to a graduate training program, that program should assess them at different times to determine their suitability for completing the degree.

_____ 12. Trainees who display rigid and dogmatic views about human behavior, and who are not responsive to remediation, should be dismissed from a training program.

_____ 13. Specialized training is necessary for those who plan to conduct online therapeutic interventions.

_____ 14. Lifelong learning is a critical component of professional competence.

_____ 15. I might not seek out workshops, seminars, courses, and other postgraduate learning activities if continuing education were not required to maintain my license to practice.

Introduction

In this chapter we focus on the ethical and legal aspects of professional competence and the ongoing education and training required for mental health professionals. We discuss issues related to professional licensing and certification as well as approaches to continuing education.

Ability is not easy to assess, but competence is a major concern for mental health professionals. Striving for competence is a lifelong endeavor. We are called upon to devote the entire span of our careers to developing, achieving, maintaining, and enhancing our competence. Competence at one point in our career does not assure competence at a later time. To remain current, we must take active steps to maintain our knowledge and skills. Continuing education is particularly important in learning about emerging areas of practice.

Barnett and Johnson (2015) remind us to consider the scope of our competence. Being competent in one area of counseling does not mean we are competent or feel comfortable handling client concerns in other areas. It is important to accurately assess each area of our practice to ensure competence. In one study examining school counselors' comfort and perceived competence in addressing student issues pertaining to spirituality, 80% of participants felt they needed to improve their competence level even though they said they were comfortable with these issues (Smith-Augustine, 2011). Practitioners and students can develop competence both as generalists and as specialists. A generalist is a practitioner who is able to work with a broad range of problems and client populations. A specialist is a worker who has developed competence in a particular area of practice such as career development, addiction counseling, eating disorders, or family therapy.

Definitions of competence center around a practitioner's ability to perform certain tasks and roles appropriately and effectively (Johnson et al., 2008). Competent practitioners have the necessary self-awareness, knowledge, skills, and abilities to provide effective services. To apply our knowledge and skills competently, we must consistently attend to our physical, emotional, mental, and spiritual well-being. As we saw in Chapter 2, self-care and wellness are basic to being able to function competently in our professional work and are considered ethical issues.

We give the education and training of mental health professionals special attention because of the unique ethical issues involved. Indeed, ethical issues must be considered from the very beginning, starting with admission and screening procedures for graduate programs. One key issue is the role of training programs in safeguarding the public when it becomes clear that a trainee has problems that are likely to interfere with professional functioning.

Therapist Competence: Ethical and Legal Aspects

LO1

In this section we examine **therapist competence**, or the skills and training required to effectively and appropriately treat clients in a specific area of practice. We discuss what competence is, how we can assess it, and what some of its ethical and legal dimensions are. We explore these questions: What ethical standards offer guidance in determining competence? What ethical issues are involved in training therapists? To what degree is professional licensing an accurate and valid measure of competence? What are the ethical responsibilities of mental health professionals to continue to upgrade their knowledge and skills?

Competence can best be considered on a continuum from incompetent to highly competent. **Competence** is both an ethical and a legal concept. From an *ethical* perspective, competence is based on the principles of beneficence and non-maleficence (Knapp, Gottlieb, & Handelsman, 2015). Ethical practitioners protect and serve their clients. Even though mental health professionals may not intend to harm clients, incompetence is often a major contributing factor in causing harm. From a *legal* standpoint, incompetent practitioners are vulnerable to malpractice suits.

Perspectives on Competence

We continue this discussion of competence with an overview of specific guidelines from various professional associations. They are summarized in the Ethics Codes box titled "Professional Competence."

ETHICS CODES: Professional Competence

American Mental Health Counselors Association (2015)
Mental health counselors recognize the boundaries of their particular competencies and the limitations of their expertise. (C.1.a.)

American Association for Marriage and Family Therapy (2015)
Marriage and family therapists do not diagnose, treat, or advise on problems outside the recognized boundaries of their competencies. (3.10.)

American Psychological Association (2010)
Psychologists provide services, teach, and conduct research with populations and in areas only within the boundaries of their competence, based on their education, training, supervised experience, consultation, study, or professional experience. (2.01.a.)

American Counseling Association (2014)
Counselors practice only within the boundaries of their competence, based on their education, training, supervised experience, state and national professional credentials, and appropriate professional experience. Whereas multicultural counseling competency is required across all counseling specialties, counselors gain knowledge, personal awareness, sensitivity, disposi-tions, and skills pertinent to being a culturally competent counselor in working with a diverse client population. (C.2.a.)

American Psychiatric Association (2013b)
A psychiatrist who regularly practices outside his or her area of professional competence should be considered unethical. Determination of professional competence should be made by peer review boards or other appropriate bodies. (2.3.)

American School Counselor Association (2016)
School counselors monitor their emotional and physical health and practice wellness to ensure optimal professional effectiveness. School counselors seek physical or mental health support when needed to ensure professional competence. (B.3.f.)

These guidelines leave several questions unanswered. What are the boundaries of competence, and how do professionals know when they have crossed them? How can practitioners determine whether they should accept a client when their experience and training are questionable? What should be the minimal degree required for entry-level professional counseling? Counselors may need to be both generalists and specialists to be competent to practice with some client populations. Many substance abuse counselors argue that if you are licensed as a generalist, you are not qualified to work in the area of treatment of addictions. To qualify as a substance abuse counselor, the CACREP (2016) standards identify specific knowledge, skills, and practices in the following areas: foundations; contextual dimensions, counseling, prevention, and intervention; diversity and advocacy; assessment; research and evaluation; and diagnosis.

Mental health professionals bear the responsibility of ensuring that we meet minimal standards of competence. Ongoing self-assessment and self-reflection are necessary throughout our careers. When unsure of our competence to provide services in a particular area of counseling practice, we consult with colleagues (Barnett & Johnson, 2015). Gathering anonymous feedback from current and former clients can be beneficial in assessing the degree to which clients experienced us as competent. It is a good practice to routinely ask clients for feedback about what is working in the sessions and how they view us as their therapist. By reflecting on some positive and unhelpful interventions, counselors can make it safe for clients to share their own critiques. Routine self-assessment and an honest appraisal of our skills provide the foundation for continued growth and positive changes that will increase our competency and benefit future clients.

Assessment of Competence

Assessing competence is an extremely difficult task. Some who complete a doctoral program lack the skills or knowledge needed to carry out certain therapeutic tasks. It is especially important for counselor trainees seeing clients as part of a practicum or internship to learn to assess their own competence. As future professionals, you need to monitor your competence and take steps to acquire the knowledge and skills required for effective practice. Kaslow and colleagues (2007) suggest that assessment approaches are most effective when they integrate both formative and summative evaluations. **Formative assessment** is a developmentally informed process that provides useful feedback during one's training and throughout one's professional career. **Summative assessment** is an end point evaluation typically completed at the end of a professional program or when applying for licensure status. Together these assessments address an individual practitioner's strengths and provide useful information for developing remedial education plans, if needed, for the person whose competence is being evaluated. Johnson and colleagues (2012) acknowledge that formative and summative assessments of trainees provide rigor and efficacy, but they note some problems associated with self-assessment. Clinicians often fail to recognize their own problems with competence, and some may be reluctant to address problems of competence in colleagues even when there is evidence that these problems exist.

Johnson and colleagues (2008) contend that those who are responsible for educating and training mental health professionals are ethically and professionally obligated to balance their roles as advocate and mentor of trainees with their gatekeeping role. One way to manage these sometimes conflicting roles is to thoroughly and accurately provide routine formative and summative assessment for trainees, carefully document these evaluations, and ensure that multiple professionals give independent evaluations of each trainee. Training faculty are ethically obligated to provide accurate, relevant, and timely feedback for all trainees throughout the program. Jacobs and colleagues (2011) address the importance of initiating difficult conversations with trainees when formative and summative feedback given to trainees has not been effective.

How do beginning counselors assess their readiness to practice independently? Is the number of supervised hours a sufficient criterion, or are other measures needed? If you are unsure of your ability to provide services in a particular area of counseling practice, you should consult with colleagues. When it becomes clear that a client's counseling needs exceed your competence, you must either develop the competence necessary to effectively treat the client or refer this client to another competent professional. The decision to refer must be made for the benefit of the client rather than for the comfort of the counselor. Self-reflection and colleague consultation are important steps in making this decision.

As a beginning counselor, if you were to refer all the clients whose problems seemed too difficult for you, it is likely that you would have few clients. You must be able to make an objective and honest assessment of how far you can safely go with clients and recognize when to refer clients to other therapists or when to seek consultations with other professionals. It is not at all unusual for even highly experienced therapists to question whether they have the personal and professional abilities needed to work with some clients. Thériault and Gazzola (2005) suggest that "many therapists continue to worry about their competence despite years of experience" (p. 11) and that "questioning one's competence is a significant aspect of being a therapist" (p. 16). It is more troubling to think of therapists who rarely question their competence. Difficulty working with some clients does not by itself imply incompetence, nor does lack of difficulty imply competence.

One way to develop or upgrade your skills is to work with colleagues or professionals who have more experience, especially when you go into new areas of practice. Seek consultation before you practice in areas where you have not received education and training, and continue to seek supervision throughout the process of developing competence in those areas. Doll (as cited in Barnett, Doll, Younggren, & Rubin, 2007) contends that practitioners must constantly build competence in new knowledge, skills, and practices, long after they leave their training programs. Doll notes that when therapists extend the boundaries of their practice, or when they branch out into an area requiring specialty competence, they should seek collegial consultation or professional supervision with acknowledged experts. Ongoing training and continuing education should be sought throughout the duration of one's career.

New skills can be learned by attending conferences and conventions, by reading books and professional journal articles, by taking additional courses in areas you do not know well and in theories that you are not necessarily drawn to, and by participating in workshops that combine didactic work with supervised practice. The feedback you receive can give you an additional resource for evaluating your readiness to undertake certain therapeutic tasks.

Making Referrals

Although you may be competent in a certain area, you still may need to refer a client if the resources are limited in the setting in which you work or if the boundaries of your professional role restrict you from effectively delivering the services your client needs. For example, a school counselor may make a referral to a mental health professional outside of the school for a student needing individual psychotherapy. The school counselor is practicing ethically by referring the student for more intensive services because these services cannot be provided within a school context. If your work setting limits the number of counseling sessions for clients, develop a list of appropriate, qualified referral resources in your area.

The counseling process can be unpredictable at times, and you could encounter situations in which the ethical path is to refer your client. For example, a school counselor was working with Quan, whose presenting problem was anxiety pertaining to academic success in college, which was within the scope of the school counselor's training. However, after meeting with Quan a few times, the counselor sensed that this student was very depressed and learned that he had engaged in self-mutilation and other forms of self-destructive behavior. Quan's counselor recognized that these symptoms and behaviors reflected a problem area that was outside the scope of his practice. Ethical practice required that he make a referral to another professional who was competent to treat Quan's problems.

Possessing the expertise to effectively work with a client's problem is one benchmark, but other circumstances can also make you wonder if a referral is in order. However, as you will recall from Chapter 3, referring a client because of a conflict with your value system is not an ethically acceptable reason for a referral. Wise and her colleagues (2015) have eloquently delivered the message that attaining competence to work with a diverse public is not optional: "students do not have the option to avoid working with particular client populations or refuse to develop professional competencies because of conflicts with their attitudes, beliefs, or values" (p. 268). Linde (2016) states that if counselors lack knowledge about clients with whom they are working, they have the obligation to seek additional training, consultation, or supervision to acquire the knowledge and skills to work with these clients. Linde acknowledges that it is ethical to make a referral in some situations: "If the client needs a higher level of care than the counselor can provide, then the counselor may refer the client" (p. 20).

You need to develop a framework for evaluating when to refer a client. It is imperative that you make skillful referrals when the limits of your competence are reached. Your clients deserve to understand the reason for the referral, and you will need to learn how to make this referral in such a manner that your client will be open to accepting your suggestion rather than feeling rejected or abandoned.

We hope you would not see referring a client with whom you have difficulty as a cure-all. If you are inclined to make frequent referrals, explore your reasons for being unwilling or unable to counsel these individuals. You may need to refer yourself for further help! Most codes of ethics have a guideline pertaining to conditions for making a referral, such as this one from the code of ethics for social workers:

> Social workers should refer clients to other professionals when the other professionals' specialized knowledge or expertise is needed to serve clients fully or when social workers believe that they are not being effective or making reasonable progress with clients and that additional service is required. (NASW, 2008, 2.06.a.)

The Case of Binh

Binh is 45 years old and has seen a counselor at a community mental health center for six sessions. She suffers from periods of depression and frequently talks about how hard it is to wake up to a new day. It is very difficult for Binh to express what she feels, and most of the time she sits silently during the session. The counselor decides that Binh's problems warrant long-term therapy, which he doesn't feel competent to provide. In addition, the center has a policy of referring clients who need long-term treatment to therapists in private practice. The counselor therefore approaches Binh with the suggestion of a referral:

Counselor: Binh, during your intake session I let you know that we are generally expected to limit the number of our sessions to six visits. Today is our sixth session, and I'd like to discuss the matter of referring you to another therapist.

Binh: Well, you did say that the agency generally limits the number of visits to six, but what about exceptions? I mean, I feel as if I've just started with you, and I really don't want to begin all over again with someone I don't know or trust.

Counselor: I can understand that, but you may not have to begin all over again. I could meet with the new therapist to talk about what we've done these past weeks.

Binh: I still don't like the idea at all. I don't know whether I'll see another person if you won't continue with me. Why can't I stay with you?

Counselor: I think you need more intensive therapy than I'm trained to offer you. As I've explained, I'm expected to do only short-term counseling.

Binh: Intensive therapy! Do you think that my problems are that serious?

Counselor: It's not just a question of you having serious problems. I am concerned about your prolonged depressions, and we've talked about my concerns over your suicidal fantasies. I think it is in your best interest to see someone who is trained to work with depression.

Binh: I think you've worked well with me. If you won't let me come back, then I'll forget about counseling.

Consider the ethical issues involved in Binh's case by addressing these questions:

- What do you think of the way Binh's counselor approached her? Would you have done anything differently?
- Was the counselor working beyond the scope of his practice, or was Binh not very sophisticated about the process of therapy?
- Is it possible that the counselor was not clear enough regarding the limitation of six visits?

- At what point would you have discussed the six session limitation with Binh?
- If you were Binh's counselor and you did not think you were competent to treat her, would you agree to continue seeing her if she refused to be referred to someone else? Why or why not?

Commentary. This exchange reflects a common problem; counselors and clients often have different perspectives on termination and referral issues. It is unethical for this therapist to continue counseling Binh, even though she opposes ending therapy with him. Continued treatment of a client's problem that is beyond the scope of the therapist's competence is a serious violation of the standard of care (Younggren & Gottlieb, 2008). When a therapist deems termination and referral to be the appropriate course of action, to do otherwise violates the fiduciary obligation to the client and the ethics code that prohibits rendering unnecessary treatment sessions. The counselor may have a duty to terminate regardless of the perception and wishes of the client. In extreme cases termination may occur over the objections of the client, yet such objections do not make termination inappropriate (Younggren et al., 2011).

How the counselor suggests the referral is critical. This counselor would have been wise to suggest a referral before the last session. With rare exceptions, a therapist should be able to determine whether he or she is competent to treat a given client by the end of the initial interview. The counselor should have stressed the short-term nature of the help he was qualified to provide during the informed consent process at the first session. Ultimately, it is the client's choice whether to accept or decline a referral. If this counselor can demonstrate that a referral is in Binh's best interest, there is a greater chance that she will accept the referral. In this case, the counselor would have been wise to consider not accepting a client like Binh whose problems would clearly be better served on a long-term basis. •

Ethical Issues in Training Therapists

Training is a basic component of practitioner competence. You will be able to assume an active role in your training program if you have some basic knowledge about policy matters that affect the quality of your education and training. Although providing adequate training is primarily the responsibility of the faculty in your program, you too have a role and a responsibility to ascertain that your training will provide you with the experiences necessary to become a competent practitioner. In this section, our discussion of the central ethical and professional issues in training is organized around questions pertaining to selection of trainees and the content of training programs.

Selection of Trainees

A core ethical and professional issue involves formulating policies and procedures for selecting appropriate candidates for a training program. Here are some issues that training program faculty need to consider:

- What criteria should be used for admission to training programs?
- Should the selection of trainees be based solely on traditional academic standards, or should it take into account factors such as personal characteristics, character, and psychological fitness?

- Is there a good fit between the candidate and the training program?
- To what degree is a candidate for training open to learning and to considering new perspectives?
- Does the candidate have problems that are likely to interfere with training and with the practice of psychotherapy?
- What are some ways to increase applications to programs by diverse groups of candidates?

Your training program has an ethical responsibility to establish clear selection criteria, and you, as a candidate, have a right to know the nature of these criteria when you apply. Although grade-point averages, scores on the Graduate Record Examination (GRE), and letters of recommendation are often considered in the selection process, relying on these measures alone does not provide a comprehensive picture of you as a candidate.

As part of the screening process, ethical practice requires that candidates be given information about what will be expected of them if they enroll in the program. Just as potential therapy clients have a right to informed consent, students applying for a program have a right to know the material they will be expected to learn and the manner in which education and training will take place. In most training programs, students are expected to engage in appropriate self-disclosure and to participate in various self-growth activities. Programs should make sure that applicants understand these requirements. The language in the informed consent document must be unambiguous, and the criteria for successful completion of the program easily understood by all concerned.

Screening can be viewed as a two-way process. Faculty screen candidates and make decisions on whom to admit, and at the same time candidates are screening the program and faculty to decide whether this is the right program for them. As students progress in a program, some may come to the realization that the counseling profession is not for them. If you have doubts about continuing in a program, discuss the matter with a faculty person whom you trust. It is easy to feel overwhelmed and come to a hasty self-assessment about being unsuitable for the profession when in fact you are simply feeling discouraged at the moment.

The Case of Leo

Julius is on a review committee in a graduate counseling program. Leo has taken several introductory courses in the program, and he has just completed an ethics course taught by Julius. It is clear to this professor that Leo has a rigid approach to human problems, particularly in areas such as interracial marriage, same-sex relationships, and abortion. Over the course of the semester, Leo appeared to be either unwilling or unable to challenge his beliefs. When challenged by other students in the class about his views, Leo responded by saying that he felt he was in a double bind. His faith gave him very clear guidelines on what is acceptable church teaching. At the same time, in this supervision class he is being asked to violate those values, so he feels conflicted no matter which decision he makes. Nobody offers him a solution. If he refers a future client with whom he has value conflicts, he is behaving unethically; if he were to accept such a client, he would be violating his church's teachings. In meeting with the committee charged with determining whether candidates should be advanced in the program,

Julius expresses his strong concern about retaining Leo in the program. His colleagues share this concern.

- What reactions do you have to this case? How would you respond to Leo's dilemma?
- Do you see any benefit to Leo expressing his values openly in his training program?
- Are any other avenues open in working with Leo short of disqualifying him from the program?
- If Leo's values reflected his cultural background, would that make a difference? Would the committee be culturally insensitive for rejecting him from the program?
- What if Leo said that when he eventually obtained his license he intended to work exclusively with people from his cultural and religious background? Should he be denied the opportunity to pursue a degree in counseling if his career goal is to work with a specific population that shares his views and values?
- If you were on the committee, how would you handle candidates who seemed to exhibit racism, homophobia, and rigid thinking?
- Are there any informed consent issues pertaining to graduate students that should be addressed in a case such as this? If so, what are they?

Commentary. Leo's case illustrates the dilemma counselor educators sometimes face when they have serious concerns about trainees who are likely to impose their values on their future clients. Ethically, the client's problems need to be explored and resolved in a way that matches the client's values, not the therapist's values. Leo will be expected to help clients understand and address the concerns they bring to therapy. Although Leo is not seeing clients now, he has the potential to do harm to clients if the rigidity of his value system is not challenged. Leo's openness about his beliefs gives the faculty and his supervisors a place to begin to work with him. The greater concern is that Leo seems unwilling to examine how his beliefs might hinder his ability to work with clients who do not share his values.

Educators and supervisors have several ethical obligations to students and trainees who may be impaired or incompetent. At least one faculty representative should meet with Leo to explore with him how his religious values might affect his work with clients. Leo has a right to his own values, but it would be unethical for him to impose them on clients. Leo must learn to bracket his values in sessions, and he should be given the opportunity to receive supervised practice in bracketing his values with mock clients. The faculty should document consistent and clear formative feedback to Leo as well as efforts to encourage remediation or personal development before deciding to dismiss him from the program.

Educators who fail to adequately orient prospective and current students regarding expectations and evaluation procedures heighten the risk of conflicts with ill-informed students (Barnett & Johnson, 2015). Leo should have been clearly oriented to the graduate program's expectations for students, including minimum competencies such as working with culturally different clients and avoiding the imposition or the intrusion of one's own values. ●

Content of a Program

It is important to ask questions about the content of your own training program and to seek ways to become as actively involved as possible in your own learning. From an ethical perspective, counselor educators and trainers are expected to present varied theoretical positions. Training programs would do well to offer students a variety of therapeutic techniques and strategies that can be applied to a wide range of problems with a diverse clientele.

Look at your program and ask how it measures up against these questions:

- Is the curriculum inclusive of many cultures, or is it culturally biased?
- What does your program tell you about imposing your values on clients? Or about referring clients with whom you have a conflict of values?
- Does the curriculum give central attention to the ethics of professional practice?
- What core knowledge is being taught in your training program?

In training programs for various mental health professions, general content areas are part of the core curriculum, which are generally outlined by CACREP (2016) standards. Content areas typically required for all students in counseling programs include professional counseling orientation and ethical practice, social and cultural diversity, human growth and development, career development, counseling and helping relationships, group counseling and group work, assessment and testing, and research and program evaluation.

Effective training programs are designed to help you acquire a more complete understanding of yourself as well as gain theoretical knowledge and develop clinical skills. Ideally, you will be introduced to various content areas, will acquire a range of skills you can utilize in working with diverse clients, will learn how to apply theory to practice through supervised fieldwork experiences, will learn a great deal about yourself personally, and will develop a commitment to acquiring or enhancing personal wellness. A good program does more than impart knowledge and skills essential to the helping process. In a supportive and challenging environment, the program will challenge you to examine your attitudes and beliefs, will encourage you to build on your life experiences and personal strengths, and will provide opportunities for expanding your awareness of self and others. An effective program also addresses the importance of self-care and emphasizes wellness throughout the program.

Although ethics is supposedly incorporated in a number of required courses, seminars, supervision, and practicum and internship experiences, we contend that the lack of systematic coverage of ethical issues will hinder students, both as trainees and later as professionals. The topics addressed in books like this deserve a separate course as well as infusion throughout all courses and supervised fieldwork experiences.

Effective programs combine academic and personal learning, weave together didactic and experiential approaches, and integrate study and practice. A program structured exclusively around teaching academics does not provide important feedback to students on how they function with clients. In experiential learning and in fieldwork, problem behaviors of trainees will eventually surface and can be ameliorated. Evaluation is an important component of this process, and we turn to this topic shortly.

Training Practitioners to Work in a Digital Culture

Technology is evolving at breakneck speed and is expanding the ways counseling services can be conceptualized and delivered. With the popularity of social media as a platform for communication in society, online counseling has garnered the attention of numerous researchers (e.g., Bradford & Rickwood, 2014; Glasheen et al., 2016; Richards, 2013; Steele, Jacokes, & Stone, 2014/2015). Online counseling services are increasingly common, and counselor preparation programs need to rise to the challenge of training their students to work in a digital culture. Anthony (2015) states that the need for training in transferring face-to-face skills to the online environment has been acknowledged for a number of years by leading professional organizations as not simply desirable but also essential. Because training in this area "is a relatively young part of the profession, certainly younger than online therapy itself . . . literature on it is scarce" (p. 37). We anticipate that research in this area will continue to increase as the use of online interventions expands.

Counselors in training must become knowledgeable about the complicated ethical and legal considerations that may apply when working with clients online. Describing the complications of working online with clients who reside in other countries, Anthony (2015) points out the need for a central database that spells out what is allowed in each country; services may be unregulated in some countries and subjected to strict regulations in others. "Where once we were able to trust our knowledge of laws and ethics within our own geographical barriers as part of our core training, we are now required to know those of all the countries in the world when approached by an international client" (p. 39). Globalization is creating new challenges that future generations of counselors will have to meet, and memorizing the intricacies of every country's code of ethics and laws is a daunting task. Instead, trainees and experienced counselors alike should learn about the *process* of finding the relevant facts they may need to work with international clients.

LO6

Evaluating Knowledge, Skills, and Personal Functioning

As a student in a counselor education program, you have a right to know how you will be evaluated, both academically and personally. If you are aware of the evaluation criteria and procedures, you are in a better position to ask key questions that can influence your degree of satisfaction and your involvement in your educational program.

Evaluation Criteria and Procedures

Every training institution has an ethical responsibility to screen candidates so the public will be protected from incompetent practitioners. Programs clearly have a dual responsibility: to honor their commitment to the students they admit and to protect future consumers who will be served by those who graduate. The criteria for selecting applicants to a program should be clear, and the criteria for successful completion and the specifics of the evaluation process need to be spelled out just as clearly and objectively. The criteria for dismissing a student should be equally clear and objective. Academic programs should have written policies that are available to students as part of the orientation to the program.

As a student you need to know that your knowledge and skills, clinical performance, and interpersonal behaviors will be evaluated at different times during the program. Ongoing evaluation of you as a trainee is crucial to determine whether you are making satisfactory progress in the various areas of the training program (Wilkerson, 2006). In addition to assessing knowledge and skills competencies, it is of vital importance to assess *personal* and *interpersonal competencies,* such as the capacity for self-awareness and self-reflection (Orlinsky, Geller, & Norcross, 2005). Consistent with the existing research on psychotherapy outcomes, Orlinsky and colleagues state that *interpersonal relatedness* is a core aspect of the therapeutic process. They emphasize the *personal* qualities of the therapist, including the therapist's emotional resonance and responsiveness, social perceptiveness, compassion, desire to help, self-understanding, and self-discipline. In our view, possessing personal characteristics such as these are the foundation for *professional competence.*

As a student, you need feedback on your progress so you can build on your strengths or remediate problem areas. It is important that you also engage in self-evaluation to determine whether you are "right" for the program and whether the program is suitable for you. The first goal of an evaluation of candidates is to assess progress and correct problems. If shortcomings are sensitively pointed out to trainees in a timely way, they can often correct them and continue in the program.

Ideally, we would like to see each professional organization develop specific guidelines pertaining to students' successful completion of a program: NASW for social worker students, AAMFT for students in marital and family therapy programs, APA for students in clinical and counseling psychology, and ACA for students in counselor education programs and clinical mental health counseling programs. Faculty in these respective professional training programs would then have the backing of their professional association in determining the evaluation procedures to be used when decisions regarding retaining or dismissing students are made.

We strongly support the standards for performance evaluation of the ACA, NASW, and APA (see the Ethics Codes box titled "Evaluating Student Performance"). In addition to evaluating candidates when they apply to a program, we favor periodic reviews to determine whether trainees should be retained.

ETHICS CODES: Evaluating Student Performance

American Counseling Association (2014)
Counselor educators clearly state to students, prior to and throughout the training program, the levels of competency expected, appraisal methods, and timing of evaluations for both didactic and clinical competencies. Counselor educators provide students with ongoing feedback regarding their performance throughout the training program. (F.9.a.)

National Association of Social Workers (2008)
Social workers who have responsibility for evaluating the performance of others should fulfill such responsibility in a fair and considerate manner and on the basis of clearly stated criteria. (3.03.)

American Psychological Association (2010)
In academic and supervisory relationships, psychologists establish a timely and specific process for providing feedback to students and supervisees. Information regarding the process is provided to the student at the beginning of supervision. (7.06.a.)

Psychologists evaluate students and supervisees on the basis of their actual performance on relevant and established program requirements. (7.06.b.)

Evaluation of Interpersonal Behavior and Personal Characteristics

Your success in a counseling program and as a future counseling professional involves a great deal more that performing well academically. Who you are as a person and your ability to develop and maintain effective interpersonal relationships during your training program are of major importance. When you begin seeing clients in a practicum, your knowledge and helping skills as well as your ability to make connections with clients will be directly related to positive outcomes. Your interpersonal style, your ability to relate to clients, and your willingness to reflect on the characteristics that either help or hinder you in working with clients are key variables.

It is of the utmost importance that your faculty evaluate your professional behavior, clinical performance, and identify interpersonal behaviors and personality characteristics that are likely to influence your ability to effectively deliver mental health services. Evaluating trainees on the basis of personal characteristics is often a challenging task. Interpersonal behaviors of trainees have a direct bearing on their clinical effectiveness, so these factors must be taken into consideration in the evaluation process. According to Sofronoff, Helmes, and Pachana (2011), assessment of *fitness to practice* (FTP) within training programs requires balancing the rights of students to pursue their career interests with the rights of their future clients.

The faculty of each training program has a responsibility to develop clear definitions and evaluation criteria for assessing the character and psychological fitness of trainees. Later in this chapter, we address some ways of evaluating students whose performance or behavior does not meet professional and ethical standards.

Scholars across disciplines are engaged in discussions about psychological fitness of trainees (Wilkerson, 2006), referring to this notion variously as problem students; inadequate, unsatisfactory, deficient, substandard behavior; and problematic student behaviors. Elman and Forrest (2007) recommend better terminology and clearer definitions and caution that the term *impairment* overlaps with a specific legal meaning in the Americans With Disabilities Act (ADA), which could create legal risks for programs. They recommend that faculty avoid using the term *impairment* to refer to trainees who are not meeting minimum standards of professional competence and instead refer to such trainees as having *problems with professional competence* or *professional competence problems*. Kress and Protivnak (2009) prefer the term *problematic counseling student behaviors*. They state that "problematic" focuses on student behaviors without labeling the student as incompetent or impaired. Possible problematic behaviors include poor clinical skills; poor interaction with faculty, supervisors, and colleagues; inappropriate self-disclosure with clients; and failure to communicate with clinical supervisors or faculty about needs and concerns.

Sometimes students have personal characteristics or problems that interfere with their ability to function effectively, yet when this is pointed out to them, they may deny the feedback they receive. The helping professions often use *DSM-5* criteria to classify mental dysfunctions of clients yet show no such clarity in defining the mental, emotional, and personal characteristics required of students entering a training program. A program has an ethical responsibility to take action rather than simply pass on a student with serious academic or personal problems. However, university administrators are often in favor of high graduation and completion rates and are fearful of lawsuits and may put pressure on faculty to pass students (Maureen Kenny, personal communication, September 25, 2016). Students who are manifesting emotional, behavioral, or interpersonal problems could be encouraged to avail themselves of services at the campus counseling center. Elman and Forrest (2004) believe training programs should have written policies describing how and when personal psychotherapy might be recommended or required with respect to the remediation of a student's problems.

> Training programs need to reduce their ambivalence about involvement in personal psychotherapy when it is used for remediation. The challenge is to provide developmentally appropriate educational experiences for trainees in a safe learning environment while protecting the public by graduating competent professionals (p. 129).

Information about remediation of a student's interpersonal problems could be put in the student handbook and given to students at the orientation session prior to admission to the program. However, addressing these policies and procedures only at the time of orientation is not sufficient. Faculty should make clear to incoming students that becoming a competent counselor involves more than acquiring knowledge and skills; a critical variable of effective counseling is the ability of trainees to establish a working alliance with their clients, which depends largely on their own personality characteristics and behavioral attributes. Ongoing discussion of these issues throughout the training program is necessary to prepare trainees for potentially difficult conversations pertaining to their own professional competence (Jacobs et al., 2011).

Letourneau (2016) describes a collaborative decision-making model for addressing problematic behaviors in counseling students. Designed to address diversity and cultural influences, students are involved in the decision-making process, which can help establish students' trust in the process. Letourneau notes that inclusion of a student during any point of the decision-making process may foster the student's commitment to the course of action taken and may contribute to the student's sense of empowerment.

Systematic Procedures in Evaluation of Student Performance

As a student you have a right to be clearly informed of the procedures that will be used to evaluate your performance. A key part of the informed consent process involves learning about the policies pertaining to the roles that personal and professional development play in the program. Informed consent requires clear statements about what constitutes ground for concerns, including when and why students may be terminated from a program (Wilkerson, 2006). Brown-Rice and Furr (2013) point out that the types of problems that result in student dismissals fall into three categories: inadequate academic or clinical skill levels, psychological or personality unsuitability, and inappropriate moral character. Your faculty has an ethical responsibility to ensure that you are qualified to enter the profession of counseling after you graduate; their ultimate ethical obligation is to protect the clients with whom you will be working by effectively executing their role as gatekeepers of the profession.

Kress and Protivnak (2009) describe a systematic plan for assisting students in remediating problematic areas. Their professional development plans (PDPs) are detailed contracts that can be used to address problematic student behaviors. PDPs systematically document and address faculty expectations of students; specific behaviors required of students; tasks students need to attend to; and consequences to students if they do not successfully address the specific tasks and engage in the required behaviors. Such concrete, simple, and explicit plans can be integrated into a program's remediation, review, dismissal, and retention policies.

Seattle University's Department of Counseling and School Psychology has developed an excellent form designed to assess students' personal and professional competencies at several junctures in their program. With the permission of the faculty and dean of this program, we are reproducing their assessment form, which is a good model for informing students about expectations of the program and for providing students with regular feedback on both their personal and professional development (see the box titled "Personal and Professional Competencies").

Personal and Professional Competencies

The counseling faculty, Department of Counseling and School Psychology, College of Education, Seattle University, believes that counseling students must be able to demonstrate basic counseling skills and be knowledgeable of a variety of counseling theories. Additionally, they must be able to integrate the learned skills with their own developed philosophical and theoretical constructs. The faculty knows the role of the school counselor, mental health counselor, and post-secondary counselor to be, and, therefore, expects students to meet the *Personal and Professional Competencies*. Each student is assessed at candidacy, prior to internship, and at the end of each quarter of the three-quarter internship. Students are aware of the *Personal and Professional Competencies* when they enter the program and know that they will be evaluated as to whether or not they meet these competencies. At the end of internship, the student must have met each competency.

Student _____ Date _____

_____ School _____ Mental Health _____ Post Secondary _____ Certification-only

_____ On-going/optional _____ Candidacy/required _____ Pre-Internship/required

MC = Meets competency **NM** = Does not meet competency **NO** = Not observed or documented Shaded column = on-going or at candidacy; non-shaded = pre-internship

A. Counseling Skills and Abilities	MC		NM		NO	
1. The student counselor creates a safe clinical setting with appropriate boundaries regarding such issues as the professional relationship, meeting times and location.						

continued

A. Counseling Skills and Abilities	MC		NM		NO	
2. The student counselor listens to the client and conveys the primary elements of the client's story.						
3. The student counselor responds to client feelings, thoughts and behaviors in a therapeutic manner using appropriate counseling responses.						
4. The student counselor communicates empathy by expressing the perspective of the client, when appropriate.						
5. The student counselor stays in the here and now, when appropriate.						
6. The student counselor is intentional by responding with a clear understanding of the therapeutic purpose.						
B. Professional Responsibility	MC		NM		NO	
7. The student counselor follows professional codes of ethics, the Seattle University Student Honesty Code, civil laws; demonstrates analysis and resolution of ethical issues; and relates to peers, professors, and clients in a manner consistent with professional standards.						
8. The student counselor demonstrates sensitivity to real and ascribed differences of client and counselor roles and manages role differences therapeutically.						
9. The student counselor demonstrates the ability to match appropriate interventions to the presenting clinical profile in a theoretically consistent manner and provides only those services and applies only those techniques for which the student is qualified, or is in the process of being qualified, through education, training, and experience.						
10. The student counselor has a commitment to social justice and demonstrates a respect for individual differences, including those related to age, gender, race, ethnicity, culture, national origin, religion, sexual orientation, disability, language, and socioeconomic status.						
11. The student counselor articulates an understanding of how and when a counselor may take a leadership role.						
12. The student counselor articulates how regional, national, and international issues affect the role of the counselor.						

C. Personal Responsibility	MC		NM		NO	
13. The student counselor demonstrates an awareness of the student's own belief systems, values, needs, and limitations and the effect of these on personal and professional behavior.						
14. The student counselor demonstrates the ability to receive, integrate, and utilize feedback from peers, faculty, teaching assistants, and supervisors.						
15. The student counselor demonstrates appropriate behavior in and out of the classroom and is dependable regarding assignments, attendance, and deadlines.						
16. The student counselor takes responsibility for personal and professional behavior.						
17. The student has an accurate assessment of personal and professional competencies.						
18. The student exhibits appropriate levels of self-assurance and confidence.						
19. The student counselor expresses thoughts and feelings effectively both orally and in writing.						
20. The student counselor demonstrates the ability to manage the stresses of a demanding profession by developing effective coping skills, that include professional and personal support systems.						

Comments (refer to specific competency):

Orientation (*to be signed at the new student orientation*)

By signing below, the student is certifying that the student understands: 1) the personal and professional competencies listed above; 2) that the student is expected to meet these competencies; and 3) that the student *may* be evaluated at any time; and *will* be evaluated at candidacy and prior to internship using this document.

_____   _____

Student   Date

_____   _____

Faculty   Date

(copy to student file)

Candidacy (*to be signed at the meeting with the student advisor at candidacy*)

By signing below, the student is certifying that the student has met with the student's advisor and 1) has discussed the student's candidacy status; 2) understands competencies that have

continued

not been meet; 2) has a strategy for meeting unmet criteria; 3) and understands that unmet competencies are expected to be met before the student finished the program.

_____   _____
Student   Date

_____   _____
Faculty   Date

Disposition or recommendation:

Pre-Internship (*to be signed at a meeting with the student advisor at the discretion of the student or the advisor prior to internship*)

By signing below, the student is certifying that the student has met with the student's advisor and 1) has discussed the student's pre-internship status; 2) understands competencies that have not been met; 2) has a strategy for meeting unmet criteria; 3) and understands that unmet competencies are expected to be met before the student finished the program.

_____   _____
Student   Date

_____   _____
Faculty   Date

Disposition or recommendations:

_____

We thank the counseling faculty, Department of Counseling and School Psychology, College of Education, Seattle University, for granting us permission to reproduce the form they use in their program.

Gatekeeper Role of Faculty in Promoting Competence

A key role of clinical training faculty is to promote and facilitate students' competence and professional behavior. A major problem faced by educators in these training programs is identifying, dealing with, and possibly dismissing students who are not making satisfactory progress toward professional competence (Oliver et al., 2004).

The academic faculty in a professional program generally has a **gatekeeper's role**, protecting consumers by identifying and intervening with graduate students who exhibit problematic behaviors or who give evidence of performance problems (Johnson et al., 2008; Letourneau, 2016; Vacha-Haase, Davenport, & Kerewsky, 2004). Counselor educators serve as gatekeepers to the profession by evaluating trainees' suitability to enter and remain in the field (ACA, 2014; APA, 2015). In a Delphi study conducted by Herlihy and Dufrene (2011) regarding critical ethical issues in counselor preparation, gatekeeping ranked second, with 89% of participants stating that this was a critical and emerging ethical issue for training faculty. This gatekeeper role is addressed in the ethics codes of most professional organizations.

Clinical training faculty also have a responsibility to protect other graduate students in their program from those trainees who are dealing with problems of professional competency. Brown-Rice and Furr's (2013) study involving 389 master's students attending CACREP-accredited programs revealed that the majority (74%) of trainees were aware of classmates who were experiencing problems of professional competency and felt frustration toward faculty for failing to address these problematic peers. More than 50% of the respondents who observing classmates with competence issues stated that "they were affected by a problematic peer or peers" (p. 227). One challenge we have found as faculty is that students may express frustration with what appears to be inaction on the part of the faculty, yet due to confidentiality issues faculty often are not permitted to share what is being done to remediate any problem behaviors with a particular student. Sometimes faculty are unaware of the scope of the student's problematic behavior or dispositions, and peers can play a role in helping to identify students who may be in need of remediation or dismissal. In some cases, the institution impedes rather than supports faculty attempts at remediation or dismissal, giving the problematic student too much power due to fear of litigation.

Historically there has been very little examination of problematic student behavior or of the evaluation and dismissal of students in professional programs, but this is now changing. With increased awareness of the damage that can be caused by mental health professionals who do not possess the personal qualities necessary for effective practice, there is an ethical imperative for training faculty to serve as gatekeepers for the profession (Johnson et al., 2008). With revisions to the ACA *Code of Ethics* in 2014 and recent litigation initiated by students dismissed for attitudes and behaviors in violation of ethical standards, gatekeeping has gained significant attention (Francis & Dugger, 2014), and the role of counselor educators as gatekeepers is expanding. Counselor educators have the responsibility for being culturally and developmentally sensitive in interpreting, applying, and enforcing ethics codes with counseling students (Letourneau, 2016).

Faculty cannot rely on screening procedures during the admissions process alone to identify students who do not have the necessary personality characteristics to become competent clinicians (Kerl, Garcia, McCullough, & Maxwell, 2002). Programs have an obligation to operationally define the personality characteristics that are likely to impede a student's ability to practice effectively. In fairness to students, counseling faculty need to develop objective evaluation procedures and processes to communicate to students both their strengths and areas needing improvement with respect to interpersonal behavior and clinical performance. This should begin as early as possible in the program so that a timely intervention might solve the problem and help the student. If a student initiates a legal challenge regarding his or her professional performance, faculty and program administrators must show documentation of the student's lack of competency (Kerl et al., 2002).

Gaubatz and Vera (2002) investigated whether formalized gatekeeping procedures and program-level training standards influence the rates at which problematic trainees are graduated from counseling programs. Their findings indicated that programs with formalized standards and procedures reduce the number of deficient students it graduates. In a later study, Gaubatz and Vera (2006) discovered that "well-designed gatekeeping procedures appear to improve the effectiveness with which [deficient students] are identified and prevented from progressing unremediated into the counseling field" (p. 41). Although Gaubatz and Vera endorse the efforts of individual training programs to address the issue of deficient trainees, they also add that these efforts "should be integrated into the professional standards that guide the field of counselor training as a whole" (p. 41).

The Case of a Discouraged Professor

Karmella was a student at a university with a 48-unit master's degree program in counseling. This core degree and a few additional classes qualified a graduate to apply for the licensed professional counselor examination once the required supervised internship hours were completed. Karmella was identified by the faculty as having a level of affect that indicated a complete lack of empathy. In counseling dyads, group process experiences, and classroom exercises, it became clear that Karmella was unable to make empathic connection. Academically, Karmella received good grades; she completed the reading, wrote satisfactory papers, and did well on the examinations. It was in the behavioral dimension—such as reflective listening, being able to establish client rapport, and demonstrating empathic understanding—that her lack of skill was noted.

Karmella progressed through most of the graduate program and entered an intensive group process course, which was a requirement of the program. The professor in this didactic training environment noted Karmella's barriers to building effective counseling relationships and made two or three interventions. These interventions included direct discussion with Karmella as well as referral and recommendation for personal counseling. At the end of the semester, Karmella's behaviors and skills had not improved, and by some measures they had actually deteriorated. The grade for the group process class was the only grade Karmella needed to complete her degree program. After many hours of soul searching, the professor decided that this student should not be allowed to advance because her lack of empathic understanding and her typically bizarre responses in counseling dyads made her, as a potential counseling professional, a risk to others. He gave Karmella a failing grade, which meant that Karmella would not receive her degree without successfully repeating the group process class.

Karmella responded by suing both the professor and the university. An investigation was completed at the university by the academic senate. In addition to the professor and the student, several members of the faculty and many individuals from the group process class were called as witnesses. The senate overruled the professor's grade and awarded a master's degree in counseling to Karmella. Today she is a licensed professional counselor.

Discouraged by the lack of support from the university, the professor reduced his teaching to part time and retired at the first available opportunity. In reflecting on this case, what implications can you draw?

- Was the professor justified in blocking her from a master's degree based on her performance in this one group process course?
- Might Karmella's lack of empathy and connection to others cause potential harm to clients?
- Does Karmella's lack of empathy and connection necessarily imply that she is incompetent? What else might explain her behaviors?
- What criteria were used to determine her fitness?
- What are your thoughts about the actions taken by the administration?
- Is it the responsibility of professional accrediting agencies to intervene in a situation such as this?

- Did other professors who had noticed Karmella's lack of empathy have an ethical responsibility to address this issue with her earlier in her graduate coursework?

Commentary. The gatekeeping function continues to present many challenges to faculty in counseling programs. In addition to possible legal issues, administrative support may be lacking for a program's decision to dismiss a student for nonacademic reasons. The welfare of future clients is paramount when evaluating students who are deemed to lack competence due to personality issues. Furthermore, students need to know that they will not be endorsed by faculty before a licensing board or for employment if they demonstrate problematic behaviors. Students should be advised as early as possible if their behavior is problematic, and they should be given direction and opportunities to ameliorate problem areas. When students are not made aware of concerns on the part of the faculty until later in the program, they have a legitimate complaint.

Students in counselor training programs are often asked to work on their personal problems as a part of their professional development. This can expose parts of the student's personal life that may make the student more vulnerable to negative evaluations. Faculty must provide space for students' growth, both personally and professionally, but students must be challenged when their personal characteristics may cause harm to future clients. This requires effort on the part of all involved, and intervention and remediation must be tailored to the individual to be beneficial.

Students should not be allowed to complete a graduate program if they do not successfully remediate personal or interpersonal problems that negatively affect their clinical performance. Karmella was unable to offer the emotional connection that many clients require to profit from therapy. In our view, the professor did the right thing in adhering to both a clear process of feedback and remediation and his obligation to serve as gatekeeper for the profession in protecting the public. When there are conflicts between ethical obligations and institutional policies (e.g., graduating incompetent students), we should make the conflict known to the institution and then stick to our ethical duties. •

Dismissing Students for Nonacademic Reasons

From our perspective, faculty who are in the business of training counselors should be credited with the ability to have accurate perceptions and observations pertaining to personality characteristics that are counterproductive to effective counseling. When a student has good grades but demonstrates substandard interpersonal behavior, action must be taken immediately. Some students may not possess the emotional maturity or interpersonal skills necessary for clinical work, but they may have other skills that may be useful in our profession. We sometimes counsel students to focus on a different area of the profession, such as research or writing, if those are their strengths. Supporting students in following a path that accentuates their areas of strength can be beneficial. Dismissal from a program is a measure of last resort and should be employed only after all other attempts at remediation have failed.

Legal Deterrents to Dismissing Students

Some of the barriers to taking the action of dismissing students from a program include difficulties in giving clear evidence to support the decision to dismiss a student; the lack of adequate procedures in place to support a dismissal decision;

concern about the psychological distress for faculty and students; concern about the heightened resistance and defensiveness in the trainee; the potential for receiving criticism from other faculty or supervisors who were not involved in the trainee's remediation; and lack of administrative support (Forrest, Elman, Gizara, & Vacha-Haase, 1999). Perhaps the major deterrent to dismissing a student is the fear of legal reprisal by that student. Bernard and Goodyear (2014) have noted that faculty in training programs traditionally have been concerned about their legal standing if they decide to dismiss a student from a program for "nonacademic" reasons. At times, both counselor educators and administrators are reluctant to dismiss students who have interpersonal or clinical skills deficits. This may be especially true if the concerns are about personal characteristics or problematic behavior, even when the faculty is in agreement regarding the lack of suitability of a given student.

If it can be demonstrated that a program failed to adequately train an individual, the university may be held responsible for the harm the graduate inflicts on clients (Custer, 1994; Kerl et al., 2002). Custer (1994) describes a lawsuit involving a master's level counselor who graduated from Louisiana Tech's College of Education. A female therapy client filed suit against Louisiana Tech, claiming that the program allowed an incompetent practitioner to graduate from the program. The client claimed that her life had been destroyed by incompetent therapy. The claim was that the program itself was inadequate in that it simply did not adequately prepare her counselor. The counselor was named in the malpractice action along with her supervisor and the university. The initial lawsuit was settled in 1994 for $1.7 million. A case such as this makes it clear that specific competency standards for retaining and graduating counseling students are not only useful, but necessary.

Court Cases on Dismissing Students From a Program

Mary Hermann summarized a court case pertaining to dismissing a student for nonacademic reasons (as cited in Remley et al., 2002). In *Board of Curators of the University of Missouri v. Horowitz* (1978), the United States Supreme Court considered a case brought by a student who had been dismissed from medical school, in spite of the fact that she had excellent grades. The decision to dismiss the student was based on the faculty's determination that she was deficient in clinical performance and interpersonal relationship skills. Prior to the dismissal, on several occasions the faculty expressed dissatisfaction with the student's clinical work and informed her that she faced dismissal if she did not exhibit clear improvement. The student continued to receive unsatisfactory evaluations on her clinical work. Prior to the student's dismissal from medical school, she was evaluated by seven independent physicians in the community, all of whom agreed with the medical school professors that her clinical skills were unsatisfactory.

After being dropped from the program, the student filed a lawsuit claiming that her dismissal from medical school violated her constitutional rights. In reviewing the case, the Supreme Court considered that the student had been informed of the faculty's dissatisfaction with her clinical performance, and the student knew that unless she made significant improvement in this area, she would be dismissed from the program. The Court held that the decision to dismiss the student from medical school was based on a careful and deliberate evaluation by the faculty, and thus the student's dismissal was not a violation of her constitutional rights.

The model described for medical students would be an excellent model for counselor education programs to adopt in dealing with a student identified as lacking the necessary qualifications to be an effective helper. Using this model, the problematic student would be evaluated both at the university and in the community, where a number of experienced practitioners would review the findings of the faculty and administration.

Kerl and colleagues (2002) describe the importance of designing systematic procedures for training programs to evaluate students' professional performance. When dismissal from a program is based on interpersonal or clinical incompetence, Kerl and colleagues underscore the importance of sound systematic academic evaluation and adherence to procedural and substantive due process. These authors argue that in counselor education programs the evaluation of students' interpersonal and clinical skills is part of the overall assessment of their academic performance. They conclude that courts have consistently viewed personal characteristics or behaviors as basic to academic performance, which makes this an academic issue. Kerl and colleagues describe an evaluation instrument, Professional Counseling Performance Evaluation (PCPE), designed by the counseling faculty at Southwest Texas State University to provide feedback to students on their progress in meeting professional standards and to document deficiencies that are serious enough to result in dismissal from the program.

The PCPE is provided to all students at admission and is discussed during program orientation. The PCPE is completed for each student in every experiential course. Students receive a copy of the evaluation and have an opportunity to discuss their ratings with the faculty member at the end of each course. Kerl and colleagues state that using the PCPE throughout the program has resulted in significantly fewer students finding out about their problematic behavior as they reach the end of their program and significantly fewer dismissals from the program.

Kerl and colleagues describe a legal challenge by a student who was dismissed from the counseling program at Southwest Texas State University. The student exhibited poor impulse and anger control, unethical behavior, and inadequate counseling skills. This student had received three completed PCPEs that identified significant reservations by faculty members regarding the student's professional performance competency. Suggestions for improvement were given to the student at the time each PCPE was shared and discussed with the student. The student failed to follow through with remediation plans and filed suit against the university and the counseling program. Kerl and colleagues describe the outcome of this case:

> The court ruled that the student was provided adequate due process, that the university had the obligation to uphold professional standards, that the university's policies and procedures were enunciated in the graduate catalog and other departmental documents, and that the faculty had followed these procedures. (pp. 330–331)

This court decision identified professional performance competence as an academic concern. The use of the PCPE (along with the clear standards, policies, and procedures developed by the faculty) played a key role in the court's judgment, which ruled in favor of the university on all counts (Kerl et al., 2002).

McAdams, Foster, and Ward (2007) and McAdams and Foster (2007) describe their experience and lessons learned from a challenge in federal court when their program dismissed a counseling student on the grounds of deficient professional performance. The student had engaged in unethical behavior during a clinical practicum and then failed to cooperate with a remedial program implemented by the program faculty. Many systematic procedures were implemented prior to making the decision to dismiss the student, who later filed a lawsuit against the counseling program faculty and the university. One of the charges was that the program and the university violated the student's constitutional right to due process. To the credit of this program, the faculty had designed a document detailing specific criteria for systematically evaluating students in their program in their Professional Performance Review Policy Standards (PPRP).

A key strength of the program's legal position rested in the steps the faculty took in formally documenting all the remedial actions taken in dealing with the student. In a federal jury trial, the court ruled in favor of the counseling program and the university by upholding the dismissal decision. This court case demonstrates that when counselor trainees are found to be deficient in their professional performance, training programs have a legal obligation to develop a just and fair remedial plan of action (McAdams & Foster, 2007). Although the faculty won the case, there was no sense of victory in the aftermath of a painful and long litigation process that had a huge impact on both the students and the faculty in the program.

Professional Licensing and Certification

Most states have established specific requirements of supervised practice beyond the receipt of a master's or doctoral degree for licensing and certification in areas such as clinical social work, clinical or counseling psychology, rehabilitation counseling, clinical mental health counseling, and couples and family therapy. In some countries, licensure and regulation do not exist and any individual can call him- or herself a counselor and establish a counseling practice. For example, Ireland has no mechanism in place to license counselors (O'Morain, McAuliffe, Conroy, Johnson, & Michel, 2012). All 50 U.S. states require licensure, but some do not have a professional scope of practice that requires an individual to be licensed prior to establishing a private practice. Prior to going into private practice, review your state's laws regarding professional scope of practice.

Purposes of Legislative Regulation of Practice

Sweeney (1995) describes credentialing as an approach to identifying individuals by occupational group, involving at least three methods: registry, certification, and licensure. In its simplest form, **registry** is generally a voluntary listing of individuals who use a title or provide a service. Registration represents the least degree of regulation of practice. Both certification and licensure involve increased measures designed to regulate professional practices.

Although licensing and certification differ in their purposes, they have some features in common. Both require applicants to meet specific requirements in terms of education and training and acceptance from practicing professionals. Both also generally rely on tests to determine which applicants have met the standards and deserve to be granted a credential.

Certification is a voluntary attempt by a group to promote a professional identity. Certification confirms that the practitioner has met a set of minimum standards established by the certification agency. Some types of certification are required for practicing in a certain setting. For example, in most states school counselors must obtain a certificate in order to practice.

Unlike certification, **licensure statutes** determine and govern professional practice. Licensure acts, sometimes called practice acts, specify what the holder of the license can do and what others cannot do (Remley, 1995). "Licensure is a governmentally sanctioned credential that regulates which professionals can be reimbursed legally by third-party and private payers for general counseling services" (Tarvydas, Hartley, & Gerald, 2016, p. 17).

Licensure and certification assure the public that practitioners have completed minimum educational programs, have had a certain number of hours of supervised training, and have gone through some type of evaluation and screening. Licenses and certifications do not, and probably cannot, ensure that practitioners will competently do what their credentials permit them to do. A degree or a license alone does not guarantee competence for rendering all psychological services to all populations. For example, clinicians need to acquire specialized knowledge and skills for the ethical practice of family therapy. The main advantages of licensure and certification are the protection of the public from grossly unqualified and untrained practitioners and the formal representation to the public that practitioners are part of an established profession. Credentialing protects counseling consumers by establishing the minimum standards of professional skills and knowledge (Tarvydas et al., 2016). However, there are limitations to ensuring competence by means of licensure, and some question whether licensure does ensure general competence, protect consumers, or promote higher standards of professional practice (Remley & Herlihy, 2016).

Licensure restricts both the use of the title and the practice of an occupation. Most licenses are generic in nature; the holder of the license is assumed to have minimal competence in the general practice of counseling or clinical work. Licenses usually do not specify the clients or problems practitioners are competent to work with, nor do they specify the techniques they are competent to use. For example, a licensed professional counselor may possess the expertise needed to work with adults yet lack the training necessary to work with children. The same person may be qualified to do individual psychotherapy yet have neither the experience nor the skills required for family counseling or group therapy. Most licensing regulations do specify that licensees are to engage only in those therapeutic tasks for which they have adequate training, but it is up to the licensee to put this rule into practice. Such a broad definition of practice also applies to many other professions.

Continuing Professional Education and Demonstration of Competence

Professionals are required to engage in ongoing study, education, training, and consultation in their areas of practice. A practitioner's level of competence may diminish over time, and changes in laws pertaining to mental health, evolving ethical standards, and new trends in professional and evidence-based practices continue to be made. Most professional organizations support efforts to make continuing professional education a mandatory condition of relicensing (see the Ethics Codes box titled "Continuing Professional Education Requirements").

ETHICS CODES: Continuing Professional Education Requirements

American Counseling Association (2014)
Counselors recognize the need for continuing education to acquire and maintain a reasonable level of awareness of current scientific and professional information in their fields of activity. Counselors maintain their competence in the skills they use, are open to new procedures, and remain informed regarding best practices for working with diverse populations. (C.2.f.)

American School Counselor Association (2016)
School counselors engage in professional development and personal growth throughout their careers. Professional development includes attendance at state and national conferences and reading journal articles. School counselors regularly attend training on school counselors' current legal and ethical responsibilities. (B.3.e.)

National Association of Social Workers (2008)
Social work administrators and supervisors should take reasonable steps to provide or arrange for continuing education and staff development for all staff for whom they are responsible. Continuing education and staff development should address current knowledge and emerging developments related to social work practice and ethics. (3.08.)

American Association for Marriage and Family Therapy (2015)
Marriage and family therapists pursue knowledge of new developments and maintain their competence in marriage and family therapy through education, training, and/or supervised experience. (3.1.)

American Mental Health Counselors Association (2015)
Mental health counselors recognize the importance of continuing education and remain open to new counseling approaches and procedures documented by peer-reviewed scientific and professional literature. (C.1.f)

American Psychiatric Association (2013b)
Psychiatrists are responsible for their own continuing education and should be mindful of the fact that theirs must be a lifetime of learning. (5.1.)

Most mental health professionals are required to demonstrate, as a basis for relicensure or recertification, that they have completed a minimal number of continuing education activities. As a condition for relicensure as a social worker, psychologist, clinical mental health counselor, or a marriage and family therapist, most states require specific courses and a minimum number of hours of continuing professional education. The most common area of mandated continuing education is professional ethics, and 32 states currently require an ethics course as a component of continuing professional development (Taylor & Neimeyer, 2016). Licensing boards often conduct random continuing education audits of their licensees. In California, if licensees fail a continuing education audit, such as not completing the total required hours of continuing education within a renewal period, or not completing the law and ethics course, they are subject to a citation and a fine (California Board of Behavioral Sciences, 2017).

A Lifelong Commitment to Maintaining Competence

A commitment to lifelong learning is a common theme in the ethics codes of most mental health professions as a way to maintain and enhance competence. Johnson and colleagues (2012) doubt whether a beginning mental health professional will have either the capacity or the determination to accurately assess his or her own competence across a lifetime of ever-changing job demands, life stressors, personal problems, and declining abilities due to aging. They recommend ongoing peer consultation and state that "periodic recertification of competence should become a requirement of licensure renewal" (p. 566). The focus of continuing education should be on *maintaining competence*, rather than simply on accumulating the required hours to maintain licensure.

To assume that our skills never deteriorate or that we know everything we need to know upon graduation is naive. Unless mental health practitioners engage in lifelong learning, their professional knowledge may decline drastically, even if they are in the early phase of their career (Neimeyer, Taylor, & Cox, 2012; Taylor & Neimeyer, 2016). A useful way to combat knowledge obsolescence and maintain competence is to be willing to consult with other professionals throughout your career, participate in peer consultation groups, engage in self-directed learning, and attend professional conferences. Learning never ceases, and new clients present new challenges. Even recent graduates may have significant gaps in their education that will require them to take workshops or courses in the future. Research in the allied health fields supports the notion that lifelong learning is a key component of professional competence, and Taylor and Neimeyer (2015) recommend that training faculty "instill a love for lifelong learning in graduate school, reinforcing the notion that lifelong learning is an ongoing endeavor that must be continued to be pursued, even after graduation" (p. 388). New areas of knowledge and practice demand ongoing education. Online classes are becoming increasingly popular because this form of continuing education delivery is convenient and economical; it is likely that online offerings will increase in years to come (Taylor & Neimeyer, 2016).

You may also need to seek supervision and consultation in working with various client populations or to acquire skills in certain therapeutic modalities. For example, your job may require you to conduct groups, yet your program may not have included even one group course in the curriculum. When continuing education is tailored to your personal and professional needs, it can keep you on the cutting edge of your profession.

Clarifying Your Stance It is important to find ways to maintain and enhance your competence over the course of your career. Use the following questions to clarify your thinking on the issues we have raised. What is your own strategy for remaining professionally competent?

- What effects on individual practitioners do you think the trend toward increased accountability is likely to have? How might this trend affect you?
- Do you think it is ethical to continue practicing if you do not continue your education? Why or why not?
- What is the rationale for stating that maintaining competence as a lifelong endeavor?
- What are some advantages and disadvantages to using continuing education programs solely as the basis for renewing a license? Is continuing education enough?
- What are your reactions to competence examinations (oral and written) for entry-level applicants and as a basis for license renewal? What kinds of examinations might be useful?
- What are your thoughts about enhancing your knowledge via online continuing education? Would you be inclined to participate in online delivery for some continuing education?
- Should evidence of continuing education be required (or simply strongly recommended) as a basis for recertification or relicensure?
- If you support mandatory continuing education, who should determine the nature of this education? What standards could be used in making this determination?
- What kinds of continuing education would you want for yourself? Through what means do you think you can best acquire new knowledge and skills and keep abreast of advances in your field?

Review, Consultation, and Supervision by Peers

Peer review is an organized system by which practitioners within a profession assess one another's services. Peer review provides some assurance to consumers that they will receive competent services. In addition to providing peer review, colleagues can challenge each other to adopt a fresh perspective on problems they encounter in their practice. Regarded as a means rather than an end in itself, peer review has as its ultimate goal not only to determine whether a practitioner's professional activity is adequate, but also to ensure that future services will be up to standard. Peer review continues a tradition of self-regulation.

Peer supervision provides a path to continue the transition from trainee to independent practitioner. It entails elements of support and is another useful route to enhancing professional competencies. The goal of peer supervision is to assist professionals in obtaining feedback on their professional work and functioning and to help them monitor their personal reactions to their cases (Shah & Rodolfa, 2016). Peer supervision groups are useful for counselors at all levels of experience. For trainees, peer supervision groups offer a supportive atmosphere and help them learn that they are not alone with their concerns. For counselors in practice, they provide an opportunity for continued professional growth. According to Shah and Rodolfa (2016), peer supervision groups provide for vicarious learning to occur. "As peers consult with each other, provide feedback, and share experiences, they can take the learning with them and apply it to future professional situations when they arise" (p. 204). Counselman and Weber (2004) contend that peer supervision groups are valuable for therapists for many reasons, some of which include ongoing consultation and support for difficult cases, networking, and combating professional isolation and potential burnout. Clinicians often recognize a renewed need for supervision at a later point in their careers because they want additional training, because of the emotional intensity of practicing therapy, or because of the stress associated with their professional work.

Chapter Summary

The welfare of clients is directly affected by ethical issues in the training of therapists and in the debate over whether professional licensure and credentialing are adequate measures of competence. To prevent obsolescence of knowledge and skills, counselors must acquire new knowledge and skills throughout their professional career. This is particularly true for practitioners wishing to develop a specialty area dealing with certain client populations or problems.

A core ethical and professional issue in training involves the question of how to develop policies and procedures for selecting the candidates who are best suited for the various mental health professions. The challenge is to adopt criteria for choosing people who have the life experiences that will enable them to understand the diverse range of clients with whom they will work. The personal characteristics of trainees, such as attitudes, beliefs, character, and psychological fitness, are critical to success, as is the ability to remain objective when working with clients with diverse values. The ability of trainees to effectively relate to others, including clients, must be assessed throughout the program, and remedial work for students with interpersonal competence problems should be addressed by faculty. The evaluation process encompasses knowledge, skills, and interpersonal relationship dimensions. Training programs have an ethical responsibility to intervene when students have major personal and interpersonal problems that interfere with their professional competence.

An ongoing commitment to continuing education is necessary for professionals to maintain competence, and practitioners have an ethical responsibility to participate in self-directed learning (reading professional literature), engage in peer consultation, participate in conferences and workshops, or seek other ways to become informed about new developments in their field. A lifelong commitment to continuing education is a hallmark of the ethics codes of most mental health professions.

Suggested Activities

1. In small groups explore the topic of when and how you might make a referral. Role-play a referral, with one student playing the client and another playing the counselor. After a few minutes the "client" and the other students can give the "counselor" feedback on how he or she handled the situation.

2. In small groups explore what you think the criteria should be for determining whether a therapist is competent. Prepare a list of specific criteria, and share it with the rest of the class. Are you able as a class to identify some common criteria for determining competence? Is it easier to determine incompetence?

3. As a class project, several students can form a committee to investigate some of the major local and state laws that apply to the practice of psychotherapy. You might want to ask mental health professionals what major conflicts they have experienced between the law and their professional practice. Look up the requirements for licensure or certification of the major mental health specializations in your state. What are some of the common elements?

4. Assume that you are applying for a job or writing a résumé to use in private practice. Write your own professional disclosure statement in a page or two. Bring your disclosure statements to class and have fellow students review what you have written. They can then interview you, and you can get some practice in talking with "prospective clients." This exercise can help you clarify your own position and give you valuable practice for job interviews.

5. Assume that you are a graduate student who is part of the interviewing team for applicants for your training program. Identify six questions to pose to all applicants. What are you hoping to learn about the applicants from your questions?

6. Interview professors or practitioners in schools, agencies, or work settings that interest you. Ask them what they most remember about their training programs. What features were most useful for them? What training do they wish they had more of and wish they had less of? How adequately did their graduate program prepare them for the work they are now doing? What continuing education experiences did they most value?

7. Review the Personal and Professional Competencies evaluation form reproduced in this chapter. Complete this evaluation form based on how you would assess your current level of competency in each area. What areas would you target for further work? Outline a plan of action to help you develop these personal and professional competencies.

8. Consider the advantages of forming a peer support group in one of your classes. Several of you could make a commitment to meet to explore ways to get the most from your training and education. Make a list of topics that you would find useful to cover in a peer support group.

Ethics in Action Video Exercises

9. Reflect on all of the role-playing situations enacted in the *Ethics in Action* video program. Putting yourself in the place of the counselor, can you think of any situations in which you would determine that a referral is in the best interests of your client? Consider situations such as a lack of multicultural competence in a particular case, a client to whom you were sexually attracted, or a client who cannot pay you because of losing employment. Select an area where you could envision yourself making a referral and role-play this with another student as the client. Assume that your client does not want to accept the referral and insists on remaining with you.

10. In video role play 4, Counselor Competence: Dealing With Delusions, the counselor (Suzanne) recognizes that she is beyond her level of competence and considers referral of a client (LeAnne) who appears to be delusional. When LeAnne reveals that others are following her, the counselor expresses her concern and attempts to convince the client to see a more qualified professional. LeAnne is not responsive to this suggestion and feels that Suzanne can help her.

As a counselor, what do you think you would do in a similar situation? How might you respond if your client flatly refuses the idea of a referral? Would you be inclined to continue seeing a client if you thought you were not competent to counsel this person, even though your client says you are helping her? Discuss in small groups your thoughts about making a referral when you lack competence.

MindTap for Counseling

Go to MindTap® for digital study tools and resources that complement this text and help you be more successful in your course and career. There's an interactive eBook plus videos of client sessions, skill-building activities, quizzes to help you prepare for tests, apps, and more—all in one place. If your instructor *didn't* assign MindTap, you can find out more about it at CengageBrain.com.

CHAPTER

9

Ethical Issues
in Supervision

LEARNING OBJECTIVES

1. Identify ethical issues in clinical supervision

2. Delineate the responsibilities of supervisees

3. Describe the roles and responsibilities of supervisors

4. Recognize ethical and effective practices in supervision

5. Clarify the meaning of becoming a competent supervisor

6. Discuss legal issues in clinical supervision

7. Understand the ethical issues unique to online supervision

8. Describe the special issues that arise when supervising school counselors

9. Examine multicultural and diversity issues in supervision

10. Understand how gender-role socialization affects clinical supervision

11. Grasp the multiple roles and relationships in the supervisory process

12. Address the ethical aspects of combining supervision and counseling

SELF-INVENTORY

Directions: For each statement, indicate the response that most closely identifies your beliefs and attitudes. Use the following code:

5 = I *strongly agree* with this statement.

4 = I *agree* with this statement.

3 = I am *undecided* about this statement.

2 = I *disagree* with this statement.

1 = I *strongly disagree* with this statement.

_____ 1. Ethical guidelines for clinical supervision are needed to protect the supervisor, the supervisee, and the client.

_____ 2. Supervisors should be held legally accountable for all of the actions of the trainees they supervise.

_____ 3. Supervisors have the responsibility to consistently monitor and assess a trainee's performance.

_____ 4. Working under supervision is one of the most important components for the development of a competent practitioner.

_____ 5. Supervisors must be sure that trainees fully inform clients about the limits of confidentiality.

_____ 6. Supervision, at its best, protects the welfare of the client and increases the competence of the supervisee.

_____ 7. Informed consent is as fundamental in the supervisory relationship as it is in the therapeutic relationship.

_____ 8. If supervisors lack multicultural and diversity competence, supervision is likely to be ineffective.

_____ 9. Supervisors should obtain regular feedback about the quality of their supervision and use that feedback to improve their supervisory competence.

_____ 10. Supervisees have a right to know what is expected of them and how they will be evaluated from the beginning of the supervisory relationship.

_____ 11. It is unethical for counseling supervisors to operate in multiple roles such as mentor, adviser, teacher, and evaluator.

_____ 12. Ethically, supervisors need to clarify their roles and to be aware of potential problems that can develop when boundaries become blurred.

_____ 13. Supervisors or counselor educators who provide therapy to current students or supervisees are behaving unethically.

_____ 14. Personal information that trainees share in supervision should remain confidential and never be shared with other faculty members.

_____ 15. Supervisors have a role in advocating for their supervisees and clients in the educational and training settings within which they practice.

Introduction

Supervision is an integral part of your professional training and is one of the ways in which you acquire the competence needed to fulfill your professional responsibilities. Textbook knowledge alone is not sufficient; you need guidance in putting your knowledge into practice. Supervision provides a forum for examining your beliefs, attitudes, personality characteristics, and behaviors as they affect your clients and the therapeutic process. Remley and Herlihy (2016) distinguish between administrative supervision and clinical supervision. *Administrative supervision* involves directions given by direct-line administrators to their employees. The purpose of administrative supervision is to see that counselors who are employed are doing their jobs competently. Administrative supervisors generally have direct control and authority over those they supervise. *Clinical supervision* involves a supervisor overseeing your professional work as a trainee with four major goals: (1) to protect the welfare of clients, (2) to promote supervisee growth and development, (3) to monitor supervisee performance and to serve as a gatekeeper for the profession, and (4) to empower the supervisee to self-supervise and carry out these goals as an independent professional (Corey, Haynes, Moulton, & Muratori, 2010; Falender, 2017). Our discussion in this chapter is primarily concerned with clinical supervision.

As future practitioners, you can never know all that you might like to know, nor can you attain all the skills required to effectively intervene with all client populations or all types of problems. This is where the processes of supervision and consultation come into play, and why supervision remains a relevant process throughout your career. As mentioned in Chapter 8, professional competence is a developmental process. Being a competent professional demands continuing education and a willingness to obtain periodic supervision when faced with ethical or clinical dilemmas. By consulting experts, practitioners at all levels of experience demonstrate responsibility in obtaining the assistance necessary to provide the highest quality of care for clients.

Ethical and professional standards and guidelines for clinical supervision are an integral part of competent supervision. This chapter explores dilemmas frequently encountered in clinical supervision and provides guidelines for ethical and legal practice. Supervision is a required component of your training program, and you will obtain the maximum benefit from your experience in supervision if you understand the roles, functions, and responsibilities of supervision. Prepare to assume an active role in your supervision and develop a collaborative relationship with your supervisor. Ethical, legal, and professional issues are of primary importance in supervision. Know your rights and responsibilities as a supervisee, and learn what you can expect from your supervisor.

In this chapter we discuss both the supervisor's and the supervisee's perspectives. We address what it takes to be an ethical and competent supervisor, what is involved in being an active supervisee, and the ethical concerns students will encounter as they gain experience and competence in the field.

Ethical Issues in Clinical Supervision

Effective and ethical supervision involves a fine balance on the supervisor's part between protecting clients' welfare and providing training for supervisees. Falender and Shafranske (2014) define effective supervision as "practice that encourages supervisee development and autonomy, facilitates the supervisory relationship, protects the client, and enhances both client and supervisee outcomes" (pp. 1031–1032). Supervisors are ethically and legally responsible to monitor the quality of care clients receive and to assist supervisees in learning the art and craft of therapeutic practice. Through supervision supervisees gain the experience necessary to become independent professionals.

The American Mental Health Counselors Association's (2015) ethics code addresses the commitment to clinical supervision:

> Clinical supervision is an important part of the mental health treatment process. This purpose is two-fold: to assist the supervisee to provide the best treatment possible to counseling clients, through guidance and direction by the supervisor regarding clinical, ethical, and legal issues; and to provide training to the supervisee, which is an integral part of counselor education. Supervision is also a gatekeeping process to ensure safety to the client, the profession and to the supervisee. (III.B.)

When we take into consideration the dependent position of the trainee and the similarities between the supervisory relationship and the therapeutic relationship, the need for guidelines describing the rights of trainees and the responsibilities of supervisors becomes obvious. The Association for Counselor Education and Supervision addressed this early in the "Ethical Guidelines for Counseling Supervisors" (ACES, 1993, 1995) and more recently in "Best Practices in Clinical Supervision" (ACES, 2011). ACES now provides a comprehensive discussion of informed consent, goal setting, ongoing feedback for supervisees, effective supervision, the supervisory relationship, diversity and advocacy considerations, documentation, supervision format, and the supervisory role. These best practice guidelines support supervisors in their work and clarify most aspects of the supervisory process. The American Psychological Association's (2015) "Guidelines for Clinical Supervision in Health Service Psychology" are referred to throughout the chapter.

Informed Consent in Supervision

Many of the ethical standards pertaining to the client–therapist relationship also apply to the supervisor–supervisee relationship. **Informed consent in supervision** is as essential as informed consent in counseling practice (see Chapter 5). It is now considered the standard of practice to incorporate clear informed consent material for supervisees, both orally and in writing. In addition, it is the responsibility of supervisors to ensure that supervisees carry out an informed consent process with their clients prior to beginning a counseling relationship.

It is beneficial to discuss the rights of supervisees from the beginning of the supervisory relationship, in much the same way as the rights of clients are addressed early in the therapy process. Supervisors are expected to engage in sound informed consent practices in the initial supervision session and to clearly state the parameters for conducting supervision (ACES, 2011). When supervisees learn what to expect in all aspects of their supervision and what they need to do to achieve success, they are empowered to express expectations, make decisions, and become active participants in the supervisory process. In addition, misunderstandings are minimized and both parties are more likely to experience satisfaction in their respective roles. Glosoff, Renfro-Michel, and Nagarajan (2016) state that one way to establish and maintain a strong supervisory working alliance is for supervisors to engage in sound informed consent practices for the duration of the supervisory relationship. Supervisors need to remember that "the goal of the initial and ongoing process of informed consent is not simply to disseminate information to supervisees but also for supervisors to foster a collaborative, egalitarian supervisory working alliance" (p. 37). Bringing the supervisee into the conversation as a partner facilitates a collaborative spirit and helps build autonomy.

Responsibilities of Supervisees

In addition to your rights as a supervisee, you have responsibilities, some of which are listed below:

- Come prepared to each supervision session. Bring your files and notes as well as a written list of questions for your supervisor.
- Be an active participant and collaborate in your supervision. Own the power you have as a trainee and learner.
- Take the initiative to ask for what you need from your supervisor.
- Do related research and reading between sessions to enhance your work with clients.
- Pay attention to your interactions with clients and with your supervisor, and be willing to address any areas of concern you have.
- If you are having trouble with colleagues or fellow supervisees, bring these matters into supervision.
- Ask for feedback about both your strengths and areas where you need to improve.
- Be open to feedback from supervisors, fellow supervisees, and your clients.
- Try to critically evaluate feedback you feel is not constructive.
- Establish healthy boundaries for yourself in terms of what is asked of you by your clients and your supervisors.
- Let your supervisor know if you are feeling overwhelmed by your work with clients.
- Be open to various forms of supervision, including live supervision and videotaping.
- Talk about insecurities and anxieties you have that pertain to your work.
- Provide feedback to your supervisor about what you find helpful or unhelpful in your supervisory relationship.

- Pay attention to possible sources of countertransference, and in supervision explore how these reactions are affecting your work with clients.
- If you are not receiving adequate supervision and your efforts to communicate with your supervisor are not effective, reach out to a professor or another trusted adviser.

The Supervisor's Roles and Responsibilities

You get the most from your supervision as a trainee when you understand the roles and responsibilities of those who supervise you. Supervisors must provide the training and supervised experiences that will enable supervisees to deliver ethical and effective services. To provide effective clinical supervision, supervisors must be competent both in the practice of supervision and in the area of counseling being supervised. Supervisors should provide supervision only after obtaining the needed education and training to ensure competence in this role, and only if they can devote the required time to provide adequate oversight (Barnett & Johnson, 2015).

Supervisors are ultimately responsible, *both ethically and legally,* for the actions of their trainees. Therefore, they are cautioned not to supervise more trainees than they can responsibly manage at one time. They must check on trainees' progress and be familiar with their caseloads. Just as practitioners keep case records on the progress of their clients, supervisors are required to maintain records pertaining to their work with trainees.

Clinical supervisors have a position of influence with their supervisees; they operate in multiple roles as teacher, mentor, consultant, counselor, adviser, administrator, evaluator, and documenter. Supervisors may serve many different functions during a single supervisory session. They might instruct a supervisee in a clinical approach, act as a consultant on how to intervene with the client, act as a counselor in helping the supervisee understand how countertransference could be affecting work with the client, and give evaluative feedback to the supervisee regarding his or her progress as a clinician. Falender (2017) states that "a skilled supervisor balances the multiple roles, giving ongoing feedback, positive and corrective, while also supporting the development of the supervisee and ensuring that the power differential is clear" (p. 213). Competent supervisors have a clear understanding of the role in which they are functioning in any given situation, why they are serving in that role, and what they hope to accomplish with the supervisee (Corey et al., 2010). It is important for supervisors to monitor their own behavior so as not to misuse the inherent power in the supervisor–supervisee relationship. Supervisors are expected to be aware of the power differential inherent in the supervisory relationship and to discuss the power dynamics in this relationship with supervisees. Supervisors should strive to minimize the power differential by establishing a collaborative relationship and encouraging open discussion, yet at the same time they must maintain appropriate authority (ACES, 2011). The complexity of the supervisory relationship and the multiple roles and inherent power differential of supervision require specialized training in clinical supervision (Falender, 2017).

Ethical supervisors seek their own supervision or consultation when faced with complex supervisory issues.

Supervisors are responsible for ensuring compliance with relevant legal, ethical, and professional standards for clinical practice (ACES, 2011). The main purposes for ethical standards for clinical supervision are to provide behavioral guidelines to supervisors, to protect supervisees from undue harm or neglect, and to ensure quality client care (Bernard & Goodyear, 2014). Supervisors can demonstrate their knowledge of these ethical guidelines through the behavior they model in the supervisory relationship.

Supervisor Responsibilities to Supervisees and Their Clients

Supervisors understand that client welfare is their main and highest responsibility (ACES, 2011; APA, 2015). Supervisors have the responsibility of monitoring each supervisee's conduct and competence. Supervisors have an ethical and legal obligation to provide trainees with timely feedback, monitor trainee's actions and decisions, teach trainees about due process and their rights, and guide their personal development as it pertains to their clinical competence (ACES, 2011). Supervisors must be fair in the process of evaluation and provide opportunities for supervisees to take remedial actions when their performance does not meet expected standards.

At times your supervisor may consult with faculty members regarding your progress, but personal information you share in supervision generally remains confidential. At the very least, you have a right to be informed about what will and will not be shared with others on the faculty. Supervisors should put ethics in the foreground of their supervisory practices, which is best done by treating supervisees in a respectful, professional, and ethical manner. One of the best ways for supervisors to model professional behavior for supervisees is to deal appropriately with confidentiality issues pertaining to supervisees.

Methods of Supervision

The ethical standards of the APA (2010), NASW (1994, 2008), ACA (2014), and ACES (2011) require that supervisors demonstrate a conceptual knowledge of supervisory methods and techniques and that they are skilled in using this knowledge to promote the development of trainees. From an ethical perspective, supervisors must have a clearly developed framework for supervision and a rationale for the methods they employ. A variety of evaluative methods are typically employed in supervision. *Self-report* is one of the most widely used supervisory methods, but it is not the best representation of a student's performance. Digital recordings can augment self-report, which is otherwise limited by the supervisee's conceptual and observational ability. Verbal exchange and direct observation are the most commonly used forms of supervision. In verbal exchange, the supervisor and supervisee discuss cases, ethical and legal issues, and personal development. Direct observation methods involve a supervisor actually observing a supervisee's practice. Direct observation, even though it demands time and effort, provides a unique reflection of the skills and abilities of the supervisee.

The quality of the supervisory relationship is an important factor in determining supervision outcomes (Falender & Shafranske, 2014). The methods and techniques supervisors use are more likely to be helpful if an effective and collaborative working relationship with supervisees has been established. In much the same way that effective therapists create a climate in which clients can explore their choices, supervisors need to establish a positive relationship that encourages trainees to reflect on what they are doing.

Philosophy and Styles of Supervision

You may require and benefit from different styles of supervision at different stages in your professional development. Although you may need more direction when you begin your training, it is a good idea to foster a reflective and questioning approach that leads to self-initiated discovery. An effective supervisor will promote autonomy without overwhelming the supervisee.

When we supervise, we focus on the dynamics between ourselves and our trainees as well as the dynamics between supervisees and their clients. We see a parallel process operating between a counseling model and a supervisory model. Supervisees can learn ways to conceptualize what they are doing with their clients by reflecting on what they are learning about interpersonal dynamics in the supervisory relationship. Although the trainee's ability to assess and treat a client's problems is important, in supervision we are equally concerned with the interpersonal aspects that are emerging.

As supervisors we oversee the work of our supervisees and help them refine their own insights and clinical hunches. We strive to help supervisees identify their own intuitions, perceptions, and struggles. Rather than using our words with clients, we expect that supervisees will find their own words and develop their own voice. Our style of supervision is reflected in the questions we explore:

- What direction do you think is most appropriate to take with your clients?
- How are you reacting to your clients? How is your behavior affecting them?
- What client issues trigger your countertransferences?
- How might our relationship, in these supervisory sessions, mirror your relationships with your clients?
- Are you feeling free enough to bring into these supervisory sessions any difficulties you are having with your clients?

Ethical and Effective Practices of Clinical Supervisors

A collaborative supervisory relationship, characterized by a strong working alliance, is a key component of effective supervision (ACES, 2011; APA, 2015; Falender, Shafranske, & Ofek, 2014; Shafranske & Falender, 2016). Supervisors regularly include constructive feedback on ethics when meeting with supervisees, and supervisors are well trained, knowledgeable, and skilled in the practice of clinical supervision. Effective supervisors recognize their responsibility to serve as role models for supervisees and conduct themselves ethically in the supervisory relationship (Barnett, as cited in Barnett, Cornish, et al., 2007). Supervisors regularly ask for feedback from their supervisees about the kind of supervision they are providing and use this feedback to improve their supervisory practices (APA, 2015).

In a study of the assessment of culturally competent supervision, counselor trainees indicated it was helpful to them when their supervisor initiated discussions of power dynamics in the supervisory relationship (Ancis & Marshall, 2010). This same study revealed that supervisors who made efforts to create a safe and open supervisory climate allowed trainees to be vulnerable and take risks that encouraged a discussion of various personal and professional issues. Many of these counselor trainees viewed their supervisors as open, accepting, and flexible throughout the supervisory experience, which enhanced both the supervisory relationship and relationships with their own clients.

Competence of Supervisors

Clinical supervisors are increasingly vulnerable and at risk for ethical and legal liability. Yet only recently has the standard for qualifying to be a clinical supervisor included formal coursework and supervision of one's work with supervisees. Currently, most psychology and counselor education programs offer a course in supervision at the doctoral level, but training for supervisors at the master's level is lacking. Many supervisors lack education and training in supervision. They may rely on their previous supervisory experience as trainees and their clinical knowledge to inform their practice as supervisors (Bernard & Goodyear, 2014; Shafranske & Falender, 2016).

From both an ethical and legal standpoint, supervisors are required to have the competence necessary to adequately carry out their roles. They provide supervision only for those supervisees and clients for whom they have adequate training and experience (ACES, 2011). The counselor licensure laws in a number of states now stipulate that licensed professional counselors who practice supervision are required to have relevant training experiences and coursework in supervision.

Competent supervisors must effectively deal with trainees who manifest problematic behaviors. Jacobs and colleagues (2011) reviewed cases in which trainees manifested problems of professional competence and found that supervisors often are not managing these situations effectively. Jacobs and colleagues contend that difficult conversations with trainees who have problems of professional competence are necessary and are an ethical responsibility.

In addition to specialized training in methods of supervision, supervisors must have an in-depth knowledge of the specialty area in which they will provide supervision. It is unethical for supervisors to offer supervision in areas beyond their scope of practice. When supervisees are working outside the area of competence of the supervisor, it is the responsibility of the supervisor to arrange for competent clinical supervision of the cases in question. It is extremely important that supervisors know their limits and accurately assess them; such self-evaluation reflects their own metacompetence (Falendar & Shafranske, 2007). In her thoughtful article about best practices in supervision, Borders (2014) emphasizes that supervisor expertise requires reflective knowledge "built during years of practice and is dependent on continual self-awareness, self-assessment, self-monitoring, and self-reflection, which are predominant characteristics of expert supervisors" (p. 161).

It is our conviction that the competence of supervisors is related to their personal qualities. Effective supervisors demonstrate the four A's—they tend to be available, accessible, affable, and able. The general picture of the good supervisor reveals an individual who is a technically competent professional with good human relations skills and effective organizational and managerial skills (Corey et al., 2010).

The Problem of Supervisor Incompetence

This discussion would not be complete without considering supervisor incompetence. At times, supervisors may be unable to effectively carry out their supervisory role due to personal or external factors or because of physical and psychological depletion. Similar to the case of incompetent therapists discussed in Chapter 2, incompetent supervisors can do harm to trainees.

Supervisor behaviors and attitudes that have the potential to be extremely damaging include boundary violations, misuse of power, sexual contact with supervisees, substance abuse, extreme burnout, or diminished clinical judgment. In some cases, supervisor incompetence may be a result of the supervisor's inexperience in the supervisory role, which can be improved with guided supervision. Other cases may reflect more serious problems such as personal or mental health issues that interfere with the supervisor's ability to competently carry out his or her supervisory duties.

According to Muratori (2001), it is critical to be aware of the reality that supervisors are in an evaluative position vis-à-vis their trainees, which limits trainees' options in deciding what to do in situations of incompetent supervision. Trainees need to consider the power differential inherent in the supervisory relationship, the personalities of both the supervisor and the supervisee, and their level of development as counselor trainees and the extent to which this influences their perceptions of their supervisor's competence. Supervisees need to carefully consider their course of action with an incompetent supervisor because of the possible consequences that could be associated with the supervisor's misuse of power.

Have you considered what you might do if you had to deal with a problematic supervisor? Put yourself in Melinda's shoes as you reflect on the following case.

The Case of Melinda

Melinda, a second year master's student, was thrilled when she found out she had been selected to do a 1-year internship at her college's counseling center. She hoped this experience would help launch her career as a college counselor upon completion of her degree. Unfortunately, a few weeks into the first semester Melinda began to suspect that her on-site supervisor, Kathy, was emotionally unstable. Although Kathy was personable at times, her mood seemed to fluctuate in an unpredictable manner. On several occasions Kathy berated Melinda during supervision for not taking her direction. Melinda was starting to develop autonomy as a counselor, which was appropriate at this point in her training. Nevertheless, whenever she expressed her own ideas, Kathy appeared to feel threatened and angry. Not surprisingly, Melinda started to question her own abilities and felt reluctant to talk openly about her cases during supervision sessions. Aware that she had an ethical responsibility to provide her clients with an acceptable standard of care, she began to worry that the inadequate supervision she was receiving might compromise her ability to provide proper services to her clients. She asked herself, "Should I confront Kathy and tell her that I need more guidance from her? If I do that, will I compromise my chances of finishing the program because Kathy has the power to fail me? If I tell anyone about what's happening, will they think I am just being a difficult and rebellious supervisee?" Ultimately, Melinda took the risk of consulting with a professor in her program and transferred to a new supervisor. Although she felt angry that she received such poor supervision from Kathy, she reported factual information only to her professor and did not vent her negative feelings. Despite some fallout from this experience, Melinda was able to complete the program and pursue her career as a college counselor.

- How do you assess the way Melinda handled the situation?
- How would you determine that a supervisor is emotionally unstable or incompetent?
- If your supervisor appeared to be ineffective, what would you do? Would you confront the person directly, discuss the problem with other supervisors or professors, or try to ignore it and make the most out of a bad situation? Explain.
- If you took action, would you have any fear of retribution from your supervisor? How could you minimize the risks associated with taking action?

Commentary. This case illustrates the vulnerability of the supervisee. It would be difficult to fault any of the steps that Melinda took to take care of her supervision problem. She consulted with a professor in the program, and it then became the professor's responsibility to take action. Melinda could have confronted Kathy directly, but her experience with Kathy suggested that this would be unlikely to yield a satisfying outcome. We think Melinda handled the dilemma well. If Melinda's final evaluation from Kathy was clearly unfair or punitive, Melinda should file a formal grievance through her training program.

Supervisees assigned to an incompetent supervisor generally have fewer options than a client who has an incompetent counselor. Counselor educators and program supervisors have a responsibility to inform students about the courses of action open to them when they encounter supervisors such as the one described in this case. Speaking up about an incompetent or ineffective supervisor can be difficult, and doing so is not an easy decision to make. If you find yourself in a similar situation, seek the counsel of your faculty supervisor. If this individual is not available, talk to a trusted professor or adviser who can help you make the decision that is best in your case. As with any ethical dilemma, do not make this decision in isolation. •

Legal Aspects of Supervision

Three legal considerations in the supervisory relationship are informed consent, confidentiality and its limits, and liability. First, supervisors must see that trainees provide the information to clients that they need to make informed choices. Clients must be fully aware that the counselor they are seeing is a trainee, that he or she is meeting on a regular basis for supervisory sessions, that the client's case may be discussed in group supervision meetings with other trainees, and that sessions may be recorded or observed.

Accountability requires an arrangement consisting of professional disclosure statements and contracts that outline the model to be used in supervision, the goals and objectives of supervision, and assessment and evaluation methods (Corey et al., 2010). Supervisors can make use of informed consent through contracting for supervision so that supervisees are informed of the potential benefits, risks, and expectations of entering into the supervisory relationship. A **supervision contract** is an explicit agreement between supervisor and supervisee, and it can prevent problems that could arise (Westefeld, 2009). The contract is not merely a checklist; it represents a vital, ongoing process of mutual understanding of the parameters of training (Shafranske & Falender, 2016). "The contract is an outgrowth of the supervisory relationship in which the supervisor is respectful, collaborative, empathic, genuine, and explicit in articulating the power differential within which supervision occurs" (Falender, 2017, p. 213).

A supervision contract plays a key role in establishing and maintaining the supervisory alliance. It is a gold standard for best supervision practices, and it provides the groundwork for an effective supervision experience. Some topics a contract may address include legal and ethical requirements, methods to be used in supervision, expectations and parameters for supervision and the training experience, procedures for evaluation of job performance, feedback procedures, supervisor and supervisee roles and responsibilities, limits of confidentiality in supervision, documentation of supervision, and expectations for supervisee disclosures (Falender, Shafranske, & Ofek, 2014; Shafranske & Falender, 2016). Falender and Shafranske (2014) state that "the contract lays out the duties of the supervisor, including protection of the client as the highest priority, clarification of the supervisor's multiple and potentially conflicting roles of client protection and gatekeeper for the profession, and [balances that] with the role of enhancing and facilitating the growth and development of competence of the supervisee" (p. 1036).

Second, supervisors have a legal and ethical obligation to respect the confidentiality of client communications. Supervision involves discussion of client concerns and review of client materials, and supervisees must respect their clients' privacy by not talking about their clients outside of the context of supervision. By their own behavior, supervisors model for supervisees appropriate ways of talking about clients and keeping information protected and used only in the context of supervision (Bernard & Goodyear, 2014). Supervisors must make sure that both supervisees and their clients are fully informed about the limits of confidentiality, including those situations in which supervisors have a duty to report or protect. The informed consent process should include information on all technology that might be used, as well as safeguards to protect the client and the supervisee (Glosoff et al., 2016).

Third, supervisors ultimately bear legal responsibility for the welfare of those clients counseled by their trainees. In addition to being ethically vulnerable, supervisors are legally vulnerable to the work performed by those they supervise. Supervisors are expected to understand the legal ramifications of their supervisory work. To carry out their ethical and legal responsibilities, supervisors are required to be familiar with all cases of every supervisee. Failure to do this invites legal action. Supervisors cannot be cognizant of all of the details of every case, but they should at least know the direction in which the cases are being taken.

Remley (2017) has identified a number of steps clinical supervisors can take to reduce their legal liability:

- Supervisors consider the relationship with a supervisee as educational rather than as being in control.
- Supervisors clarify their role with the supervisee and with other supervisors.
- Supervisors provide a written contract and discuss it with the supervisee.
- Supervisors communicate any concerns with the supervisee.
- Supervisors monitor the work of the supervisee.
- Supervisors instruct supervisees to follow the directives of the job supervisor.
- Supervisors provide suggestions for improvement rather than giving directives.
- Supervisors defer to the on-site supervisor's authority.

Bernard and Goodyear (2014) indicate that supervisors bear both direct liability and vicarious liability. **Direct liability** can be incurred when the actions of supervisors are the cause for harm. For example, supervisors may give trainees inappropriate direction about treatment or give tasks to trainees that exceed their competence. **Vicarious liability** pertains to the responsibilities supervisors have to oversee the actions of their supervisees. Supervisors are liable for the actions of their supervisees due to their professional relationship with supervisees. From both a legal and an ethical standpoint, trainees are not expected to assume final responsibility for clients; rather, their supervisors are legally expected to carry the decision-making responsibility and liability.

Polychronis and Brown (2016) broaden the concept of vicarious liability by addressing the legal doctrine of strict liability as it applies to clinical supervision. The doctrine of **strict liability** holds clinical supervisors responsible for supervisees' actions in a professional realm without any need to establish that supervisors were negligent or careless. "What is problematic about the strict liability standard is that it holds clinical supervisors responsible for unforeseeable and professionally indefensible actions of supervisees even if deliberately concealed from supervisory oversight" (p. 141). Even supervisors who provide exemplary supervision may bear legal responsibility for any wrong caused by a supervisee. This level of liability may contribute to the reluctance of some professionals to become supervisors. Supervisors who practice in jurisdictions that apply the strict liability standard to clinical supervision are especially vulnerable and need to engage in vigorous risk management strategies to protect themselves.

Corey and colleagues (2010) recommend an organized approach to managing the multiple tasks in the supervisory process. They identify the following risk management practices for supervisors:

- Don't supervise beyond your competence.
- Evaluate and monitor supervisees' competence.
- Be available for supervision consistently.
- Formulate a sound supervision contract.
- Maintain written policies.
- Document all supervisory activities.
- Consult with appropriate professionals.
- Maintain a working knowledge of ethics codes, legal statutes, and licensing regulations.

- Use multiple methods of supervision.
- Have a feedback and evaluation plan.
- Verify that your professional liability insurance covers you for supervision.
- Evaluate and screen all clients under your supervisee's care.
- Establish a policy for ensuring confidentiality.
- Incorporate informed consent in practice.

Supervisors rely on their supervisees to provide clear and truthful reporting of client progress and associated clinical issues. Just as therapists are vulnerable to clients who may decide to press forward with malpractice actions, supervisors are open to malpractice litigation against them by the supervisees' clients. Documentation of supervisory activity is of the utmost importance; if a supervisor is involved in a legal action, accurate documentation is necessary for a supervisor's defense. The APA (2015) guidelines state: "Supervisors maintain accurate and timely documentation of supervisee performance related to expectations for competency and professional development" (Guideline 5.). Supervisors should practice risk management in supervision much as they would in working with their own counseling clients.

Ethical Issues for Online Supervision

Few would argue that the recent proliferation of technology has truly changed the way people interact and communicate with each other. It may come as no surprise that the field of clinical supervision has been affected by these technological advances and trends as well. The number of technological innovations being used in clinical supervision has exploded in the past decade. Due to an international movement toward integrating technology into clinical supervision around the world, Renfro-Michel, Rousmaniere, and Spinella (2016) find that supervisors are independently experimenting with using technology to improve the breadth and depth of services offered to supervisees and clients. As cybersupervision and the use of electronic media in supervision have become more prevalent, ethical issues regarding confidentiality, informed consent, and the supervisory relationship have taken on added dimensions. A number of authors have addressed these issues in counseling and supervision (Barros-Bailey & Saunders, 2010; Chapman, Baker, Nassar-McMillan, & Gerler, 2011; Glosoff et al., 2016; Gordon & Luke, 2012; Haberstroh & Duffey, 2016; McAdams & Wyatt, 2010; Renfro-Michel et al., 2016; Rousmaniere, Abbass, & Frederickson, 2014).

Confidentiality in online supervision is fraught with potential problems such as the possibility of people hacking into confidential communications between a supervisor and supervisee and the risk of confidential content being sent to others in error. Although safeguards are often in place to secure electronic exchanges, such as encryption software or virtual private networks (VPNs), it cannot be assumed that the technology is foolproof and that confidentiality can be absolutely guaranteed. "Technology experts warn that even encryption-protected telecommunications systems remain highly vulnerable to intrusion and that cybertheft has reached epidemic proportions" (McAdams & Wyatt, 2010, p. 180). Therapists or trainees who are working with a supervisor online must clearly convey to clients the potential for inadvertent breaches of confidentiality. Despite ongoing philosophical debates about the legitimacy of technology-assisted practices in the field of counseling and clinical supervision, McAdams and Wyatt (2010) recognize that these new technologies are inexorably tied to the future of the counseling profession. As Rousmaniere and colleagues (2014) point out, "making the assumption that the 'old methods are best' may do the field a disservice by blinding us to new opportunities and alienating a younger generation of supervisees who identify with technology being integrated into every part of their lives" (p. 1092).

Haberstroh and Duffey (2016) emphasize that effective supervision involves supervisors and supervisees mutually integrating feedback and working through conflict. The maturity of both supervisees and supervisors has a great deal to do with the quality of the supervisory relationship and the success of the supervision experience. Haberstroh and Duffey believe that distance technologies can facilitate effective supervisory relationships: "When supervisors establish clear guidelines for distance communication, seek to be honest and compassionate, and take risks, supervisees who are invested in the process can certainly benefit from supervisory relationships at a distance" (p. 99).

LO8

Special Issues in Supervision for School Counselors

Faced with increasing threats of violence on school campuses and achievement gap issues that disproportionally affect students from low socioeconomic backgrounds, today's school counselors have a greater responsibility than ever before to meet the academic, social, and emotional needs of children and adolescents. As Wood and Rayle (2006) have observed, existing clinical/mental health models of supervision fail to meet the needs of school counseling trainees because these models do not address all of the tasks required of school counselors, which include leadership and advocacy. Schools must carefully examine ways to develop effective clinical supervision programs. Many school systems hire administrators to serve as the supervisors for school counselors; however, these administrators have no counseling background. Clinical supervisors for school counselors should be appropriately trained as both clinicians and clinical supervisors.

An excellent way to build supervision opportunities in school settings is to establish community linkages between local schools and university faculty. Faculty in counselor preparation programs are in a good position to advise and educate school counselors on innovations in counseling that can be applied to schools. Swank and Tyson (2012) point out that counselor education programs are well placed to help school systems understand the difference between supervision and evaluation. These programs explain how supervision can enhance the professional development, identity, and competency of both the school counseling supervisee as a prospective candidate for employment and the practicing school counselor as a site supervisor.

Few school counselors have received formal preparation in supervision, and web-based supervision training modules are now being designed to inform those functioning as on-site supervisors (Swank & Tyson, 2012). Even in cases where the clinical supervisor is appropriately prepared, he or she may not work in the same site as the counselor being supervised. This situation does not allow for direct observation of the counselor's performance. Most schools have only one counselor, or even a part-time counselor, which raises the issue of how realistic it is to hire a counseling supervisor.

School counselors generally do not choose their clinical supervisors. From a legal vantage point, it is unlikely that school counselors would be held accountable if a supervisor were to inappropriately disclose information about school-age children to teachers or administrators. However, in such situations school counselors have an ethical responsibility to address concerns they have about their supervisor's actions. If a supervisor has evaluative authority with counselors, this can place these counselors in a vulnerable position.

Boundary issues in the supervisory relationship need to be considered. An example of a multiple relationship might involve the clinical supervisor also serving as the administrative supervisor for the school counselor. Another boundary issue pertains to including a discussion of the supervisee's personal concerns in the supervisory sessions. At times it may be necessary to address a supervisee's personal life, especially if these concerns are having an impact on his or her ability to work effectively with clients. When helping the supervisee to identify and understand how personal issues may be interfering with effectively delivering services, the challenge is to maintain appropriate boundaries so that the supervisory relationship does not become a therapy relationship.

LO9

Multicultural and Diversity Issues in Supervision

Multicultural and diversity competence is an ethical imperative in clinical supervision (APA, 2015; Falender, Shafranske, & Falicov, 2014). A lack of diversity competence is likely to result in ineffective supervision (Falender, Shafranske, & Ofek, 2014). Diversity competence is an inseparable and basic component of supervision and involves relevant knowledge, skills, and values/attitudes (APA, 2015). Supervisors should include cultural and advocacy competencies in the supervisory contract and intentionally address these topics throughout the supervisory process. Furthermore, supervisors should encourage supervisees to infuse diversity and advocacy considerations in their work with clients (ACES, 2011). Barnett (as cited in Barnett, Cornish, et al., 2007) makes three key points:

- Attention to diversity issues in the supervision process is critically important.
- Effective supervisors are aware of their impact on the attitudes and beliefs of supervisees; they use the supervisory relationship to promote attention to, and respect for, the range of diversity of those they serve.
- Supervisors strive to increase their supervisees' awareness of how diversity is a factor with all their clients; diversity concerns become a major focus of discussion in the supervision sessions.

Multicultural supervision encompasses the full range of cultural factors, including race, ethnicity, socioeconomic status, ability status, privilege, sexual orientation, spirituality and religion, values, gender, family characteristics and dynamics, country of origin, language, and age (ACES, 2011). Supervisors have an ethical responsibility to become aware of the complexities of a multicultural society (see Chapter 4). Ethical and competent supervision involves recognizing and addressing the salient issues that apply to multicultural supervision. Supervision involves an inherent power differential, and supervisors need to address power and privilege issues with supervisees. A supervisor's lack of awareness of the power, privilege, diversity issues, and multiple identities that operate in the supervisory relationship is likely to negatively influence the supervisory process (Falender, Shafranske, & Falicov, 2014).

Ancis and Marshall (2010) found that discussing and attending to cultural variables in the supervisory relationship results in a higher degree of satisfaction with supervision and an enhanced working alliance between supervisor and supervisee. If supervisors include multicultural issues in supervision sessions, Ancis and Marshall contend that trainees will have a basis from which to develop multicultural competence. Furthermore, supervisees tend to view such discussions as having a positive influence on their work with clients. The modeling of a supervisor is one of the best ways to give supervisees an appreciation for attending to cultural variables in their work with clients.

Supervisors need to ensure that all assessments, diagnostic formulations, counseling interventions, and the supervisory process itself are sensitive to the range of diversity that supervisees may encounter (Barnett & Johnson, 2015). In this section we take a closer look at some of these issues as they relate to supervision.

Racial and Ethnic Issues

There is a price to be paid for ignoring racial and ethnic factors in supervision. If supervisors do not assist supervisees in addressing racial and ethnic issues, their clients may be denied the opportunity to explore these issues in their therapy. The supervisor's recognition of racial issues can serve as a model for supervisees in their counseling relationships. Reflecting on racial interactions in supervision offers a cognitive framework for supervisees to be inclusive in their counseling practices.

When supervisors are working with trainees from a different ethnic or cultural background, it is important for supervisors to acquire knowledge and skills in culturally congruent methods and styles of supervision. Supervisors must use culturally appropriate modes of social interaction, and they need to recognize how their position of authority is likely to play out in the supervisory relationship.

Multicultural Competence in Supervision Westefeld (2009) urges supervisors to be concerned with multicultural competence in the supervisory process. He encourages supervisors to directly address multicultural issues as a way to help trainees achieve true multicultural competence in their professional practice. It is a mistake to assume that students will learn the skills they need in the single diversity course. Supervisors should integrate sensitivity to and understanding of diversity issues in all of their supervisory sessions and in all training activities.

To develop the knowledge and skills to work effectively in multicultural counseling situations, trainees need to understand their own level of racial and cultural identity. Furthermore, they need to recognize how their attitudes and behaviors affect their clients. Good supervision will enable trainees to explore the impact that diversity issues may have on their counseling style. Ancis and Marshall (2010) found that counselor trainees were more likely to engage in self-disclosure and discussion about their cultural background and values when their supervisors took the lead in being open and genuine in sharing something of their own cultural background, experiences, and biases. Being open, accepting, and flexible fosters a positive relationship with supervisees. In addition, multicultural discussions in supervision positively affect client outcomes.

Butler-Byrd (2010) emphasizes the importance of self-knowledge in the development of competence as multicultural counselors. In her view, self-knowledge consists of understanding one's historical and current cultural context and the numerous aspects of one's identity such as ethnicity, social location, class, gender, and ability. It also includes being cognizant of the impact one's behavior has on others and the need to change behaviors that are no longer promoting growth or healthy relationships. In helping trainees to increase their self-knowledge and develop multicultural competence, Butler-Byrd supports students' "deliberate strengths-based preparation in multicultural counseling skills and consciousness-raising around critical social justice issues" (p. 12).

All of this occurs in the context of balancing the growth and development of the supervisee with competent and ethical treatment for the client. The issues to be addressed by supervisors increase in complexity when a conflict arises between a supervisee's culturally derived learning or communication style and the need of direct intervention with a client who is in crisis. Supervisors strive to be sensitive to the individual needs of their supervisees. However, in situations of immediate crisis, client welfare and safety are primary.

Spiritual Issues in Supervision

Spirituality, which is an aspect of culture, plays an important role in the lives of some clients and supervisees. Clients are oftentimes faced with spiritual matters as they go through the various stages of life, experience loss, and have chronic pain or other disabling conditions. Supervisors must be prepared to address spirituality or religious matters important to clients or supervisees in a culturally sensitive manner; however, supervisors often receive little training in these areas, which can be problematic. As noted by Shafranske (2016), "agreement with the client's spiritual worldview is not required to appreciate the role it serves; however, cultural humility is necessary to be receptive to client perspectives that are in variance with the supervisee's beliefs and ontological commitments" (p. 19). Supervisors must be mindful of their own spiritual or religious beliefs and values to ensure that they do not impose them on either supervisees or clients. It is an ethical imperative that mental health professionals be well prepared to understand, honor, and address spirituality and religious diversity.

Gender Issues in Supervision

Gender bias of supervisees and the supervisor is often overlooked. Differences in culture, ethnicity, religion, age, gender, and sexual orientation could have a negative influence on the supervisory relationship if not understood and integrated (Russell-Chapin & Chapin, 2012).

Implications of Feminist Supervision Theory With Male Supervisees
MacKinnon, Bhatia, Sunderani, Affleck, and Smith (2011) write about the intersection of feminist supervision theory and masculine psychology and state that supervisors need to open a dialogue regarding the impact of gender on the supervision process. More specifically, MacKinnon and colleagues believe supervisors who lack awareness of masculine psychology are at risk of providing ineffective supervision with male supervisees, which can have detrimental effects on their professional development. Many men place a high value on personal achievement and individual success, and during supervision discussions male supervisees are likely to focus on cases in which they are succeeding. This tendency may deprive male supervisees of the opportunity to explore the ways they may be struggling with clients. Thinking that they are surrendering their power, male supervisees may not be willing to engage in a conversation with their supervisor on clinical and relationship issues and may be unreceptive to feedback from the supervisor.

These principles and ideas apply equally with female supervisees. All supervisees should feel that it is appropriate for them to raise any concerns they have about gender differences in the supervisory relationship, issues of power, and how their gender-role socialization influences their ability to get fully involved in the supervision process. Regardless of the model a supervisor operates from, it is important to make the supervision relationship safe so trainees can gain the maximum benefit from clinical supervision. One way to create this safety is for supervisors to take the initiative in discussing gender issues that are operating in the supervisor–supervisee relationship.

Multiple Roles and Relationships in the Supervisory Process

The ACES (2011) "Best Practices in Clinical Supervision" state that clinical supervisors are expected to possess the personal and professional maturity to play multiple roles. **Multiple-role relationships in supervision** occur when a supervisor has concurrent or consecutive professional or nonprofessional relationships with a supervisee in addition to the supervisor–supervisee relationship. For example, your supervisor may be a clinician at your training site and also hold an administrative or leadership position wherein she or he makes employment decisions. The AMHCA (2015) ethical standard cautions supervisors to "avoid all dual relationships that may interfere with the supervisor's professional judgment or exploit the supervisee" (III.B.2.i.). The AAMFT (2015) code addresses exploitation: "Therapists, therefore, make every effort to avoid conditions and multiple relationships that could impair professional objectivity or increase the risk of exploitation" (IV.4.1.).

Multiple roles and relationships are common in clinical supervision; some may be unavoidable and most can be beneficial (Falender, 2017). However, these relationships also have the potential to be problematic, and it is the ethical responsibility of supervisors to carefully manage these relationships so they do not result in harm to or exploitation of supervisees. It is critical for supervisors to possess both the personal and professional maturity to serve as effective role models in establishing and maintaining appropriate boundaries (Austin, Austin, Muratori, & Corey, 2017). Both faculty and supervisors play critical roles in helping counselor trainees understand how to balance multiple roles and manage multiple relationships. Dickens, Ebrahim, and Herlihy (2016) investigated doctoral students' experiences with multiple roles and relationships. All the doctoral students in their study acknowledged that multiple roles and relationships are an inevitable part of counselor education. Participants recognized both positive and negative effects of multiple roles and relationships on personal and professional levels. Many participants reported struggling with role confusion and emphasized a desire for ongoing, open conversations with faculty members. This study underscores the importance of faculty and supervisors providing clarity *before* students are asked or required to engage in multiple roles and relationships.

Barnett and Johnson (2015) believe going too far in avoiding all nonprofessional relationships (multiple relationships) may limit opportunities for appropriate relationships with supervisees and students. Kozlowski, Pruitt, DeWalt, and Knox (2014) claim that supervisors who maintain rigid boundaries run the risk of depriving their trainees of deeper mentoring relationships as well as authentic emotional relationships that can assist supervisees in learning how to provide therapy. Although measures must be taken to avoid role confusion, some positive boundary crossings (PBC) can enhance the supervisory relationship (Kozlowski et al., 2014). One study showed that supervisees who experienced a PBC within the context of the supervisory relationship felt increased comfort and camaraderie and felt understood and cared for (Kozlowski et al., 2014). The participants of this study also reported that the PBC enhanced their training.

Supervisors need to clarify their roles and to distinguish between flexible and rigid boundaries. If the supervisor does not maintain objectivity, the supervisee will not be able to make maximum use of the process. As Herlihy and Corey (2015b) point out, unless the nature of the supervisory relationship is clearly defined, both the supervisor and the supervisee may find themselves in a difficult situation at some point in their relationship. The core issue of multiple-role relationships in the training and supervisory process is the potential for abuse of power. Like therapy clients, students and supervisees are in a vulnerable position and can be harmed by an educator or supervisor who exploits them, misuses power, or crosses appropriate boundaries. Both feminist supervision and multicultural supervision pay attention to the power dynamic in the supervisory relationship and try to reduce its impact. For example, instead of the supervisor telling supervisees what to do, the supervisor can help supervisees think about their clients in new ways, formulate their own interpretations, and devise their own interventions.

Sexual Intimacies During Professional Training

In their national survey on sexual intimacy in counselor education and supervision, Miller and Larrabee (1995) found that counseling professionals who were sexually involved with a supervisor or an educator during their training later viewed these experiences as being more coercive and more harmful to a working relationship than they did at the time the actual sexual involvement occurred. Perceptual changes took place over time with respect to how students were affected by becoming sexually involved with people who were training them, which raises questions about their willingness to freely consent to such relationships and how prepared they were to deal with the ethics of such intimacies. Moreover, it seems clear that educators and supervisors have professional power and authority long after direct training ends.

When supervisees first begin counseling, they are typically naive and uninformed with respect to the complexities of therapy. They frequently regard their supervisors as experts, and their dependence on their supervisors may make it difficult to resist sexual advances. Supervisees may disclose personal concerns and intense emotions during supervision, much as they might in a therapeutic situation. The openness of supervisees and the trust they place in their supervisors can be exploited by supervisors who choose to satisfy their own psychological or sexual needs at the expense of their supervisees. If the supervisory relationship evolves into a romantic one, the supervisory process will be ineffective, and sooner or later the supervisee will likely allege exploitation.

McMurtery, Webb, and Arnold (2011) examined the perceptions and attitudes of intimate behaviors in clinical supervision among licensed professionals in three fields: counselors, social workers, and psychologists. Although none of the participants in this self-report study admitted to engaging in a sexual relationship with a supervisee or supervisor during the supervisory relationship, a few respondents endorsed high-risk behaviors that could potentially lead down the slippery slope to sexual behavior. Engaging in sexual behavior with students and supervisees is contrary to the ethics codes of the various professional organizations and educational institutions (see the Ethics Codes box titled "Sexual Relations Are Prohibited Between Supervisor and Trainee").

ETHICS CODES: Sexual Relations are Prohibited Between Supervisor and Trainee

---

American Counseling Association (2014)
Sexual or romantic interactions or relationships with current supervisees are prohibited. This prohibition applies to both in person and electronic interactions or relationships. (F.3.b.)

Commission on Rehabilitation Counselor Certification (2010)
Rehabilitation counselors do not engage in sexual or romantic interactions or relationships with current supervisees or trainees. (H.3.b.)

American Association for Marriage and Family Therapy (2015)

Marriage and family therapists do not engage in sexual intimacy with students or supervisees during the evaluative or training relationship between the therapist and student or supervisee. (4.3.)

American Mental Health Counselors Association (2015)

All forms of sexual behavior with supervisees, students, or employees are unethical. (III.A.3.)

American Psychological Association (2010)

Psychologists do not engage in sexual relationships with students or supervisees who are in their department, agency, or training center or over whom psychologists have or are likely to have evaluative authority. (7.07.)

The American Psychiatric Association (2013b)

Sexual involvement between a faculty member or supervisor and a trainee or student, in those situations in which an abuse of power can occur, often takes advantage of inequalities in the working relationship and may be unethical because:

a. Any treatment of a patient being supervised may be deleteriously affected.

b. It may damage the trust relationship between teacher and student.

c. Teachers are important professional role models for their trainees and affect their trainees' future professional behavior. (4.14.)

Not only is sexual behavior in the supervisory relationship against the ethics codes, but it also creates a climate in which the supervisee can justify breaches in his or her own actions with clients or future supervisees. Just as counselors are prohibited from crossing sexual boundaries with their clients, supervisors must model appropriate behaviors and boundaries with their supervisees. Supervisors are in a position of power, and acting on sexual attractions with supervisees can lead to a multitude of negative outcomes for the supervisee, both personally and professionally. Supervisory relationships have qualities in common with instructor–student and therapist–client relationships. In all of these professional relationships, it is the professional who occupies the position of power. Thus, it is the professional's responsibility to establish and maintain appropriate boundaries and to explore with the trainee (student, supervisee, or client) ways to prevent potential problems associated with boundary issues. If problems do arise, the professional has the responsibility to take steps to resolve them in an ethical manner.

Assume that you are a trainee. During your individual supervision sessions the supervisor is frequently flirtatious with you. You get the distinct impression that your evaluations will be more favorable if you respond positively to these advances. What course of action would you take in such a situation? Is there a difference between sexual harassment and consensual sexual relationships, or are all sexual advances in unequal power relationships really a form of sexual harassment? Can there ever be consensual sex in such a situation? Explain your answers.

The Case of Augustus

Augustus meets weekly with his supervisor, Amy, for individual supervision. With only 3 weeks remaining in the semester, Augustus confesses to having a strong attraction to Amy and says he finds it difficult to maintain professional distance with her. Amy discloses that she, too, feels an attraction. But she is sensitive to the professional boundaries governing their relationship, and she tells him it would be inappropriate for them to have any other relationship until the semester ends. She lets him know that she would be open to further discussion about a dating relationship at that point. Even though he will still be in the program, Amy says that she will no longer have a supervisory role with him, nor will she be evaluating his status in the program.

- Do you think Amy handled her attraction to Augustus in the most ethical way? Explain your response.

- If you were a colleague of Amy's and heard about this situation from another student, what would you do?

- Is the fact that Amy will no longer be supervising Augustus sufficient to eliminate the imbalance of power in the relationship?

- Do you think it would be appropriate for them to date each other while Augustus is still a student in the program? What about after he graduates? Why or why not?

Commentary. We wonder how Amy's sexual attraction toward Augustus affected her supervision. We also wonder about her motivation for disclosing her attraction. In our view, it is inappropriate for therapists to disclose their sexual feelings toward clients; in a like manner, we consider it inappropriate for supervisors to reveal their sexual attraction to a supervisee, especially given that they are role models.

Amy should have sought consultation once she became aware of her attraction. Amy's willingness to initiate a romantic relationship with Augustus immediately following the current supervisory rotation is contrary to guidelines in most ethics codes, which prohibit sexual relationships between professors and trainees as long as the trainee is enrolled in the graduate program. Even after Augustus has graduated, Amy will have to show that the relationship is not exploitive or harmful to Augustus in any way.

This case has implications for what supervisors teach their supervisees through what they model in the supervisory sessions. Trainees need to have a safe environment in which they can discuss sexual attractions they may be having for their clients. They need to be reassured that these feelings in themselves are human and harmless but that acting on them is always inappropriate and unethical. Supervisors who model clear personal and professional boundaries can competently address sexual attraction and boundary issues with supervisees. Supervisees can be encouraged to discuss reactions they have to clients with trusted colleagues. Seeking consultation from colleagues is a good practice to begin early in one's career and to continue throughout one's professional life. •

The Case of Chun Hei

Chun Hei, a counseling psychology student, is attending graduate school in the United States to become a psychologist. Her family in Korea is proud of her for being accepted as a doctoral candidate at a prestigious American university. Being in a competitive educational environment, Chun Hei feels much pressure to do well in her program.

Chun Hei's recent interactions with her clinical supervisor have increased her feelings of anxiety. For the past few weeks, Chun Hei's supervisor, an older male faculty member who is supervising her practicum, has been making sexually inappropriate comments to her. Chun Hei has been taught to respect authority, which has left her feeling confused about how to handle her supervisor's comments. At first Chun Hei appreciated the attention she was receiving. She thought her supervisor liked her and was pleased with the progress she was making in developing her clinical skills. Because she comes from a different culture, Chun Hei wonders if she may be misinterpreting her supervisor's behavior. However, as her supervisor's comments became more overt and sexually explicit, she became very uncomfortable. Chun Hei wonders what her options are for dealing with this situation. She is afraid of jeopardizing her status as a graduate student in the program, and yet she is becoming aware that her supervisor is being inappropriate and is crossing some ethical boundaries.

- If you were in Chun Hei's position, how would you handle this situation?
- What might the consequences be if Chun Hei decides to report being sexually harassed by her supervisor?
- If Chun Hei decides to take no action at all, what consequences might result from her decision?
- If you were enrolled in the same practicum as Chun Hei and witnessed the supervisor making sexually inappropriate comments to her, what would you be inclined to do? As a bystander and a peer, what are your ethical responsibilities?

Commentary. Without question, this doctoral student is faced with a difficult decision. Chun Hei is forced to deal with the pain of being betrayed by someone she should be able to trust and respect. She is in training to learn how to create a safe space for clients' personal self-explorations, and the person who is supposed to be her mentor and role model is teaching her through his actions that he cannot be trusted. Chun Hei is left confused and disenchanted as a result of the unethical behavior of her supervisor.

Our concern is that out of fear of retribution Chun Hei may be inclined to tolerate this abusive behavior and say nothing about being sexually harassed. Once again, the power differential between supervisor and supervisee is a critical factor.

Our hope is that Chun Hei will reach out to people she considers safe and with whom she has established a trusting relationship. It is important that Chun Hei feel empowered to reach a decision about how to respond without feeling pressured. If Chun Hei decides to report her supervisor, with help, she can devise a plan for reporting him and for dealing with the potential repercussions she fears. •

Ethical Issues in Combining Supervision and Counseling

Supervisors play multiple roles in the supervision process, and the boundaries between therapy and supervision are not always clear. In the literature on supervision, there seems to be basic agreement that the supervision process should concentrate on the supervisee's professional development rather than on personal concerns and that supervision and counseling have different purposes. However, there is a lack of consensus and clarity about the degree to which supervisors can ethically deal with the personal issues of supervisees. Supervisory relationships are a complex blend of professional, educational, and therapeutic aspects. This process can become increasingly complicated when supervisors are involved in certain multiple roles with trainees. It is the supervisor's responsibility to help trainees identify how their personal dynamics are likely to influence their work with clients, yet it is not the proper role of supervisors to serve as personal counselors for supervisees. Supervisors play a key role in modeling the personal factors (beliefs, attitudes, life experiences, personality and interpersonal styles, and countertransference) that can affect a supervisee's professional practice. Developing awareness of these personal factors should be included in the supervision contract (Falender & Shafranske, 2014), and exploring supervisee's personal reactivity, or countertransference, should focus on the impact that has for engagement with the client (Shafranske & Falender, 2016).

In general, supervision should address trainees' personal dynamics to bring to their awareness any limitations or unresolved problems that could negatively affect their working relationships with clients. It is inappropriate to turn supervisory sessions into therapy sessions, but the supervisory process can be *therapeutic* in the sense that supervision involves dealing with supervisees' personal limitations so that clients are not harmed (Austin et al., 2017). Supervision could involve assisting the supervisee in identifying personal factors so that these concerns do not become the client's problem. The purpose is to facilitate the trainee's ability to work successfully with clients. When personal concerns, such as countertransference reactions, are discussed in supervision, the goal is to reinforce a supervisee's efforts to bring countertransference into awareness, not to solve the trainee's problem. A more in-depth exploration of the dynamics of countertransference is called for in personal therapy, which is beyond the scope of supervision. If the trainee needs or wants personal therapy to explore the dynamics of countertransference, the best course for a supervisor to follow is to make a referral to another professional. The supervisor also may want to normalize this process and explain that this can be common for beginning counselors. We now consider two specific cases.

The Case of Hartley

During a supervision hour, Hartley confides to his supervisor that his 5-year personal relationship has just ended and that he is in a great deal of pain. As he describes in some detail what happened, he becomes very emotional. Hartley expresses his concern about his ability to work with clients, especially those who are struggling with relationships. Here are four options for dealing with Hartley's concerns during supervision:

Supervisor A: I'm sorry you're hurting, but I feel the need to use this time to help you work with your clients. I can see no way for you to refer your clients at this point without serious repercussions for them.

Supervisor B: [*After listening to Hartley for some time and acknowledging his pain*] I know it is difficult for you to work with your clients. I know you are in therapy, and I encourage you to consider increasing the frequency of your sessions to give yourself an opportunity to deal with your own pain.

Supervisor C: That must be very painful. Do you want to talk about it? What is going on with you interferes with your ability to be present with clients, so I think it is essential that we work with your pain. [*The more the supervisor works with Hartley, the more they tap into other problems in his life. Three weeks later the supervision time still involves Hartley's hurt and crisis.*]

Supervisor D: You are obviously very affected by the changes in your life. I am glad that you can see how this may affect your work with clients. Can we spend a little time discussing how your experience may affect your dealings with clients? What specifically are you afraid may happen with you when helping clients with similar problems?

- Which of the four responses comes closest to your own, and why?
- How might you have responded to Hartley?
- Do you think any of these four responses crossed the boundary between supervision and personal therapy? Explain.

Commentary. All of the supervisors acknowledge Hartley's struggle, yet their strategies differ with respect to how they address his emotional pain in supervision. Supervisor B is not replacing supervision with therapy, but he is making sure that Hartley is working on his problems in his personal therapy. Supervisor D is allowing some time in supervision to explore how Hartley's struggle is likely to affect his clinical work, without converting supervision into therapy. We are inclined to attend to Hartley's pain, without exploring the historical roots of his problem. The supervisor in this case should continue to carefully monitor Hartley's clinical work during supervision and take appropriate action should Hartley's emotional state begin to affect his ability to work with his clients effectively.

All of us are likely to experience personal problems and crisis situations from time to time. We must be able to recognize and manage aspects of our personal life so that these problems do not influence our ability to work effectively with clients. Although trainees may experience personal problems such as a relationship breakup, it is incumbent on them to seek resources to help them effectively cope with such personal difficulties. Having problems is not the problem; not dealing with our problems is the problem.

The Case of Greta

Ken is a practicing therapist as well as a part-time supervisor in a counseling program. One of his supervisees, Greta, finds herself in a personal crisis after she learns that her mother has been diagnosed with terminal cancer. Much of her internship placement involves working with hospice patients. She approaches Ken and lets him know that she feels unable to continue doing this work. He is impressed with her therapeutic skills and thinks it would be most unfortunate for her to interrupt her education at this point. He also assumes that he can more effectively deal with her personal crisis because of their trusting relationship. For the next four supervision sessions, Ken focuses almost exclusively on Greta's personal problems. As a result of his help, Greta recovers her stability and is able to continue working with the hospice patients, with no apparent adverse effects for either them or her.

- What are your thoughts on the problem and the solution Ken chose? Explain.
- What are your reactions to Ken blending the roles of supervisor and counselor?
- What potential ethical issues, if any, would you see if Ken had recommended that Greta temporarily discontinue her field placement and enter therapy with him in his private practice?
- If Ken recommended that Greta see another therapist for her personal therapy but she refused on the ground that he knew her best, would that make a difference?
- Do you see another way of dealing with this situation?
- Is it ever appropriate for supervisors to blend the roles of supervisor and therapist? Why or why not?

Commentary. Attending to the personal dynamics of trainees is a necessary part of supervision, and addressing countertransference is one of the central tasks of supervision. Greta is vulnerable to countertransference if she continues to see her clients at this time. If countertransference is not recognized and not managed, it will have a negative impact on both therapeutic and supervisory relationships. The exploration of countertransference is best accomplished on the foundation of a well-established supervisory relationship in which consideration of personal factors is encouraged and modeled by the supervisor. The counselor should attend to the pain that is triggered by Greta's work but not explore unfinished business Greta might have with her mother. Supervision typically focuses on the here and now. Past concerns are more appropriately explored in personal therapy.

Supervision sessions are generally time limited and often need to cover administrative, legal, ethical, and clinical issues. These time constraints pose a challenge for supervisors who are asked to deal with personal concerns that supervisees may want to address. Although Ken decided to flex the customary time boundary for a few sessions to help Greta address her personal crisis, he did so without neglecting supervision of her work. In our view, Ken could also have encouraged Greta to pursue personal therapy to more fully address her personal crisis. •

Educators and Supervisors Who Counsel Students

Many ethics codes address the inadvisability of educators and supervisors offering their services as therapists to current students and supervisees. For example, the AMHCA (2015) code states: "Mental health counselors do not engage in ongoing counseling relationships with current supervisees, students, or employees" (III.A.2.). The ACA (2014) code states: "Counselor educators do not serve as counselors to current students enrolled in a counseling or related program over whom they have power and authority" (F.10.e.). Although the practice of faculty members' providing counseling for current students for a fee is unethical, some situations are not so clear-cut. Once students complete a program, for example, what are the ethics of a psychology professor taking them on as clients? Can it still be argued that the prior role as educator might negatively affect the current role as therapist? If the former student and the professor/therapist agree that there are no problems, is a therapeutic relationship ethically justified? To clarify your position on this issue, reflect on the following two cases.

The Case of Brent

A psychology professor, Hilda, teaches counseling classes, supervises interns, and provides individual therapy at the university counseling center. One of her graduate students, Brent, approaches her with a request for personal counseling. Even though she tells him of her concern over combining roles, he is persuasive and adds that he trusts her and sees no problem in being both her student and her counselee.

- What are your reactions to this request?

- What issues, if any, ethical or otherwise, do you see in this case?

- Would it make a difference if Brent had approached her for counseling after he had completed the course with her?

- Would the situation take on a different dimension if the professor had a private practice and charged Brent a fee for her service?

- Assume that Hilda was leading a therapy group during the semester and that Brent wanted to join the group. Is being a client in a group different from being an individual client?

- Do you see any potential for exploitation in this case?

- Would it make a difference if there was a lack of availability of other counseling resources in the area?

Commentary. The code of ethics of both the ACA (2014) and the APA (2010) clearly state that educators, or those who have an evaluative role, do not serve as counselors to current students or supervisees, unless this is a brief role associated with a training experience. Regardless of how persuasive a student or supervisee is about requesting personal therapy from an educator or supervisor, it is the professional's responsibility to avoid surrendering to this pressure. In Brent's case, the professor would be acting unethically if she agreed to provide personal counseling for Brent. •

The Case of Laura

Laura, a master's level graduate student in a counseling program, has completed a "Social and Cultural Foundations of Counseling" course that was very personal and required a lot of self-reflection and journaling. During this course, she had the opportunity to listen to and talk with two lesbian women who had been living in an open, committed relationship for 15 years. In meeting these people, she decided it was time for her to "come out" too. She started with a close friend who had known her all her life, but it did not go well. Her friend was shocked and very disapproving, and they have not talked to each other since the disclosure. She is also wondering whether she should now tell her parents because she is afraid her former friend will say something to someone in the small town in which they live, and it will get back to her parents anyway.

Laura is now failing her "Methods of Research" course because she has missed a lot of classes struggling with this issue. She needs more time and help to catch up, but her instructor is unsympathetic. She does not want to tell him what is going on for fear of his reaction. Laura has been confiding in one professor, a licensed professional counselor, who is both a supervisor of her practicum and an instructor in her courses. The professor acknowledges what a difficult decision Laura is facing with regard to telling her parents and others, and the professor lets Laura know that she is available to talk to her any time the student needs a friendly ear. She also tells Laura about a lesbian counselor who has a private practice in the area. Laura is not ready to see someone she does not know, and she is reluctant to be seen going to a counselor who is known to be gay or lesbian.

The professor does nothing to persuade her differently and reminds Laura that she is available at any time. She also inquires whether Laura would like her to talk to the "Methods of Research" instructor—without disclosing more than the fact that the student is having a hard time right now and could use some help and understanding. Laura accepts this offer.

- Do you approve or disapprove of how the professor worked with Laura?
- What are the multiple relationship issues involved here, and how would you resolve them?
- Do you think the professor/counselor was engaged in appropriate social activism or in boundary violations?
- What ethical issues are raised in this case?
- If Laura were your student, how would you have dealt with this situation?

Commentary. When supervisees require personal counseling, supervisors should provide appropriate referrals. We like how the professor in Laura's case offered empathy, support, and practical assistance without agreeing to engage Laura as a client or otherwise blur the professor–student relationship in a way that could be harmful. It is up to counselor educators and supervisors to provide a rationale to students or supervisees when it is necessary that they seek personal therapy outside of the teaching or supervisory relationship and to assist them in finding an appropriate referral. •

Chapter Summary

Counselors are often asked to assume the role of a supervisor. It is clear that special training is needed to effectively perform the many supervisory functions required in these activities. Some of the key ethical issues associated with supervision involve carrying out professional roles and responsibilities, maintaining clear boundaries between roles, and avoiding the problems created by dual or multiple relationships.

Supervision is one way in which trainees learn how to apply their knowledge and skills to particular clinical situations. It is essential that supervisees receive regular feedback so that they have a basis for honing their skills. Effective supervision deals with the professional as a person and as a practitioner. It is not enough to focus only on the trainee's skills. The supervisory relationship is a personal process, and the supervisee's dynamics are equally important in this process. Although supervision aims at honing the skills of trainees, the welfare of the clients served by trainees is the primary consideration. Supervisors must balance protection of client welfare with the secondary responsibility of increasing competence and professional development of the supervisee (APA, 2015). Supervisors have both legal and ethical responsibilities to clients, who have a right to competent service regardless of the supervisee's level of training (Welfel, 2016).

Supervisors must not exploit students and trainees or take unfair advantage of the power differential that exists in the context of training. Managing multiple roles ethically is the responsibility of the supervisor. Supervisors have a much better chance of managing boundaries in their professional work if they are able to take care of their boundaries in their personal lives. Supervisors who are able to establish appropriate personal and professional boundaries are in a good position to teach students how to develop appropriate boundaries for themselves.

Suggested Activities

1. Role-play a situation that involves a supervisor asking supervisees to get involved in therapeutic situations that are beyond the scope of their training and experience. One student in class can play the role of a persuasive supervisor who thinks students will learn best by "jumping into the water and learning how to swim." The supervisor can ask trainees to work with a family, lead a therapy group alone, or work with abused children. After the role play, discuss the ethical and clinical issues involved with a focus on ways to deal with inadequate supervision.

2. Set up another role-playing situation. In this case, the supervisor is difficult to reach and rarely keeps his or her appointments with supervisees. One student can play the inaccessible supervisor, and several others can assume the roles of students who need to meet with their supervisor to discuss difficult cases. What are some ways of dealing with this type of supervisor?

3. Investigate some of the community agencies in your area to learn what supervision they offer to interns and to newly hired practitioners. Several students can form a panel to share the results.

4. Form an ethics committee in class to review these situations dealing with supervision:

   - A supervisor has made sexual overtures to several supervisees.
   - A supervisor is accepting supervisees as clients in his or her private practice.
   - A supervisor frequently cancels supervision sessions.
   - A supervisor appears intoxicated during supervision sessions on several occasions.

   The ethics committee can present its case in class with appropriate courses of action for each problem area.

5. In dyads or triads, explore your thoughts about the ethical issues raised in the following situations. What would be your course of action in these situations?

   - You are aware that a clinical supervisor has made it a practice to have sexual relationships with several of his supervisees. Some of these students are friends of yours, and they tell you that they felt pressure to comply because they were in a vulnerable position. What would you do?
   - Several of your friends tell you that a clinical supervisor at the university makes it a practice to date former supervisees. When colleagues confronted him in the past, he maintained that all of these trainees were adults, that none of them were his supervisees when he dated them, and that what he did in his private life was strictly his own business. What are your reactions to his behavior?
   - Imagine yourself as a supervisee in an internship placement in a community agency. Your supervisor at this agency makes inappropriate advances to you. How might you react? What would you do?
   - You determine that your supervisor is incompetent. How could you deal with this situation?
   - A supervisor has determined that a supervisee is not meeting the expectations of the training site due to not being fully truthful regarding interventions with clients, minimizing client presenting issues, and not responding to supervisory feedback. How should the supervisor best approach the supervisee with these concerns?

6. Assume that you are in a field placement as a counselor trainee in a community agency. The administrators tell you that they do not want you to inform your clients that you are a student intern. They explain that your clients might feel that they were getting second-class service if they found out that you were in training. What would you say to these administrators? Might you accept the internship assignment under the terms outlined if you could not find any other field placements?

7. Interview one or two clinical supervisors to determine what they consider to be the most pressing ethical and legal issues in the supervisory relationship. Here are some questions you might ask supervisors: What are the rights of trainees? What are the main responsibilities of supervisors? To what degree should supervisors be held accountable for the welfare of the clients who are counseled by their trainees? What kind of specialized training have they had in supervision? Who is the primary focus of supervision—the client? the trainee? What are some common problems faced by supervisors in effectively carrying out their duties?

8. What are the ethical issues involved in delivering clinical supervision online? As a trainee, what would it be like for you if you could not meet face to face with your supervisor?

9. Identify the potential ethical and legal issues raised in the following brief scenarios, and consider how you would address them:

- Your supervisor does not provide what you consider to be adequate supervision. He sometimes cancels supervision sessions. You are left mainly on your own with a difficult caseload. The staff members where you work also have overwhelming caseloads. When you do get time with your supervisor, he also seems overwhelmed with responsibilities. Thus, you do not get enough time to discuss your cases. What would you do?
- You have a conflict with your supervisor over the most ethical way to deal with a client. What would you do?
- You do not get adequate feedback on your performance as a trainee. At the end of the semester your supervisor gives you a negative evaluation. What potential ethical and legal issues might be involved? How would you deal with the situation?
- Do you think it is unethical for supervisors to initiate social or romantic relationships with trainees after they have graduated (and when the supervisors have no professional obligations to the trainees)? Explain your position.
- If during the course of your supervision you became aware that personal problems are interfering with your ability to work effectively with clients, what would be your solution to the problem?
- What are the main problems with multiple relationships in supervision? What potential problems do you see, and how might you resolve them? Do you think all such relationships in supervision should be minimized or even avoided entirely?
- What possible benefits, if any, do you see when supervisors combine a multiplicity of roles such as teacher, mentor, counselor, consultant, evaluator, and supervisor?

Ethics in Action Video Exercises

10. Reflect on all of the role-playing situations enacted in the *Ethics in Action* video. Put yourself in the place of the counselor. Would you seek input from a supervisor in any of these situations? Consider situations such as working with a pregnant teenager who urges you not to tell her parents; becoming aware of countertransference with a client; having a sharp value difference between you and your client; finding yourself attracted to a client; dealing with a client that expresses a sexual attraction to you; having difficulty establishing and maintaining boundaries with a client; considering a situation involving bartering; accepting a gift from a client. Select the one vignette in the video that you would find most challenging. A small group of students can offer you peer supervision as you play the role of a counselor struggling with a particularly difficult ethical situation. Ask another student to role-play the counselor with an ethical issue you would find challenging. Assume the role of the supervisor of this counselor. What questions would you ask of the counselor? What kinds of suggestions might you offer?

MindTap for Counseling

Go to MindTap® for an eBook, videos of client sessions, activities, practice quizzes, apps, and more—all in one place. If your instructor didn't assign MindTap, you can find out more information at CengageBrain.com.

CHAPTER

Issues in Theory and Practice

LEARNING OBJECTIVES

1. Articulate how developing a counseling style relates to ethical practice

2. Understand the ethical issues involved in using techniques

3. Grasp the ethical, clinical, and cultural issues in assessment and diagnosis

4. Describe the theoretical perspectives on assessment and diagnosis

5. Explain the arguments for diagnosis

6. Clarify the arguments against diagnosis

7. Identify ethical and legal issues in diagnosis

8. Examine cultural issues in assessment and diagnosis

9. Understand the practice of using tests in counseling

10. Comprehend the ethical issues pertaining to evidenced-based therapy practice

SELF-INVENTORY

Directions: For each statement, indicate the response that most closely identifies your beliefs and attitudes. Use the following code:

5 = I *strongly agree* with this statement.

4 = I *agree* with this statement.

3 = I am *undecided* about this statement.

2 = I *disagree* with this statement.

1 = I *strongly disagree* with this statement.

_____ 1. I would rather combine insights and techniques derived from various theoretical approaches to counseling than base my practice on a single model.

_____ 2. People are capable of and can be responsible for finding their own solutions to their problems.

_____ 3. I would find it difficult to work for an agency that expected me to perform functions I didn't think were appropriate to counseling.

_____ 4. I should have the power to define my own role and professional identity as a mental health practitioner.

_____ 5. Clients should always select the goals of counseling.

_____ 6. I would be willing to work with clients who did not seem to have any clear goals or reasons for seeking counseling.

_____ 7. Competent diagnosis is necessary for planning appropriate treatment.

_____ 8. The drawbacks associated with diagnosis in counseling outweigh the benefits.

_____ 9. Testing can be a very useful adjunct to counseling.

_____ 10. The medical model of mental health can be applied effectively in counseling and psychotherapy.

_____ 11. Skill in using a variety of techniques is one of the most important assets of a therapist.

_____ 12. Counselors should develop and modify their own theory of counseling as they practice.

_____ 13. There are major shortcomings in applying most of the contemporary counseling theories to diverse ethnic and cultural groups.

_____ 14. It is unethical for practitioners to fail to do some type of assessment and diagnosis, especially with high-risk (suicidal or dangerous) clients.

_____ 15. It is critical to take cultural factors into consideration in assessment and diagnosis if the therapist hopes to gather accurate data and come up with a valid perspective on a client.

Introduction

Ethical practice requires a solid theoretical framework. Therapists' theoretical positions and conceptual views influence how they practice. Ideally, theory helps practitioners make sense of what they hear in counseling sessions. In this chapter we address a variety of interrelated ethical issues, such as why a theory has both practical and ethical implications, the goals and techniques that are based on a theoretical orientation, the role of assessment and diagnosis in the therapeutic process, issues in psychological testing, and issues surrounding evidence-based practices (EBPs).

Clinicians must be able to conceptualize what they are doing in their counseling sessions and why they are doing it. Sometimes practitioners have difficulty explaining why they use certain counseling interventions. When you first meet a new client, for example, what guidelines would you use in putting into a theoretical perspective what clients tell you? What do you want to accomplish in this initial session? Can you explain your theoretical understanding of how people change in a clear and straightforward way? Think about how your theoretical viewpoint influences your decisions on questions such as these:

- What are your goals for counseling?
- What techniques and interventions would you use to reach your goals?
- What value do you place on evidence-based treatment techniques?
- What is the role of assessment and diagnosis in the counseling process?
- How do you make provisions for cultural diversity in your assessment and treatment plans?
- Does the client's presenting problem influence the specific assessments you choose to use?
- How does your theoretical viewpoint influence the specific assessment measures you choose to use with clients?
- How flexible are you in your approach?
- What connections do you see between theory and practice?
- Do you consult with colleagues on matters pertaining to theory and practice?

Developing a Counseling Style

Theories of counseling are based on worldviews, each with its own values, biases, and assumptions of how best to bring about change in the therapeutic process. Contemporary theories tend to be oriented toward individual change and are grounded in values that emphasize choice, the uniqueness of the individual, self-assertion, and ego strength (see Chapter 4). Many of these assumptions are inappropriate for evaluating clients from cultures that focus on interdependence, de-emphasize individuality, and emphasize being in harmony with the universe. In some cultures, basic life values tend to be associated with a focus on inner experience and an acceptance of one's environment. Within cultures that focus more on the social framework than on development of the individual, a traditional therapeutic model has limitations. In addition, it is not customary for many client populations to seek professional help, and they will typically turn first to informal systems such as family, friends, and the community.

Developing a counseling approach is more complicated than merely accepting the tenets of a given theory. Ideally, the theoretical approach you use to guide your practice is the result of intensive study, reflection, and clinical experience. Furthermore, because a theory of counseling is often an expression of the personality of the theorist and of the therapist, it is worthwhile to take a critical look at the theorist who developed it and try to understand why it appeals to you. Uncritically following any single theory can lead you to ignore some of the insights that your life and your work open up to you. This is our bias, of course, and many would contend that providing effective therapy depends on following a given theory. Ultimately, your counseling orientation and style must be appropriate for the unique needs of your clients and for the type of counseling you do. Developing an approach to counseling is an ongoing and fluid process. It is common for counselors in training to be drawn to a particular theory initially but to modify it as they gain more experience and evaluate what seems to be working or not working with their clients.

When developing or evaluating a theory, a major consideration is the degree to which that perspective helps you understand and organize what you are doing with clients. Does your framework provide a broad base for working with diverse clients in different ways, or does it restrict your vision and cause you to ignore variables that do not fit the theory? Does your theory address all types of problems? Does your theory take into consideration how cultural differences operate? It is important to evaluate what you emphasize in your counseling work. The following questions may help you make this evaluation:

- At this point in your training, how would you describe your theory?
- Do you anticipate that your theoretical approach will change as you gain clinical experience?
- What does your approach emphasize and/or de-emphasize, and why does it appeal to you?
- What are some of the techniques associated with your theoretical approach?
- To what extent does your theory address multicultural and diversity factors?
- Does your theory have research to support its effectiveness?
- Is your theory a good fit with the community standards where you practice?
- How would you present your theoretical model in your informed consent document?
- Have your life experiences caused you to modify your theoretical viewpoint in any way?
- How does your theory explain how change happens?
- Does your theory view client's problems as being more individually or more systemically based?
- How does your theory affect how power is used in sessions and in the counselor–client relationship?
- In what ways does your theory influence the way you see the roles of counselor and client?

Your assumptions about the nature of counseling and the nature of people have a direct impact on the way you practice. The goals you think are important in therapy, the techniques and methods you employ to reach these goals, the way in which you see the division of responsibility in the client–therapist relationship, your view of your role and functions as a counselor, and your view of the place of assessment and diagnosis in the therapeutic process are all largely determined by your theoretical orientation—and all of these factors have implications for ethical practice.

Practicing counseling without an explicit theoretical rationale is somewhat like trying to sail a boat without a rudder. Just as a good sailor can adjust to the movement of the wind, a good therapist goes along with the movement of the client. A theoretical orientation is not a rigid structure that prescribes specific steps of what to do in a counseling situation; rather, it is a set of general guidelines that counselors can use to make sense of what they are hearing and what needs to change. Some practitioners favor an integrative approach rather than relying on a single theoretical model (Corey, 2013a, 2017). An integrative approach is not a "catch all" style but a purposeful and intentional integration of theoretical models that resonate with you (Kristin Vincenzes, personal communication, October 14, 2016).

The Division of Responsibility in Therapy

Beginning mental health practitioners often burden themselves with too much responsibility for client outcomes. They may be critical of themselves for not knowing enough, not having the necessary skill and experience, or not being sensitive enough. Overly anxious counselors frequently fail to include clients in the therapeutic work, focusing too much on the interventions, treatment plans, and goals rather than being present with their clients during sessions (Kristin Vincenzes, personal communication, October 14, 2016).

The question of responsibility is an integral part of the initial sessions and includes involving clients in thinking about their part in their own therapy. One way to clarify the shared responsibility in a therapeutic relationship is by a **contract**, which is based on a negotiation between the client and the therapist to define the therapeutic relationship. A contract (which can be an extension of the informed consent process discussed in Chapter 5) encourages both client and therapist to specify the goals of the therapy and the methods likely to be employed in obtaining these goals. For clients who have little or no knowledge of what the counseling process involves, this discussion may be limited. Legal and ethical considerations need to be taken into account in designing the contract and the treatment plan, and this is especially true when dealing with vulnerable populations such as children, the elderly, and clients with disabilities. A contract can be written, or it may be part of an ongoing discussion between therapist and client regarding treatment goals, progress, and outcomes. Therapists who work within a managed care context need to discuss with clients how managed care will influence the division of responsibility between the health management organization (HMO), the client, and the therapist. These providers may determine what kinds of problems are acceptable for treatment, how long treatment will last, the number of sessions, and the focus of the work. Under this system, practitioners must be accountable to the managed care company by demonstrating that specific objectives have been met.

From our own perspective, therapy is a collaborative venture of the client and the therapist. Both have serious responsibilities for the direction of therapy, and this needs to be clarified from the very beginning of counseling. Lambert (2013) notes that "learning how to engage the client in a collaborative process is more central to positive outcomes than which process (theory of change) is provided" (p. 202). Most probably the therapist has the greater responsibility in the initial phase of therapy, especially in exploring the presenting problem and designing the treatment plan. In essence, the therapist has the responsibility to create the environment that allows change to take place. However, as therapy progresses, the responsibility generally shifts more to the client.

Clinicians who typically decide what to discuss and are overdirective run the risk of imposing their own views and perpetuating their clients' dependence. Clients should be encouraged to assume responsibility from the beginning of the relationship. This is especially true of the cognitive-behavioral approaches, which emphasize client-initiated contracts and homework assignments as ways in which clients can fulfill their commitment to change. These devices help to keep the focus of responsibility on clients by challenging them to decide what they want from therapy and what they are willing to do to get what they want. It also keeps the therapist more active in the process.

As you consider the range of viewpoints on the division of responsibility in therapy, think about your own position on this issue. How has your position changed over time? What are the ethical implications of taking responsibility for the direction of the therapy process?

Deciding on the Goals of Counseling

Therapy without a goal is unlikely to be effective, yet practitioners may fail to devote enough time to thinking about the goals they have for their clients and the goals clients have for themselves. The initial task of therapy is to identify a client's problems and concerns, which leads directly to establishing goals with the client. The therapist's theory will greatly influence the types of goals established as well as the methods used to reach those goals. Both the therapist and the client should clearly understand the goals of their work together and the desired outcomes of their relationship. In this section we discuss possible aims of therapy, how goals are determined, and who should determine them.

When considering therapeutic goals, it is important to keep in mind the cultural determinants of therapy. The aims of therapy may be specific to a particular culture's definition of psychological health. An effective theory considers the person-in-relation and the cultural context as essential aspects in developing appropriate goals for the helping process (see Chapter 4).

Clinicians should not impose goals, but some practitioners may persuade their clients to accept certain goals. Others are convinced that the specific aims of counseling ought to be determined entirely by their clients. Who sets the goals of counseling is best understood in light of the theory you operate from, the type of counseling you offer, the setting in which you work, the problems of the client, and the characteristics of your clients. Your theoretical orientation influences general goals, such as insight versus behavior change. If you are not clear about your general goals, your techniques and approach may be random and arbitrary.

Other factors can also affect the determination of goals. For example, if you work with clients in a managed care system, the goals will need to be highly specific, limited to reduction of problematic symptoms, and often aimed at teaching coping skills. When you work in crisis intervention, goals are likely to be short term and functional, and you may be much more directive. Working with children in a school, you may combine educational and therapeutic goals. As a counselor to the elderly in an assisted living facility, you may stress coping skills and ways of relating to others in this environment. Working with veterans, you may intertwine career counseling, psychoeducation, and therapeutic goals. What your goals are and how actively you involve your client in determining them will depend to a great extent on the type of counseling you provide and the type of client you see.

The Case of Leon

Leon, a 45-year-old aeronautical engineer, has been laid off after 20 years of employment with the same company. He lives with his partner of 10 years, and they have three children together. Leon shows signs of depression, has lost weight, and was referred to you by his primary care physician. He has had no previous history of depression, but his father committed suicide at age 50. Leon is not close to his mother or siblings and describes his relationship with his partner as lackluster at best. He expresses, without much affect, feelings of abandonment at being terminated after so many years of dedicated service. How would you assess and work with Leon if he were your client? Consider these questions:

- What specific goals would you have in mind as you develop a treatment plan for Leon?
- What theoretical approach would you use and why?
- Would your approach include a suicide assessment? Why or why not?
- Would you recommend a medical evaluation? Why or why not?
- Would you assess Leon's use of alcohol and other substances?
- Would you explore Leon's support system, and how significant would that be in setting goals? Explain.
- Would you consider bringing Leon's partner in for some couples sessions? Why or why not?
- To what degree would you involve Leon in creating goals?
- Would you consider Leon's unemployment a significant factor in this case? Would your goals include dealing with that reality?
- How would you assess the outcomes of your work with Leon? What would need to change for you to deem your work with Leon successful? In what ways could you involve Leon in assessing outcomes?

Commentary. Leon shows signs of having serious emotional problems that he is not fully expressing. Some indicators are his lackluster relationship, depression, the suicide of his father, and his lack of affect. In Leon's case, assessment is crucial to the process of identifying goals for therapy. An initial goal is to discover Leon's purpose in seeking therapy. One of our immediate goals would be to assess for possible suicidal ideation, especially because of his father's suicide. We suspect that Leon's low affect is an indicator of much unexpressed emotional pain, which we would want to pursue with him. As part of the assessment process, we would ask about his use of alcohol or other substances to gauge whether these may be contributing to or exacerbating his presenting issue. Leon was referred by his physician, so we might ask for a release of information to learn of any medical conditions that may be contributing to Leon's presenting problems. Our theoretical orientation will guide how we conceptualize Leon's case and the interventions we make with him. •

The Use of Techniques in Counseling

Your use of techniques in counseling is closely related to your theoretical model. What techniques, procedures, or intervention methods would you use, and when and why would you use them? Out of anxiety, counselors may feel pressured to try technique after technique in an indiscriminate fashion. Practitioners must have a clear understanding of the techniques they use and why they are using them. From an ethical perspective, practitioners should have a rationale for using a particular technique and have training in the interventions they use. In a legal proceeding, a counselor may be required to provide an explicit rationale and evidence-based documentation to substantiate the interventions used with a particular client.

Empirical research consistently supports the centrality of the therapeutic relationship as a primary factor contributing to the psychotherapy outcome (Angus, Watson, Elliott, Schneider, & Timulak, 2015; Cain, 2016; Crits-Christoph, Gibbons, & Mukherjee, 2013; Elkins, 2016; Lambert, 2011, 2013; Norcross, 2010). The therapeutic alliance enhances the quality of the working relationship, and this alliance is the product of the collaborative efforts of both client and therapist (Cain, 2016; Keenan & Rubin, 2016). Researchers have repeatedly confirmed that a positive alliance and a collaborative therapeutic relationship are the best predictors of a positive therapy outcome (Elkins, 2016; Keenan & Rubin, 2016; Kottler & Balkin, 2017; Miller, Hubble, Duncan, & Wampold, 2010). Practitioners would do well to pay attention to the way they interact with clients and the manner in which they participate in the therapy, providing high levels of empathy, respect, and collaboration. Lambert (2013) believes too much attention is sometimes devoted to studying techniques rather than focusing on therapists as people and their interactions with clients. The techniques counselors employ, although important, are less crucial to therapy outcomes than are the interpersonal factors operating in the client–counselor relationship.

Your techniques cannot be separated from your personality and your relationship with your client. When practitioners fall into a pattern of mechanically employing techniques, they are not responding to the particular individuals they are counseling. To avoid this pitfall, you must pay attention to the ways you use techniques. The purpose in using a technique is to facilitate movement. You may try a technique you have observed someone else using very skillfully only to find that it does not work well for you. In essence, your techniques need to fit your therapeutic style, your level of training, and the specific needs of your client. When working with culturally diverse client populations, it is clinically and ethically imperative that you use interventions that are consistent with the values of your client. With all clients, it is best to adapt your techniques to the needs of your clients rather than expecting your clients to fit your techniques.

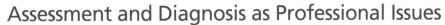

Assessment and Diagnosis as Professional Issues

Assessment and diagnosis are an integral part of the practice of mental health counseling and psychotherapy. No matter what their theoretical orientation, all competent mental health practitioners use some type of assessment to arrive at a client's diagnosis. This assessment is subject to revision as the clinician gathers further data during the therapy sessions; assessment is an ongoing part of the therapeutic process.

Assessment consists of evaluating the relevant factors in a client's life to identify themes for further exploration. **Diagnosis**, which is sometimes part of the assessment process, consists of possibly identifying a specific mental disorder based on a pattern of symptoms that leads to a specific diagnosis described in the *Diagnostic and Statistical Manual of Mental Disorders*, fifth edition (American Psychiatric Association, 2013a), the official guide to a system of classifying psychological disorders and generally referred to as the *DSM-5*. Both assessment and diagnosis are intended to provide direction for the treatment process.

Psychodiagnosis (or **psychological diagnosis**) is a general term covering the process of identifying an emotional or behavioral problem and making a statement about the current status of a client. Psychodiagnosis might also include identifying a syndrome that conforms to a diagnostic system such as the *DSM-5*. This process involves identifying possible causes of the person's emotional, cognitive, physiological, and behavioral difficulties, leading to some kind of treatment plan designed to ameliorate the identified problem. The clinician must carefully assess the client's presenting symptoms and think critically about how this particular conglomeration of symptoms impairs the client's ability to function in his or her daily life. Practitioners often use multiple tools to assist them in this process, including clinical interviewing, observation, psychometric tests, and rating scales. They also may make a referral for a medical evaluation.

Differential diagnosis is the process of distinguishing one form of mental disorder from another by determining which of two (or more) disorders with similar symptoms the person is suffering from. The *DSM-5* is the standard reference for distinguishing one form of mental disorder from another; it provides specific criteria for classifying emotional and behavioral disturbances and shows the differences among the various disorders. The *DSM-5* deals with a variety of disorders pertaining to developmental stages, learning and cognition, trauma, personality, substance abuse, moods, anxiety, sex and gender identity, eating, sleep, impulse control, and adjustment.

Some dispute that diagnosis should be part of the psychotherapeutic process; others see diagnosis as an essential step leading to a treatment plan. Some approaches stress the importance of conducting a comprehensive assessment of the client and see it as the initial step in the therapeutic process. The rationale is that specific counseling goals cannot be formulated and appropriate treatment strategies cannot be designed until a thorough picture of the client's past and present functioning is formed. Furthermore, evaluation of progress, change, improvement, or success may be difficult without an initial assessment. Those who oppose a diagnostic model claim that the *DSM* labels and stigmatizes people.

In performing psychodiagnosis of any type, it is crucial that clinicians consider cultural factors and how these may influence the client's current behaviors, feelings, thoughts, and symptom presentation. Dadlani, Overtree, and Perry-Jenkins (2012) emphasize the importance of addressing clinicians' and clients' experiences with privilege and oppression as a basic aspect of diagnostic assessment. They call for a reformulation of diagnostic assessment that puts culture at the center of the assessment process. The multicultural and social justice perspective on assessment and treatment focuses on client strengths within a cultural and historical framework. Later in this chapter we address more fully the cultural dimensions of diagnosis.

Nystul (2016) believes the clinical interview is a useful tool in the assessment and diagnostic process because it provides a structure for organizing information. The clinical interview serves many purposes, some of which are providing information on a client's presenting problems, giving glimpses of historical factors that may be contributing to the client's condition, and providing a framework for making a differential diagnosis to determine whether an individual suffers from a particular mental disorder. Because most therapy settings require a clinical interview, familiarity with this form of assessment is essential. Nystul claims that the clinical interview can be structured to suit both the counselor's theoretical orientation and the unique needs of the client.

Theoretical Perspectives on Assessment and Diagnosis

Depending on the theory from which you operate, a diagnostic framework may occupy a key role or a minimal role in your therapeutic practice. Practitioners using a cognitive-behavioral approach and the medical model may place heavy emphasis on the role of assessment as a prelude to the treatment process. Many practitioners using relationship-oriented approaches view the process of assessment and diagnosis as external to the immediacy of the client–counselor relationship. They feel that it distracts the therapist from concentrated attention on the subjective world of the client.

The developmental, multicultural, and social justice theoretical model emphasizes client strengths (Ivey, Ivey, Meyers, & Sweeney, 2005; Zalaquett et al., 2008). The individual develops within a family in a community and cultural context, and this model places greater attention on environmental and contextual issues. By establishing an egalitarian therapeutic relationship, clients can be actively involved in diagnosis and case formulation, with the goal of fostering their psychological liberation (Crethar, Torres Rivera, & Nash, 2008; Duran et al., 2008).

Understanding differences among theoretical models has relevance for ethical practice because the way in which diagnosis is practiced rests on theoretical foundations. Regardless of the particular theory espoused by a therapist, both clinical and ethical issues are associated with the use of assessment procedures and diagnosis as part of a treatment plan. Practitioners within the same theoretical model often differ with respect to the degree to which they employ a diagnostic framework in their clinical practice. The box titled "Assessment and Diagnosis and Contemporary Theories of Counseling" provides a summary of the way each model addresses assessment and diagnosis.

Assessment and Diagnosis and Contemporary Theories of Counseling

Psychoanalytic Therapy

Some psychoanalytically oriented therapists, though certainly not all, favor psychodiagnosis. This is partly due to the fact that for a long time in the United States psychoanalytic practice was largely limited to people trained in medicine.

Adlerian Therapy

Assessment is a basic part of Adlerian therapy. The initial session focuses on developing a relationship based on a deeper understanding of the individual's presenting problem. A comprehensive assessment involves examining the client's lifestyle. The therapist seeks to ascertain the faulty, self-defeating beliefs and assumptions about self, others, and life that maintain the problematic behavioral patterns the client brings to therapy.

Existential Therapy

The main purpose of existential clinical assessment is to understand the personal meanings and assumptions clients use in structuring their existence. This approach is different from the traditional diagnostic framework because it focuses on understanding the client's inner world, not on understanding the individual from an external perspective.

Person-Centered Therapy

Like existential therapists, person-centered practitioners maintain that the best vantage point for understanding another person is through his or her subjective world. They believe that traditional assessment and diagnosis are detrimental because they are external ways of understanding the client.

Gestalt Therapy

Gestalt therapists attend to interruptions in the client's here-and-now awareness and encourage clients to explore what they are experiencing in the present. The emphasis on the present moment is viewed as being more important than interpretations or any diagnosis.

Behavior Therapy

The behavioral approach begins with a comprehensive assessment of the client's present functioning, with questions directed to past learning that is related to current behavior. Practitioners with a behavioral orientation generally favor a diagnostic stance, valuing observation and other objective means of appraising both a client's specific symptoms and the factors that have led up to the client's malfunctioning. Such an appraisal, they argue, enables them to use the techniques that are appropriate for a particular disorder and to evaluate the effectiveness of the treatment program.

Cognitive-Behavioral Approaches

The assessment used in cognitive-behavioral therapy is based on getting a sense of the client's pattern of thinking using a collaborative approach. Once self-defeating beliefs have been identified, the treatment process involves examining specific thought patterns and substituting constructive ones.

continued

Reality Therapy

Reality therapists do not make use of psychological testing and traditional diagnosis. Instead, through the use of skillful questioning, the therapist helps clients make an assessment of their current behavior. This informal assessment encourages clients to focus on what they want from life and to determine whether what they are doing is working for them.

Feminist Therapy

Feminist therapists have criticized the *DSM* classification system, claiming it emphasizes the individual's symptoms and ignores the social factors that cause dysfunctional behavior. The feminist assessment process emphasizes the cultural context of clients' problems, especially the degree to which clients possess power or are oppressed. They contend that as traditionally practiced, diagnostic systems such as the *DSM* reflect the dominant culture's definitions of psychology and health. Misdiagnosis and blaming the victim may occur when sociopolitical factors are minimized or ignored.

Postmodern Approaches

Solution-focused brief therapy and narrative therapy are two examples of postmodern therapies that do not emphasize formal diagnosis or categorization of individuals. Postmodern approaches do not highlight a client's deficits, problems, failures, and what is wrong with people. Instead, emphasis is placed on an individual's competencies, accomplishments, skills, strengths, and successes. The therapist's assessment and provisional diagnosis are generally arrived at by collaborative conversations with a client.

Systemic Therapies

Family systems therapists believe that many symptoms stem from problems within the system, rather than originating in the individual. In most systemic approaches, both therapist and client are involved in the assessment process. Some systemic therapists assist clients in tracing the key events of their family history and identifying issues in their family of origin. As a part of the assessment process, individuals may be asked to identify what they learned from interacting with their parents, from observing their parents' interactions with each other, and from observing how each parent interacted with each sibling.

Source: *Case Approach to Counseling and Psychotherapy* (Corey, 2013b).

DSM-5 Assessment

Although you may not yet have had to face the practical task of diagnosing a client, you will need to come to terms with this reality at some point in your work. Many state licensing boards require applicants to demonstrate competence in the use of diagnostic tools including the *DSM-5*. Regardless of your theoretical orientation, you will most likely be expected to work within the *DSM* framework if you are practicing in a community mental health agency or in any other agency in which insurance companies pay for client services. Because you will need to think within the framework of assessing and diagnosing clients, it is important that you become familiar with the diagnostic categories and the structure of the

DSM-5. The Council for Accreditation of Counseling and Related Educational Programs (CACREP, 2016) emphasizes the need for counseling students to acquire the competencies that will enable them to effectively use *DSM-5* assessment in their practices.

Important advances in neurology, genetics, and the behavioral sciences over the past two decades have increased our understanding of mental illness. In the *DSM-5*, considerable attention has been given to developmental issues, gaps in the current system, disability and impairment, neuroscience, and cross-cultural issues (American Psychiatric Association, 2012a, 2013a). Cultural factors are included in assessment by using the Cultural Formulation Interview, a semistructured interview with 16 questions. Comas-Diaz and Brown (2016) contend that this cultural formulation is limited because "the American Psychiatric Association's cultural formulation is medically oriented and is, consequently, based on clients' deficits and psychopathology instead of focusing on clients' strength and resilience" (p. 250).

The *DSM-5*, like its predecessors, has attracted broad criticism and debate (Pickersgill, 2014). Vanheule and Devisch (2014) point out that the *DSM-5* lacks an operational framework for assessing distress when diagnosing a mental disorder. Other scholars have also been critical of the contents of the *DSM-5*, but Cosgrove and Wheeler (2013) focus on the firestorm of controversy surrounding *DSM-5* panel members' ties to the pharmaceutical industry. It was reported that 69% of task force members who oversaw development of the revised manual had ties to the pharmaceutical industry, an increase of 21% over previous edition task force members who had such relationships (Cosgrove & Krimsky, 2012). Blumenthal-Barby (2014) believes this emphasis will have consequences: an increasing number of phenomena that were previously considered "clinically unremarkable" (p. 531) are now labeled as mental disorders and are likely to be treated pharmacologically.

"The authors of the DSM-IV have critiqued the authors of the *DSM-5* for expansions that they believe will cause harm from over-diagnosis and false-positives in practice" (Blumenthal-Barby, 2014, pp. 531–532). Reflecting on lessons they learned from working on the previous edition of the manual, the authors of that edition cited examples of diagnoses such as Asperger's and bipolar II, which were added to the *DSM-IV*, that ultimately were "wildly overused in ways that were never intended" (p. 532). They expressed their concerns that the *DSM-5* could potentially provoke several more epidemics.

Another controversy emerged prior to publication of the *DSM-5* when the National Institute of Mental Health (NIMH) announced plans to develop its own psychiatric nosology, the Research Domain Criteria (RDoC), which would classify mental disorders based on specific functional analysis of certain cells, genes, neural circuits, and behaviors (Pickersgill, 2014; Sisti, Young, & Caplan, 2013). With the aim of informing future editions of the *DSM* and the International Classification of Diseases (ICD), another widely used classification system, the RDoC rests on the premise that the only objective way to classify disorders is to start with biology and work back to symptoms. The NIMH hopes to create *biosignatures* for mental conditions and, through the creation of the RDoC, suggests that mental disorders can be explained through a value-neutral combination of genetics, imaging, and neuroscience.

Advocates of an exclusively biomedical model strive to minimize the role of values in a classification of psychiatric conditions, but some argue that values infuse medical categories in a variety of ways:

> Values can drive practical considerations about where and how to divide up constellations of already agreed upon symptoms. Or they might operate at a more fundamental level and influence what is considered to be dysfunctional or disordered behavior in the first place. (Sisti et al., 2013, p. 2)

Sisti and colleagues (2013) concluded that values and objectivity are compatible, as can be seen in many psychiatric cases. The idea that the RDoC classification system "will be somehow value-free and objective because it begins with genes instead of behavior is to impose a value on crude reductionism that will not lead to any more objectivity than can be found in the pages of the DSM-5" (p. 4).

The Case For Psychodiagnosis

Practitioners who favor the use of diagnostic procedures argue that such procedures enable the therapist to identify a particular emotional or behavioral disorder, which helps in designing an appropriate treatment plan. Diagnosis stems from the medical model of mental health, which holds that different underlying causal factors, some of which are biological, produce different types of disorders. Proponents of traditional diagnosis often make the following points:

- Therapists have a legal, professional, and ethical obligation to assess whether clients may pose a danger to themselves or to others. They also need to screen for disorders that might respond best to a combination of medication and psychotherapy. Diagnosis may alert them to the need for a referral to a physician or a psychiatrist for a medical diagnosis, or for the treatment of a possible neuropsychological problem.
- Practitioners must be skilled in understanding and utilizing diagnostic procedures in order to function effectively in most mental health agencies.
- In working with a professional team, diagnosis is essential so that all team members have a common language and a common frame of reference.
- A diagnosis may be helpful to the therapist who wants to consult with other therapists about a given client.
- Diagnosis can assist in conceptualizing a case.
- It may be difficult to formulate a meaningful treatment plan without clearly defining the specific problems that need to be addressed. Diagnosis can help clinicians identify treatment possibilities, as they clearly specify particular symptoms and difficulties the client is experiencing.
- Diagnosis can provide information about possible causal factors associated with different types of mental disorders.
- Diagnosis can provide a framework for research on diagnostic categories and into various treatment approaches.
- A diagnosis may be critical to determine therapeutic success, which can be defined as the reduction of symptoms or the absence of the disorder as a consequence of treatment.

- Practitioners who work in an agency seldom have a choice about diagnosis. In many cases, they are required to make a diagnosis, often in the first session.
- Diagnosis may be a minimum standard of care for some licensed professionals. The failure to formulate a diagnosis may result in legal and credential consequences.
- There often is no insurance reimbursement without an acceptable diagnosis.
- Diagnosis can help to normalize a client's situation. Some clients find reassurance in knowing they are not alone and that there is a name for their condition.

The Case Against Psychodiagnosis

Some mental health professionals believe *DSM* diagnosis has many limitations and that it can harm clients. Some voices in the field have been critical of the broader philosophy behind this diagnostic and medical model, and we include their concerns here. Carl Rogers (1961) consistently maintained that diagnosis was detrimental to counseling because it tended to pull clients away from an internal and subjective way of experiencing themselves and to foster an objective and external conception of themselves. The result was an increased tendency toward dependence, with clients acting as if the responsibility for changing their behavior rested with the expert and not with themselves.

Feminist therapists have challenged the *DSM* system and proposed alternatives for making meaningful assessments. Therapists who question the usefulness of traditional diagnosis make these observations:

- Diagnosis is typically done by an expert observing a person's behavior and experience from an external viewpoint, without reference to what they mean to the client.
- Diagnostic categories can minimize the uniqueness of the client. When clients are categorized, it can lead to imposing labels on them in such a way as to not see their complexity or individuality.
- Reducing people to the sum of their symptoms ignores natural capacities for self-healing.
- Because the emphasis of the *DSM* model is on pathology, deficits, limitations, problems, and symptoms, individuals are not encouraged to find and utilize their strengths, assets, competencies, and abilities.
- Diagnosis can lead people to accept self-fulfilling prophecies or to despair over their condition.
- Diagnosis can narrow therapists' vision by encouraging them to look for behavior that fits a certain disease category. A diagnostic framework is based on a medical model that is not congruent with many counselors' core values and beliefs (Zalaquett et al., 2008).
- *DSM* diagnoses do not adequately consider contextual, social, and cultural factors.
- *DSM* diagnoses are based on the assumption that distress in a family or social context is the result of individual pathology, whereas a systemic approach views the source of the distress as being within the entire system.

- The best vantage point for understanding another person is through his or her subjective world, not through a general system of classification.
- Some disorders, especially those associated with children, depend on adults in homes and schools to give subjective reports that are often self-serving in terms of trying to control the child or to protect themselves.
- A diagnosis assigned to clients can have implications for their employment and future employability status.
- Many of the warnings against diagnosis speak to social justice issues. Often the person with the least power is the one being labeled, which can further silence oppressed clients and communities.

Carlos Zalaquett, a counselor educator, contends that some professionals assume they understand a particular person by knowing his or her diagnosis (personal communication, January 29, 2009). In reality, *DSM* diagnoses do not capture the uniqueness of the individual. A diagnosis is a label with no capacity to describe the totality of a human being. Therefore, it is always important to learn how the specific diagnosis is expressed in a particular client. Zalaquett adds that, once formulated, a diagnosis can follow an individual even if the assigned diagnosis no longer fits the person. For example, a college student diagnosed with a major depressive disorder associated with difficulties in college may not be accepted in a work-related position at some later time. Even though the person is no longer depressed, he or she may still carry the stigma of being labeled as depressed, which could have long-term implications.

Our Position on Assessment and Psychodiagnosis

Both assessment and diagnosis, broadly construed, are legitimate parts of the therapeutic process. The kind of diagnosis we have in mind is the result of a collaborative effort by the client and the therapist, also referred to as co-diagnosis. Both should be involved in discovering the nature of the client's difficulty, a process that commences with the initial sessions and continues until therapy is terminated. Even practitioners who oppose conventional diagnostic procedures and terminology unavoidably make an assessment of clients based on questions such as these:

- What brought the client into therapy?
- What are the client's resources for change?
- What are the client's strengths and vulnerabilities?
- Has the client had previous success in dealing with a similar problem?
- What does the client want from therapy, and how can it best be achieved?
- What should be the focus of the sessions?
- What environmental factors are contributing to the client's problems, and what can be done to alleviate these external factors?
- In what ways can an understanding of the client's cultural background shed light on developing a plan to deal with the client's problems?
- What role does the client's spirituality play in assessing and treating the problem?
- What specific family dynamics might be relevant to the client's present struggles and interpersonal relationships?

- What kind of support system does the client have?
- What are the prospects for meaningful change?

From our perspective, assessment and diagnosis (either formal or informal) help the practitioner conceptualize a case, implement treatment, and evaluate outcomes. The clinician and the client can discuss key questions as part of the therapeutic process. Clinicians will develop hypotheses about their clients, and they can talk about these conjectures with them. Diagnosis does not have to be a matter of categorizing clients; rather, practitioners can think more broadly, describe behavior, and think about its meaning. In this way, diagnosis becomes a process of thinking *about* the client *with* the client. Diagnosis can be viewed as a general descriptive statement identifying a client's style of functioning. The therapist can develop hunches about a client's behavioral style and perhaps even share these observations with the client as a part of the therapeutic process.

Comas-Diaz and Brown (2016) suggest that a process-oriented clinical assessment can be appropriate for culturally diverse clients. The first task in this assessment is to engage clients in treatment by inviting them to tell their story. Comas-Diaz and Brown recommend "that cultural similarities and differences be explored during the initial stages of assessment and then continuously throughout treatment" (p. 249).

As we emphasized earlier, we favor a collaborative approach to assessment that includes the client as a therapeutic partner. After the initial assessment of the client is completed, a decision can be made whether to refer the individual for alternative or additional treatment. The assessment information can be used in exploring the client's difficulties in thinking, feeling, and behaving and in establishing treatment goals. Assessment and diagnosis can be linked directly to the therapeutic process, forming a basis for developing methods of evaluating how well the therapist's procedures are working to achieve the client's goals.

Using diagnostic nomenclature is a reality that most practitioners must accept, especially if they work within a managed care system or with a third-party reimbursement system. For therapists who are required to work within a diagnostic framework, the challenge is to use diagnosis as a means to the end of providing quality service to clients rather than as an end in itself that leads to a justification for treatment. We concur with Herlihy, Watson, and Patureau-Hatchett (2008) that it is possible to work within a diagnostic framework in an ethical and diversity-sensitive manner. They offer the following suggestions for diversity-sensitive diagnosis. Reflecting on their recommendations can be a useful route to avoiding bias in one's diagnostic practices.

- Counselor self-awareness is the starting point for culturally sensitive diagnosis.
- Rather than assess only symptoms of behavior, strive to gather information about the context in which clients live and the meaning of their life experiences.
- Do not assume that differences between the counselor and the client are necessarily barriers to effective counseling.
- If symptoms are identified, consider reframing them as coping mechanisms as opposed to signs of pathology.
- Consider the benefits of making diagnosis a collaborative process.

Herlihy, Watson, and Patureau-Hatchett conclude that the *DSM* system is here to stay, at least for the foreseeable future. The question for mental health practitioners is not *whether* to use the *DSM* system but *how* to use it while being culturally sensitive in a way that can benefit clients.

Clarifying Your Position What is your position on diagnosis? The following questions may help you clarify your thinking on this issue:

- After reviewing the cases for and against psychodiagnosis, what position makes the most sense to you and why?
- Some contend that clients have a right to know their diagnoses as part of informed consent. What do you think of this practice? What client variables would you consider when discussing a diagnosis with a client?
- Some maintain that clients should not be told their diagnoses because of the possibility of their living up to a self-fulfilling prophecy. What is your thinking on this matter?
- If you were working for an agency that relied on managed care programs, how would you deal with the requirement of quickly formulating a diagnosis and a treatment plan, generally within the initial session? How would you work with the limitations of being able to see clients for no more than six visits?
- What are your thoughts about the right of clients to decide whether information will be released to third-party payers?
- Do you agree or disagree that therapists who do not accept the medical model, yet who provide diagnoses for reasons of third-party payments, are compromising their integrity?
- What ethical, legal, and professional issues can you raise pertaining to diagnosis? In your view, what is the most critical issue?
- What cultural critique can you offer about the diagnostic system and therapists being expected to diagnose clients?

Diagnosis Within an Insurance Context

Ethical dilemmas are often created when diagnosis is done strictly for insurance purposes, which often entails arbitrarily assigning a client to a diagnostic classification, sometimes merely to qualify for third-party payment. Some practitioners who are opposed to a diagnostic framework take the path of least resistance and give every client the same diagnosis. Clients who consult therapists regarding problems that do not fit a standard "illness" category may not be reimbursed for their psychotherapy. Some therapists may agree to see a couple or a family but submit a claim for an individual as the "identified patient," using an acceptable *DSM* diagnosis. Although it may be tempting for a clinician to present an "acceptable" but inaccurate diagnosis, this is both unethical and fraudulent. Braun and Cox (2005) note that the intentional misdiagnosis of mental disorders for the purpose of seeking insurance reimbursement constitutes health care fraud, which can lead to legal censure and court action at the local, state, and federal level.

Many insurance carriers will not pay for treatment that is not defined as an "illness" for which treatment is medically necessary. If a therapist treats a couple for marital difficulties and submits a claim to a managed care organization for couples therapy, chances are that the claim will be rejected. Although some family and couples counselors may view assigning certain diagnoses antithetical to their practice because they believe dysfunctional behaviors are manifestations of a faulty family system, they are aware that "utilization reviews typically require *DSM* diagnoses of individuals rather than of relationships" (Braun & Cox, 2005, p. 428). Practitioners must always be cognizant of their ethical responsibilities and use their best clinical judgment when making decisions involving diagnosis.

With some managed care mental health companies, a therapist may call the company with a diagnosis. A technician may then look up "appropriate" treatment strategies to deal with the identified problem (if, indeed, the diagnosis meets the criteria for reimbursement). This raises significant ethical issues as important treatment decisions may be made by a nonprofessional who has never seen the client and who lacks a depth of understanding of mental health issues.

Ethical and Legal Issues in Diagnosis

Under no circumstances should clinicians compromise themselves regarding the accuracy of a diagnosis to make it "fit" criteria accepted by an insurance company. If therapists do not understand how to work within some kind of diagnostic and assessment framework, and if they do not have a clear picture of the client's problem, it is possible that they will not help the client. We also think it is an ethical (and sometimes legal) obligation of therapists to be mindful that a medical evaluation is many times indicated. This is especially true in dealing with problems such as dementia, schizophrenia, bipolar disorder, and depression with suicidal ideation. Students need to learn the clinical skills necessary to do this type of screening and referral, which is a form of diagnostic thinking.

Practitioners may cause harm to clients if they treat them in restrictive ways because they have diagnosed them on the basis of a pattern of symptoms. Therapists may then behave toward clients in ways that make it very difficult for clients to change. If practitioners do not possess the competence to use *DSM* diagnosis appropriately, this raises an ethical issue. Practitioners who use the *DSM-5* must be trained in its use. This training requires learning more than diagnostic categories; it involves knowing personality theory, psychopathology, and seeing how they relate to therapeutic practice. Zalaquett and colleagues (2008) recommend reframing the way counselors are trained to use the *DSM* model. They write about the benefits that can be derived from building a collaborative relationship with clients in ways that result in meaningful case formulations, diagnoses, and treatment planning.

Now let us look at two specific cases where diagnosis and treatment options had to be evaluated.

The Case of Irma

Irma has just accepted her first position as a counselor in a community agency. An agency policy requires her to conduct an intake interview with each client, determine a diagnosis, and establish a treatment plan—all in the first session. Once a diagnosis is established, clinicians have a maximum of five more sessions with a given client. After 3 weeks, she lets a colleague know that she is troubled by this timetable. Her colleague reassures her that what she is doing is acceptable and that the agency's aim is to satisfy the requirements of the HMO. Irma does not feel reassured and cannot justify making an assessment in so short a time.

- What are your reactions to Irma's concern? Are there ethical difficulties with this agency's policies? Explain.
- Is it justified to provide a person with a diagnosis mainly for the purpose of obtaining third-party payment? Explain.
- If Irma retains her convictions, is she ethically obliged to discontinue her employment at this agency? What other alternatives, if any, do you see for her situation?
- In the course of a client's treatment, if the original diagnosis no longer applies, would you continue to use that diagnosis simply because your client wishes to see you?

Commentary. Before accepting the position, Irma should have done some research and assessed whether the expectations of the agency were congruent with her beliefs about the helping process. Irma cannot simply take the opinion of a colleague as an answer to her concerns now and should contact the HMO administration to see whether other options are open to her, such as requesting additional sessions. Although Irma may take issue with the requirement to diagnose each client, she will need to balance this theoretical concern with the ethical and legal standards requiring professionals to carefully assess and accurately diagnose clients before commencing any intervention.

In addition to advocating for her clients if more time is required for diagnoses and treatment in some cases, Irma has an obligation to recognize the limits of her own competence. As a relatively new counselor, Irma may require more time to arrive at accurate diagnoses. She must take the initiative to request supervision of her work, allow more senior clinicians to conduct intake and diagnostic interviews, or consider working in a different agency. •

The Case of Bob

Bob displays symptoms of insomnia, sadness, lethargy, and hopelessness. He has also been diagnosed with a substance abuse disorder. After 12 weeks of treatment, Felicita realizes that her client has all the symptoms of a major depression and that he is showing no improvement. She is inclined to double the number of weekly sessions to accelerate her client's progress.

- What do you think of Felicita's plan? Is it justified?
- Should she have done a more thorough assessment earlier in the treatment? What assessment strategies could she have used? Might the results have indicated alternative treatments?
- Is Felicita obligated to refer Bob for a psychiatric evaluation to determine whether antidepressant medication is indicated? Is she obliged to refer him if he so desires? Explain.
- What are her ethical obligations if he refuses to see a psychiatrist?
- What other ethical issues do you see in this case?

Commentary. Felicita is limited in her scope of practice, and Bob may need more help than she can provide. She cannot prescribe medication, which may be indicated in this case. Because of her assessment of Bob as being seriously depressed, it is important that she conduct an assessment for suicidality. Felicita should refer Bob for a medical and psychiatric evaluation as well. Because of his problems with substance abuse and his depression, Bob may benefit from an intensive outpatient treatment program. Felicita may help her client most by exploring adjunct treatment options with Bob and making any informed and clinically necessary referrals. •

Cultural Issues in Assessment and Diagnosis

The *DSM* system tends to pathologize clients, perpetuating the oppression of clients from diverse groups (Remley & Herlihy, 2016). Durodoye (2013) notes that "because of biases in mental health treatment, diverse populations have been psychiatrically mislabeled and treated on the basis of mainstream definitions of what is normal" (pp. 299–300). La Roche, Fuentes, and Hinton (2015) argue that the *DSM* is based on Western American assumptions (such as individualism and universalism), which limits its usefulness among different cultural groups. They also contend that the cultural contexts of clients must be included in the assessment process to prevent misconstruing the meaning of symptoms. For example, it is a mistake to assume that a Mexican American woman who resides at home with her parents until she marries is enmeshed. Instead, her living situation may be a result of gender-role expectations in her family. Zalaquett and colleagues (2008) acknowledge that cultural biases exist in both traditional helping models and the *DSM* model, yet they do not suggest that either should be discarded from a counselor's practice. Instead they emphasize the responsibility of counselors to use these models in more culturally competent ways. Cultural sensitivity is essential in making a proper diagnosis, and a range of factors need to be considered in interpreting the assessment process. See the Ethics Codes box titled "Cultural Sensitivity in Assessment" for some professional guidelines regarding culturally sensitive diagnosis.

ETHICS CODES: Cultural Sensitivity in Assessment

American Counseling Association (2014)
Counselors recognize that culture affects the manner in which clients' problems are defined and experienced. Clients' socioeconomic and cultural experiences are considered when diagnosing mental disorders. (E.5.b.)

American Mental Health Counselors Association (2015)
Mental health counselors consider multicultural factors (including but not limited to gender, race, religion, age, ability, culture, class, ethnicity, sexual orientation) in test interpretation, in diagnosis, and in the formulation of prognosis and treatment recommendations. (I.D.2c.)

American Psychological Association (2010)
When interpreting assessment results, including automated interpretations, psychologists take into account the purpose of the assessment as well as the various test factors, test-taking abilities, and other characteristics of the person being assessed, such as situational, personal, linguistic, and cultural differences, that might affect psychologists' judgments or reduce the accuracy of their interpretations. They indicate any significant limitations of their interpretations. (9.06.)

Commission on Rehabilitation Counselor Certification (2010)
Proper Diagnosis. If within their professional and individual scope of practice, rehabilitation counselors take special care to provide proper diagnosis of mental disorders. Assessment techniques (including personal interviews) used to determine care of clients (e.g., focus of treatment, types of treatment, or recommended follow-up) are carefully selected and appropriately used. (G.3.a.)

Cultural Sensitivity. Rehabilitation counselors recognize that culture affects the manner in which the disorders of clients are defined. The socioeconomic and cultural experiences of clients are considered when diagnosing. (G.3.b.)

Clearly, it is important to consider cultural and other diversity factors in both the assessment process and when formulating a diagnosis. If clinicians fail to consider ethnic and cultural factors in certain patterns of behavior, a client may be subjected to an erroneous assessment, diagnosis, and course of treatment. Failure to give adequate weight to cultural factors can result in misdiagnoses that perpetuate stereotypes based on race, ethnicity, gender, and sexual orientation (Comas-Diaz & Brown, 2016). Culturally diverse clients may prematurely drop out of treatment during the assessment process. Rather than focusing on pathology during the assessment phase, Comas-Diaz and Brown suggest using the initial session as a consultation meeting with the aim of negotiating mutually satisfactory goals for treatment and engaging clients in treatment. The goal should be to promote client agency and foster a collaborative therapeutic relationship. Nystul (2016) believes that it is critical that therapists be aware of the cultural context of language when differentiating mental health from mental illness. What is considered healthy can vary greatly from one culture to the next. Nystul maintains that a comprehensive assessment helps therapists better understand clients in terms of cultural, gender, religion or spirituality, and other aspects of diversity.

Barnett and Johnson (2015) suggest that practitioners think twice before they render a diagnosis. They point out that accurate assessment and diagnosis involves taking into consideration the realities of discrimination, oppression, and racism in society and also in the mental health disciplines. Barnett and Johnson caution counselors to give extra attention to avoid misdiagnosing and pathologizing certain cultural groups who have traditionally been disadvantaged by the mental health system. They emphasize carefully considering the ways in which clients' socioeconomic and cultural experiences can influence behavior, including the presentation of symptoms.

Whenever clinicians assess clients from culturally diverse populations, it is important for them to be aware of unintentional bias and to keep an open mind to the possibility of distinctive ethnic and cultural patterns. Kress, Eriksen, Rayle, and Ford (2005) maintain that clinicians need to strive toward diversity-sensitive diagnostic practices because doing so is ethically required and integral to effectively delivering services to diverse client groups. They encourage counselors to conduct a thorough assessment of their clients' cultural realities and to acquire an understanding of the complexity of the nature of the *DSM-5*. La Roche and colleagues (2015) point out that we all live in cultural contexts that shape our way of being in the world, so it is essential for all of us to assess and address cultural meanings and contextual variables.

LO9

Using Tests in Counseling

Testing is different from assessment, although tests may be used in the process of assessment. A test generates a score that represents a sample of behavior on a particular day. An assessment is an integrated process that yields a comprehensive picture of the client's functioning using multiple measures in multiple settings. Clinicians do not interpret test scores; rather, they interpret assessment batteries to produce a comprehensive, holistic picture of the client's psychological functioning as it applies to the referral question. It is important to understand the common assessment tools used in your profession, even if you choose not to use these tools in your practice.

As is true of diagnosis and assessment, the proper use of psychological testing in counseling and therapy is the subject of some debate. Generally, those who use therapeutic approaches that emphasize an objective view of counseling are inclined to use testing procedures as tools to acquire information about clients or as resources that clients themselves can use to help them in their decision making. Therapists who employ person-centered and existential approaches tend to view testing in much the same way that they view diagnosis—as an external frame of reference that is of little use to them in counseling situations.

We think the core issue is not whether you will use tests but rather under what circumstances and for what purposes. Tests are available that measure aptitude, ability, achievement, intelligence, values and attitudes, vocational interests, or personality characteristics. Unfortunately, these tests are often misused, and when this occurs, ethical concerns are raised. Tests may be given routinely, given without providing feedback to clients, used for the wrong purposes, interpreted without consideration for cultural factors, or given by unqualified testers. Clinicians may choose measures based on what is available or easy to give rather than on which measure will best provide information to address the referral question or the reason for the testing in the first place. Here are some guidelines that will help you think about the circumstances under which you might want to use tests for counseling purposes and how to use them in an ethical manner.

- It is important for clinicians to be familiar with any tests they use and preferably to have taken these tests themselves. It is essential to know the purpose of each test and how it measures what it purports to measure. Sometimes mental health workers find that they are expected to give and interpret tests as a basic function of their job. If they have not had adequate training in this area, they are in an ethical bind. In-service training and continuing education programs are ways of gaining competence in using some psychological assessment devices.
- Familiarize yourself with the standards pertaining to testing in the ethics code of your profession. Recognize the limits of your competence to use and interpret tests. Know when you need to refer clients to a specialist in testing.
- Select tests that are appropriate for your client given his or her unique cultural, social, and cognitive factors. If others who are similar to your client in terms of demographics are not included in the standardization sample of the instrument you have chosen to use, it is highly probable that the test you have chosen is inappropriate for your client.
- Clients from culturally diverse backgrounds may react to testing with suspicion if tests have been used to discriminate against them in schools and employment. To minimize such negative reactions, it is a good practice to explore a client's views and expectations about testing and to work with him or her in resolving attitudes that are likely to affect the outcome of a test.
- Involve your clients in the selection of tests. Clients need to understand what information the tests are designed to provide. Before administering tests, obtain your client's informed consent.

- Know why you want to use a particular test. Does your agency require that you administer certain tests? Are you giving tests because they will help you understand a client better? Do you administer tests mainly when clients request them?
- Assume a stance of critically evaluating tests you may use. Know their limitations, and keep in mind that a test can be useful and valid in one situation but inappropriate in another.
- Explore why clients want to take a battery of tests, and teach clients the values and limitations of testing. If that is done, there is less chance tests will be undertaken in a mechanical fashion or that unwarranted importance will be attributed to the results. Clients need to be aware that tests are merely tools that can provide useful information they can then explore in their counseling sessions.
- In general, it is best to give clients test *results*, not simply test *scores*. In other words, explore with your clients the meaning the results have for them. Integrate the test results with other information, such as clients' developmental, social, and medical history. Evaluate your clients' readiness to receive and accept certain information and be sensitive to the ways in which clients respond to the information provided.
- How well do your assessment results parallel what the client is reporting in his or her own subjective experience? Have you adequately investigated all salient areas of the client's life in your current assessment process?
- It is critical to maintain the confidentiality of test results. Results may be handled in different ways, depending on the purpose and type of each test or on the requirements of the agency where you work. Nevertheless, your clients need to feel that they can trust you and that test results will neither be used against them nor revealed to people who have no right to this information.

Paying attention to the above points when considering administrating or interpreting testing is one way to increase the likelihood that you are practicing in a culturally sensitive manner. From a social justice perspective, clinicians can use their power to bring to light the misuses and inaccurate applications of assessment, especially with those from underserved and oppressed communities.

Clients being tested should know what the test is intended to discover, how it relates to their situation, and how the results will be used. Perhaps the most basic ethical guideline for using tests is to keep in mind the primary purpose for which they were designed: to provide objective and descriptive measures that can be used by clients in making better decisions. It is wise to remember that tests are tools that should be used in the service of clients.

Evidence-Based Therapy Practice

Mental health practitioners are frequently expected to make decisions about what they believe to be the best therapeutic approaches or interventions with a particular client. Clinical practice should be based on the best available research integrated with a practitioner's expertise within the context of a particular client (Norcross, Hogan, & Koocher, 2008). For many therapists the choice of interventions they make in their practice is based on their theoretical orientation. Over the past couple of decades, however, a shift has occurred toward promoting the use of specific interventions for specific problems or diagnoses based on empirically supported treatments (APA Presidential Task Force, 2006; Cukrowicz et al., 2005; Deegear & Lawson, 2003; Edwards, Dattilio, & Bromley, 2004; Lazarus & Rego, 2013; McCloskey, 2011; Tarvydas, Addy, & Fleming, 2010). Treatment manuals were developed for a wide range of psychological disorders, and they yielded impressive research results. Lazarus and Rego (2013) state that this success ushered in the movement toward empirically supported treatments and evidence-based practice.

Increasingly, clinicians who practice in a behavioral health care system are encountering the concept of evidence-based practice (Bride, Kintzle, Abraham, & Roman, 2012; Norcross et al., 2008). **Evidence-based practice** (EBP) is "the integration of the best available research with clinical expertise in the context of patient characteristics, culture, and preferences" (APA Presidential Task Force, 2006, p. 273). This idea encompasses more than simply basing interventions on research. Norcross and colleagues (2008) advocate for inclusive evidence-based practices that incorporate each of the three pillars of EBP: best available evidence, clinician expertise, and client characteristics.

Evidence-based practice is often associated with cognitive-behavioral approaches. These approaches are the most extensively researched psychotherapies, with hundreds of studies supporting their effectiveness for a wide range of emotional and behavioral problems (Antony, 2014). Hollon and Beck (2013) report that cognitive-behavioral interventions have generated powerful evidence of success in treating depression, anxiety disorders, panic disorders, social phobia, posttraumatic stress disorders, eating disorders, substance abuse, personality disorders, and childhood depression and anxiety disorders. Although abundant research has been conducted on cognitive-behavior therapies, it is a mistake to conclude that these approaches have a monopoly on evidence-based therapy practice.

In their extensive review of research on humanistic psychotherapy from 1990 to 2015, Angus and colleagues (2015) concluded that "humanistic psychotherapy researchers have made significant contributions to innovative advancements in the field of psychotherapy methods and research findings over the past 25 years" (p. 338). Angus and colleagues also contend that humanistic psychotherapies " are supported by multiple lines of scientific evidence and should therefore be included in clinical guidelines and lists of evidence-based psychotherapy" (p. 339). Elliott, Greenberg, Watson, Timulak, and Freire (2013) compiled a comprehensive review of the humanistic-experiential psychotherapies and report that a substantial and rapidly growing body of data supports these approaches with a wide range of client problems including depression, relationship problems, anxiety disorders, eating disorders, coping with chronic medical conditions, psychotic disorders, and substance abuse.

The movement toward grounding psychotherapy practice on a scientific foundation led to the concept of **empirically supported treatments** (EST). "Proponents of ESTs believe that each form of therapy needs to be tested in carefully controlled experimental research. The results would show which therapies actually worked and which, though well intended, did nothing to help the patient or, worse, were harmful" (Pope & Wedding, 2014, p. 576).

Managed care companies and other third-party insurance companies embrace the concept of ESTs and tend to restrict payments to therapies that demonstrate evidence of being effective and efficient (Pope & Wedding, 2014). Increasing the availability and use of ESTs has become a focus of public policy, and some individuals have concentrated their efforts on discovering the best ways to train practitioners in the use of these treatments and to disseminate this information (Godley, Garner, Smith, Meyers, & Godley, 2011; McCloskey, 2011; Vismara, Young, Stahmer, Griffith, & Rogers, 2009).

However, there is another side to the EST issue. In his extensive review of the efficacy and effectiveness of psychotherapy, Lambert (2013) states that identifying lists of empirically supported treatments for specific disorders is controversial and puts too much emphasis on small differences in outcomes associated with certain treatments. Lambert concludes, "to advocate empirically supported therapies as preferable or superior to other treatments is probably premature" (p. 205).

Basing one's psychotherapeutic practices on interventions that have been empirically validated may seem to be the ethical path to take, but business considerations do enter into this picture. In seeking to specify the treatment for a specific diagnosis as precisely as possible, health insurance companies are concerned with determining the minimum amount of treatment that can be expected to be effective. There is a pressure for ESTs to be both short and standardized. Treatments are operationalized by reliance on a treatment manual that identifies what is to be done in each therapy session and how many sessions will be required (Edwards et al., 2004). Bolen and Hall (2007) note that organizations competing for managed care contracts are assessed by their capacity to manage programs and costs as well as by their skill in implementing focused and brief methodologies.

Some practitioners believe that this approach is mechanistic and does not take into full consideration the relational dimensions of the psychotherapy process. Indeed, relying exclusively on standardized treatments for specific problems may raise another set of ethical issues. One of these issues is the reliability and validity of these empirically based techniques. Human change is complex and difficult to measure unless researchers operationalize the notion of change at such a simplistic level that the change may be meaningless. Not all clients come to therapy with clearly defined psychological disorders. Many clients have existential concerns that do not fit in any diagnostic category and do not lend themselves to clearly specified symptom-based outcomes. Evidence-based practice has significant limitations for practitioners working with individuals who want to pursue meaning and fulfillment in their lives. Lazarus and Rego (2013) raise this key question: What should therapists do when clients do not respond to manualized treatments or present with a problem for which no treatment manual exists?

Treatment manuals focus on methods and procedures but lack consideration of the client–therapist relationship as a basic element in therapy. If there is not a working alliance, which calls for the genuine meeting of client and therapist, then the effects of the application of empirically established methods and the best of manuals will be diluted, if not erased (Lazarus & Rego, 2013).

Norcross, Beutler, and Levant (2006) remind us that many aspects of treatment— the therapy relationship, the therapist's personality and therapeutic style, the client, and environmental factors—contribute to the success of psychotherapy and must be taken into account in the treatment process. Proponents of the common factors approach point out that EBPs tend to emphasize only one of these aspects: interventions based on the best available research. Bohart and Wade (2013) argue that substantial research supports the position of the *client* accounting for more of the treatment outcome than either the relationship or the method employed. "There is evidence that clients make the single strongest contribution to outcome" (p. 219).

Norcross and his colleagues (2006) acknowledge that mental health professionals are challenged by the mandate to demonstrate the efficiency, efficacy, and safety of the services they provide. Although the goal of EBP is to enhance the effectiveness of client services and to improve public health, Norcross and his colleagues show that there is a great deal of controversy and discord when it comes to EBP. They stress the value of informed dialogue and respectful debate as a way to gain clarity and to make progress.

Elmore (2016) reports that ESTs have come to represent an accepted standard of care in many circles, but the EST movement has been the source of much controversy since its inception. Proponents of the common factors perspective have argued that the narrow focus of the EST movement neglects key dimensions of effective psychotherapy, including the emphasis on the therapeutic alliance and an accurate explanation of the client's presenting difficulties. Miller, Duncan, and Hubble (2004) are critical of the EST movement and argue that the best hope for integration of the field is a focus on using data generated during treatment to inform the process and outcome of treatment. "Significant improvements in client retention and outcome have been shown where therapists have feedback on the client's experience of the alliance and progress in treatment. Rather than EBP, therapists tailor their work through practice-based evidence" (p. 2). One private practitioner collected data on his own effectiveness over 45 years of practice. Clement (2013) analyzed outcome data on 1,599 cases and demonstrated that his effectiveness did not improve across the years. In addition, he found that the "years with the largest patient caseloads or the greatest proportion of patients with managed care insurance tended to show the poorest outcomes" (p. 23). Clement's goal in publishing his own practice-based evidence was to encourage his colleagues to follow suit. In his own words, "I have shown you my practice-based evidence. Now you show me yours" (p. 42).

EBP involves far more than simply employing interventions based on the best available research. The APA Presidential Task Force on Evidence-Based Practice (2006) emphasize that psychotherapy is a collaborative venture in which clients and clinicians develop ways of working together that are likely to result in positive outcomes. The involvement of an active, informed client is crucial to the success of therapy services. Based on their clinical expertise, therapists make the ultimate judgment regarding particular interventions, and they make these decisions in the context of considering the client's values and preferences. Bohart and Wade (2013) found that research on clients' perspectives supports the idea of the client as an active agent in the therapy process.

For further reading on the topic of EBPs, we recommend APA Presidential Task Force (2006), Duncan, Miller, Wampold, and Hubble (2010), Norcross, Beutler, and Levant (2006), and Norcross, Hogan, and Koocher (2008).

Findings From Psychotherapeutic Research

Just as clinicians sometimes underuse theory, some do not see the practical value of understanding how psychotherapy research can enhance their practice. Without understanding how to translate current research findings into their practices, therapists limit themselves in their ability to help clients. Clinicians need to understand how theory and research contribute to more effective and therefore more ethical practice.

Most of the questions we have raised in this chapter have a direct relationship to a therapist's therapeutic approach. Specialized techniques, the balance of responsibility in the client–therapist relationship, the functions of the therapist, and the goals of treatment are all tied to a therapist's theoretical orientation. But at some point you will probably ask: Does my psychotherapeutic approach or these specific techniques work? To answer this question, you may need to rely on the findings of psychotherapeutic research.

Boisvert and Faust (2003) examined leading international psychotherapy researchers' views on psychotherapy outcome research. Participants in the study rated level of research evidence for or against various assertions about psychotherapy process and outcomes. Their study revealed some interesting conclusions.

Experts showed strong agreement that research *did support* the following assertions:

- Therapy is helpful to the majority of clients.
- Most people achieve some change relatively quickly in therapy.
- People change more due to "common factors" than to "specific factors" associated with therapies.
- In general, the various therapeutic approaches achieve similar outcomes.
- The relationship between therapist and client is the best predictor of treatment outcome.
- Most therapists learn more about effective therapy techniques from their experience than from the research.
- Approximately 10% of clients get worse as a result of therapy.

Experts showed strong agreement that research *does not support* the following assertions:

- Placebo control groups and waitlist control groups are as effective as psychotherapy.
- Therapist experience is a strong predictor of outcome.
- Long-term therapy is more effective than brief therapy for the majority of clients (p. 511).

In his review of the effectiveness of psychotherapy, Lambert (2013) supports most of the conclusions of the Boisvert and Faust study. Lambert notes that the theme derived from meta-analyses of the large body of psychotherapy research clearly shows that "psychotherapy has proven to be highly beneficial" (p. 176).

What are the primary determinants of the effectiveness of psychotherapy? Elkins (2012, 2016) cites evidence showing that personal and interpersonal factors are the major determinants of effectiveness. The humanistic elements of psychotherapy, which include the client, the therapist, and the therapeutic alliance, are powerful factors in psychotherapy outcome. Although specific theories and techniques are important, they are not the crucial factors that account for outcome. Most psychotherapy research, training, and practice are based on the assumption that a therapist's theory and techniques—not personal and interpersonal factors—are the primary instruments of change. Elkins (2012) proposes a change in the focus of training students to provide less emphasis on theory and techniques and more emphasis on the therapist as a person. The aim of this training is to cultivate the trainee's capacity to connect with clients on a deep level so clients will feel understood, supported, and accepted. In short, Elkins asserts that we need to rethink many of our assumptions and beliefs about clinical research, training, and practice and make significant changes in these areas to bring the profession into alignment with the findings of contemporary science. Angus and colleagues (2015) also point to ample evidence to suggest that therapeutic training should emphasize the person of the therapist and "the development of empathic communication skills, the capacity to enhance clients' emotional expression and self-regulation, and the capacity to develop a secure and productive therapeutic alliance for the facilitation of client narrative disclosure and productive meaning-making in therapy sessions" (p. 340). Angus and colleagues emphasize that the collaborative nature of the therapeutic relationship is key to the process of therapy unfolding. It is clear that the authentic personal relationship is central to effective therapeutic practice.

Chapter Summary

Issues in theory and practice are necessarily interrelated. From an ethical perspective, therapists need to anchor their practices to theory. Without a theoretical foundation, practitioners are left with little rationale to formulate therapeutic goals and develop techniques to accomplish these goals. Practitioners are sometimes impatient when it comes to articulating a theory that guides practice. Some rely on a limited number of techniques to deal with every conceivable problem clients may present. However, a good theory helps clinicians understand what they are doing.

We do not advocate that you subscribe to one established theory. Therapeutic techniques from many theoretical approaches may be useful in your practice. By developing an integrative approach to counseling practice, you can adjust your approach to fit your clients' needs. Ideally, your theoretical orientation will serve as a basis for reflecting on matters such as goals in counseling, the division of responsibility between the client and the counselor in meeting these goals, the techniques that are most appropriate with specific clients in resolving a variety of problems, and the approach that will be most beneficial for the client.

The use of assessment and diagnosis and testing in counseling is related to a practitioner's theoretical orientation. Regardless of the theory a therapist employs as a basis for practice, assessment and diagnosis are matters that will need to be addressed. It is important that cultural considerations be attended to in conducting an assessment, in formulating a diagnosis, and in deciding whether specific tests are appropriate.

Practitioners are increasingly being faced with providing services within the framework of evidence-based practice. Broadly interpreted, there are three pillars of evidence-based practice: looking for the best available research, relying on clinical expertise, and taking into consideration the client's characteristics, culture, and preferences. Despite this trend, personal and interpersonal factors remain the most powerful determinants of psychotherapy outcome. Although a therapist's theoretical orientation and use of techniques are important, they have not been shown to be critical to outcome.

Suggested Activities

1. In dyads, describe your theoretical stance. How do you see your theory influencing the way you counsel? If you are in the process of selecting a theory or theories, talk about what parts of the different theories appeal to you most and least and why.
2. Make a list of the pros and cons of using assessment and testing with diverse populations and discuss in small groups or have a debate in class: those *for* assessment and diagnosis and those *against* assessment and diagnosis.
3. If you were applying for a job as a counselor and were asked, "What are the most important goals you have for your clients?" how would you respond? How would you respond if you were asked, "Do you have any questions about our agency?"
4. Suppose a client came to you and asked you to administer a battery of interest, ability, and vocational tests. How would you respond? What questions would you ask the client before agreeing to arrange for the testing?
5. Interview at least one practicing therapist and discuss how his or her theoretical orientation influences his or her practice. Ask the practitioner questions raised throughout this chapter. Bring the results of your interview to class.
6. In dyads or triads, discuss the position that a thorough assessment and diagnosis is a necessary step in effective counseling practice. Also, discuss the ethics of using a diagnosis exclusively for the purpose of insurance reimbursement. What factors need to be taken into account when diagnosing and assessing clients?
7. As a small group activity, explore how you would go about getting to know your client during your initial contact. How would you structure future sessions? Explore the following questions:

   - Are tests important as a prerequisite to counseling? Would you decide whether to test, or would you allow your client to make this decision?
   - Would you develop a contract with your client specifying what the client could expect from you and what the client wanted from counseling? Why or why not?
   - Would you be inclined to use directive, action-oriented techniques, such as homework assignments? Why or why not?

8. In small groups, discuss the advantages and limitations of evidence-based practice or have a debate in class with one side arguing for EBP and the other side arguing against it.
9. Hold a mock trial and have a student role-play a therapist who is subpoenaed to discuss his or her treatment plan for a client.

MindTap for Counseling

Go to MindTap® for an eBook, videos of client sessions, activities, practice quizzes, apps, and more—all in one place. If your instructor didn't assign MindTap, you can find out more information at CengageBrain.com.

Ethical Issues in Couples and Family Therapy

LEARNING OBJECTIVES

1. Understand the basic premises involved in the systems theory perspective

2. Identify key ethical standards in working with couples and families

3. Understand the role of informed consent in couples and family therapy

4. Describe some contemporary professional issues in couples and family therapy

5. Clarify how therapist values can be an ethical issue in couples and family work

6. Explain the themes involved in gender-sensitive couples and family therapy

7. Recognize and understand the responsibilities of couples and family therapists

8. Appreciate the complexity of confidentiality in family therapy

SELF-INVENTORY

Directions: For each statement, indicate the response that most closely identifies your beliefs and attitudes. Use the following code:

5 = I *strongly agree* with this statement.

4 = I *agree* with this statement.

3 = I am *undecided* about this statement.

2 = I *disagree* with this statement.

1 = I *strongly disagree* with this statement.

_____ 1. A person who comes from a dysfunctional family is generally unlikely to become a good family therapist.

_____ 2. In working with couples or families, from the outset I would explain what a "no secrets" policy means and the reasons for such a policy.

_____ 3. In practicing couples counseling, I would be willing to see each of them for individual sessions in addition to conjoint therapy.

_____ 4. Counselors have an ethical responsibility to encourage spouses to leave partners who are physically or psychologically abusive.

_____ 5. I would not be willing to work with a couple if I knew that one of the individuals was having an affair.

_____ 6. It is ethical for family therapists to use pressure and sometimes even coercion to get a reluctant client to participate in family therapy.

_____ 7. Therapists who feel justified in imposing their own values on a couple or a family can cause considerable harm.

_____ 8. In couples or family therapy, confidentiality needs to be thoroughly addressed from the outset.

_____ 9. Most family therapists, consciously or unconsciously, work to keep the family together.

_____ 10. There are ethical problems in treating only one member of a family.

_____ 11. I would be willing to work with a single member of a family and eventually intend to bring the entire family into therapy.

_____ 12. Before accepting a family for treatment, I would obtain supervised training in working with families.

_____ 13. Before working with families, I need to know my struggles with my own family of origin.

_____ 14. Skill in using family therapy techniques is far more important to success in this area than knowing my own personal dynamics.

_____ 15. I support requiring continuing education in the field of couples and family therapy as a condition for renewal of a license in this area.

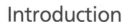

Introduction

Many of the ethical issues we discuss in this chapter take on special significance when therapists work with more than one client. Most graduate programs in couples and family therapy now require a separate course in ethics and the law pertaining to this specialization, with an increased emphasis on ethical, legal, and professional issues unique to a systems perspective. The professional practice of couples and family therapy is regulated by legal statutes, professional specialty guidelines, peer review, continuing education, managed care, consultation, and is self-regulated by ethics codes (Goldenberg, Stanton, & Goldenberg, 2017). A growing body of research has demonstrated the efficacy of family therapy (Lebow & Stroud, 2016). Specific areas of ethical concern for couples and family therapists that we discuss in this chapter include ethical standards of practice, therapist values, gender sensitivity, therapist roles and responsibilities, confidentiality, informed consent, and the right to refuse treatment.

The Systems Theory Perspective

Much of the practice of couples and family therapy rests on the foundation of **systems theory**, which views psychological and relational problems as arising from within the individual's present environment and the intergenerational family system. Symptoms are believed to be an expression of dysfunctions within the system, which can be passed along through numerous generations. Using a systems perspective, problems are defined as interactional, and professionals who conduct family therapy generally adopt a systemic perspective as the foundation of their practice. Psychotherapy traditionally focused on the individual, but family therapy has broadened this scope to include the family and larger social systems (Lebow & Stroud, 2016).

The systems perspective views the family as a functioning entity that is more than the sum of its members. The family provides the context for understanding how individuals behave. Actions by any individual member influence all the other members, and their reactions have a reciprocal effect on the individual. For instance, a child who is acting out may be expressing deep conflicts between the parental figures and may actually be expressing the pain of an entire family. Family therapists often work with individuals, the couple, and parents and children to get a better understanding of patterns that affect the entire system and to develop strategies for change. Even when the focus is on an individual, Wilcoxon, Remley, and Gladding (2012) point out that the individual's actions are analyzed in terms of how they affect other members of the relationship system, as well as how other members' actions reciprocally affect and shape the individual. Operating from a family relational perspective, the therapist is primarily concerned with the transactional patterns expressed by a family or a couple.

The idea that the identified client's problem might be a symptom of how the system functions, not just a symptom of the individual's maladjustment and psychosocial development, was a revolutionary notion. For therapists accustomed to Western cultural ideals, the family systems perspective demands a major paradigm shift away from the values associated with individualism, autonomy, and independence (Bitter, 2014). Key concepts such as collectivism, interdependence, family embeddedness and connectedness, hierarchies of relationship, and multigenerational perspectives are more familiar concepts in non-Western cultures. Harway and Kadin (Harway, Kadin, Gottlieb, Nutt, & Celano, 2012) argue in support of a paradigm shift in the field of psychology to accommodate the changing needs of service recipients. Systemic approaches must be taught side by side with individualistic approaches because many cultural groups are collectivistic.

Goldenberg and colleagues (2017) encourage family therapists to view all behavior, including the symptoms expressed by the individual, within the context of the family and society. Although traditional approaches to treating the individual have merit, expanding the perspective to consider family, community, and societal dynamics can enhance therapists' understanding. Family therapists with a systems orientation are concerned with understanding *what* is occurring (such as conflict between individuals), *how* it occurs (noting repetitive patterns of behavior), and *when* it occurs (instances when power and control arise). Systems-oriented therapists focus on the *process* rather than the *content* of these transactions. A systems orientation does not preclude dealing with the individual, but it does broaden the traditional emphasis to address the roles individuals play in the family.

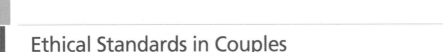

Ethical Standards in Couples and Family Therapy

The AAMFT *Code of Ethics* (2015) provides a framework for many of the ethical issues we consider in this chapter, but practitioners are required to know and follow the ethics codes of their own professional affiliation on matters related to couples and family therapy. In addition, many states have their own professional organizations that outline ethical standards for the practice of couples and family therapy.

We begin our discussion by considering the AAMFT's (2015) code in each of nine core areas, followed by a brief discussion of what this means for therapists.

Responsibility to Clients

> Marriage and family therapists advance the welfare of families and individuals and make reasonable efforts to find the appropriate balance between conflicting goals within the family system. (Standard I.)

As the focus of therapy shifts from the individual to the family system, a new set of ethical questions arises: Whose interests should the family therapist serve? To whom and for whom does the therapist have primary loyalty and responsibility: the client identified as being the problem, the separate family members as individuals, or the family as a whole? By agreeing to become involved in family therapy, the members can generally be expected to place a higher priority on the goals of the family as a unit than on their own personal goals. Balancing the rights and well-being of the individuals with the family as a whole is one of the most challenging aspects of ethical family practice.

Confidentiality

> Marriage and family therapists have unique confidentiality concerns because the client in a therapeutic relationship may be more than one person. Therapists respect and guard the confidences of each individual client. (Standard II.)

The principle of confidentiality, as it applies to couples and family therapists, entails that practitioners not disclose what they have learned through the professional relationship except (1) when mandated by law, such as in cases of physical or psychological child abuse, incest, child neglect, abuse of the elderly, or abuse of people with a disability; (2) when it is necessary to protect clients from harming themselves or to prevent a clear and immediate danger to others; (3) when the family therapist is a defendant in a civil, criminal, or disciplinary action arising from the therapy; or (4) when a waiver has previously been obtained in writing. If therapists use any material from their practice in teaching, lecturing, and writing, they take care to preserve the anonymity of their clients. For therapists who are working with families, any release of information must be agreed to by all parties. However, there is an exception to this policy when a therapist is concerned that a family member will harm him- or herself or will do harm to another person. Another exception occurs when the law mandates a report.

How would you explain confidentiality and its limits to a couple or family you are counseling? What challenges might you face in dealing with confidentiality matters in working with couples and families?

Professional Competence and Integrity

> Marriage and family therapists maintain high standards of professional competence and integrity. (Standard III.)

Responsible clinicians keep abreast of developments in the field through continuing education and clinical experiences. A single course or two in a graduate counseling program is inadequate preparation for functioning ethically and effectively as a couples or family practitioner. Competence in working with couples and families comes with years of training and supervision. Practitioners continue to improve their skills through interactions with other therapists and with ongoing continuing education. Practitioners who hope to specialize in couples and family therapy are advised to seek out postgraduate opportunities to receive more advanced training at a family therapy institute, if feasible, or at workshops or conferences sponsored by relevant professional organizations such as AAMFT.

How likely are you to recognize when your own personal or family-of-origin issues begin to interfere with your professional work with couples and families? What could you do if you discovered these issues? What steps can you take to maintain your level of competence in couples and family therapy after earning your degree?

Responsibility to Students and Supervisees

> Marriage and family therapists do not exploit the trust and dependency of students and supervisees. (Standard IV.)

Practitioners are cautioned to avoid multiple relationships, which are likely to impair clinical judgment. As you saw in Chapters 7 and 9, perspectives differ on how best to handle dual relationships and avoid exploiting the trust and dependency of clients, students, and supervisees. Most family therapy training programs encourage genogram work and other processes designed to engage students with their own family-of-origin issues. In such programs, trainers inevitably engage in therapeutic interventions with their students from time to time. Faculty need to clearly provide information about program requirements ahead of time so students are aware they will be expected to be personally involved in their training program.

Research and Publication

> Marriage and family therapists respect the dignity and protect the welfare of research participants, and are aware of applicable laws, regulations, and professional standards governing the conduct of research. (Standard V.)

Researchers must carefully consider the ethical aspects of any research proposal, making use of informed consent procedures and explaining to participants what is involved in any research project. At universities and in clinical settings, researchers are required to follow certain rules and regulations, which include procedures for meeting HIPAA requirements. Even when functioning outside of a university or clinical setting, marriage and family therapists must meet standards of ethical research practice when working with couples or families.

Technology-Assisted Professional Services

> Therapy, supervision, and other professional services engaged in by marriage and family therapists take place over an increasing number of technological platforms. There are great benefits and responsibilities inherent in both the traditional therapeutic and supervision contexts, as well as in the utilization of technologically-assisted professional services. This standard addresses basic ethical requirements of offering therapy, supervision, and related professional services using electronic means. (Standard VI.)

Marriage and family therapists are expected to determine which, if any, technology-assisted professional services are appropriate for clients or supervisees. Clients and supervisees must be made aware of both the risks and the responsibilities associated with technology-assisted professional services. Moreover, Wilcoxon (2015) states that couples and family therapists need to think about the potential use and misuse of technology—not only by clients but by themselves. Confidentiality and the limitations and protections of using technology must be addressed at the beginning of therapy or supervision services. Marriage and family therapists must be competent in the use of all chosen technology-assisted professional services prior to engaging in these services.

How would you determine the appropriateness of using any form of technology in your work with therapy clients or supervisees? How could you assess your level of competence in using technology? What would you want to include in the informed consent process regarding the use of technology? What are the main benefits and disadvantages inherent in using technology-assisted services?

Professional Evaluations

Marriage and family therapists aspire to the highest of standards in providing testimony in various contexts within the legal system. (Standard VII.)

Informed consent is essential in performing forensic services. This includes obtaining written consent from the people being evaluated. Marriage and family therapists avoid conflicts in roles in legal proceedings and disclose potential conflicts. As therapy begins, it is essential to clarify roles and the extent of confidentiality when legal systems are involved. In addition, if therapists do not wish to be custody evaluators, it is important to state this in the informed consent so clients are aware of this prior to beginning services.

Financial Arrangements

Marriage and family therapists make financial arrangements with clients, third party payors, and supervisees that are reasonably understandable and conform to accepted professional practices. (Standard VIII.)

Couples and family therapists do not accept payment for making referrals and do not exploit clients financially for services. They are truthful in representing facts to clients and to third parties regarding any services rendered. Ethical practice dictates a disclosure of fee policies at the onset of therapy.

Advertising

Marriage and family therapists engage in appropriate informational activities, including those that enable the public, referral sources, or others to choose professional services on an informed basis. (Standard IX.)

Ethical practice dictates that practitioners accurately represent their competence, education, training, and experience in couples and family therapy. How would you advertise your services? How would you promote yourself as a couples and family practitioner?

Special Ethical Considerations in Working With Couples and Families

A number of ethical considerations are unique to couples and family therapy. Because most couples and family therapists focus on the family system, potential ethical dilemmas needing immediate clarification can arise even in the first session. Therapists who work with cohabitating couples or multiple family members, for example, often encounter dilemmas that involve serving one member's best interest at the expense of another member's interest. When counseling couples or families, therapists need to be mindful of working primarily for the good of the relationship rather than solely for the good of one individual.

Therapists can respond to ethical dilemmas over conflicting interests of multiple individuals by identifying the couple or family system rather than a single individual as the "client" (Kleist & Bitter, 2014; Wilcoxon et al., 2012). Therapists who function as an advocate of the system avoid becoming agents of any one partner or family member. Fisher (2009) proposes that we stop asking, "Who is the client?" and reframe this question to consider our ethical responsibilities to everyone involved. Working within a framework that conceptualizes change as affecting and being affected by all family members, practitioners are able to define problems and consider plans for change in the context of the family system and all its members.

Wilcoxon and colleagues (2012, p. 103) ask a number of ethical questions couples and family counselors may face:

- In what ways are ethical principles unique for the practice of marriage and family therapy?
- Can therapists automatically assume the right to define presenting problems of couples and families in terms of their own therapeutic orientation?
- How much concerted effort can therapists exert in bringing together all the significant family members for therapy sessions?
- Under what situations, if any, should therapists impose their control on couples and families? If so, to what extent should they impose it in seeking change in the relationship pattern?
- What nontraditional family structures raise unique ethical concerns for marriage and family therapists?

Informed Consent in Couples and Family Therapy

Informed consent is a critical ethical issue in individual psychotherapy (see Chapter 5), and it is also a necessary part of the practice of couples and family therapy. Before each individual agrees to participate in family therapy, family practitioners are expected to provide information about the purpose of therapy, typical procedures, the risks of negative outcomes, the possible benefits, the fee structure, the rights and responsibilities of clients, the option that a family member can withdraw at any time, what can be expected from the therapist, and the limits of confidentiality. Family members are then in a position to decide whether to participate in therapy and how much to disclose to the therapist.

Couples and family therapists are obligated to explain their work from the beginning and to revisit information at later sessions as new interventions are made (Shaw, 2015). Specific applications of confidentiality and its limitations must be discussed early and frequently during the course of family therapy (Kleist & Bitter, 2014; Goldenberg et al., 2017). The family therapist and the family members need to agree to the specific limitations of confidentiality mandated by law and also to those the family practitioner may establish for effective treatment.

Informed consent can be more complex than it appears. Many times families enter counseling with one person in the family being perceived as the one with the problem or as the "identified patient." When therapy commences, however, the entire family is the focus of the therapist's intervention. Family members should have opportunities to raise questions and know as clearly as possible what they are getting involved in when they enter family therapy. Therapists might do well to consider the following ethical question: "What are my ethical responsibilities to each of the parties in this case?"

The informed consent document should include the conditions for family therapy to begin. For instance, some family therapists will conduct family sessions even if certain members refuse to attend. Other family therapists require that all members of the family participate in the therapy process. Should willing family members seeking assistance be denied family therapy because one individual refuses to participate? According to Wilcoxon and colleagues (2012), this is one of the most common ethical issues facing therapists who refuse treatment to a family unless all the members of that system become involved in the therapy. Many therapists strongly suggest that a reluctant family member participate for a session or two to determine what potential value there might be in family therapy. Some lack of cooperation can arise from a family member's feeling that he or she will be the main target of the sessions or that the member will face negative consequences from having divulged certain information.

There is no professional agreement on whether it is necessary to see all the family for change to take place, but we believe it is particularly important when it comes to therapy with children. The child is often the first family member presented for therapy, which can put an inordinate burden on the child. Including the whole family in therapy provides more protection for the child, and as the whole system corrects itself, the family can become a source of support for the child. In addition, family systems issues that may be contributing to the child's difficulty can be explored.

Contemporary Professional Issues

In this section we identify a few of the current professional issues in the practice of couples and family therapy. These include the personal, academic, and experiential qualifications necessary to practice in the field.

Personal Characteristics of the Family Therapist

The personal characteristics of the therapist are a major factor in creating an effective therapeutic alliance (see Chapter 2). Bitter (2014) identifies the following personal characteristics and attitudes of effective family practitioners: presence; acceptance, interest, and caring; assertiveness and confidence; courage and risk-taking; adaptability; appreciating the influence of diversity; tending to the spirit of the family and its members; and involvement, engagement, and satisfaction in working with families.

Self-knowledge with regard to family-of-origin issues is particularly critical for family therapists. Harway and Kadin (Harway et al., 2012) note that the dynamics of couples therapy often involve matters such as infidelity, separation and divorce, gender inequality, emotional abuse, cultural biases, and parenting styles. Therapists may have a blind spot that can affect the course of therapy. Specialized training, ongoing self-reflection, and supervision are required to become aware of and manage emotional reactions.

When we conduct therapy with a couple or a family, or with an individual who is sorting out a family-of-origin issue, our perceptions and reactions are likely to be influenced by our history in our family. If we are unaware of our own vulnerabilities, we might misinterpret our clients' comments or steer them in a direction that will not arouse our own anxiety. If we are aware of our emotional issues, we are less likely to get entangled in the problems of our clients, and we stand a better chance of working with them objectively and effectively. Couples and family therapists must manage many emotional challenges, and emotional competence is crucial to effective practice (Shaw, 2015).

Many trainers of family therapists believe that a practitioner's mental health, as defined by relationships with his or her family of origin, has implications for professional training. It is assumed that trainees can benefit from an exploration of the dynamics of both their family of origin and their present family because this exploration enables them to relate more effectively to the families they will meet in their clinical practice. From an ethical perspective, training programs must inform students prior to admission of the personal nature of their training.

Educational Requirements for Family Therapy

Family therapy practitioners must make a paradigm shift from an individual context to a systemic way of thinking. Many master's programs in counseling offer a specialization in relationship counseling or couples and family therapy. Components of the training program include the study of systems theory, an examination of family of origin, and an emphasis on ethical and professional issues specific to working with couples and families. Clinicians trained to deliver individual psychotherapy are not competent to make interventions from a systemic perspective without further training (Harway et al., 2012). The efficacy of systemic interventions for marriage and family counseling is increasingly noted in the literature. All couples and family training programs acknowledge that conceptual knowledge, clinical skills, and an understanding of ethical and professional issues are necessary to become a competent family therapist. According to Scher and Kozlowska (2012), like other helping professionals, many family therapists interact with clients in a "closed, private setting with no other professionals to notice, one way or the other, what actually transpires. . . . In this kind of setting, the best (and arguably only) way of promoting ethical professional conduct is by doing whatever is possible to ensure that the therapist is properly trained and that she acts in good faith and with good intentions" (p. 103).

As training programs have evolved, major didactic and experiential components have been identified. If you intend to work with families, you will need to gain experience in working with a variety of families from different ethnic and socioeconomic backgrounds who present a range of problems. A program offering both comprehensive coursework and clinical supervision provides the ideal learning environment.

Experiential Qualifications for Family Therapy

In training couples and family therapists, primary emphasis needs to be given to the quality of supervised practice and clinical experience. Academic knowledge comes alive in supervised practicum and internship experiences, and trainees learn how to use and apply their intervention skills. Clinical experience with families is of limited value without regularly scheduled supervisory sessions, especially during the early stages of training. It is through direct clinical contact with families, under close supervision, that trainees develop their own styles of interacting with families.

Experiential methods include both personal therapy and working with issues of one's own family of origin. Students are often expected to provide their own genogram as part of the coursework in a family therapy program. A rationale for personal therapeutic experiences is that such exploration enables trainees to increase their awareness of transference and countertransference, which enables trainees to relate more effectively to the families they meet in their clinical practice.

If clinicians are seeing families as part of their work, and if their program did not adequately prepare them for competence in intervening with families, they are vulnerable to a malpractice suit for practicing outside the boundaries of their competence. Those practitioners who did not receive specialized training in their program need to involve themselves in postgraduate in-service training or supervision. The AAMFT (2015) *Code of Ethics* offers this guideline regarding competence:

> Marriage and family therapists pursue knowledge of new developments and maintain their competence in marriage and family therapy through education, training, and/or supervised experience. (3.1.)
>
> While developing new skills in specialty areas, marriage and family therapists take steps to ensure the competence of their work and to protect clients from possible harm. Marriage and family therapists practice in specialty areas new to them only after appropriate education, training, and/or supervised experience. (3.6.)

Whether you are just beginning or are an experienced family therapist, you will need to periodically upgrade your skills through continuing education. There are many paths to the lifelong learning required of family practitioners.

The Case of Ludwig

Ludwig is a counselor whose education and training have been exclusively in individual counseling. Ella comes to him for counseling. After more than a dozen sessions with Ella, Ludwig realizes that much of her difficulty lies not just with her but with her entire family system. By this time Ludwig has established a strong working relationship with Ella. Because he has no experience in family therapy, he decides to refer Ella to a colleague who is trained in family therapy, but he realizes that doing so could have a detrimental effect on her. One of Ella's problems has been a sense of abandonment by her parents. He wants to avoid giving her the impression that he, too, is abandoning her. He decides to stay with her and work with her individually. Much of the time is spent trying to understand the dynamics of the family members who are not present.

- Do you agree with Ludwig's clinical decision? Do you agree with his rationale?
- From your perspective, would it have made a difference if he had consulted with Ella? Would it have made a difference if he had consulted with or obtained supervision from a colleague?
- Would it have been ethical for Ludwig to see the entire family and attempted to do family therapy for the benefit of his client, even though he was not trained as a family therapist?
- What if Ludwig had been trained in family systems but, when he suggested family sessions to Ella, she refused?

Commentary. Once Ludwig determined that Ella needed family therapy, which he was not qualified to provide, he had an ethical responsibility to refer her for family therapy. Whenever a therapist makes a referral, it is important to communicate to the client that the referral is related to the therapist's limitations rather than making the client responsible for the difficulty. If Ludwig shares his concerns with Ella about her possibly seeing his referral as a rejection or abandonment, Ella may be able to see that Ludwig's intentions come from a place of wanting what is best for her. Ludwig could suggest that he continue to see Ella for individual therapy for the problems not involving the family if Ella chose to do so. By supporting Ella in this way, her feelings of abandonment may be abated. Alternatively, Ludwig might suggest including a family therapist in a session with Ella, if doing so is feasible. This could help Ella to feel safe with the new therapist and lessen any feelings of abandonment. •

Values in Couples and Family Therapy

In Chapter 3 we talked about the impact of the therapist's values on the goals and direction of the therapeutic process. We now consider how values take on special significance in counseling couples and families. Ethical issues are raised in establishing criteria of psychosocial dysfunction, assessing the problems of the identified patient in the family context, and devising treatment strategies. Values pertaining to marriage, the preservation of the family, divorce, same-sex marriages, gender roles and the division of responsibility in the family, child rearing, adoption of children by same-sex couples, and extramarital affairs can all influence therapists' interventions. Therapists may take sides with one member of the family against another; they may impose their values on family members; or they may be more committed to keeping the family intact than are the family members themselves. Conversely, therapists may have a greater investment in seeing the family dissolve than do members of the family.

The value system of the therapist influences the formulation and definition of the problems the therapist sees in a family, the goals and plans for therapy, and the direction the therapy takes. It is an ethical mandate for therapists to be aware of how their values affect their work. The California Association of Marriage and Family Therapists' (CAMFT, 2011a) code of ethics states:

Marriage and family therapists make continuous efforts to be aware of how their cultural/racial/ethnic identity, values, and beliefs affect the process of therapy. Marriage and family therapists do not exert undue influence on the choice of treatment or outcomes based on such identities, values, and beliefs. (3.7.)

Counselors who, intentionally or unintentionally, impose their values on a couple or a family can do considerable harm. It is not the function of a therapist who works with couples and families to decide how members should change. We believe that the role of the therapist is to help all members see more clearly what they are doing, to help them make an honest evaluation of their present patterns, and to encourage them to make the changes they deem necessary. Couples and family therapists assist couples and families in negotiating the values they want to retain, modify, or discard.

What values and experiences of yours are likely to influence how you would work with couples and families? As you study the following two cases, reflect on how your sexual attitudes and values might influence your interventions. Then consult the ethics codes of various helping professions to identify standards that validate the responses given by the counselors in these cases.

The Case of Virginia and Tom

Virginia and Tom find themselves in a marital crisis when Virginia discovers that Tom has had several affairs during the course of their marriage. Tom agrees to see a marriage counselor. Tom says that he cannot see how his affairs necessarily got in the way of his relationship with his wife, especially since they were never meaningful. He believes that what is done is done and that it is pointless to dwell on past transgressions. He is upset over his wife's reaction to learning about his affairs. He says that he loves his wife and that he does not want to end the marriage. His involvements with other women were sexual in nature rather than committed love relationships. Virginia says that she would like to forgive her husband but that she finds it too painful to continue living with him knowing of his activities, even though they are in the past. She is not reassured by Tom's reactions to his past activities and fears that he might continue to rationalize these activities.

Counselor A. This counselor tells the couple at the initial session that from her experience extramarital affairs add many strains to a marriage, that people get hurt in such situations, and that affairs do pose problems for couples seeking counseling. However, she adds that affairs sometimes have positive benefits for both the wife and the husband. She says that her policy is to let the couple find out for themselves what is acceptable to them. She accepts Virginia and Tom as clients and asks them to consider as many options as they can to resolve their difficulties.

- Is this counselor neutral or biased? Explain.
- Is this counselor imposing her values by stating her stance on extramarital affairs at the first session? Explain.
- How practical and realistic does this approach seem to you? Explain.

Counselor B. From the outset this counselor makes it clear that she sees affairs as disruptive in any marriage or committed relationship. She maintains that affairs are typically started because of a deep dissatisfaction within the marriage and are symptomatic of other real conflicts. The counselor says she can help Tom and Virginia discover these conflicts in couples therapy. She further says that she will not work with them unless Tom's affairs are truly in the past, because she is convinced that counseling will not be effective unless Tom is fully committed to doing what is needed to work on his relationship with Virginia.

- Is this counselor imposing her values? Explain.
- Is it appropriate for the counselor to openly state her conditions and values from the outset? Why or why not?
- To what degree do you agree or disagree with this counselor's thinking and approach?

Counselor C. This counselor views the affairs much as Tom does. She points out that the couple seems to have a basically sound marriage and suggests that with some individual counseling Virginia can learn to get past the affairs.

- With her viewpoint, is it ethical for this counselor to accept this couple for counseling? Should she suggest a referral to another professional? Explain.
- Should the counselor have given more attention to the obvious pain expressed by Virginia?
- Should the counselor have kept her values and attitudes to herself so that she would be less likely to influence this couple's decision?

Commentary. Each of the three therapists' responses indicates definite values regarding infidelity in a committed relationship. By stating their personal values to Virginia and Tom, all three therapists are standing on shaky ethical ground. It is critical that therapists possess awareness of their personal values, but they should not impose their values either directly or indirectly. Not only do therapists need to recognize how their values pertaining to a committed relationship might influence their work, but they also need to be cognizant of any countertransference elicited by affairs. The therapist's job is to help this couple explore their own values to determine what they hope to accomplish from counseling and how committed they are to their relationship. The therapist might explore this question: Is it possible for this couple to reconcile their differing views on affairs? •

The Case of Emily and Lois

Emily and Lois, a same-sex couple, were married and now find themselves scorned and discriminated against by their neighbors. In addition, Emily had a child through in vitro fertilization, and Emily's parents have filed a petition in court to obtain custody of the child. The parents believe that the two women are unfit to raise a child because of their sexual/affectional orientation. Emily and Lois recognize that they need a support system that works for them, and they hope a counselor can help them sort out what is best for their family.

Counselor A. This counselor says that she cannot even imagine what it must be like for them to have to face the reactions of the neighbors and of Emily's parents on a daily basis. She indicates that she will make every effort to support and assist them in working through their situation.

- What are your reactions to this counselor's approach?
- Do you think the support the counselor is offering is enough in this case?

Counselor B. This counselor lets Emily and Lois know that they must have seen the problems inherent in returning home to a community that has a very strong antigay bias. He informs them that the best approach to the problem is to relocate to a more liberal community, at least for the sake of the child.

- What, if any, ethical issues do you see in this response? Is this counselor imposing his values?

- What interventions made by the counselor do you agree with? What are your areas of disagreement?
- What do the counselor's interventions suggest about how he is defining the problem?

Counselor C. This counselor feels a bit overwhelmed, especially in trying to define the problem. Is it a marriage problem? A problem pertaining to their sexual orientation? A community problem? A problem of oppression and discrimination?

- What are your reactions as you read the counselor's questions?
- Is the counselor feeling overwhelmed a sign that he is incompetent or a sign of his lack of skill or ability to wrestle with complexity?
- If you felt overwhelmed with this situation, how would you handle it?

Commentary. This case demonstrates the necessity for counselors to be prepared to deal with complex situations. Counselors should establish relationships for consultation in advance and know what resources are available to them. Counselor A's approach involves expressing empathy, validation, and support. Counselor B's advice places the burden of change on the clients rather than exploring what it feels like to be the victims of discrimination. Counselor C is wrestling with some very important questions and can discuss them with the clients to help them formulate an appropriate treatment plan.

In counseling this couple, we would begin by recognizing the complexity of the case and showing our support for the difficulty Emily and Lois are facing. We may choose to explore how the couple has navigated similar situations in the past. We would ask their permission to consult with legal, ethical, and clinical experts so that we could better assist them. We would probably ask Emily and Lois's thoughts on having a family session with the extended family of each of them. If Emily and Lois expressed an interest in family therapy, we would make an appropriate referral.

Same-sex marriage, even though legal in all states, continues to be hotly debated in both the political and personal spheres, but mental health counselors are required to avoid discrimination and to provide competent services to all couples. We still have a long way to go in training counselors to understand and work competently with clients in same-sex relationships. Evaluate how well prepared you think you are to work with a same-sex couple. Consider the following questions:

- How familiar are you with the current controversies pertaining to same-sex marriage?
- Where do you stand on the issue of same-sex marriage? Do you have any personal experiences or values that might hinder or help you in working with a same-sex couple?
- How effective is your graduate program in addressing key issues same-sex couples often face?
- To what degree do you think you are aware of heterosexual privilege and how this affects same-sex couples?
- How comfortable would you be discussing sexuality or sexual behaviors with a same-sex couple that was dealing with problems related to physical intimacy?
- How confident would you be in discussing sexuality or sexual behaviors with a heterosexual couple?

Gender-Sensitive Couples and Family Therapy

Gender-sensitive couples and family therapy attempts to help both women and men move beyond stereotyped gender roles. Sexist attitudes and patriarchal assumptions are examined for their impact on family relationships. With this approach, family therapy is conducted in an egalitarian fashion, and both therapist and client work collaboratively to empower individuals to choose roles rather than to be passive recipients of gender-role socialization.

All therapists need to be aware of their values and beliefs about gender. In Chapter 4 we discussed the importance of being aware of how your culture has influenced your personality. Likewise, the way you define gender issues has a great deal to do with your cultural background. A challenge to all family therapists is to be culturally sensitive, gender sensitive, and to avoid imposing their personal values on individuals, couples, and families. Lebow and Stroud (2016) view culture and gender as being central in family therapy practice: "Today, most family therapy methods emphasize an understanding of gender, adaptation to client culture, and full equal regard for all family forms" (p. 341).

Counselors who work with couples and families can practice more ethically if they are aware of the cultural history, the effects of heterosexism, and the impact of gender stereotyping as these are reflected in the socialization process in families, including their own. All practitioners must continually evaluate their own beliefs about appropriate family roles and responsibilities, child-rearing practices, sexual orientations, multiple roles, and nontraditional vocations for women and men. Counselors also must have the knowledge to help their clients explore educational, vocational, and emotional goals that they previously deemed unreachable. The principles of gender-aware therapy are of great importance to counselors as they help clients identify and work through gender concepts that may have limited them.

Feminist Perspective on Family Therapy

Some feminist therapists have been critical of the clinical practice of family therapy, contending that it has been filled with outdated patriarchal assumptions and grounded on a male-biased perspective of gender roles and gender-defined functions within the family. Feminists assert that our patriarchal society subjugates women and blames them for inadequate mothering. Feminists remind us that patriarchy has negative effects on both women and men. They assert that gender and cultural issues need to be taken into account in the practice of family therapy and when people are engaged in ethical decision making (Kleist & Bitter, 2014).

A **feminist view of family therapy** focuses on gender and power in relationships and encourages a personal commitment to challenge gender inequity. They espouse a vision of a future society that values equality between women and men. Examining the power differential in their relationships often helps partners demystify differences between them. Feminist family therapists share a number of roles, each of which is based on a specific value orientation; they make their values and beliefs explicit so that the therapy process is clearly understood; they strive to establish egalitarian roles with clients; they work toward client autonomy and client empowerment; and they emphasize commonalities among women.

Feminist therapists contend that all therapists have values and that it is important to be clear with clients about these values. This is different, however, from imposing values on clients. An imposition of values is inconsistent with viewing clients as their own best experts. Clients should be encouraged to make their own choices; their choices can be challenged but need to be supported by their therapist. It is clear that feminist therapists do not take a neutral stance with respect to gender roles and power in relationships. They advocate for definite change in the social structure, especially in the area of equality, power in relationships, the right to self-determination, freedom to pursue a career outside the home, the right to an education, and social justice for all races, cultures, and sexual orientations.

These feminist values may not conform to the values people in other cultures hold. Values such as equality and self-determination may not be prized as much in some cultures as honoring one's extended family and putting the welfare of the family before one's personal agenda. Above all, the therapist must be respectful of the client's value system.

A Nonsexist Perspective on Family Therapy

Regardless of their particular theoretical orientation, family therapists must take whatever steps are necessary to account for gender issues in their practice and to become nonsexist family therapists. In a classic article, Margolin (1982) provides a number of recommendations (that still have relevance today) on how to be a nonsexist family therapist and how to use the therapeutic process to challenge the oppressive consequences of stereotyped roles and expectations in the family. One recommendation is that family therapists examine their own behavior for comments and questions that imply that women and men should perform specific roles and hold a specific status. For example, a therapist can show bias in subtle and nonverbal ways, such as looking at the woman when talking about rearing children or addressing the man when talking about any important decisions that need to be made. Further, Margolin contends that family therapists are particularly vulnerable to the following biases: (1) assuming that remaining married would be the best choice for a woman, (2) demonstrating less interest in a woman's career than in a man's career, (3) encouraging couples to accept the belief that child rearing is principally the responsibility of the mother, (4) showing a different reaction to a wife's affair than to a husband's, and (5) giving more attention to the husband's needs than to the wife's needs. She raises two important questions dealing with the ethics of doing therapy with couples and families:

- How does the therapist respond when members of the family seem to agree that they want to work toward goals that (from the therapist's vantage point) are sexist in nature?
- To what extent is the therapist culturally sensitive, especially when a family member's definition of gender-role identities differs from the therapist's view?

As you read the case examples below, think about your own values. What are your views pertaining to gender, and how might your values affect your way of counseling others?

The Case of Marge and Al

Marge and Al come to marriage counseling to work on the stress they are experiencing in rearing their two adolescent sons. The couple directs the focus of treatment toward how little their sons are doing to contribute to the family. In the course of therapy, the counselor learns that both Marge and Al have full-time jobs outside the home. In addition, Marge has sole responsibility for all the household chores and management as well. Her husband refuses to share any domestic responsibilities. Marge doesn't question her dual career. Neither of them shows much interest in exploring the division of responsibilities in their relationship. Instead, they focus the sessions on getting advice about how to handle problems with their sons.

- What would you do with their presenting problem—their trouble with their sons? What might the behavior of the sons imply?
- Is it ethical for the therapist to focus only on the expressed concerns of Marge and Al? Does the therapist have a responsibility to challenge this couple to look at how they have defined themselves and their relationship through assumptions about gender roles, and how their values and actions may be influencing the behavior of their sons?
- If you were counseling this couple, what would you do? How would your interventions reflect your values in this case?

Commentary. This case represents a fairly frequent dilemma for family therapists. These overextended parents may have little time to give to their children, yet the children are presented as the problem. This needs to be explored without blaming the parents. By working with the entire family, we can make an accurate assessment of the nature of the problem. It is often the family system that requires intervention, not the child or parent alone. We agree with the systems perspective that a "problem child" often reflects problems within the family system.

This case illustrates how critical it is for therapists to be aware of their values pertaining to gender as well as being aware of their own gender bias. For example, a more egalitarian therapist will have to resist imposing his or her values regarding the distribution of domestic duties within the marriage, especially if strong cultural or religious values underlie the couple's practices. The therapist could explore with the couple how satisfied they are with the way they have defined their relationship and challenge them to come up with their own solutions. If they could change anything about their roles in the relationship, what might that look like? •

As you think about this case and the following two cases, ask yourself how your values regarding traditional roles for wives and mothers might affect your work with clients like Melody and Naomi.

The Case of Melody

Melody, 38, is married and has returned to college to obtain a teaching credential. During the intake session she tells the counselor that she is experiencing conflicting feelings and is contemplating some major changes in her life. She has met a man who shares her interest and enthusiasm for school as well as many other aspects of her life. She is considering leaving her husband and children to pursue her own interests.

Which of the following reactions, if any, reflect your thinking? If you were Melody's counselor, would you be inclined to bring up any of these points with your new client?

- "Perhaps this is a phase you are going through. It happens to a lot of women who return to college. Maybe you should slow down and think about it."
- "You may have regrets later on if you leave your children in such an impulsive fashion."
- "Many women in your position would be afraid to do what you are thinking about doing."
- "I hate to see you divorce without having some marriage counseling first to determine whether that is what you want."
- "Maybe you ought to look at the prospects of living alone for a while. The idea of moving out of a relationship with your husband and right into a new relationship with another man concerns me."

Think about how your values would influence your interventions with Melody.

Commentary. The therapist's role is to facilitate a process that provides Melody with the opportunity to arrive at her own answers—ones that are congruent with her values. All of the therapists' statements above represent legitimate issues to explore with Melody, but the statements come from assumptions made by the therapist and reflect his or her own values. These statements all fall in the giving advice category rather than in helping Melody find her own way. To aid Melody in making this decision, we might ask her questions such as "What is it like for you to be considering this decision?" "What scares you the most, or makes you most excited, as you think about your course of action?" or "Are there any aspects of your decision that you want to explore more fully?" It is important for therapists to assist clients in achieving their long-term interests by carefully exploring potential outcomes of major life decisions. In this case, it may be relevant to explore Melody's cultural and societal expectations of women and family. •

The Case of Naomi

The White family (consisting of wife, husband, four children, and the wife's parents) has been involved in family therapy for several months. During one of the sessions, Naomi (the wife) expresses the desire to return to her career as an athletic coach. This wish causes tremendous resistance on the part of every member of her family. Her husband says that he wants her to continue to be involved in his professional life and that, although he admires her ambitions, he simply feels that it would put too much strain on the entire family if they were both to work outside of the home. Naomi's parents are shocked by their daughter's desire, viewing it as selfish, and they urge her to put the family's welfare first. The children express their desires for a full-time mother. Naomi feels great pressure from all sides, yet she seems committed to following through with her professional plans. She is aware of the sacrifices that would be associated with her going back to work, but she is asking for everyone in the family to make adjustments so she can fulfill her professional dreams. She is convinced that her plans would not be detrimental to the family's welfare. The therapist shows an obvious bias by giving no attention or support to Naomi's desires and by not asking the family to consider making any basic adjustments.

- Do you think this therapist is guilty of furthering gender-role stereotypes?
- Do his interventions show an interest in the well-being of the entire family?
- What are other potential ethical issues in this case?
- Being aware of your own bias regarding gender roles, how would you work with this family?

- Should the therapist's goal be to help everyone in the family be content with a particular decision or to help them navigate the decision-making process without focusing on a set outcome?

- Assume that the therapist had an obvious bias in favor of Naomi's plans and advised the family to learn to accept her decision. Do you see any potential ethical issues in this approach? Do you think a therapist can remain neutral in this kind of case? Explain your stance.

Commentary. This therapist's values are influencing identification and exploration of the family's problems. This case illustrates how critical it is that therapists understand their personal beliefs and values and guard against imposing them in work with clients. The lack of support for Naomi's aspirations should be a key focus for exploration in therapy for this family. Yet Naomi is without support from her therapist, just as she is without support from her husband, children, and parents. The therapist is not listening to Naomi's concerns. Instead, he is colluding with the family by subtly discouraging her from following through with her plans.

Couples fall into habits regarding roles and responsibilities, so it may be useful to ask how their roles were negotiated and whether they want to reevaluate their roles as their responsibilities have shifted. It is not uncommon for one partner to feel resentful about his or her duties while the other person may feel that the status quo is acceptable. It is possible to question the couple without pushing an agenda. The goal of the inquiry should be to help the couple achieve greater insight about their situation rather than to reach a specific outcome influenced by the therapist's values. •

Responsibilities of Couples and Family Therapists

In her seminal article, Margolin (1982) argues persuasively that difficult ethical questions confronted in individual therapy become even more complicated when a number of family members are seen together. She observes that the dilemma with multiple clients is that in some instances an intervention that serves one person's best interests could burden another family member or even be countertherapeutic. Therapists avoid becoming agents of any one family member, believing that all family members contribute to the problems of the whole family. Ethical practice demands that therapists be clear about their commitments to each member of the family.

Therapist Responsibilities in Counseling Couples

Therapist responsibilities are also a crucial issue in counseling with couples. This is especially true when the partners do not have a common purpose for seeking counseling. How do therapists carry out their ethical responsibilities when one partner comes for divorce counseling and the other wants to work on saving the marriage?

A key consideration is whether to treat a couple's conflict and relationship issues in individual therapy or in conjoint therapy. Individual therapy is common, but Chambers, Solomon, and Gurman (2016) note that conjoint therapy is the treatment of choice in addressing problems encountered by a couple. Couples therapy has become the main practice within the broad field of family therapy, and the efficacy of couples therapy is well established in hundreds of randomized controlled trials. "Specifically, research has found that 70% of couples show improvement with couple therapy" (p. 321). Therapists who conduct conjoint therapy have the professional responsibility of receiving training in couples therapy and practicing ethically. They must be competent in addressing the special considerations involved in working with couples.

Therapist Responsibilities in Intimate Partner Violence

Intimate partner violence is a well-recognized mental health issue that affects people from all ethnic and socioeconomic backgrounds. Women are more often the target of domestic violence, but men may also be victims. Intimate partner violence occurs in both same-sex and heterosexual relationships. Under current law, mental health providers generally are not required to report intimate partner violence. It is assumed that clients would not be forthcoming about their abuse, either as victims or perpetrators, if they knew the situation would be reported. Counselors working with clients experiencing intimate partner violence need to make difficult decisions regarding how to intervene in such cases if reporting is not done. The therapist's goal is to protect victims from any further harm, including protecting any children the couple may have at home. In most states, counselors are required to report a situation of child abuse if children are known to have witnessed domestic violence because they may be psychologically damaged.

As you begin to explore this difficult subject, examine your own responses to the complex issues pertaining to intimate partner violence by answering these questions:

- Do you agree with the law that counselors are not mandated to report all incidences of intimate partner abuse in their clients? Why or why not?
- What are some potential clinical benefits of not having to report the existence of domestic violence in a relationship?
- What drawbacks or risks exist to the counselor, the perpetrator, and the victims by not reporting intimate partner violence?
- Because counselors are not mandated reporters, are they part of the problem?
- What personal experiences do you have that might be triggered by working with a client who is either the perpetrator of, or a victim of, intimate partner violence? How might this affect your ability to work effectively with this client?

In the case of domestic violence, clinicians agree that conducting couples therapy while there is ongoing domestic violence presents a potential danger to the abused and is therefore unethical. The failure to recognize domestic violence can have disastrous consequences for both the family and the therapist. Lebow and Stroud (2016) point out that it may be unsafe to bring individuals together for family therapy or conjoint sessions in cases involving family violence or high conflict. The therapist is responsible for determining when there is a potential for physical or emotional danger. If the abuser has completed a course of treatment, there may be a possibility of doing therapy with the couple, depending on the assessment provided by the treatment facility. In situations involving domestic violence, there are both ethical and legal issues to consider. In cases where there are conflicts between ethical and legal dimensions of practice, it is especially important for couples therapists to seek consultation.

The Case of Willa

Roselle, an experienced school counselor, has been working with 16-year-old female student Willa, who recently disclosed that she is in an "abusive" relationship with her 17-year-old boyfriend, Sawyer. Willa said she would deny everything if Roselle reports it or tells Willa's parents. To make things more complicated, Willa's mother is a physical education teacher at the school, and Roselle often runs into her in meetings and in the staff lounge. Willa's mother had given her consent for Roselle to meet with her daughter and had remarked in a sarcastic tone, "If she tells you anything awful, I don't want to know about it!" Roselle's concerns for her client are growing as Willa has shown up to sessions with bruises and has stopped sharing any information about her relationship with Sawyer. Roselle decides not to break confidentiality at this point. She continues to work with Willa to gain her trust, and she hopes to find out more about the kind of "abuse" that is occurring between the teenagers.

- What legal and ethical obligations does the school counselor have in this situation?
- Is this a case of child abuse or domestic violence, or both? Based on your answer, what are your obligations regarding reporting?
- What clinical concerns would you have about working with Willa if you were to tell her mother or make a report?
- Would you consider meeting with Willa and her mother? Why or why not?
- Would you consider bringing Sawyer in for a session? Why or why not?

Commentary. We agree that Roselle needs to gather more information from Willa before determining whether she needs to involve Willa's mother. The fact that Willa's mother works in the same school does not give Roselle the right to talk more openly with her than she would with another client's parent. However, because Willa is a minor, her parents have the right to information regarding Willa's sessions if they ask for it.

Initially, we would not bring Sawyer or Willa's parents into sessions. We would focus on working closely with Willa to get a better picture of her situation and to determine if she or her partner is in any danger. We would try to find out if Sawyer is a student at the same school or a different school and if he is indeed only 17 years old. If he is much older than Willa, this may be a case of child abuse rather than intimate partner abuse. We would not bring Sawyer in at this point because this could increase Willa's risk if she is the victim. We would also check the laws in our state regarding abuse between minors to determine how to proceed. •

LO8

Confidentiality in Couples and Family Therapy

Confidentiality assumes unique significance in the practice of couples and family therapy. The challenges to confidentiality increase exponentially, say Kleist and Bitter (2014), when practitioners work with multiple people in one room. They add that ethical issues regarding confidentiality become more complex and extremely difficult in the practice of family therapy. Some of these ethical concerns involve conceptualizing the client(s) served, providing informed consent, and handling relational matters in an individual context.

Adding an online component makes a challenging situation even more complicated in cases of couples and family therapy (Wilcoxon, 2015). Confidentiality tends to be less reliable in online therapy than in face-to-face therapeutic encounters. Hackers, online viruses, and other problems that can occur during online exchanges pose threats to confidentiality. The Ethics Codes box titled "Confidentiality in Counseling Couples and Families" provides some guidelines for best practices.

ETHICS CODES: Confidentiality in Counseling Couples and Families

American Association for Marriage and Family Therapy (2015)
Marriage and family therapists disclose to clients and other interested parties at the outset of services the nature of confidentiality and possible limitations of the clients' right to confidentiality. Therapists review with clients the circumstances where confidential information may be requested and where disclosure of confidential information may be legally required. Circumstances may necessitate repeated disclosures. (2.1.)

American Counseling Association (2014)
In couples and family counseling, counselors clearly define who is considered 'the client' and discuss expectations and limitations of confidentiality. Counselors seek agreement and document in writing such agreement among all involved parties regarding the confidentiality of information. In the absence of an agreement to the contrary, the couple or family is considered to be the client. (B.4.b.)

International Association of Marriage and Family Counselors (2011)
Couple and family counselors inform clients that statements made by a family member to the counselor during an individual counseling, consultation, or collateral contact are to be treated as confidential. Such statements are not disclosed to other family members without the individual's permission. However, the couple and family counselor should clearly identify the client of counseling, which may be the couple or family system, and inform clients in writing who(m) the intended client is. Couple and family counselors should inform clients that they do not maintain family secrets, collude with some family members against others, or otherwise contribute to dysfunctional family system dynamics. If a client's refusal to share information from individual contacts interferes with the agreed goals of counseling, the counselor may terminate treatment and refer the clients to another counselor. Some couple and family counselors choose to not meet with individuals, preferring to serve family systems. (Section B.)

Differing Perspectives on Confidentiality with Multiple Clients

Couples and family therapists must clarify what confidentiality means for the couple or the family group and how it will be maintained. Issues of confidentiality with multiple clients tend to arise around dealing with secrets (Wilcoxon et al., 2012). Should the therapist attempt to have families explore all of their secrets?

What are the pros and cons of revealing a family secret if some members are likely to suffer from extreme discomfort if the secret is disclosed? Some couples therapists will not see the couple (or will stop seeing the couple) if an affair is going on and the person is unwilling to terminate it.

Therapists have differing perspectives on the role of confidentiality when working with couples or families. One view is that therapists should not divulge in a family session any information given to them by individuals in private sessions. In the case of couples counseling, some practitioners are willing to see each spouse for individual sessions. Information given to them by one spouse is kept confidential. Others refuse to see any member of the family separately, claiming that doing so fosters unproductive alliances and promotes the keeping of secrets. Some therapists tell family members that they will exercise their own judgment about what to disclose from an individual session in a couples or family session.

Some therapists who work with couples or entire families go further. They have a policy of refusing to keep information secret that was shared individually. Their view is that secrets are counterproductive for effective couples or family therapy. Hidden agendas are seen as material that should be brought out into the open during a couples or family session. Some therapists inform their clients that any information given to them during private sessions will be divulged as they see fit in accordance with the greatest benefit for the couple or the family. Benitez (2004) takes the position that a "no secrets" policy is essential for therapists who offer couples counseling. According to Benitez, this policy should state that information shared with the therapist by one member of the couple outside of the presence of the other might be disclosed to the partner at the therapist's discretion. Such a policy frees the therapist from being put in the position of keeping a secret of a client participating in conjoint therapy. However, each person must be informed of this policy in advance and also agree to it. Couples may need to be reminded of this policy frequently. Therapists who have not promised confidentiality are not free of problems and thus must carefully consider the therapeutic ramifications of their actions.

A good example of a potential problem involves one member of a couple informing the therapist during an individual session that he or she is involved in an extramarital affair. This person asks, or even demands, that the therapist not divulge the "secret." Shaw (2015) contends if the therapist and one of the individuals hold a secret between them, collusion is the result. Secrecy such as this "can undermine a therapeutic goal of secure attachment, and compromise the duty to provide equal advocacy for all parties" (p. 513). The late Jay Haley, a noted family therapist, used to say that once a secret is told to the therapist without the other partner's knowledge, "you've already colluded." This provides the rationale that some family practitioners have for making it a policy to only see the couple or family as a unit.

Therapists should explain, negotiate, and set the parameters of services from the very beginning of therapy. This includes getting all parties to agree to limits to confidentiality within the couple–therapist system and putting this in writing (Butler, Seedall, & Harper, 2008). Echoing this view, attorney Richard Leslie (as cited in Riemersma, 2007) states that therapists need to inform their clients from the beginning of the professional relationship of the limits of confidentiality. Leslie contends that this disclosure should involve explaining a "no secrets" policy, both verbally and in writing, including why such a policy is necessary. The main reason for this policy is to clearly inform the participants that the therapist's primary obligation is to appropriately and effectively treat the couple or the family unit. The client needs to know that this policy is designed to prevent a conflict from arising between an individual participant and the unit being treated. According to Leslie, the bottom line is that therapists should make it clear that they reserve the right to use their best clinical judgment as to what is necessary to share with the client so that effective treatment can occur.

A Case of a Therapist's Quandary

A man is involved in individual therapy to resolve a number of personal conflicts, of which the state of his relationship is only one. Later, his girlfriend comes in for some joint sessions. In their joint sessions much time is spent on how betrayed the girlfriend feels over having discovered that her boyfriend had an affair in the past. She is angry and hurt but has agreed to remain in the relationship and to come to these therapy sessions as long as the boyfriend agrees not to resume the past affair or to initiate new ones. The boyfriend agrees to her requests. The therapist does not explicitly state her views about confidentiality, nor does she explain a "no secrets" policy, but the boyfriend assumes that she will keep to herself what she hears in both the girlfriend's private sessions and his private sessions. During one of the conjoint sessions, the therapist states that maintaining or initiating an affair is counterproductive if they both want to work on improving their relationship.

In a later individual session the boyfriend tells the therapist that he has begun a new affair. He brings this up privately with his therapist because he feels some guilt over not having lived up to the agreement. But he maintains that the affair is not negatively influencing his relationship with his girlfriend and has helped him to tolerate many of the difficulties he has been experiencing in his relationship. He also asks that the therapist not mention this in a conjoint session, for he fears that his girlfriend will leave him if she finds out that he is involved with another woman. Think about these questions in deciding on the ethical course of action:

- The therapist has not explicitly stated her view of confidentiality and has not discussed her "no secrets" policy. Is it ethical for her to bring up the boyfriend's new affair in a conjoint session?

- How does the therapist handle her conviction regarding affairs in light of the fact that the boyfriend tells her that it is actually enhancing, not interfering with, the relationship?

- Should the therapist attempt to persuade the boyfriend to give up the affair? Should she persuade the client to bring up this matter himself in a conjoint session? Is the therapist colluding with the boyfriend against the girlfriend by not bringing up this matter?

- Should the therapist discontinue therapy with this couple because of her strong bias? If she does suggest termination and referral to another professional, what reasons would she give for doing so? What might the therapist say if the girlfriend is upset over the suggestion of a referral and wants to know the reasons?

- Should the therapist have initiated couples therapy when she had already taken the role of an individual therapist for the boyfriend?

Commentary. It was crucial for this therapist to clearly state her stance on secrets when she began working with the couple, especially how she would deal with secrets pertaining to affairs. This case is a good example of what can happen when a therapist fails to clearly inform her clients from the outset about the limits of confidentiality. Because of her failure to provide for informed consent by stipulating a "no secrets" policy, this therapist is limited in her ability to work with this couple therapeutically.

Ethical standards do not mandate that affairs must be disclosed. As a clinical issue, however, such secrets can pose a real challenge to the therapist's work and may influence the outcomes with couples. Shaw (2015) aptly states this challenge: "A practice policy about disclosure of secrets is both crucial and simultaneously fraught with tensions about competing accountabilities in relationship work" (p. 513). If therapists fail to make clear to couples how secrets will be handled when they are revealed by one of the partners, this issue takes on ethical dimensions. Unless the secrets are brought to the surface and explored, progress will likely be impeded in the therapy sessions. ●

Chapter Summary

The challenges of meeting the needs of multiple clients can be daunting but also can reap great rewards. A systems approach to therapy can encourage deeper growth on the part of clients and the relationships that are significant to them. The field of couples and family therapy is rapidly expanding and developing. With an expansion in educational programs comes the need for specialized training and experience. A thorough discussion of ethical issues must be part of all such programs. A few of these issues are determining who is the primary client, dealing with confidentiality, policies on handling secrets, providing informed consent, counseling with minors, and exploring the role of values in family therapy.

The task of the therapist is to help a couple or a family explore and clarify their own values, not to influence them to accept the therapist's value system. Likewise, a key ethical issue is the impact of the therapist's life experiences on his or her ability to practice effectively and objectively. As is true regarding all ethical issues, there is a significant relationship between sound ethical practices and clinical decision making. Family therapists may experience confusion, for example, regarding the ethical aspects of deciding who will attend family sessions. It is obvious, however, that such decisions cannot be made without a solid foundation in clinical theory and methodology. With increased knowledge and practical experience, therapists can make these ethical decisions with greater certainty. Being open to periodic supervision, seeking consultation when necessary, and being willing to participate in one's own therapy are some ways in which couples and family therapists can refine their clinical skills and maintain their competence.

Suggested Activities

1. In the practice of couples and family therapy, informed consent is especially important. As a class discussion topic, explore some of these issues: What are the ethical implications of insisting that all members of a family participate in family therapy? What kind of information should a family therapist present from the outset to all those involved? Are there any ethical conflicts in focusing on the welfare of the entire family rather than on what might be in the best interests of a family member?

2. Investigate the status of regulating professional practice in couples and family therapy in your state, including the academic and training requirements, if any, for certification or licensure in this field.

3. In a small group, discuss the major ethical problems facing couples and family therapists. Consider issues such as confidentiality, enforced therapy involving all family members, qualifications of effective family therapists, denying therapy for a family member, imposing the values of the therapist on a family, and practicing beyond one's competence.

4. Design a project to study your own family of origin. Interview as many relatives as you can. Look for patterns in your own relationships, including problems you currently struggle with, that might stem from your family of origin. What advantages do you see in studying your own family as one way to prepare yourself for counseling families?

5. This exercise is from Jim Bitter's (2014) text, *Theory and Practice of Family Therapy and Counseling*. Reflect on your own family of origin. What are some of the perspectives on family, culture, and gender that were contained in your upbringing? How many kinds of families and cultural perspectives have you been exposed to in your lifetime? What experiences, if any, did your family of origin have of discrimination or oppression based on cultural differences?

6. Imagine that you are participating on a board to establish standards—personal, academic, and experiential—for family therapists. What qualifications would you establish as necessary conditions for becoming an effective family therapist? What do you think the minimum requirements should be to prepare a trainee to work with families? What would your ideal training program for couples and family therapists look like?

7. Review the cases in this chapter and select the one case you find most interesting. Envision yourself as the couples or family therapist in this particular case. Apply the ethical decision making model (introduced in Chapter 1) to the case by showing the steps you would take in addressing the issues (ethical, clinical, cultural, legal) involved.

8. Discuss in dyads or triads how you would navigate the issue of dealing with secrets in couples and family therapy?

MindTap for Counseling

Go to MindTap® for digital study tools and resources that complement this text and help you be more successful in your course and career. There's an interactive eBook plus videos of client sessions, skill-building activities, quizzes to help you prepare for tests, apps, and more—all in one place. If your instructor *didn't* assign MindTap, you can find out more about it at CengageBrain.com.

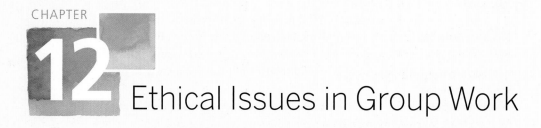

Ethical Issues in Group Work

LEARNING OBJECTIVES

1. Grasp the key ethical aspects in the training and supervision of group leaders

2. Explain ethical issues in diversity training for group workers

3. Describe guidelines for multicultural and social justice competence in group work

4. Recognize some ethical considerations involved in coleadership of groups

5. Discuss ethical issues in forming a group

6. Identify ethical issues in screening and selecting members of a group

7. Clarify ethical issues in working with involuntary group members

8. Delineate some psychological risks involved in group participation

9. Understand the role and limitations of confidentiality in groups

10. Summarize privacy and confidentiality issues involved with social media in group work

11. Describe what is involved in ethical and effective termination in group work

12. Differentiate between evidence-based practice and practice-based evidence in group work

SELF-INVENTORY

Directions: For each statement, indicate the response that most closely identifies your beliefs and attitudes. Use the following code:

5 = I *strongly agree* with this statement.

4 = I *agree* with this statement.

3 = I am *undecided* about this statement.

2 = I *disagree* with this statement.

1 = I *strongly disagree* with this statement.

_____ 1. If I am qualified to practice individual therapy, I can effectively conduct group therapy.

_____ 2. Ethical practice requires that prospective group members be carefully screened and selected.

_____ 3. It is important to prepare members so that they can derive the maximum benefit from the group.

_____ 4. Requiring people to participate in a therapy group raises special ethical issues.

_____ 5. It is unethical to allow a group to exert any kind of pressure on one of its members.

_____ 6. Confidentiality is less important in groups than it is in individual therapy.

_____ 7. Socializing among group members is almost always undesirable.

_____ 8. One way of minimizing psychological risks to group participants is to negotiate contracts with the members.

_____ 9. A group leader has a responsibility to teach members how to translate what they have learned in the group to their outside lives.

_____ 10. It is unethical for counselor educators to lead groups of their students in training.

_____ 11. Group psychotherapy cannot be conducted in an ethical manner online except in very limited circumstances.

_____ 12. It is the group leader's responsibility to make prospective members aware of their rights and responsibilities and to demystify the process of a group.

_____ 13. Group members should know that they have the right to leave the group at any time.

_____ 14. Before people enter a group, it is the leader's responsibility to discuss the personal risks involved, especially potential life changes, and help them explore their readiness to face these risks.

_____ 15. It is a sound practice to provide written ethical guidelines to group members in advance and discuss them in the first meeting.

Introduction

Practitioners are creating a multitude of groups to fit the needs of a diverse clientele in schools and community mental health agencies. In many agencies and institutions, group work is the primary form of treatment, and the types of groups that can be designed are limited only by one's imagination. Group work is not a second-rate modality; it is a treatment of choice for many clients (M. Corey, Corey, & Corey, 2018). Along with the increased use of group therapy has come a rising ethical awareness. Practitioners who work with groups face a variety of ethical quandaries that differ from those encountered in individual therapy. We are giving group work special attention, as we did with couples and family therapy, because it raises unique ethical concerns.

Our illustrations of important ethical considerations in this chapter are drawn from a broad spectrum of groups, including therapy groups, counseling groups, personal-growth groups, and psychoeducational groups. Obviously, these groups differ with respect to their member population, purpose, focus, and procedures, as well as in the level of training required for the facilitators of these groups. Although these distinctions are important, all groups face some common ethical concerns: leader values, screening and orientation of group members, informed consent, voluntary and involuntary group membership, training group leaders, confidentiality, multiple relationships in group work, diversity and multiculturalism, and procedures concerning termination and follow-up (Rapin, 2014).

LO1

Ethical Issues in Training and Supervision of Group Leaders

For competent group leaders to emerge, training programs must make group work a priority. With adequate training and through participating in a group as a member, you will have opportunities to acquire competence in facilitating a range of groups. Group workers must remain current and increase their knowledge and skills through activities such as continuing education, supervision, and participation in various personal and professional development activities (ASGW, 2008). Familiarize yourself with referral resources and refrain from working with client populations that need special assistance beyond your level of competence.

Barlow (2008) maintains that groups can be used effectively for both prevention and education. Barlow emphasizes the importance of adequate training for practitioners who are interested in conducting groups so that they can effectively and ethically maximize the unique group properties in their work.

Our Views on the Ethical Training of Group Workers

Professional codes, legislative mandates, and institutional policies alone will not assure competent group leadership. Group counselor trainees need to understand and reflect on some of the typical ethical dilemmas they will face in practice. This can best be done by including ethics in the trainees' academic program as well as discussing ethical issues that grow out of the students' experiences in practicum, internship, and fieldwork. One effective way to teach ethical decision making is by presenting trainees with case vignettes of typical problems that occur in group situations and encouraging discussion of the ethical issues and pertinent guidelines. We tell both students and professionals who attend our workshops that they will not always have the answers to dilemmas they encounter in their groups. Ethical decision making is an ongoing process that takes on new forms and increased meaning as practitioners gain experience. Group leaders need to be receptive to self-examination and to questioning the professionalism of their group practice if they hope to become competent, ethical group practitioners.

In addition to learning about ethical decision making regarding dilemmas encountered in group work, we highly recommend four other experiences as adjuncts to a training program for group workers: (1) personal experience in an experiential group, (2) personal (individual) psychotherapy, (3) group supervision, and (4) observing group therapy sessions.

Self-Exploration and Experiential Groups The CACREP (2016) standards require students to gain at least 10 hours of experience in a small group as a group member. This requirement is typically met by including an experiential group as part of a group counseling course; however, to avoid conflicts, some programs ask students to participate in a group outside of the program and document their hours. In an experiential group, students often have an opportunity to be part of a group experience and at times to facilitate the process of this group. In an experiential learning environment that involves extensive self-disclosure and dual relationships between instructors and students, students need to know they can trust their instructor's skill, ethics, and professionalism.

Students engaged in experiential training must be willing to engage in self-disclosure, to become active participants in an interpersonal group, and to engage themselves on an emotional as well as a cognitive level. Instructors can do a great deal to create a sense of safety and trust among the group members by explaining to them ways to avoid breaching confidentiality. It is important to clarify with students throughout the course how to talk about their own work with people outside of the group without revealing the identity or self-disclosures of other members (Corey, Corey, Muratori, Austin, & Austin, 2017). McCarthy, Falco, and Villalba (2014) stress the importance of structuring experiential growth groups in a manner that "supports growth and minimizes potential ethical risks" (p. 188). Among the measures instructors may take to minimize risk to student participants are discussions about the depth of self-disclosure appropriate to the context, explaining students' rights to decline answering questions that make them particularly uncomfortable, and providing options for continued emotional support outside of the experiential group (Julia Whisenhunt, personal communication, October 5, 2016).

Group leaders need to demonstrate the willingness to do for themselves what they expect members in their groups to do: expand their awareness of self and the effect that self has on others. As an adjunct to formal coursework and internship training, participation in a therapeutic group is extremely valuable. One of the best ways to learn how to assist group members in their struggles is to be a member of a group yourself. Learning about group counseling through coursework and didactic instruction alone is not considered sufficient. A survey of 82 master's-level counseling programs suggests that experiential group training is alive, evolving, and an accepted form for training group leaders (Shumaker, Ortiz, & Brenninkmeyer, 2011). Supporting this view, McCarthy and colleagues (2014) point out that the use of experiential groups for counselor trainees is found in the *Ethics Code* of the American Counseling Association (2014) and the "Best Practice Guidelines" of the Association for Specialists in Group Work (2008). In addition to enhancing personal growth, they note that such training provides participants with a solid understanding of the stages of group work, group dynamics, and group techniques that facilitate meaningful interactions.

If a self-exploration group or an experiential group is a program requirement, it is ethically imperative that students are made aware of this requirement at an orientation meeting during the admission process or prior to the time they enroll in a program. When participation in an experiential group is part of a program, it is important that safeguards are in place to manage boundaries and to reduce the risk of harm to students. Shumaker and colleagues' (2011) survey of experiential group training in counseling master's programs resulted in them recommending systematic instructor self-reflection, informed consent of students, and self-disclosure training as "the most promising and critical safeguard elements dedicated to promoting a positive experiential group experience" (p. 127).

Goodrich and Luke (2012) have written about the ethical issues in dealing with students who exhibit problematic behavior in an experiential group. When this situation arises, the group counselor-educator has multiple responsibilities: to the individual student who displays problematic behavior, to the other students in the experiential group, and to the training program. It is important for the group member to understand the impact his or her behavior has on others, and the group format provides many opportunities for learning to deal with problematic behaviors. One effective intervention is to invite other members to provide here-and-now feedback to the member exhibiting the problematic behavior. The instructor or group facilitator is responsible for blocking unproductive interactions while this feedback is being delivered to prevent the group member from being scapegoated or overwhelmed with negative feedback. As challenging as it might be in the moment, everyone in the group can benefit from the experience of successfully working through difficult situations. What students learn in an experiential group can be invaluable when they lead groups in school or community settings.

Personal Psychotherapy Sometimes issues that surface in a group are more appropriately explored in personal (individual) therapy. We also encourage individual therapy as a way of enhancing trainees' abilities to understand both themselves and others, which is essential for ethical practice. Personal therapy enables us to identify and explore countertransference reactions we may have toward certain group members, recognize our blind spots and biases, and use our personal attributes effectively in our work as a group facilitator. Psychotherapy can be a vital part of our self-care program by helping us maintain a sense of balance in our life.

Group Supervision Supervision is a key component in training group leaders. Group supervision offers unique advantages for observing group process in action; it is also an efficient supervision model given that several group leaders can be supervised at the same time. Some research confirms that group supervision has value with respect to increasing the skill development of trainees (Riva, 2010, 2014). Group supervision is of paramount importance in training group leaders as well as in monitoring the quality of care of those who participate (Riva, 2014). Group supervision provides trainees with many experiential opportunities to learn about the process and development of a group and creates the foundation for future ethical practice. Workshops that provide supervision for group trainees help them to develop the necessary skills for effective and ethical intervention. Also, this format helps interns learn a great deal about their response to criticism, competitiveness, need for approval, concerns over being competent, and power struggles. Participation in a supervision group enables trainees to learn not only from the supervisor who conducts the group but from others in the group as questions are raised and answered.

Observation of Group Therapy Sessions Although reading about group counseling is useful, watching videos of group sessions and observing groups *in vivo* make academic learning more meaningful. Weiss and Rutan (2016) surveyed trainees who sat off to one side in the group room and observed group therapy participants. The trainees consistently stated that observing a live group and having an opportunity to process the session with the leaders was one of their best training experiences. There are many benefits from observing group therapy as a teaching method. Among the lessons trainees could translate into their work with individual and couple clients were how to:

- Tolerate intense emotions and learn to trust the group process
- Identify and use group themes, metaphors, and group dynamics
- Understand ways of working with transference and countertransference
- Use techniques to highlight themes emerging in the group
- Promote immediacy and the value of working in the here and now

Weiss and Rutan conducted an observed psychodynamic therapy group for 5 years and noted that this experience increased trainees' desire to lead therapy groups. Weiss and Rutan conclude: "Observing an ongoing therapy is an exceptionally effective mode of learning for the students and provides ongoing learning and stimulation for senior leaders as well" (p. 257).

(LO2)

Ethical Issues in the Diversity Training of Group Workers

"Three-quarters of the world come from collectivistic group-oriented cultures," and Bemak and Chung (2015) assert that "as the world becomes more globalized it is inevitable that group counseling will be a major choice of healing and psychological intervention internationally" (p. 6). Group counseling and other kinds of group work are alive and well in the United States, but group work is also finding a home internationally (Hohenshil, Amundson, & Niles, 2013). An integral part of the training of group leaders is promoting sensitivity and competence in addressing diversity in all forms of group work.

Not surprisingly, the development of multicultural and cross-cultural competence for group psychotherapists has emerged as an ethical imperative. *Cultural competence* refers to the knowledge and skills required to work effectively in any cross-cultural encounter (Comas-Diaz, 2014). Merely possessing knowledge and skills, though necessary, is not sufficient for effective group work. Becoming a diversity-competent group worker involves self-awareness and an open stance on the leader's part to the diversity issues that emerge in a group. To fail to address these diversity issues is to fail the group members (Debiak, 2007). Attending to and addressing diversity is not only an ethical mandate, but this practice is also a route to more effective group work. It is the responsibility of training programs to create safe opportunities for a trainee's cultural self-explorations.

If you possess cultural tunnel vision (see Chapter 4), you are likely to misinterpret patterns of behavior displayed by group members who are culturally different from you. Unless you are clearly aware of your own cultural values and understand the values of other cultures, you may misunderstand clients from diverse backgrounds. If you are in doubt about what a group member is saying or doing, ask this person for an explanation. One technique endorsed by leading multicultural scholars is *broaching* the subjects of race, ethnicity, and culture with clients (Cardemil & Battle, 2003; Day-Vines et al., 2007). Day-Vines and colleagues (2007) state: "Counselors who display advanced levels of broaching and possess heightened levels of racial identity functioning are likely to promote trusting and open relationships with their clients that accommodate a range of social and cultural experiences" (p. 408). If you are able to appreciate cultural differences, you have opportunities to use this knowledge in effectively working with the various forms of diversity in your group.

Effective group interventions are adapted to the needs of the individual member rather than attempting to fit the member to the leader's usual interventions. In working with culturally diverse client populations, leaders may need to modify interventions to suit the client's cultural and ethnic background. Leaders can respect the cultural values of members and at the same time encourage them to think about how these values and their upbringing have a continuing effect on their behavior (Corey, Corey, Callanan, & Russell, 2015).

Social Justice Practice and Training in Group Work

Social justice refers to "the fair and equitable distribution of power, resources, and obligations in society to all people, regardless of race, gender, ability, status, sexual orientation, and religious or spiritual background" (Hage, Mason, & Kim, 2010, p. 103). Multiculturalism and social justice concepts are often intricately linked (see Chapter 4). The ASGW (2012) addresses both concepts in their guidelines for training group workers, conducting research, understanding how multiculturalism and social justice affect group process, and assisting group workers in various settings to increase their knowledge and skills in developing competence in addressing multicultural and social justice themes in group work. The guidelines emphasize the acquisition of awareness, knowledge, and skills that will equip group leaders to work ethically and effectively with the diversity within their groups. Trainees and counselors need to be mindful of multicultural and social justice themes at all times when interacting with individuals in groups. Moreover, Bemak and Chung (2015) stress the need for counselors to redefine ethics and boundaries when working in an international context. Adaptation, modification, and changes to Western traditional group counseling practices may need to be considered. For instance, it is regarded as good manners "to give and receive gifts on auspicious holidays or at special celebrations in many societies. For a group counselor to reject thoughtful personal gifts for a New Year's celebration would be considered rude and disrespectful" (p. 14).

Social justice practice, training, and research are interdependent. Effective training is necessary if group workers hope to understand and address the multiple layers of complexity involved in social justice group work (Hays, Arredondo, Gladding, & Toporek, 2010). Trainees require more than a conceptual understanding of social justice principles to develop competence; group leaders need "concrete strategies for infusing social justice in their work" (p. 181). Some strategies Hayes and colleagues recommend include values clarification, empowerment of gender and ethnicity statuses, consciousness raising, self-disclosure, social and gender-role analyses, structure to maximize group cohesion, and bibliotherapy. Additional training in international group counseling strategies may be needed for those interested in facilitating group work abroad.

Group work, perhaps more than any other counseling intervention, has the potential to further a social justice agenda (Hage et al., 2010). According to Hayes and her colleagues (2010), "the social justice movement and group work have been, and still are, a natural marriage . . . it is difficult to see social justice becoming pervasive in society without the sophisticated use of groups" (pp. 195–196). Experiences members have had with social injustices will inevitably surface when people from diverse backgrounds participate in a group. MacNair-Semands (2007) claims that group workers need to search for ways to expand their competence in addressing social justice issues that emerge regularly in groups, such as unfair treatment or inequities that result from racism, sexism, socioeconomics, sexual orientation, ableism, and other forms of "isms" that affect the quality of life. Group members can be invited to talk about their pain from the social injustices they have encountered. Group practitioners must work toward healing experiences within the group rather than allowing potentially harmful interactions to occur.

Power and privilege dynamics operate in a group just as in the wider world, and the imbalance of power can be addressed and explored in group work. In any group, some members may come from power and others may have been denied power; these power dynamics should be discussed as they emerge in a group. Social inequalities often arise from an intolerance for differences that result in discrimination, oppression, prejudice, and, at times, interpersonal violence. If these issues are not addressed, members are deprived of an opportunity to explore cultural values and biases, to raise their awareness of these injustices, and to learn to confront them.

Guidelines for Multicultural and Social Justice Competence

Most of the ethics codes of the various professional organizations now give increasing attention to applying cultural perspectives when working with diverse client populations (see Chapter 4). The ACA (2014) *Code of Ethics* addresses multicultural perspectives in every section, and the ASGW (2012) competency principles address broad areas of race, ethnicity, socioeconomic class, age, gender, sexual orientation, religion, and spirituality. The Association for Multicultural Counseling and Development (2015) highlights taking action to promote social justice and emphasizes teaching clients how to advocate for themselves. The following ethical guidelines for acquiring diversity and multicultural competence in group practice can be found in these codes.

- Group counselors strive to increase their awareness of their own multicultural identity and how their race, ethnicity, socioeconomic class, migration status, ability, age, gender identity and expression, sexual orientation, and religion and spirituality are influenced by their life experiences and histories.
- Group counselors conduct a cultural assessment of each group member within the context of their presenting concerns. They assess members' cultural identity, acculturation level, and the role that oppression and culture played in the development and evaluation of symptoms.
- Group counselors consider the impact of adverse social, environmental, and political factors in assessing problems and designing interventions. They realize that an individual's problems cannot be isolated from their societal context.
- Group counselors address issues of status, privilege, and oppression as they arise in group work facilitation.
- Group counselors increase their awareness of how myths, stereotypes, and assumptions they learned by living in society influence their work in facilitating groups.
- Group counselors are committed to expanding their services in schools, agencies, community centers, churches, temples, synagogues, shelters, and political milieus to create new ways of developing groups and identifying members to promote equity, access, harmony, and participation.
- Group counselors acquire the knowledge and skills necessary for effectively working with the diverse range of members in their groups. They seek consultation, supervision, and further education to fill any gaps and to become more fluent with culturally based practices.
- Group counselors model relationship skills that are basic to establishing and maintaining connections between multicultural group members while planning, performing, and processing groups.
- Group counselors establish norms that accept, value, and respect cultural differences. Leaders encourage open discussion of dynamics related to cultural issues early in the life of a group.
- Group counselors respect the roles of family and community hierarchies within a client's culture.

- Group counselors with a social justice orientation are aware that individual change occurs through social change, and they advocate with clients and on behalf of clients both in the group and across other systems.
- Group counselors discuss why social justice and advocacy issues are important in a group and how these issues influence the practice and outcomes of group work.
- Group counselors inform members about basic values that are implicit in the group process (such as self-disclosure, reflecting on one's life, and taking risks).
- Group counselors expand the concept of being a client to include systems and communities when they are examining change.

If group counselors do not understand how their own cultural background influences their thinking and behavior, there is little chance they can teach group members much about their cultural thinking and behavior. The characteristics of the culturally competent counselor discussed in Chapter 4 are equally relevant for practitioners who work with groups. Although it is not realistic to assume that leaders will have knowledge about every culture, it is important that counselors understand that each person participates in a group from his or her own unique perspective.

For a description of social justice and advocacy competencies that can be applied to group work, see *ACA Advocacy Competencies: A Social Justice Framework for Counselors* (Ratts, Toporek, & Lewis, 2010).

As you read the following case, consider how you could increase your own sensitivity to individuals from cultural groups different from your own.

The Case of John

John comes from an impoverished neighborhood in an eastern city, has struggled financially to get a college degree, and has finally attained a master's degree in counseling. He is proud of his accomplishments and considers himself to be sensitive to his own background and to those who struggle with similar problems. He has moved to the west coast and has been hired to work in a high school with a culturally diverse student population.

As a high school counselor, John starts a group for at-risk adolescents. His goals for this group are as follows: (1) to instill pride so that group members will see their present environment as an obstacle to be overcome, not suffered with; (2) to increase self-esteem and to challenge group members to fight the negativism they may encounter in their home and school environments; (3) to teach group members to minimize their differences in terms of the larger community (for example, he points out how some of their idioms and ways of speaking separate them from the majority and reinforce differences and stereotypes); and (4) to teach group members how to overcome obstacles in a nonsupportive environment.

John does not work very closely with teachers, administrators, or other school counselors in the district. He views them as being more interested in politics and red tape and as giving very little energy to personal counseling in the school. He has little to do with the families of the adolescents because he sees them as being too willing to accept handouts and welfare and as not being very interested in becoming self-sufficient and independent. He tells his group members: "What you have at home with your families has obviously not worked for you. What you have in this group is the opportunity to change."

- Do John's background and experiences qualify him as a culturally competent group counselor? Why or why not?
- Do you think it is helpful or damaging for John to define the problem for the group members?
- What might John be missing by coming into the group as an expert instead of doing a needs assessment?
- If John had become familiar with the environment of this particular group, would he have expressed the same goals?
- If you were John's supervisor, how would you work with him?
- If you were a group member, how might you feel toward John?

Commentary. We disagree with John's axiom that simply because he could obtain a graduate degree (against difficult odds) anybody could have the same success. John is a well-intentioned school counselor who disregarded the particular needs of the students in his school and his group. He did not conduct a needs assessment with his group. Instead, he imposed his personal agenda in terms of language and upward mobility on the group. This is a situation where one size does not fit all. In many ways John has an encapsulated view of his group and is not taking into consideration the perspectives and worldviews of the members.

John made no attempt to become aware of the unique struggles or values of the high school students he serves. He stereotyped the parents of his group members in a very indirect, but powerful fashion and set up potential conflicts between group members and their families. John acted insensitively to the families of his group members. Most ethics codes require therapists to respect community and family traditions and to utilize these as potential resources in therapy when appropriate. John failed to pay attention to the potential healing power of the community, which can be a powerful therapeutic force for change.

John seems to lack specific training that could assist him in developing multicultural competence as a group worker. In working with groups characterized by diversity, it is critical that John be aware of the assumptions he makes about people from diverse ethnic and cultural groups, and from an ethical standpoint, he should adapt his practices to the needs of the members in his group. John needs to make sure that the goals and processes of his group match the cultural values and personal goals of the members of the group. To be able to make interventions that are appropriate for members' unique cultural backgrounds, John must have an understanding of the ways diversity influences group process. John needs to become aware of his own cultural bias and be willing to reflect on the assumptions underlying his methods and practices. ●

LO4

Ethical Considerations in Coleadership

If you lead groups, you will probably work with a coleader at some time. Coleader relationships can either enhance or complicate the group process and raise a multitude of potential ethical issues. The group can benefit from the insights and feedback of two leaders. Coleaders who complement and balance each other can provide useful modeling for members. Furthermore, coleaders can share the responsibilities and provide mutual support.

Along with the advantages of coleadership, there are some disadvantages that can raise ethical concerns. Luke and Hackney (2007) found that one of the primary disadvantages involves relationship difficulties between the leaders, such as one leader having an exaggerated need for approval. Other potential drawbacks to the coleadership model include ineffective communication, competition between leaders, and overdependence on the coleader. Group members may attempt to triangulate the coleaders by pitting one against the other. Conflicts between the leaders can result in splitting within the group. Luke and Hackney emphasize the necessity for group leaders to attend to their own individual development, their development as a coleading team, and the development of the group they are facilitating. It is challenging for group leaders to divide their time between these multiple areas of development, yet doing so is essential for a successful group.

When differences between leaders result in conflict between them, it can be a source of anxiety for both members and leaders. Conflicts that are ineffectively managed place an unfair burden on the members and can be harmful to the group process and outcome. If the leaders model healthy conflict resolution for group members, showing nondefensiveness and a willingness to challenge and be challenged, this conflict can prove to be a valuable learning opportunity. It is up to the leaders to determine whether the issue is best addressed in the moment with the group members or in private between the leaders. There are pros and cons to both of these approaches. If the members witnessed the conflict, we prefer to deal with it in the group.

At this point, clarify your own position on coleadership in group work:

- What personal characteristics would you most want in a coleader?
- Would you prefer working alone to coleading a group, and why?
- Have you been in a group where the coleaders clashed on certain issues and approached group facilitation very differently? If so, what impact did this have on your participation in the group?
- What ethical implications may be involved when there are overt power struggles and conflicts between coleaders?
- In what ways could you be most helpful to your coleader?
- What do you know about yourself that would make it difficult for your coleader to work with you?
- Have you been in a group where the coleaders functioned at a high level? If so, what did they do that you particularly appreciated?

Ethical Issues in Forming and Managing Groups

How can group leaders make potential members aware of the services they are providing? What information do clients have a right to expect before they decide to attend a group? **Informed consent** is a process of presenting basic information about group treatment to potential group members to enable them to decide whether or not to join a group. Leaders have the responsibility of ensuring that members become aware of their rights (as well as their responsibilities) as group participants.

It is a good policy to provide a professional disclosure statement to group members that includes written information on a variety of topics pertaining to the nature of the group, including the therapists' qualifications, techniques often used in the group, the rights and obligations of group members, and the risks and benefits of participating in the group. Special attention needs to be given to the nature and limitations of confidentiality and the specific situations that would require breaching confidences. Although informed consent is an ethical and legal mandate, group members should not be overwhelmed with too much information at one time. It is a good practice to tell members at the outset that informed consent is an ongoing process and that various aspects of the consent process will likely be revisited at different stages of a group. When informed consent is handled effectively, it helps promote individual autonomy, engages members in a collaborative process, and reduces the likelihood of exploitation or harm (Barnett, Wise, et al., 2007; Wheeler & Bertram, 2015). The section on informed consent in Chapter 5 applies to both individual and group counseling; refer to that discussion for further details.

Screening and Selection of Group Members

Not everyone will benefit from a therapeutic group experience, and some people may be psychologically harmed by certain group experiences. Therefore, group leaders are faced with the difficult task of determining who should be included in a group and who should not.

Unless careful selection criteria are employed, Yalom (2005) argues that group therapy clients may end up discouraged and may not be helped. He maintains that it is easier to identify the people who should be excluded from group therapy than those who should be included. Citing clinical studies, he lists the following as poor candidates for a heterogeneous outpatient intensive therapy group: people with traumatic brain injuries, paranoid individuals, hypochondriacs, acutely psychotic individuals, and antisocial personalities. In terms of criteria for inclusion, he contends that the client's level of motivation to work is the most important variable. From his perspective, groups are useful for people who have problems in the interpersonal domain, such as loneliness, inability to make or maintain intimate contacts, feelings of unlovability, fears of being assertive, and dependency issues. Clients who lack meaning in life, who suffer from generalized anxiety, who are searching for an identity, who fear success, and who are compulsive workers could also profit from a group experience.

The ACA (2014) identifies the counselor's ethical responsibility for screening prospective group members as follows:

> Counselors screen prospective group counseling/therapy participants. To the extent possible, counselors select members whose needs and goals are compatible with goals of the group, who will not impede the group process, and whose well-being will not be jeopardized by the group experience. (A.9.a.)

As a general ethical guideline, we think that some type of screening, involving interviewing and evaluating potential members, should be employed to select group members. The type of group should determine the kind of members accepted. In addition, what is best for the group as a whole needs to be considered in selecting members for that group. More specifically, the question can be framed thusly: Is it appropriate for *this* person to become a participant in *this* type of group, with *this* leader, at *this* time? Screening should not be done for the comfort of the group leader, nor should it be done arbitrarily to unfairly discriminate against certain members (M. Corey et al., 2018).

Many group leaders do not screen participants, for various reasons. Some practitioners are theoretically opposed to the notion of using screening as a way of determining who is suitable for a group, and some maintain that they simply do not have the time to carry out effective screening, or doing so is not realistic in their work setting. Not all theoretical orientations favor or agree with the notion of screening, nor would they view screening as an ethical mandate. For example, some Adlerians believe screening does not fit with the democratic spirit of their theory. Some maintain that screening is done more for the comfort of the group leader than for the good of the client.

Others believe that ethical practice demands careful screening and preparation of all candidates. We are concerned that failing to evaluate the suitability of a group member could lead to harm for other group members. Even minimal screening can lessen the potential harm to group members. The need for screening members depends in part on the type of group you are forming. A person who can work well in a psychoeducational group designed to teach social skills might not be ready for an intensive therapy group. Individuals with severe emotional trauma would probably be excluded from an interpersonal process group, but they might benefit from a weekly group for outpatients at a mental health center. Screening is less important for a psychoeducational group, but potential members should be clearly informed of the purposes of this kind of group and what will be expected of them.

The Case of Angela

Angela is a counselor in a busy community agency that is understaffed, and counselors are increasingly expected to design groups as a way to meet the diverse needs of clients in the agency. Angela decides to organize a personal-growth group by sending colleagues a memorandum asking for candidates for her group. There are no provisions for individual screening of potential members, no written announcement informing the members of the goals and purposes of the group, and no preparation for incoming members. No information is given to the members about the leader's background, possible techniques to be used, expectations for participation, or how to get the most from the group experience. Angela asks the receptionist to admit the first 10 people who come to enroll, assuming that the interest of these people is a sign that they are ready for a group experience. The receptionist puts people into the group as they inquire, irrespective of the nature of their problems, and they are told when to come in for the first meeting.

- Can Angela's failure to screen members for her group be justified on ethical and clinical grounds?
- What are some alternatives to screening, if doing so formally is impractical?
- What potential problems do you see in the way Angela formed her group?
- What issues pertaining to informed consent do you believe Angela needs to address before the group begins?

Commentary. We realize that in some settings it is impractical to screen members prior to forming a group. In Angela's agency, if it is not possible to conduct screening interviews, one alternative is to use the initial session to provide orientation for the participants and to present informed consent guidelines. We think Angela was remiss in not doing any kind of screening to determine whether those who were applying were ready for this kind of group experience. Simply filling the group by admitting the first 10 people who wanted to sign up is not an effective way to form a group and raises concerns about the fit and readiness of potential members. At the very least, she could have made provisions for candidates to meet with her briefly to ask questions about the group. In addition, Angela could have created a written document containing information to help potential new members determine whether the group was appropriate for them. •

Preparing Group Participants

To what extent are group counselors ethically responsible for helping participants to benefit from their group experience? Many practitioners do very little to prepare members for a group and are opposed to preparation on the grounds that it could inhibit a group's spontaneity and autonomy. Others take the position that members need to be provided with some structure to derive maximum gains (M. Corey et al., 2018).

Yalom (2005) advocates exploring group members' misconceptions and expectations, predicting early problems, and providing a conceptual framework that includes guidelines for effective group behavior. He views this preparatory process as more than the dissemination of information. He contends that it reinforces the therapist's respect for the client, demonstrates that therapy is a collaborative venture, and shows that the therapist is willing to share his or her knowledge with the client. This cognitive approach to preparation has the goals of providing a rational explanation of the group process, clarifying how members can best participate, and raising expectations about what the group can accomplish.

The Case of Elida

Elida assumes that the more information about group process she provides to group members, the more the members will attempt to please her. To avoid this, Elida does not give information out before members actually meet, either in writing or orally, nor does she establish group rules and group norms. This leader is convinced that informed consent is not really possible, and she prefers to have an open discussion in the group that allows members to formulate rules that make sense to them. If members flounder in defining goals, Elida believes this is part of the group process; therefore, she does not expect members to identify specific goals to guide their participation in a group. Elida thinks members should follow their own spontaneous paths rather than learning about group norms and other expected group behavior from the group leader.

- Do you think an argument could be made for not giving information to potential members before they decide to join a group? Explain.
- What do you think of Elida's approach to formulating group rules and norms with the group members?
- If you were forming a group, how would you take care of the informed consent process?

Commentary. Different leaders have different leadership styles. Some leaders prefer a structured approach, whereas others prefer giving the group members maximum freedom to decide how they will function as a group. Elida's approach is to allow the group to define its own direction; she assumes that the members can formulate their own norms governing behavior in the group. We do not think Elida is behaving unethically with respect to allowing group members to formulate the group rules and norms for their group. However, by not providing any information about the group before it begins, Elida is not attending to the informed consent process. Most codes of ethics agree on the importance of providing informed consent so that clients know what they are agreeing to before they make a commitment. Although we support creativity and thinking outside of the norm, it is necessary to practice within ethical parameters. ●

In our experience in working with groups, we have found that providing members with basic information about group process tends to eliminate some of the difficulties typically encountered in the early stages of a group. Our preparation procedures apply to most types of groups, with some modifications. At both the screening session and the initial group meeting, we explore the members' expectations, clarify goals and objectives, discuss procedural details, explore the possible risks and values of group participation, and discuss guidelines for getting the most from a group experience.

As part of member preparation, we include a discussion of the values and limitations of groups, the psychological risks involved in group participation, and ways of minimizing these risks. We also allow time for dealing with misconceptions that people have about groups and for exploring the fears or reservations the members may have. In most of our groups, members do have certain fears about what they will experience. Acknowledging these fears and talking about them provides a foundation for productive group work. We also ask members to spend time before they come to the group defining what they most want to achieve and formulating personal goals that will guide their participation.

Write down some things you might do to prepare people for a group. What ethical concerns do you have regarding preparation? What do you think would occur if you did little in the way of preparing group members?

Involuntary Participation

LO7

Voluntary participation is an important beginning point for a successful group experience. Members will make significant changes only to the extent that they actively seek something for themselves. Unfortunately, not all groups are composed of clients who have chosen to be there. Are there situations in which it is ethical to require or mandate people to participate in a group? How is informed consent especially critical in groups where attendance is mandatory? Can involuntary groups be successful?

Mandatory participation in a group raises a different set of ethical issues. The negative attitudes of some members can contaminate the entire group experience. Skilled leaders often are able to change negative attitudes of some involuntary members by showing them how they might benefit from a group experience (M. Corey et al., 2018). With involuntary members, greater effort needs to be directed toward fully informing members of the nature and goals of the group, procedures to be used, the rights of members to decline certain activities, the limits of confidentiality, and what effect their level of participation in the group will have on critical decisions about them outside of the group. Group leaders should strive to help involuntary members understand their choices and the consequences of lack of compliance with the treatment program (Rapin, 2014). When attendance at group sessions is required, group leaders need to be certain that group members understand their rights and their responsibilities, and counselors must at all times show their respect for these mandated members.

Consider these questions on the ethics of involuntary membership:

- Do you think members can benefit from a group experience even if they are required to attend? Why or why not?
- From an ethical perspective, is it required that members of an involuntary group give consent? To what degree should members be informed about the consequences of their level of participation in a group?

Freedom to Withdraw From a Group

Once members make a commitment to be a part of a group, do they have the right to leave at any time they choose? Procedures for leaving a group should be explained to all members during the initial session. We tell our members that they have an obligation to attend all sessions and to inform us if they decide to withdraw. Ideally, the leader and the member cooperate to determine whether a group experience is proving to be productive or counterproductive. We take the position that clients have a responsibility to the leader and to other members to explain why they want to leave. There are several reasons for this policy. It can be psychologically damaging to members to leave without having been able to discuss what they considered threatening or negative in the experience. Further, it is unfortunate if members leave a group because of a misunderstanding about some feedback they have received. Such a termination can be harmful to group cohesion, for the members who remain may think that they caused a particular member's departure. Although members have a right to withdraw from a group, we ask them to talk about it out of respect for the needs of the remaining members as well as for their own safety and well-being. However, we do not think it is ethical to use undue pressure to keep these members, and we are alert to other members' pressuring a person to stay.

Psychological Risks

LO8

The fact that groups can be powerful catalysts for personal change means that they can also be risky. Ethical practice demands that group practitioners inform prospective participants of the potential risks involved in the group experience. Our goal is to create a safe environment where members can take risks and explore their discomfort. Group leaders have an ethical responsibility to take precautionary measures to reduce unnecessary psychological risks. AMHCA's (2015) guideline reinforces this responsibility: "In a group setting, mental health counselors take reasonable precautions to protect clients from physical, emotional, and psychological harm or trauma" (1B.3f.).

Group leaders have a significant role in preventing damaging group experiences. Smokowski, Rose, and Bacallao (2001) remind us that group leaders have a great deal of power, prestige, and status within their groups and caution that "many leaders are not able to responsibly manage, or even recognize, their power and influence" (p. 228). The outcomes of a group are very much related to what leaders bring to a group and to their actions. Smokowski and colleagues studied damaging experiences in therapeutic groups and identified a variety of factors or events that result in members having a negative group experience, some of which include lack of leader support; an aggressive and harshly confrontational leadership style; premature pressure to disclose; passive leadership style; misuse of a leader's power and influence; lack of acceptance for diverse points of view; lack of clarity about group norms; and negative norms that coerce participation or encourage excessive confrontation. Group members are often more willing to be challenged when they know they will be supported in the group.

Although all risks cannot be eliminated, certain safeguards can be taken during the course of a group to avoid negative outcomes. Here are some of the risks that participants should know about (M. Corey et al., 2018):

- Members may experience some disruptions in their lives as a result of their work in the group.
- Group participants are often encouraged to be completely open. In this quest for self-revelation, privacy is sometimes inappropriately surrendered.
- A related risk is group pressure. The participants' right not to explore certain issues or to stop at a certain point should be respected. Also, members should not be coerced into participating in an exercise.
- Scapegoating is another potential hazard in groups. Unchallenged projection and blaming can have dire effects on the target person and can have a negative impact on the progress of a group.
- Confrontation can be used or misused in groups. Harmful attacks on others should not be permitted.
- If safety is lacking in a group, members who have been subjected to social injustices may be revictimized if they are subjected to a similar kind of injustice when they explore their experiences in the group.
- Even though a counselor may continue to stress the necessity not to discuss with outsiders what goes on in the group, there is no guarantee that all members will respect the confidential nature of their exchanges.

One way to minimize psychological risks in groups is to use a contract, in which leaders specify what their responsibilities are and members specify what their commitment to the group is by declaring what they are willing to do. If members and leaders operate under a contract that clarifies expectations, there is less chance for members to be exploited or damaged by a group experience.

Of course, a contract approach is not the only way to reduce potential risks, nor is it sufficient in itself to do so. One of the most important safeguards is the leader's training in group process. Group counselors have the major ethical responsibility for preventing needless harm to members. To fulfill this role, group leaders should have a clear grasp of the boundaries of their competence. Leaders should conduct only those types of groups for which they have been sufficiently prepared. Working with an experienced coleader and supervisor is a good way to learn and also a way to reduce potential risks.

A group leader's actions have a great deal to do with setting a constructive tone in a group. The leader's behavior can minimize the risks of negative outcomes. Leaders can reduce the chances of creating a toxic climate within a group by:

(a) assuming a nonjudgmental stance toward the members;
(b) avoiding responding to sarcastic remarks with sarcasm;
(c) being honest with members rather than harboring hidden agendas;
(d) avoiding judgments and labeling of members, and instead describing the behavior of members;
(e) stating observations and hunches in a tentative way rather than dogmatically;
(f) letting members who are difficult know how they are affecting them in a non-blaming way;
(g) detecting their own countertransference and managing these reactions;
(h) avoiding misuse of their power;
(i) providing both support and caring confrontations; and
(j) avoiding meeting their own needs at the expense of the members (M. Corey et al., 2018).

Confidentiality in Groups

The ethical, legal, and professional aspects of confidentiality (discussed in Chapter 6) have a different application in group situations. Are members of a group under the same ethical and legal obligations as the group leader not to disclose the identities of other members or the content of what was shared in the group? The legal concept of privileged communication is generally not recognized in a group setting, unless there is a statutory exception. However, protecting the confidentiality of group members is an ethical mandate, and it is the responsibility of the counselor to address this at the outset of a group. The group therapist is expected to safeguard the members' right to privacy by judiciously protecting the identity of the members and protecting information of a confidential nature. Group leaders also have the ethical responsibility of informing members of the limits of confidentiality within the group setting, their responsibilities to other group members, and the absence of legal privilege concerning what is shared in a group (Wheeler & Bertram, 2015).

From the beginning of a group we discuss with members the purpose and limits of confidentiality. The ethics codes of several professional organizations address a group practitioner's role in ensuring confidentiality in a group setting. The ASGW (2008) "Best Practice Guidelines" state the following regarding confidentiality:

> Group Workers define confidentiality and its limits (for example, legal and ethical exceptions and expectations; waivers implicit with treatment plans, documentation, and insurance usage). Group Workers have the responsibility to inform all group participants of the need for confidentiality and potential consequences of breaching confidentiality; and that legal privilege does not apply to group discussions (unless provided by state statute). (A.7.d.)

In individual psychotherapy, the therapist can ensure the client's confidentiality, yet in group therapy leaders cannot prevent other members from disclosing personal information about members in the group. Group leaders are themselves ethically and legally bound to maintain confidentiality, yet a group member who violates another member's confidences faces no legal consequences (Lasky & Riva, 2006). Although confidentiality in a group cannot be guaranteed, group leaders are responsible for educating members regarding how easy it is to unintentionally breach confidentiality, as well as the importance and advantages of keeping information private that pertains to the group (Rapin, 2014).

If you were to lead a group, which of the following measures might you take to ensure confidentiality? Check any of the statements that apply:

_____ 1. I would periodically reinforce the importance of confidentiality at group meetings.

_____ 2. I would require group members to sign a statement saying that they fully understand their commitment to maintain the confidential character of the group.

_____ 3. I would let members know that they would be asked to leave the group if they violated confidentiality.

_____ 4. I would leave it up to group members to decide how they want to deal with confidentiality issues in their group.

_____ 5. I would talk with group members about the role they have in maintaining each other's confidentiality.

The Case of Pierre

Pierre briefly discusses confidentiality at the first group session, saying "Anything that happens here, stays here." He tells members that it is not necessary to go into detail in talking about confidentiality "because everyone in here already knows that confidentiality is a given." Pierre does not let members know that confidentiality cannot be guaranteed in his group, nor does he inform them of the limitations of confidentiality in a group setting. Pierre does not invite members to raise questions they might have about confidentiality because he is anxious for his group to start working.

- How do you evaluate the ethical appropriateness of Pierre's approach to discussing confidentiality in his group?
- What specific aspects of confidentiality would you most want to inform group members about?
- What potential problems, if any, do you see in the way Pierre explained confidentiality to group members?
- Given that confidentiality cannot be guaranteed in a group, what guidelines could you set as a group leader to help assure confidentiality?

Commentary. We think Pierre is guilty of oversimplification in stating that confidentiality is a given and that members are familiar with its importance. Members may be mistaken in their assumption that confidentiality can be guaranteed in a group setting. It would be wise for

Pierre to encourage members to raise any concerns they have about confidentiality at any point during the course of the group. In discussing the importance of confidentiality in the group, Pierre could point out how confidentiality can be violated in subtle ways and how confidences are often divulged without malice. Most people do not maliciously attempt to hurt others by talking with people outside the group about specific members. However, it is tempting for members to share their experiences with other people, and in so doing they sometimes make inappropriate disclosures. Because of this tendency to want to share with outsiders, we caution participants about how easily and unintentionally the confidentiality of the group can be compromised. We tell members that they are less likely to break confidentiality if they talk only about their own personal insights. •

It is our position that leaders need periodically to reaffirm to group members the importance of not discussing with outsiders what has occurred in the group. We talk with each prospective member about the necessity of maintaining confidentiality to establish the trust and cohesion required if participants are to reveal themselves in significant ways. We discuss this point during the screening interviews, again during the pregroup or initial meetings, at times during the course of a group when it seems appropriate, and again at termination.

Exceptions to Confidentiality in Groups Although group leaders are expected to stress the importance of confidentiality and set a norm, they also are expected to inform members about its limits. For example, if members pose a danger to themselves or to others, the group therapist has an ethical and legal obligation to take appropriate steps to protect the group member and society in general (AGPA, 2006). The other limitations of confidentiality discussed in Chapter 6 also apply to group work.

Therapists who lead groups must become familiar with the state laws that have an impact on their practice. For instance, all states have had mandatory child abuse reporting laws since 1967. Most states also have mandatory elder abuse and dependent adult abuse reporting laws. The great majority of states currently have laws requiring counselors to report clients' threats to harm themselves or others.

If you lead a group at a correctional institution or an inpatient facility, you may have to record in a member's chart certain behaviors or verbalizations that he or she exhibits in the group. At the same time, your responsibility to your clients requires you to inform them that you are documenting their verbalizations and behaviors and that this information is accessible to other staff.

Confidentiality With Minors Encouraging confidentiality is a special challenge for counselors who offer groups for children and adolescents in school settings. On this matter, ASCA's (2016) *Ethical Standards for School Counselors* provides an important guideline:

> School counselors communicate the aspiration of confidentiality as a group norm, while recognizing and working from a protective posture that confidentiality for minors in schools cannot be guaranteed. (A.7.e.)

Group leaders have a responsibility in groups that involve children and adolescents to take measures to increase the chances that confidentiality will be kept. It is important to work cooperatively with parents and legal guardians as well as to enlist the trust of the young members. It is also useful to teach minors, using a vocabulary they understand, about the nature, purposes, and limitations of confidentiality. It is a good idea for leaders to encourage members to initiate discussions on confidentiality whenever this becomes an issue for them.

Do parents or legal guardians have a right to information that is disclosed by their children in a group? The answer to that question depends on whether we are looking at it from a legal, ethical, or professional viewpoint. State laws differ regarding counseling minors. It is important for group leaders to be aware of the laws related to working with minors in the state in which they are practicing. Circumstances in which a minor may seek professional help without parental consent, defining an emancipated minor, or the rights of parents (or legal guardians) to have access to the records regarding the professional help received by their minor child vary according to state statutes.

Before any minor enters a group, it is a good practice to obtain written permission from the parents. Such a statement should include a brief description of the purpose of the group, the importance of confidentiality as a prerequisite to accomplishing these purposes, and your intention not to violate any confidences. Although it may be useful to give parents information about their child, this can be done without violating confidences. At the first session it is helpful to inform and discuss with minors their concerns about confidentiality and how it will be maintained. Such practices can strengthen the child's trust in the counselor.

Social Media in Group Work: Confidentiality and Privacy Considerations

LO10

Confidentiality and issues of privacy take on added dimensions when group members and their therapists interact with each other in online group counseling and when group members communicate via social media. Online platforms such as Facebook, Twitter, and Instagram have become widely used and are increasing in popularity. Kozlowski and Holmes (2014) state that "the vast majority of what the field understands about group counseling has been learned from groups that take place in face-to-face group environments . . . a gap exists in the literature concerning the experiences of members in online counseling groups" (p. 276). The implications of using online social networking sites for group counseling and group psychotherapy warrant greater attention by scholars and researchers.

Wheeler and Bertram (2015) note that there is an increased risk of breach of confidentiality when members of a counseling group engage in social media. Group counselors should address the parameters of online behavior through informed consent and should establish ground rules regarding members' commitment to avoid posting pictures, comments, or any type of confidential information about other members online. Developing these rules needs to be part of the discussion about norms governing the group. One way for members to share their experience with others outside the group is for them to talk about their own experience, reactions, and insights without describing other members or mentioning others in the group by name. Members can be educated to talk about themselves rather than telling stories about other group members.

Breaches of confidentiality or privacy may occur when members share their own information online, especially if they struggle with poor boundaries. Others may lack the technological skills and knowledge to protect information that is intended to remain private. Zur and Zur (2011) point out that some therapists who have Facebook profiles use privacy settings to protect their personal information, but others do not. They add, "those who do not use the privacy settings do not because they either do not know about these options, do not know how, or do not understand what other people can see or not see on their profiles" (p. 12). The same is true for group members. In a small study, master's-level counseling students who were part of an online (videoconferencing) process group reported experiencing a lack of trust in the other members, which was compounded by a lack of trust in the technology (Kozlowski & Holmes, 2014). According to the investigators, "members' sense of safety in the group appeared to be inversely proportional to their awareness of the capabilities of technology. The seemingly technology-savvy members were more mistrusting of how technology could be used to break confidentiality" (Kozlowski & Holmes, 2014, p. 292). Some members reported being hyperaware of the ability of other members to take screen shots and videos.

Wilson, Gosling, and Graham (2012) discovered that there is "a disparity between reported privacy concerns and observed privacy behaviors [on Facebook]" (p. 212) but that "the sheer online ubiquity of Facebook is astounding. As of February 2012, Facebook had over 845 million users (more than the population of Europe) who spent more than 9.7 billion minutes per day on the site" (p. 203). By December 2016, Facebook reported 1.23 billion daily active users and 1.86 billion monthly active users (Facebook Newsroom, 2017). It seems inevitable that mental health professionals and clients will be among those users, and they will grapple with the same concerns other users of social media encounter.

Spotts-De Lazzer (2012) comments that practitioners will have to translate and maintain traditional ethics when it comes to social media. For example, "in California, there are currently no explicit ethics or regulations regarding therapists' use of social networking sites" (p. 19). Spotts-De Lazzer believes therapists must address ethical issues dealing with boundary concerns, assessing dual relationships, maintaining impartiality and judgment as a therapist, and using Facebook to announce or market one's professional practice. Spotts-De Lazzer offers the following recommendations to help manage your presence on Facebook:

- Limit what you share online.
- Familiarize yourself with the privacy policy and take time to maximize and customize your privacy settings.
- Include clear and thorough social networking policies in your informed consent process.
- Regularly update your protective settings because Facebook's privacy options are constantly changing.

Group workers need to prepare themselves to receive a "Friend Request" from either current or former members of the groups they lead. Zur and Zur (2011) have outlined a number of questions that therapists should reflect on before responding to these requests:

- What is on the Facebook profile?
- Does the psychotherapist have a Facebook page or only a Facebook profile?
- Does he or she use privacy controls to control access?
- What can the client view on the therapist's profile?
- What is the context of psychotherapy?
- Who is the client?
- Why did the client post the request?
- What is the meaning of the request?
- What is the nature of the therapeutic relationship?
- Where is psychotherapy taking place? What is the community like where therapy is taking place?
- What does being a "Friend" with this client mean for the therapist?
- What is the potential effect on other potential clients (or group members)?
- What are the ramifications of accepting a Friend Request from a client for confidentiality, privacy, record keeping, and HIPAA compliance?
- Does accepting a Friend Request from a client constitute a dual relationship?
- How will accepting the request affect treatment and the therapeutic relationship?

As you can surmise by reviewing this extensive list of questions, a seemingly straightforward request (whether or not to accept a client or group member's Friend Request) is quite complex and requires a great deal of reflection. To read more about this topic, visit the Zur Institute website (www.zurinstitute.com).

Ethical Issues Concerning Termination

The final phase in the life of a group is critical, for this is when members have the task of consolidating their learning. At this time members need to be able to express what the group experience has meant to them and to state where they intend to go from there. Neglecting the process of termination can easily leave the members with unfinished work and will limit opportunities for them to conceptualize what they learned from a group experience. For many group members endings are difficult because they realize that time is limited in their group. The ending of a group often triggers other losses that members have experienced. Thus, the termination of a group may involve a grieving process. It is important for leaders to help members identify and explore these feelings of loss, even though they may not be completely alleviated. Members need to face the reality of termination and learn how to say good-bye. If the group has been truly therapeutic, the members will be able to extend their learning outside the group despite experiencing a sense of sadness and loss as the group ends.

The Termination Phase in a Closed Group

Generally, *closed groups* have time limitations, with the group meeting for a predetermined number of sessions. Members are typically expected to remain in the group until it ends, and new members are not added. In a closed group the task of leaders is to help members review their individual work and the evolving patterns from the first to the final session. Informed consent involves talking with group members from the beginning of a group experience about the ending and how to terminate productively.

The termination phase of a group provides an opportunity for members to clarify the meaning of their experience, to consolidate the gains they have made, and to make decisions about the new behaviors they want to carry away from the group and apply to their everyday lives. The following questions address the leaders' responsibilities during the termination of a group:

- What ethical responsibilities do group leaders have for assisting participants to develop a conceptual framework that will make sense of, integrate, and consolidate what they have learned in their group?
- To what degree is it the leader's responsibility to ensure that members are not left with excessive unfinished business at the end of the group?
- How can group leaders help participants translate what they have learned as a result of the group into their daily lives?
- How can group leaders help members use termination in a group as a way of dealing with loss and grief?
- In what ways can group leaders incorporate members' cultural beliefs and practices in the termination process?

The final phase of group work may be the one that leaders handle most ineptly, possibly owing to their lack of training or partly because of their own resistance to termination. Avoiding acknowledgment of a group's termination may reflect discomfort on the leader's part in dealing with endings and separations. A group facilitator who does not have a clear picture of his or her own vulnerabilities pertaining to loss or endings will likely find it difficult to facilitate members' expressions of their feelings about endings. When termination is not dealt with, the group misses an opportunity to explore concerns that may affect many members, and the members' therapy is jeopardized. When learning is not conceptualized, the ability to bring the meaning of the experience to real life is diminished. Thus, a discussion of endings is crucial to adequate closure.

Termination of Members in an Open Group

In an *open* group, members leave the group and new members are incorporated into the group at various times. Here are some tasks to be accomplished with a person who is leaving an open group:

- It is important to teach members in an open group to give adequate notice when they decide it is time to terminate. This policy will ensure that members have time to address any unfinished business with themselves or others in the group.
- An ideal termination is one that has been mutually agreed upon by the member and the leader and for which there is sufficient time to work through the process of loss and separation (Fieldsteel, 2005).
- Remaining group members often have reactions about the loss of a member, and it is important that they have an opportunity to express their thoughts and feelings.

- It is a good policy to ask those members who are leaving to review what they have learned in the group and, specifically, what they intend to do with this learning.

Follow-Up and Evaluation

This phase of group work can provide you with helpful feedback on the value of a group experience from the perspective of members and can be done in a variety of ways. Throughout the life of a group, group leaders assist members in assessing their progress and monitor their style of modeling. In this sense, evaluation is an ongoing process whereby members are taught how to determine whether the group is helping them attain their personal goals. But group counselors also must assess both the process and the outcomes of their groups. Once a group has ended, follow-up group sessions provide an opportunity to do this. In our opinion, follow-up activities are useful for members as well as for the group counselor and can be invaluable measures of accountability.

How to Determine What Works in a Group

Evaluating how well group psychotherapy works is not an easy task. Group practitioners operate from diverse theoretical models and possess unique individual characteristics and therapeutic styles. In addition, group members themselves have much to do with the therapeutic outcomes of any group. Practitioners who adhere to the same approach are likely to use techniques in different ways.

Evidence-Based Practice in Group Work

Although it is clear that therapy works, there are no simple explanations of how it works. Lambert's (2011, 2013) review of psychotherapy research makes it clear that the similarities rather than the differences among models account for the effectiveness of psychotherapy. Clinical practice should be based on the best available research integrated with a practitioner's expertise within the context of a particular client (see Chapter 10). However, group practitioners working in agency settings increasingly need to demonstrate the efficacy of their group procedures. One way to do this is to rely exclusively on an evidence-based practice (EBP) approach to evaluation, which considers the best research evidence in light of therapist and client factors (APA Presidential Task Force on Evidence-Based Practice, 2006).

Norcross, Hogan, and Koocher (2008) advocate for inclusive EBPs that incorporate these three pillars: best available evidence, clinician expertise, and client characteristics. It can be difficult to employ the EBP model in the practice of group work because involvement of active and informed group members is crucial to the success of a therapy group. Based on their clinical expertise, group therapists make the ultimate judgment regarding particular interventions in the context of considering the members' values, needs, and preferences. For group leaders to base their practices exclusively on interventions that have been empirically validated may seem to be the ethical and competent path to take, yet some view this model as mechanistic and failing to take into full consideration the relational dimensions of the therapeutic process.

An Alternative: The Practice-Based Approach to Group Work

Many group practitioners do not think matching techniques that have been empirically tested with specific problems is a meaningful way of working with the problems presented by group members. Duncan, Miller, and Sparks (2004) suggest an alternative to evidence-based practice; they propose the approach of *practice-based evidence* (PBE), which uses data generated from clients during treatment to inform the process and outcome of treatment.

Group practitioners with a relationship-oriented approach (such as person-centered therapy and existential therapy) emphasize understanding the world of the group members and healing through the therapeutic relationship. Norcross, Beutler, and Levant (2006) remind us that many aspects of treatment—the therapy relationship, the therapist's personality and therapeutic style, the client, and environmental factors—contribute to the success of psychotherapy and must be taken into account in any evaluation. Duncan and colleagues (2004) argue that the most significant improvements in client retention and outcome have been shown when therapists regularly and purposefully collect data on clients' experiences of the alliance and progress in treatment.

Miller, Hubble, Duncan, and Wampold (2010) emphasize the importance of enlisting the client's active participation in the therapeutic venture. They argue that you do not need to know ahead of time what approach to use for a given diagnosis. What is most important is to systematically gather and use formal client feedback to inform, guide, and evaluate treatment. Members could complete a very brief anonymous form at the end of each group session, and their ratings on specific items can be tallied as a way to get a sense of the progress of the group as a whole. Ideally, evaluation is an ongoing process throughout the life of a group that monitors the progress of both the members and the group as a whole. Monitoring group progress by collecting data from each member can help leaders make adjustments to their interventions and enhance the group process (Corey & Corey, 2016).

Inviting feedback from the group members about their experience in the group is of the utmost importance. **Feedback-informed treatment** (FIT) is an evidence-based practice that monitors client change and identifies modifications needed to enhance the therapeutic endeavor (Miller, Hubble, & Seidel, 2015). FIT involves consistently obtaining feedback from clients regarding the therapeutic relationship and their clinical progress, which is then used to tailor therapy to their unique needs. If group leaders learn to listen to members' feedback at all phases of a group, members can become full and equal participants in all aspects of their therapy (Miller et al., 2015).

Jensen and colleagues (2012) recommend that group clinicians integrate PBE into their therapy groups. They point to the benefits of taking the pulse of groups by relying on systematic measures to gather client-generated data to supplement clinical judgment. "PBE tools allow clinicians to periodically take the 'vital signs' of the group and make any needed adjustments" (p. 389). Jensen et al. contend that collecting data directly from members about their group experience is a significant part of developing an evidence-based group therapy practice. "Group psychotherapists could benefit from a structured way to check in with group members about how they are doing, as well as globally demonstrate the efficacy of their psychotherapy groups" (p. 391).

The PBE approach can help therapists assess the value of a group for its members throughout the life of the group as well as provide a tool to aid evaluation of the group experience during the termination phase. Group practitioners have an ethical responsibility to determine how well a group is working and need to be willing to use the feedback they receive from group participants to refine their interventions.

Chapter Summary

As the demand for mental health services increases, group counseling is an evidence-based alternative to individual counseling. Along with the growing popularity of group approaches to counseling and therapy comes a need for ethical and professional guidelines for those who lead groups. There are many types of groups, and there are many possible uses of groups in various settings. In this chapter we have discussed some ethical issues that are related to most groups. To become competent group leaders, counselors require adequate education and supervised experience in facilitating a group. Meeting the professional training standards for group workers is essential. As is true in any form of counseling, achieving multicultural and diversity competence is basic to becoming an ethical and effective group worker.

We also looked at the advantages and disadvantages of a coleadership model of group work. Coleadership can enhance what members learn in a group, but it is essential that the coleaders work well together and model a respectful relationship.

Conducting a group entails attending to a host of ethical issues, including providing informed consent, screening and selecting group members, and preparing members for a meaningful group experience. Leaders working with involuntary groups have the tasks of establishing procedures for members who want to leave the group, addressing psychological risks of group participation, and exploring members' concerns about confidentiality. In addition, we discussed some ethical issues pertaining to dealing with values in group counseling, addressed the use of social media in the practice of group work, and discussed how to deal ethically and effectively with termination of members in both a closed group and an open group. There are various approaches to evaluating a group experience, and practitioners do not agree on the efficacy of any one model. The evidence-based practice model is often viewed as the standard for evaluating therapeutic experiences, but we presented an alternative approach to the evaluation of a group—a *practice-based evidence* approach. Consistently obtaining feedback from group members enables the group practitioner to adjust and accommodate to maximize the beneficial outcomes for the members of a group throughout all of the group stages.

With respect to these and other issues, we have stressed the importance of formulating your own views on ethical practice in leading groups, after carefully considering the ethics codes of your professional organization. You can find guidance on becoming a more effective group worker from several documents: the "Best Practice Guidelines" (ASGW, 2008), the *Multicultural and Social Justice Competence Principles for Group Workers* (ASGW, 2012), and the *Multicultural and Social Justice Counseling Competencies* (AMCD, 2015).

Suggested Activities

1. Replicate the initial session of a group. Two students can volunteer to colead and approximately eight other students can become group members. Assume that the group is a personal-growth group that will meet for a predetermined number of weeks. The coleaders' job is to orient and prepare the members by describing the group's purpose, giving an overview of group process concepts, and talking about ground rules for effective group participation. If time allows, members can express any fears and expectations they have about being involved in the group, and they can also raise questions they would like to explore. Allow ample time at the end to process the experience and to provide feedback to the coleaders.

2. Practice conducting screening interviews for potential group members. One person can volunteer to conduct interviews, and another student can role-play a potential group member. Allow about 10 minutes for the interview. Afterward, the prospective client can talk about what it was like to be interviewed, and the group leader can share his or her experience.

3. As part of your job, you are expected to lead a group consisting of involuntary members. How will this fact affect your approach? What might you do differently with this group compared with a group of voluntary members? Have several students play the reluctant members while others practice interacting with them.

4. You are leading a counseling group with high school students. A member comes to the group obviously incoherent and disruptive. How do you deal with him? Discuss in class how you would deal with this situation, or demonstrate how you might respond by having a classmate play the part of the disruptive adolescent.

5. Again, assume that you are leading a high school counseling group. An angry father who gave written permission for his son's participation comes to your office and demands to know what is going on in your group. He is convinced that his son's participation in the group is an invasion of family privacy. As a group leader, how would you deal with his anger?

6. Selecting a good coleader for a group is important, for not all matches of coleaders are productive. Form dyads and negotiate with your partner to determine whether the two of you would be effective if you were to lead a group together. You might discuss your different counseling styles and how they might complement or interfere with each other, and any other issues that you think would have a bearing on your ability to work as a team.

7. Discuss how social justice themes can be explored within the context of a group. How can you become a culturally competent social justice group worker?

8. When members of a counseling group engage in social media there are certain risks. As a class, discuss the potential pitfalls of group members using online sites to communicate with each other. As a leader, how might you address these risks?

MindTap for Counseling

Go to MindTap® for an eBook, videos of client sessions, activities, practice quizzes, apps, and more—all in one place. If your instructor didn't assign MindTap, you can find out more information at CengageBrain.com.

Community and Social Justice Perspectives

LEARNING OBJECTIVES

1. Define the concept of the community as client

2. Articulate why a community perspective is important to the counselor

3. Describe the types of community and client interventions

4. Explain what is required by the social justice perspective

5. Understand the goals of the social justice perspective

6. Enumerate the advocacy competencies

7. Recognize the main responsibilities of helping professionals in a community setting

8. Identify alternative roles in a community perspective

9. Examine ways to become involved in the community and promote change

10. Explore ways of working within a system

11. Clarify how to be an advocate for change in a system

12. Appreciate the relationships between community worker and agency

SELF-INVENTORY

Directions: For each statement, indicate the response that most closely identifies your beliefs and attitudes. Use the following code:

5 = I *strongly agree* with this statement.

4 = I *agree* with this statement.

3 = I am *undecided* about this statement.

2 = I *disagree* with this statement.

1 = I *strongly disagree* with this statement.

_____ 1. It is important to include people from the client's environment in his or her treatment.

_____ 2. Community workers need to take an active role in seeking solutions to the social and political conditions related to human suffering.

_____ 3. Mental health experts need to devote more of their energies to preventing emotional and behavioral disorders rather than just treating them.

_____ 4. The use of unlicensed workers is a valuable, cost-effective, and ethical way to deal with the shortage of professional help and budget constraints.

_____ 5. I want to take steps to educate community members about the work done by mental health professionals.

_____ 6. Community workers need to be skilled in out-of-office strategies and roles such as change agent and outreach.

_____ 7. It is possible to work within the framework of a system and still be effective.

_____ 8. I frequently have good ideas and proposals, and I see myself as being willing to do the work necessary to translate these plans into actual programs.

_____ 9. Ethical practice requires that we look for ways to involve and mobilize resources and assets in the community to identify problems and find solutions.

_____ 10. Meaningful contact with colleagues prevents us from becoming excessively narrow in our thinking.

_____ 11. It would be unethical to accept a position with an agency if the community worker disagreed with the agency's counseling goals.

_____ 12. Human-service workers should be able to identify indigenous leaders in the community and work with them to improve local conditions.

_____ 13. A central role in human services is the development of leadership among community members.

_____ 14. One of the goals of a professional working in the community is to empower people to become increasingly self-reliant.

_____ 15. A counselor is part of a system and has an ethical responsibility to work toward changing those aspects of the system that are ineffective and are harming clients.

Introduction

When the community mental health movement came into existence, it took the family systems perspective discussed in Chapter 11 a step further to include the entire community as the focus of treatment. By looking at the whole community, it is possible to discover strengths within the community and to develop ways to bring these strengths to work for the community and the individual. Feminist therapy likewise addresses the need to consider the social, cultural, historical, political, and economic context that contributes to a person's problems in order to understand and help that person. Working with people in individual, couples, family, and group therapy are some key ways for professionals to promote mental and emotional health. Working in the community requires an expansive focus that embraces the total milieu of people's lives and fosters real and lasting community change.

Making a Difference in the Community

To be effective and practice ethically, we must be aware of the broader context of human problems no matter what setting we choose for our work. In much the same way family therapists think beyond the child to the needs and strengths of the whole family, we must think beyond the needs of the individual to the needs and strengths of the community at large. As we lean into our discomfort to examine systemic issues in the larger context of the community, we will face tough choices regarding changes in our profession and our role.

Chung and Bemak (2012) view courage in dealing with fear as a cornerstone of doing multicultural social justice work and point out that "social change and improvements in human rights have never taken place without individuals taking risks" (p. 164). For social transformation to occur, Waller (2013) feels he must be willing to get out of the office and get involved with the community: "My social justice action tends to focus on changing policies within a system that impact the community rather than just an individual" (p. 93). Bemak and Conyne (2018) discuss the issue of transforming roles in their book *Journeys to Professional Excellence: Stories of Courage, Innovation, and Risk-taking*. The authors document the importance and challenges of incorporating innovation, risk-taking, and courage in the lives of well-known mental health professionals.

To illustrate how a counselor might work with both an individual client and also address societal factors that are exacerbating a personal problem, consider this scenario:

> A school counselor begins working with a young teen struggling with depression and suicidal ideation. Upon further questioning, it becomes evident that his anxiety is related to "coming out" to his friends and family. His fear of discrimination and bullying are being expressed as feelings of hopelessness and isolation. As the counselor works with the teen on his emotions and suicidal ideation, she also works to create an environment in the school that makes it safer for all LGBTQ teens to be who they

are without fears of retaliation or bullying. To create this supportive environment, the counselor creates safe spaces for open dialogue, imparts information, gives voice to the LGBTQ community within the school, and invites guest speakers to various classes.

The Community as Client

The foundation of all ethical practice is promoting the welfare of clients. Overlooking the abilities, strengths, and resources within the community does a great disservice to the individuals we serve. If we hope to bring about significant changes for individuals and communities, Homan (2016) believes we need to change the conditions that affect people rather than change the people affected by these conditions.

Many homeless veterans of war struggle to function in society due to immobilizing PTSD symptoms, substance abuse, and low social support. Not only have they experienced trauma related to combat during their military service, but they continue to experienced traumatic events outside of the military (Carlson, Garvert, Macia, Ruzek, & Burling, 2013). Consider Tommy's circumstances:

> Stressed to the maximum after having a leg amputated, Tommy is plagued with survivor's guilt and nightmares after witnessing friends being killed in Afghanistan. Upon returning home, Tommy found it difficult to get through each day without drinking heavily and lashing out angrily at his family. Frightened by the intensity of his anger, Tommy's wife took their two small children and filed for divorce, which was devastating to him. Tommy knew he needed help and understandably felt disillusioned, disappointed, and frustrated when he was unable to get the mental health services that he desperately needed through the local VA hospital. As his mental health deteriorated and his PTSD symptoms spiraled out of control, Tommy could not handle simple tasks and ended up homeless.

What community-level interventions could help veterans and spouses and children of returning veterans feel supported and accepted in their communities? What community changes are needed to help those who are struggling to thrive? How might community members benefit from these interventions even though they are not the primary focus of the interventions?

The ethical issues we discuss in this chapter are faced by many workers in community agency settings. We use the term **community agency** broadly to include any institution—public or private, nonprofit or for-profit—designed to provide a wide range of social and psychological services to the community. Likewise, when we speak of a **community worker**, we refer to a diverse pool of human-service workers whose primary duties include serving individuals within the community in a variety of community groups. Community workers include social workers, community organizers and developers, clinical mental health counselors, psychologists, psychiatrists, nurses, counselors, couples and family therapists, artists, activists, clergy persons, human-service workers with varying degrees of education and training, and residents involved in the community.

Examine your own commitment to working in the community by thinking about these questions:

- Which communities that you belong to are most important to you? What makes you regard these communities as special or meaningful?
- What are the key problems or issues facing each of these communities? What forces within or surrounding these communities exacerbate the issues individuals and groups are experiencing?
- What are some resources available to empower people in these communities?
- In what ways have historical or current issues of oppression, discrimination, and poverty affected these communities?
- Who holds the power in each of these communities? Who are the decision makers? Who is most likely to support or thwart change?

This chapter also examines how the system affects the counselor, the ethical dimensions of practice, and how to survive and thrive while working in the system. If practitioners are limited in their ability to adapt their roles to the needs of the community, they are not likely to be effective in reaching those who most need assistance. Likewise, if the community does not understand what community mental health workers can do, they are less likely to use their services.

Why a Community Perspective Is a Concern for Counselors

Chung and Bemak (2012) suggest that by adhering to traditional roles, practitioners are maintaining and reinforcing the status quo, which results in passively supporting the social injustices, inequalities, and discriminatory treatment of certain groups of people. Chung and Bemak contend that advocacy is an ethical and moral obligation for an effective mental health professional. The community approach is relevant to all communities, but it is particularly relevant to underserved communities. By addressing the cause of the problem within the community, we can help change the lives of many individuals—not just the one person sitting in our office or clinic—as the following story demonstrates.

Moving Upstream

While walking along the banks of a river, a passerby notices that someone in the water is drowning. After pulling the person ashore, the rescuer notices another person in the river in need of help. Before long the river is filled with drowning people, and more rescuers are required to assist the initial rescuer. Unfortunately, some people are not saved and some people fall back into the river after they have been pulled ashore. At this time, one of the rescuers starts walking upstream. "Where are you going," the other rescuers ask disconcerted. The upstream rescuer replies, "I'm going upstream to see why so many people keep falling into the river." As it turns out, the bridge leading across the river upstream has a hole through which people are falling. The upstream rescuer realizes that fixing the hole in the bridge will prevent many people from ever falling into the river in the first place. (Cohen & Chehimi, 2010, p. 5)

We rarely look beyond the individual in examining how the community and the system contribute to the client's problem, and this individual focus may limit our effectiveness. How would you answer these questions:

- In what ways are your own struggles a by-product of societal ills?
- What social justice issues do you feel passionate about or have a particular interest in supporting?
- What is your sphere of influence? To what groups or communities do you belong, and what kind of power or influence do you have in those arenas?
- What role would you like to play in improving your community? What are the first steps you might take in this role as a social change agent?

If we narrowly define what it means to be a counselor, we limit ourselves and the assistance we can provide to our clients. Advocating for systemic changes can bring about positive changes in the lives of our clients. A colleague, who is a social justice advocate and counseling practitioner, often observed overt and or covert racist practices in the elementary school system. She had noticed that the same few African American boys were consistently being sent to the principal's office for disciplinary reasons. She found this troubling and brought it to the attention of the school psychologist. She used her knowledge as a clinician, along with being a member of the school community, to engage in a dialogue that led to systemic change, increased awareness, and more effective interventions. This is an illustration of how we can use our professional knowledge and skills to advocate for changes that help others in our community.

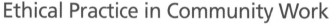

Ethical Practice in Community Work

The ethics codes of professional practice reinforce the practitioner's responsibility to the community and to society (see the Ethics Codes box titled "Responsibilities to Community and Society"). It is left to community workers to identify strategies for becoming more responsive to the community.

ETHICS CODES: Responsibilities to Community and Society

National Organization for Human Services (2015)
Human service professionals stay informed about current social issues as they affect the client and the community. They share that information with clients, groups and community as part of their work. (Standard 13.)

   Human service professionals provide a mechanism for identifying *unmet client needs*, calling attention to these needs, and assisting in planning and mobilizing to advocate for those needs at the individual, community, and societal level when appropriate to the goals of the relationship. (Standard 15.)

   Human service professionals advocate for social justice and seek to eliminate oppression. They raise awareness of underserved populations in their communities and with the legislative system. (Standard 16.)

American Mental Health Counselors Association (2015)
Mental health counselors recognize they have a moral, legal, and ethical responsibility to the community and to the general public. Mental health counselors are aware of the prevailing community and cultural values, and the impact of professional standards on the community. (V.)

American School Counselor Association (2016)
School counselors attempt to establish a collaborative relationship with outside service providers to best serve students. School counselors request a release of information signed by the student and/or parents/guardians before attempting to collaborate with the student's external provider. (A.6.f.)

One of the primary objectives of community practice is constituency self-determination. Community organizers must first determine the primary recipient of their interventions. Is the client an individual, a group of people, or society in general? Practitioners need to acquire adequate skills to deal effectively with the ethical challenges unique to community work. For instance, suppose a program is established to nurture the abilities of bright students from disadvantaged backgrounds and to assist them in getting into top colleges. On the surface this seems straightforward, but a number of assumptions underlie the stated goal. Donors are placing a high value on attendance at a top-ranked school and discounting as trivial any inconvenience travel to a distant city may cause these students and their families. Students and their families may place a high value on keeping the family intact and so would prefer the student attend the nearby college and continue to live at home. The community worker might be concerned that the best interests of certain students would not be optimally served by encouraging them to leave home to attend a college far away from their families. Although some students might adapt well, others might not for any number of reasons. This could result in them dropping out of school and returning home. On the other hand, the worker might also be concerned that the donors would stop funding the program if students forfeited the opportunity to study at a top-ranked university. Without the funding, those students who could potentially be well served by the program would lose out on this opportunity. If you were in this community worker's position, how might you navigate this ethical dilemma?

In talking about social justice, community activism, and outreach, our students are sometimes uncertain about where to begin or how they can make a difference. A good starting place is to list the communities to which you belong and describe your spheres of influence within these various systems. For example, you may be a member of a religious organization, a book club, an athletic team, or a creative arts circle. Pay attention to the issues that arise in the organizations to which you belong and ask yourself these questions:

- What sociocultural issues can you identify within the systems, organizations, groups, and communities you belong to or have frequent contact with? (Some examples might be discriminatory practices, poverty, lack of support, lack of diversity, negative influence of media, crime, and lack of access to power or resources.)
- What roles can you take in bringing about awareness, change, or confirmation of these issues?
- What do you see as potential barriers to raising awareness or bringing about change?

- What is one thing (at the macro or micro level) that you could actively do to bring about awareness of the issues harming the members of these communities? How willing are you to do this?
- What do you tell yourself that keeps you from acting as a change agent?

One of our students talked about his work as a high school football coach and how his own multicultural training helped him to identify changes that needed to be made in the language coaches and team players used. After learning about heterosexism firsthand from his college classmates, this student used his position as coach to model less sexist and homophobic language in the locker rooms. His goal was to create an environment in which a team member who might be gay would not be subject to constant verbal assaults and daily microaggressions. This seemingly small change opened the door to other important conversations among his players. What began with a change in language later was integrated into cultural sensitivity training with the staff and athletic team at the school.

The Community Mental Health Orientation

The community orientation is based on the premise that the community itself is the most appropriate focus of attention, rather than the individual, and the community also is the most potent resource for solutions. Even when counseling individuals, consider how these individuals have been influenced by the community, how they might draw on community resources to help meet their goals, and ways that the community is presently influencing them. Homan (2016) reminds us: "Just like an individual or a family, a community has resources and limitations. Communities have established coping mechanisms to deal with problems. To promote change in a community, the community must believe in its own ability to change and must take responsibility for its actions or inactions" (p. 27).

The need for diverse and readily accessible treatment programs has been a key factor in the development of the community mental health orientation. Environmental factors cause or contribute to the problems of many groups in society, and a process that considers both the individual and the environment is likely to benefit everybody. The focus of community work is on preventing rather than remediating problems.

Types of Client and Community Interventions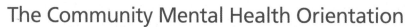

Community counseling is "a comprehensive helping framework that is grounded in multicultural competence and oriented toward social justice" (Lewis, Lewis, Daniels, & D'Andrea, 2011, p. 9). A comprehensive community counseling model described by Lewis and colleagues is based on two activities:

- *facilitating human development* by providing direct interventions with clients and community members, and
- *facilitating community development* through advocacy interventions that break down external barriers to client well-being.

Human development activities include both focused strategies (such as outreach activities) and broad-based strategies (such as developmental and preventive programs aimed at educating members of the community). Community development activities also include both focused strategies (such as advocating for clients and preparing clients to be their own advocates) and broad-based interventions (such as counselors acting as change agents in systems through social and political advocacy).

Another way of conceptualizing the community counseling model is through the various forms of services provided to clients: direct client services, indirect client services, direct community services, and indirect community services (Lewis et al., 2011).

Direct Client Services These service providers focus on outreach activities to a population that might be at risk for developing mental health problems. Community counselors provide help to clients either facing crises or dealing with ongoing stressors that overwhelm them. By reaching out to schools and communities that are receptive to help, community workers can offer a variety of personal, career, family, and counseling services to at-risk groups. This population also would include referrals from the courts, churches, mosques, synagogues, probation departments, VA centers, and drug and alcohol treatment centers. Direct client service providers empower clients with skills, knowledge, and understanding that will help them cope with external stressors (Toporek et al., 2009).

Indirect Client Services Client advocacy and consultation are at the heart of these services, and community workers create partnerships by working *with* groups in a collaborative way rather than merely providing services *for* these groups. Counselors identify factors that negatively affect their clients and take action, often in collaboration with others, to bring about needed changes (Lewis et al., 2011). If a community worker is advocating on behalf of clients with physical disabilities who are constantly overlooked for jobs they are capable of performing, the community worker might organize a campaign to educate employers and raise their awareness about people with physical disabilities. If the client community conducts the research, prepares the materials to be distributed, participates in presentations, and evaluates the success of the campaign, their abilities and strengths will be showcased to employers. In addition, the client population will be empowered by participating in their own advocacy.

Direct Community Services Community counselors serve their communities by offering *preventive education programs* geared to the population at large. Examples of these programs include life planning workshops, value clarification seminars, interpersonal skills training, and teaching parents about their legal rights and responsibilities. Because the emphasis is on prevention, these programs help people develop a wider range of competencies. The focus of preventive programs is on teaching effective living and problem-solving competencies.

Indirect Community Services Community workers strive to change the social environment to reduce the mental and physical health problems of the population as a whole by influencing public policy. The focus is on promoting systemic change by working closely with those in the community who develop public policy. For example, a community worker might focus on helping to shape policies at the local, state, or national level that support people with disabilities in finding satisfactory employment and that safeguard their rights in the workplace. Another community agent might work closely with stakeholders to develop effective community interventions and new public policies to assist people suffering with an opiate addiction in getting the treatment they need to recover.

Community work is not easy; there are institutional obstacles to getting meaningful work done. Bemak (2013) comments that "being effective in community work requires a rigorous focus on the goals of the work and a profound understanding that the process of achieving these goals may be fraught with challenges and complications" (p. 193). He believes that a main challenge for counselors is to take action and do what is necessary to meet their goals by drawing on their passion and commitment to make the world a better place.

Social Justice Perspective

Broadly constructed, "**social justice** involves access and equity to ensure full participation in the life of a society, particularly for those who have been systematically excluded on the basis of race/ethnicity, gender, age, physical or mental disability, education, sexual orientation, socioeconomic status, or other characteristics of background or group membership" (Lee, 2013a, p. 16). Counseling from a social justice perspective involves addressing the realities of oppression, privilege, and social inequities.

Social justice and advocacy have become areas of major concern for all counselors, and indeed, social justice is referred to as a **fifth force** that entails a paradigm shift beyond the individual. The *fifth force* represents a proactive concern with advocacy and social change and focuses on changing systems and policies on multiple levels (Chung & Bemak, 2012). "Social justice counseling with marginalized groups in our society is most enhanced (a) when mental health professionals can understand how individual and systemic worldviews shape clinical practice and (b) when they are equipped with organizational and system knowledge, expertise, and skills" (Sue & Sue, 2013, pp. 108–109). From this perspective, the helping professional's role includes advocate, consultant, psychoeducator, change agent, and community worker.

Counselors with a community orientation are committed to making society a better place by challenging systemic inequities. Although not all counselors will have the time or energy to effect major institutional change, all have the capability of working toward some kind of social change. For example, counselors might strive for social change by challenging colleagues who have made erroneous assumptions regarding marginalized client populations. Hogan (2013) believes we need to recognize that our own cultural framework is the starting point for how we engage the world. Understanding ourselves as cultural beings powerfully influences our perceptions, as well as the methods we use in our professional work.

Social Justice Advocacy as an Ethical Mandate

Counselors who base their practice on aspirational ethics oppose all forms of discrimination and oppression. Some of the ethics codes refer to the role of social justice advocacy as an ethical mandate (see the Ethics Codes box titled "Social Justice Advocacy").

ETHICS CODES: Social Justice Advocacy

National Association of Social Workers (2008)
(a) Social workers should engage in social and political action that seeks to ensure that all persons have equal access to the resources, employment, services, and opportunities that they require in order to meet their basic human needs and to develop fully. Social workers should be aware of the impact of the political arena on practice, and should advocate for changes in policy and legislation to improve social conditions in order to meet basic human needs and promote social justice.

(b) Social workers should act to expand choice and opportunity for all persons, with special regard for vulnerable, disadvantaged, oppressed, and exploited persons and groups.

(c) Social workers should promote conditions that encourage respect for cultural and social diversity within the United States and globally. Social workers should promote policies and practices that demonstrate respect for difference, support the expansion of cultural knowledge and resources, advocate for programs and institutions that demonstrate cultural competence, and promote policies that safeguard the rights of and confirm equity and social justice for all people.

(d) Social workers should act to prevent and eliminate domination of, exploitation of, and discrimination against any person, group, or class on the basis of race, ethnicity, national origin, color, sex, sexual orientation, gender identity or expression, age, marital status, political belief, religion, immigration status, or mental or physical disability. (6.04.)

American Mental Health Counselors Association (2015)
Mental health counselors may serve as advocates at the individual, institutional, and/or societal level in an effort to foster sociopolitical change that meets the needs of the client or the community.

Ethical dilemmas may arise when the cultural values of the community are not congruent with the values of the community worker. Practitioners need to think about the cultural values of the community where they work and the degree to which their intervention strategies are likely to advance the mental health of clients in the community (Pack-Brown, Thomas, & Seymour, 2008). What is the practitioner to do when there is a conflict between a community agency's program and the personal values of the practitioner? Reflect on the following case of a social worker who is seeking advice.

The Case of Lupe

Lupe is a social worker in a community mental health agency that is sponsoring workshops aimed at preventing the spread of HIV. The agency has attempted to involve the local churches in these workshops. One church withdrew its support because the workshops encouraged "safer" sexual practices, including the use of condoms, as a way of preventing HIV. A church official contended that the use of condoms is contrary to church teachings. Being a member of this church, Lupe finds herself struggling with value conflicts. She believes the teachings of her church and thinks the official had a right to withdraw his support of these workshops. But she also is aware that many people in the community she serves are at high risk for contracting HIV because of both drug use and sexual practices. In an attempt to resolve this value conflict, Lupe seeks out several of her colleagues, each of whom provides some advice.

Colleague A: I hope you tell your clients and others in the community that you have value conflicts between agency practice and your religious beliefs and, for that reason, you are voluntarily resigning from the agency.

Colleague B: Be up front with the people you come in contact with by telling them of your values and providing them with adequate referrals so they can get information about prevention of this disease. You do owe it to them not to steer them in the direction you think they should move.

Colleague C: It is best that you not disclose your values or let clients know that you agree with the church's views. Instead, focus on the underlying causes of their behaviors and work toward helping clients become more aware of how they are engaging in self-destructive behaviors.

If Lupe were to seek you out and ask for your advice, consider what you would say to her. In formulating your position, answer these questions:

- Which of her colleagues comes closest to your thinking, and why?
- With which colleague do you find yourself disagreeing the most, and why?
- Would it be ethical for Lupe not to disclose her values to her clients? Why or why not?
- What are the potential consequences if Lupe imposes her moral beliefs on the population she is serving? Is it her ethical and moral duty to the community to develop a program aimed at prevention of HIV? Explain.

Commentary. This case highlights a conflict between the social worker's personal values and her agency's requirements in a community context. Lupe should identify any conflicts between her ethical duty to avoid harm and promote her clients' best interests and the church's teachings, and then abide by the ethical mandate. We would remind Lupe that just as in individual counseling, she is committed to working for the best interests of her client, in this case, the community as a whole. Lupe's failure to provide necessary information to members of the community puts the community at risk of harm. Because the teachings of the church prevent such a partnership, Lupe may need to enlist other community groups in her efforts to provide outreach regarding methods of safer sex. Even though Lupe's values are congruent with the church's position, ethically she cannot replace community values with her personal values. Johnson, Barnett, Elman, Forrest, and Kaslow (2012) have encouraged the profession to modify and amplify the principle of beneficence to incorporate qualities of caring and compassion. This case illustrates the need for practitioners to demonstrate care and compassion in their work in the community. •

The Goals of Social Justice and Advocacy

Advocacy can help create a better world that goes beyond an individual client (Chung & Bemak, 2012). The goal of counseling from a social justice perspective is to promote the empowerment of people who are marginalized and oppressed in our society (Herlihy & Watson, 2007). Stone and Dahir (2016) claim that "the basic principles of advocacy are helping socially devalued groups gain the tools, confidence, political clout, and skills needed to move away from oppression" (p. 125).

Chung and Bemak (2012) state that "being an advocate requires the core counseling skills and multicultural competencies, along with energy, commitment, motivation, passion, persistence, tenacity, flexibility, patience, assertiveness, organization, resourcefulness, creativity, a multisystems and multidisciplinary perspective, and the ability to deal with conflict and negotiate and access systems" (p. 175).

Counselors must be willing to work outside of traditional school and agency settings to lower societal barriers that impede optimum human functioning (Steele, 2008; Stone & Dahir, 2016). Some of these societal barriers include limited access to health care and a quality education, poverty, segregation, racism, sexism, and discrimination, all of which are conditions that contribute to oppressive societal practices and create barriers to participating fully in society. Tensions in American society related to social injustice have increased in recent years. Although some progress has been made, society remains polarized. Stories about police brutality directed toward Black males, mass shootings and acts of terrorism both on American soil and abroad, xenophobia, and intolerance toward the LGBTQ community, religious minorities, and other vulnerable populations abound. Global issues such as terrorism, war, radicalization, political dissension, and economic instability may have an impact on our lives and on the lives of our clients in ways that we cannot yet imagine. Through the ubiquitous presence of technology and social media in our lives today, we can access news anywhere in the world as it is occurring, which certainly makes the world seem smaller. Some may find the sheer amount of information available to be overwhelming and stressful.

In this age of globalization, counselors and other helping professionals need to be prepared to deal with demands that previously may have seemed to be beyond the scope of their training. For instance, a counselor working with refugees who escaped unthinkable conditions in war-torn countries may be dealing with the trauma of experiencing or witnessing atrocities in the client's country of origin as well as the trauma of leaving one's home and loved ones behind; finding appropriate housing and employment; learning a new language and navigating a new culture; and dealing with xenophobic attitudes from others in the community. Working on issues such as self-actualization must, by necessity, take a backseat to these higher priorities.

Refugees and other clients who have been oppressed may need assistance with a variety of tasks, and it is imperative that the counselor and the client establish goals in a collaborative manner. Community-oriented counselors must adopt a flexible approach and be willing to assist clients in finding resources that will help them make a positive adjustment. During my (Cindy's) work with Sudanese refugees, it was not uncommon for me to conduct home visits. Although I provided mental health services, my clients often needed basic information such as how to get a driver's license, apply for college classes, find jobs, use kitchen appliances, and sort through mail that was important versus "junk." Although this may not seem like counseling, it was a basic part of establishing trust and was necessary in order for my clients to feel ready to begin to talk about the deeper issues of trauma that accompanied them when they entered the country.

Social justice and advocacy competencies are necessary for counselors to work effectively on a systemic level. Counselor education programs must include skills training to intervene effectively on both individual and community levels. Lewis,

Toporek, and Ratts (2010) point out that "more and more counselors have begun to use the wide-angle lens in their work. The counseling profession has come to accept the idea that advocacy strategies and a social justice perspective belong at the center of good practice" (p. 243).

Advocacy Competencies

Counselors function as **advocates** when they use their skills in helping clients challenge institutional barriers that impede their personal, social, academic, or career goals (Lee & Hipolito-Delgado, 2007). Counselors who have a social justice advocacy perspective demonstrate leadership abilities and understand the importance of speaking out to empower individuals, families, and their community (Ratts & Hutchins, 2009). A primary focus for school counselors who assume an advocacy role is to become the voice for students who lack educational opportunities. All students deserve equal access to a quality education (Stone & Dahir, 2016), and Lee and Rodgers (2009) point out that school counselor advocates are risk-takers and often take on causes that are unpopular. They assert that it takes courage "to intervene not only into the lives of clients but also into the larger social/political arena for the benefit of an individual client as well as to foster social justice for all" (p. 286).

Ethical practice requires counselors to assume an advocacy role that is focused on affecting public opinion, public policy, and legislation (ACA, 2014; Lee & Rodgers, 2009). Practitioners also need to develop an awareness of their own beliefs and attitudes regarding social issues and marginalized populations, the scope of their knowledge, and their level of skill at intervening within the different domains of advocacy. Finally, multicultural competence is essential in understanding the cultural relevance and appropriateness of advocacy interventions as counselors bring their own attitudes and beliefs to the sociopolitical history of their communities. For comprehensive discussions of social justice and systems changes as applied to working with diverse client populations, see *ACA Advocacy Competencies: A Social Justice Framework for Counselors* (Ratts et al., 2010) and *Social Justice Counseling: The Next Steps Beyond Multiculturalism* (Chung & Bemak, 2012).

Social Justice Advocacy in School Counseling

The role of school counselors is expanding to include advocating for social justice on a broader scale (Lee & Rodgers, 2009). Stone and Dahir (2016) devote a chapter to the topic of school counselors as advocates, and their ideas are represented in this discussion. Raising hopes and expectations and empowering students are critical roles for school counselors to play in supporting a better future for students. However, a proactive stance goes beyond working with individual students to advocating for change throughout the school system when inequities and discriminatory practices are found. Stone and Dahir list some guiding principles for effective advocacy:

- Counselors demonstrate a willingness to be passionate advocates and risk-takers who assist students in finding a voice.

- Counselors believe that they can make a significant difference by relentlessly and collaboratively pursuing an advocacy role. They recognize that they can affect change, and they accept and celebrate their small successes.
- Counselors believe in their students and do not allow others to sidetrack them with negativity. School counselors can help foster a vision and a belief in the development of high aspirations for every student.

Roles of Helpers Working in the Community

As we indicated in Chapter 4, to meet the needs of many ethnic and culturally diverse clients, traditional counselors must have a different vision and master different skills. Providing services in nontraditional settings outside the office may be clinically and ethically indicated and may be most beneficial to clients.

Outreach Interventions

The outreach approach may include both developmental and educational efforts, such as skills training, stress management, and consultation. Outreach activities also include family preservation services, the goal of which is to develop a treatment plan with a family to maintain children's safety in their own homes. For instance, during a series of home visits to a parent with poor coping skills, an outreach worker teaches, models, and reinforces parenting strategies that can be used to effectively navigate challenging parent–child interactions. Community counselors also attempt to change the dysfunctional system that is producing problems for individuals, families, and communities. The focus is on looking at the problem in its community context rather than dealing only with the problem within the individual.

MacLeod and McMullen (2016) suggest that counselors also can reach out to the community outside of the counseling setting by volunteering at nonprofit organizations in their local area. Providing outreach beyond the counseling setting is one way to combat stigma and stereotypes regarding mental health concerns; outreach interventions can teach people about wellness and the benefits of counseling. "Outreach and volunteer work allows counselors to use their skills in new and useful ways, while providing the public with an experience of what counselors do and what they value" (p. 78).

Alternative Counselor Roles

Community-oriented counseling emphasizes the necessity for recognizing and dealing with environmental conditions that often create problems for ethnically diverse client groups. In this psychosocial approach, community workers focus on alternative ways of helping clients that embody fundamental principles of social justice and activism aimed at client empowerment. Atkinson (2004) suggests these alternative roles for counselors who work in the community: *advocate, change agent, consultant, adviser, facilitator of indigenous support systems,* and *facilitator of indigenous healing methods.* Counselors who adopt these alternative roles base their work on a developmental foundation rather than on a service approach. The role of community workers as advocates and change agents has been described; now let's take a look at some other alternative counselor roles.

Consultant Operating as **consultants**, counselors encourage clients from diverse cultures to learn skills they can use to interact successfully with various forces within their community. In this role, client and counselor cooperate in addressing unhealthy forces within the system. Consultants work with clients from diverse racial, ethnic, and cultural backgrounds to design preventive programs aimed at eliminating the negative impacts of racism and oppression. The role of consultant can be seen as the role of a teacher.

Adviser The counselor as **adviser** initiates discussions with clients about ways to deal with environmental problems that contribute to their personal problems. In many ways, this is a social work approach that considers the person-in-the-environment rather than simply addressing problems within the individual. For example, recent immigrants may need advice on immigration paperwork, coping with problems they will face in the job market, or problems that their children may encounter at school. Veterans transitioning out of the military also may need help finding a job, accessing education benefits, finding a place to live, and identifying local supports for their family.

Facilitator of Indigenous Support Systems Many ethnically diverse clients, people in rural environments, and older people would not consider seeking professional help in the traditional sense. However, they may be willing to put their faith in family members or close friends, or turn to other social support systems within their own communities. Community workers need to be aware of cultural factors that may be instrumental in contributing to a client's problem or resources that might help alleviate or solve the client's problem. Counselors can play an important role by encouraging clients to make full use of **indigenous support systems** (such as family and friendship networks) within their own communities.

Facilitator of Indigenous Healing Systems Mental health practitioners need to learn what kinds of healing resources exist within a client's culture. In many cultures, individuals with problems are more likely to put their trust in traditional healers. For that reason, counselors need to be aware of **indigenous healing systems** (such as religious leaders and institutions, energy healers, and respected community leaders) and be willing to work collaboratively with them when it is to the benefit of the client. Ignoring these indigenous resources can have a negative effect on the client's welfare, and therefore, has ethical implications.

In summary, we see it as ethically incumbent on practitioners who work in the community to assume some or all of the alternative roles described above when needed to benefit their clients and provide optimal and at times alternative care. We are not discounting the efforts of practitioners primarily engaged in individual counseling as they also contribute significantly toward creating a more actualized community.

Educating the Community

There are many reasons for the underuse of available mental health resources. Clients may be unaware of their existence; they may not be able to afford the services; they may have misconceptions about the nature and purpose of counseling; they may be reluctant to recognize their problems; they may harbor the attitude that they should be able to solve their own problems; they may feel a social stigma attached to seeking professional help; or they may perceive that these resources are not intended for them because the services are administered in a culturally insensitive way. Services are not always easily accessible, which discourages some from making use of resources in the community. A major barrier for clients is that access to social and psychological services can be confusing, and those providing services may not be receptive or friendly.

One goal of the community approach is to educate the public and attempt to change the attitudes of the community about mental health and the attitudes toward those who deliver mental health services. Many people still cling to a very narrow definition of mental illness. Widespread misconceptions include the notion that once people suffer from any kind of emotional disturbance they can never be cured, the idea that people with emotional and behavioral disorders are merely deficient in "willpower," and the belief that the mentally ill are always dangerous and should be separated from the community lest they "contaminate" or harm others. Professionals face real challenges in combating these misconceptions, but unless this is done many people will not seek professional help. Practitioners are ethically bound to actively work at presenting mental health services in a way that is understandable to and respectful of the community at large. Counselors can assume an advocacy role for the counseling profession by informing the public and potential clients about psychological services. Community education can open doors for people who previously would not have sought these services due to their misconceptions or preconceived notions about the mental health profession (MacLeod & McMullen, 2016).

Influencing Policymakers

The challenges facing community workers can be overwhelming, especially with current constraints on funding and the bureaucratic malaise. How can dedicated community workers continue to develop social programs if they are constantly faced with the possibility that their programs will be cut back or canceled? There is little room for staff members to initiate innovative social programs when the agencies themselves are concerned with mere survival.

One way community workers can initiate change is by organizing within an agency or even several agencies and developing a collective voice. Practitioners can empower a community to organize political action to influence the state and national government to fulfill their responsibilities. This action may involve providing funds, technical assistance, legal protection, or other support a smaller community requires to flourish (Homan, 2016).

The Case of a Nonprofit Agency Designed to Educate the Community

The Coalition for Children, Adolescents and Parents (CCAP) is a community agency aimed at the prevention of adolescent pregnancy. This small grassroots agency in Orange County, California, applies outreach strategies to educate the community as a way to meet a critical need in the community (Hogan-Garcia & Scheinberg, 2000). CCAP has served as a model for how to involve the community in a project to enhance the community. From its inception, a high priority has been given to hiring a multiethnic staff that could serve and mirror the community. The staff is committed to understanding each other, rather than allowing their differences to separate them, and staff members meet frequently for cultural sharing. Those who work at the agency have opportunities to critically examine their ethnocentric assumptions about the world and the community. All the members of the agency staff are committed to clarifying and understanding personal values, beliefs, and behaviors.

One of the early projects designed by CCAP involved outreach and education in the Latino community to prevent the spread of HIV. A Latina staff member conducted interviews with 30 mothers in the community regarding their understanding of HIV, human sexuality, and teen pregnancy. From this contact with these mothers, a group of leaders (*comadres*) was formed to educate the community. The women who served as leaders met for monthly meetings, which were held at a neighborhood center. Eventually, the women invited their husbands into the classes. This project was funded by an external source, and the agency was required to report to the funders about the outcomes of the project. Hogan-Garcia and Scheinberg (2000) summarize these outcomes as follows:

> By the end of the contract year, the agency had exceeded the expectations of funders with the project and the Comadres Project had spread the word about HIV prevention to friends, neighbors, and family members. The empowerment of disenfranchised women and men continued beyond the contract term. CCAP staff continued to meet with and follow this special group of friends. Three women went back to school, a group of the women formed a Spanish-speaking PTA group, and one went on to become a school board member. (p. 28)
>
> In 2000 the agency served more than 12,000 clients, providing after-school recreational services, tutoring, academic enrichment programs, physical examinations, parenting education, conflict resolution, cultural-diversity training, school-based group counseling, a homeless shelter, drug abuse prevention, and child care training.

Commentary. This agency is an example of an effective collaboration committed to ensuring that the members of the community have a full voice in determining the nature of community services. Because the individuals on the staff believe in the value of understanding cultural diversity, they are able to serve as a bridge between the mainstream and minority communities. This is also a good example of *developing* leadership rather than simply providing leadership. •

Promoting Change in the Community

Effective community workers encourage community members to discover their own strengths and to build on these resources. Homan (2016) poses a question that has significant implications for community work: "Are you willing to honestly examine who owns the project?" From Homan's perspective, if we are just doing things we think are right *for* people, rather than the project really being theirs to take charge of, we may be unconsciously reasserting a form of social control. Although some client/constituent groups do not have the immediate skills, or even the time to take care of every aspect of a change project, they can learn skills and receive support for their work. Thus the matter of "who owns" the project is an important ethical concern.

A Developmental Versus a Service Approach Homan (2016) compares the functions of community workers who operate within a developmental approach with those who rely on a service orientation. The **developmental approach** is grounded on strengths, focuses on assets and capacities, promotes capability and power, changes conditions, and is aimed at prevention. This approach builds on identifying resources within the individual, the group, or the community that can be more fully activated. In contrast, a **service approach** focuses on problems to be solved and holes to fill. It is concerned more with maintaining rather than changing conditions and is oriented toward fixing problems rather than preventing them. A service orientation relies on experts and reinforces power imbalances, whereas a developmental approach relies on partnerships and equalizes power relationships.

Ways to Involve Yourself in the Community

If you want to bring about change within the community, you need to be willing to get involved. Here are some things you might do to link individuals to the environment in which they live. Rate each of these activities, using the following code:

A = I would do this on a *regular basis.*

B = I would do this *occasionally.*

C = I would do this *rarely.*

_____ 1. I would work with agencies to assess community needs.

_____ 2. I would familiarize myself with available community resources so that I could refer people to appropriate sources of further help.

_____ 3. With my clients' permission, I would enlist people who had a direct influence on their lives.

_____ 4. I would connect my clients to both formal and informal support systems and resources that are already available in the community.

_____ 5. I would work actively with groups committed to bringing about change in the community.

_____ 6. I would bring together clients who are affected by a common condition and help them work out strategies to change the condition that affects them.

_____ 7. I would encourage efforts to make the community's helping network more responsive.

_____ 8. I would provide training to key people from various cultural groups in peer-counseling skills so that they could work with those people who might not seek professional services from an agency.

_____ 9. I would work with politicians and community stakeholders who were actively involved in helping the community.

If you plan on going into one of the mental health professions, you are likely to spend some time working in a community agency setting, and you will be working with many different facets of the community. If you were to work in such a setting at this time, consider the following questions:

- What skills do you already have that can be applied to community change?
- What concerns do you have of working in the community?
- How would you translate your ideas into a practical set of strategies aimed at community change?
- How aware are you of your beliefs and attitudes toward the people you serve, and how might this affect the way you work?

For an excellent treatment of the community perspective, see *Promoting Community Change: Making It Happen in the Real World* (Homan, 2016).

Working Within a System

One of the major challenges for counselors who work in the community is to learn how to make the system work for the clients they serve and, secondarily, work for themselves so that in the process they do not lose their ability to be effective. Working in a system can put an added strain on the counselor due to the monumental amount of paperwork required to justify continued funding, high caseloads, and a multitude of policy directives. Another source of strain is the counselor's relationships with those who administer the agency or institution. Practitioners who deal with clients directly may have little appreciation for the intricacies with which administrators must contend in managing and funding their programs. If communication is poor and problem solving is inadequate, tension and problems are inevitable. The ultimate challenge is to empower the community to address its own problems.

The Challenge of Maintaining Integrity in an Agency Environment

Many professionals struggle with the issue of how to work within a system while retaining their integrity and vitality. Although working in an organization is oftentimes frustrating, counselors need to examine their attitude, which might be part of the problem. Blaming others does not effect change. Focusing on the things that can be changed fosters a sense of personal power that may allow for progress.

Homan (2016) suggests that simply putting up with problems within a system is rarely gratifying and that workers gain professional satisfaction by actively taking steps to promote positive changes. Recognizing the need for action is the first step toward responding to unacceptable circumstances. Once a problem has been identified, you have four options:

- You can change your perception by identifying the situation as acceptable.
- You can leave the situation, either by emotionally withdrawing or by physically leaving.
- You can recognize the situation as unacceptable and then decide to adjust to the situation.
- You can identify the situation as unacceptable and do what you can to change it. (pp. 108–109)

Each of these actions has consequences for both you and your clients. If you recognize that you do have choices in how you respond to unacceptable situations, you may be challenged to take action to change these circumstances. From an ethical perspective, you are expected to alert your employer to circumstances that may impair your ability to reach clients.

By creating and participating in support groups, those who work in an agency might find ways to collectively address problems in the system of which they are a part. A case can be made for the value of support groups in agency settings. These groups create an internal subculture that provides some support in dealing with bureaucratic pressure. Workers alone will likely have difficulty in changing large organizations, but when they unite, they have a greater opportunity for effecting change.

The Case of Toni

For over 20 years Toni has worked with women in recovery in a community agency that is funded by a grant. To prevent burnout, she and her coworkers organized a support group among the community workers in the agency. Her group consists of about 15 people, some of whom are case managers, treatment counselors, nurses, social workers, and supervisors. They meet at the agency during work hours twice a month for up to 2 hours. During these sessions the workers have opportunities to talk about difficult clients or stressful situations they are facing on the job, such as cutbacks and increased workloads. Personal concerns sometimes have an impact on workers' abilities to function professionally, and members are able to use the support within the group as a way to deal with personal issues.

- If you worked in an agency, would you want this kind of support group that Toni describes?
- To what extent do you think members of this group could effect change in the agency?
- How might you deal with the demands of an increased workload due to cutbacks?

Commentary. Toni's case represents a familiar scenario that mental health workers will increasingly face in effectively working in an agency. Workers in community agencies will increasingly be expected to meet the demands placed upon them with fewer staff and resources to accomplish the tasks expected of them. Those who work with client populations with high needs can experience compassion fatigue and can quickly burn out. Self-care is extremely important in this situation. One way Toni found to take care of herself was by finding ways to meet with colleagues in the agency to discuss how others were dealing with the demands of their work situation. ●

Being an Advocate and Working in a System

Counselors walk a fine line when trying to support causes of equity, justice, and fairness while keeping their jobs. Bemak and Chung (2008) and Chung and Bemak (2012) identify some strategies and skills counselors can use to be effective advocates within a system, especially in an educational setting:

- Define your role.
- Emphasize equal opportunity.
- Reach out to the larger community with intervention strategies.
- Provide clients with tools that will promote constructive change.
- Formulate partnerships with clients who may lack the skills to self-advocate.
- Learn about organizational systems.
- Work with individuals within a system who will work toward social change.
- Form collaborative relationships with other mental health professionals.
- Promote social action within a sociopolitical context.
- Generate team support by collaborating with community agencies.

As social justice counselors, we cannot preach social justice values in our work setting unless we are willing to practice what we teach (Chung & Bemak, 2012). "It demands that we question ourselves about, if, how, and when we are willing to take risks which are fundamental to multicultural social justice counseling" (p. 266).

For thoughtful discussions of community action, many case examples of social justice programs, and re-visioning clinical practice, we highly recommend *Helping Beyond the 50-Minute Hour: Therapists Involved in Meaningful Social Action* (Kottler, Englar-Carlson, & Carlson, 2013).

Relationships Between Community Worker and Agency

The ethical violations in a community agency are more complex and difficult to resolve than violations pertaining to individual counseling. If a worker is not motivated, the system may tolerate this lack of motivation. If the system violates the rights of the client (community), then this is a real challenge to address. There is no easy solution to systemic problems, but clearly the people seeking help are vulnerable and need to be protected. Correcting systemic abuse demands the willingness of those involved in the system to practice aspirational ethics and take action.

Moving Toward Empowerment Think about how you can empower yourself to help create systemic change in your community. Imagine yourself in each of these situations, and ask yourself how you could increase your effectiveness within the system:

- What would you do if the organization for which you worked instituted a policy to which you were opposed?
- What would you do if you believed strongly that certain changes needed to be made in your institution but your colleagues disagreed with you?
- What do you think you would do if members of the staff seemed to work largely in isolation from one another?

- What are some steps you can think of to promote change within an agency?
- What do you consider to be the ethics involved in staying with a job after you have done everything you can to bring about change, but to no avail?

The Case of Adriana

Adriana works in a community mental health clinic, and most of her time is devoted to dealing with crisis situations. The more she works with people in crisis, the more she is convinced that the focus of her work should be on preventive programs designed to educate the public. Adriana comes to believe strongly that there would be far fewer clients in distress if people were effectively contacted and motivated to participate in growth-oriented educational programs. She develops detailed, logical, and convincing proposals for programs she would like to implement in the community, but these proposals are consistently rejected by the director of her center. Because the clinic is partially funded by the government for the express purpose of crisis intervention, the director feels uneasy about approving any program that does not relate directly to this objective.

If you were in Adriana's place, which of the following courses of action would you choose?

_____ 1. I would do what the director expected.

_____ 2. I would continue to work toward a compromise and try to find some way to make room for my special project.

_____ 3. If I could not do what I deemed important, I would have to consider looking for another job.

_____ 4. I would involve clients in setting the direction for the proposal and providing the necessary support to secure approval.

_____ 5. I would get several other staff members together, pool our resources, and look for ways to implement the program as a group.

_____ 6. With my director's approval, I would try to obtain a grant for a pilot program in the community.

Commentary. Adriana has tried repeatedly to convince the director of the center that preventive programs would help to avert crises and improve community health. One alternative role open to her is to advocate for policy changes in government regulations. At the local level, Adriana could join forces with others in her agency to work toward an expanded definition of crisis intervention that includes preventive measures. At the state level, Adriana could reach out to colleagues in her state's counseling association to identify peers who may be interested in helping to advocate for policy changes in government regulations specifically in relation to preventive programs for crisis interventions. •

As a mental health practitioner, you may need to decide how you will work within a system and how you can be most effective. Study the agency's philosophy before you accept a position, and determine whether the agency's norms, values, and expectations coincide with what you expect from the position. If you are not able to support the philosophy and policies of that agency, you are almost certain to experience conflicts, if not failure. It will be up to you to find your own answers to questions such as these:

- To what degree is my philosophy of helping compatible with the agency where I work?

- How can I meet the requirements of an institution and at the same time do what I most believe in?
- What can I do to bring about change in a particular system?
- What special ethical obligations am I likely to face in working in a system?

The Case of Ronnie

Ronnie, an African American student, moved with his family into a mostly White community and attends high school there. Almost immediately he was on the receiving end of racial jokes and experienced social isolation. A teacher noticed his isolation and sent him to the school counselor. It is evident to the counselor that Ronnie is being discriminated against, not only by many of the students but also by some of the faculty. The counselor has no reason to doubt the information provided by Ronnie because she is aware of racism in the school and in the community. She determines that it would be much more practical to help Ronnie learn to ignore the prejudice than to try to change the racist attitudes of the school and the community.

- How do you evaluate this counselor's decision? What are its ethical ramifications? Does she have an obligation to work to change community attitudes?
- If you were consulted by this counselor, what suggestions would you make?
- Does a school system have an ethical obligation to attempt to change attitudes of a community that discriminates against some of its citizens?
- What are the risks of not addressing the problem of racism?

Commentary. This counselor is struggling with the nature of the challenge and seems ill equipped to take it on. She may fear reprisals if she acts on values that are not shared by many in the community. She may want to do what is needed to promote the well-being of her client, yet she may be struggling with self-doubts and with anxiety about not being accepted by some faculty members. Although this counselor seems unwilling or perhaps is unable to confront racism within the school setting, she has an ethical duty to advocate for change in the school community. By talking with the teacher who sent Ronnie to her, she may be able to begin to gather a coalition for change in the school community. She might consider presenting workshops and classroom guidance activities on racism in the school. The counselor also may be able to gain the support of the school administration if she approaches the problem in a noncombative manner. In this case, the client is the school community, and Ronnie's troubles will not be resolved without community change. •

As mental health professionals, we are expected to translate our awareness of inequities and societal conditions into various forms of social action. Part of our ethical and moral obligation is to advocate with the aim of creating a just society in which all people have equal opportunities and resources to strive toward their personal goals. Chung and Bemak (2012) capture the essence of this message in this way: "We must move forward and beyond the traditional approach of focusing solely on the intrapsychic, accept and recognize the impact of sociopolitical factors on our clients and their families, and determine how our advocacy can effectively address those issues" (p. 182).

Chapter Summary

The primary focus of this chapter has been on the importance of working in the community as a change agent. The community mental health orientation is one way to meet the increasing demand for a variety of services. Too often mental health professionals have been denied the opportunity to devise programs that address the diverse needs of the community. Over the past few years some alternatives to conventional therapy have arisen, creating new roles for counselors who work in a community agency setting. If you seek a full-time career in an agency, consider how you can work *with* the system for the benefit of you and your clients. Counselors also need to be aware of social justice issues that are manifested in the community. Becoming increasingly aware of how oppression and discrimination operate in the lives of our clients is a fundamental part of ethical practice.

We challenge you to think of ways to accept the responsibility of working effectively in an organization and thus increasing your effectiveness as a professional. Being a social change agent does not require that you focus on macro-level changes. MacLeod and McMullen (2016) contend that advocacy can be done at a micro level by adjusting how counselors promote the counseling profession in common interactions with clients, agencies, community stakeholders, and other mental health providers. If you decide to assume a social advocacy role, facilitating change within your agency or local community is a significant first step. We also recommend that you make efforts to educate community members about what community practitioners actually do. Finally, we ask you to reflect on the major causes of disillusionment that often accompany working in a system and to find creative ways to retain your vitality, both as a person and as a professional.

Suggested Activities

1. Retake the self-assessment at the end of Chapter 1, which surveys your attitudes about ethical and professional issues. Cover your initial answers when you complete the self-assessment, and compare your responses now to see whether your thinking has changed. In addition, circle the 10 questions that are most significant to you or that you are most interested in pursuing further. Bring these to class and discuss them in small groups. Write down a few of the most important things you have learned in this course and from this book. You might also write down some questions that remain unanswered for you. Exchange your ideas with other students.

2. In small groups discuss your thoughts about the relationship between the social justice advocacy perspective and ethical practice. What relationship do you see between social justice advocacy competencies and multicultural competencies? Which of the advocacy competencies would you most want to incorporate in your practice in the community?

3. Reflect on and discuss alternative roles human-service professionals might play when working in the community. Identify which of the following roles you think you could assume as a community worker: (a) advocate, (b) change agent, (c) consultant, (d) adviser, (e) facilitator of indigenous support systems, (f) facilitator of indigenous healing systems, or (g) all of the above roles. In small groups discuss in which of these roles you would feel least comfortable functioning, and why. How could you learn to

carry out professional roles in the community different from those in which you were trained?

4. An issue you may well face in your practice is how to get through the hesitation people have toward asking for professional assistance. How would you respond to clients who have questions such as these: "What will people think if they find out that I am coming for professional help?" "Shouldn't I be able to solve my problems on my own? Isn't it a sign of weakness that I need others to help me?" "Will I be able to resolve my problems by consulting you?" Share your responses in dyads or in small groups.

5. Suppose you were applying for a job in a community mental health center. How would you respond to the following questions during the interview?

   • Many of our clients represent a range of diverse cultural and ethnic backgrounds. To what degree do you think you will be able to work with them?

   • How much do you understand about your own acculturation process? How will this help or hinder you in working with our clientele?

   • What will be your biggest challenge in forming trusting relationships with clients who are culturally different from you?

6. Several students can interview a variety of professionals in the mental health field about the major problems they encounter in their institution. What barriers do they meet when they attempt to implement programs? How do they deal with obstacles?

7. After recognizing that a problem exists within the organization for which you work, identify skills you would need to make the desired changes. How might you go about developing strategies for getting support from coworkers if you were interested in changing an agency?

8. As noted in this chapter, Chung and Bemak (2012) identify a characteristic of a social justice counselor as being a courageous risk-taker. Discuss with a partner how courageous you consider yourself to be when faced with opposition from others. Do you think of yourself as a risk-taker? If not, how can you become more of a risk-taker? What can you do to prepare yourself to be a social justice advocate for your clients?

9. Discuss the ways in which you can be a social justice advocate in the communities to which you belong. What gaps or needs do you see in your local community, and how might you help bridge these gaps?

10. If social justice is not a topic you often reflect on, discuss the privileges you possess that make social justice less visible to you. What identities do you possess that keep you from having to look more closely at issues of social justice in your own community?

MindTap for Counseling

Go to MindTap® for digital study tools and resources that complement this text and help you be more successful in your course and career. There's an interactive eBook plus videos of client sessions, skill-building activities, quizzes to help you prepare for tests, apps, and more—all in one place. If your instructor *didn't* assign MindTap, you can find out more about it at CengageBrain.com.

Authors' Concluding Commentary

Throughout this book, we have raised some of the ethical and professional issues that you may encounter in your counseling practice and have encouraged you to think about your own guidelines for professional practice. If one fundamental question can serve to tie together all the issues we have discussed, it is this: "Who has the right to counsel another person?" This question can be the basis for self-examination whenever you have concerns about clients. At times you may be troubled and believe that you have no right to counsel others. This may be because you are not doing in your own life what you are challenging your clients to do. Occasional self-doubt is far less damaging, in our view, than a failure to question. Complacency will stifle your growth as a practitioner. Your commitment to ongoing self-exploration and self-care can make you a more effective helper. The great challenge of life itself is the struggle to live a meaningful life and to find new and significant ways to stimulate whole communities to better their existence.

Developing a sense of professional and ethical responsibility is a task that is never really finished. There are no final or universal answers to many of the questions we have posed. For ourselves, we hope never to reach the point where we think we have figured it all out and no longer need to reexamine our assumptions and practices. The issues raised in this book demand periodic reflection and an openness to change. Give careful thought to your own values and ethics. Be willing to rethink your positions as you gain more experience. When you are interested in what you do and in the people you serve, you are in a good position to become a responsible and an ethical practitioner. Some of our most trusted mentors have taught us the importance of asking ourselves whether we have left the relationships and the systems we are a part of better than how we found them. Have our attitudes and beliefs been challenged, changed, or confirmed through our learning? If the answer is no, then there is work left for us to do.

References and Suggested Readings

*Books and articles marked with an asterisk are suggested for further study.

American Association for Marriage and Family Therapy. (2015). *Code of ethics.* Washington, DC: Author.

American Counseling Association. (2005). *Code of ethics.* Alexandria, VA: Author.

American Counseling Association. (2014). *Code of ethics.* Alexandria, VA: Author.

American Group Psychotherapy Association. (2006). *Guidelines for ethics.* New York, NY: Author.

American Mental Health Counselors Association. (2015). *Code of ethics of the American Mental Health Counselors Association.* Alexandria, VA: Author.

American Mental Health Counselors Association. (2016). *AMHCA standards for the practice of clinical mental health counseling.* Alexandria, VA: Author.

American Music Therapy Association. (2015). *Code of ethics.* Retrieved from www.musictherapy.org/ethics.html

American Psychiatric Association. (2000). *Diagnostic and statistical manual of mental disorders: Text revision* (4th ed.). Washington, DC: Author.

American Psychiatric Association. (2012a). *DSM-5 development. Frequently asked questions.* Retrieved from www.dsm5.org/about/Pages/faq.aspx

American Psychiatric Association. (2013a). *Diagnostic and statistical manual of mental disorders* (5th ed.). Washington, DC: Author.

American Psychiatric Association. (2013b). *The principles of medical ethics with annotations especially applicable to psychiatry.* Washington, DC: Author.

American Psychological Association. (1985). *White paper on duty to protect.* Washington, DC: Author.

American Psychological Association. (1993a). Guidelines for providers of psychological services to ethnic, linguistic, and culturally diverse populations. *American Psychologist, 48*(1), 45–48.

American Psychological Association. (1993b). Record keeping guidelines. *American Psychologist, 48,* 984–986.

American Psychological Association. (2003a). Guidelines on multicultural education, training, research, practice, and organizational change for psychologists. *American Psychologist, 58*(5), 377–402.

American Psychological Association. (2003b). Report of the ethics committee, 2002. *American Psychologist, 58*(8), 650–657.

*American Psychological Association. (2007). Record keeping guidelines. *American Psychologist, 62*(9), 993–1004.

American Psychological Association. (2010). *Ethical principles of psychologists and code of conduct.* Retrieved from www.apa.org/ethics/code/index.aspx

American Psychological Association. (2015). Guidelines for clinical supervision in health service psychology. *American Psychologist, 70*(1), 33–46.

*American Psychological Association, Division 44. (2000). Guidelines for psychotherapy with lesbian, gay, and bisexual clients. *American Psychologist, 55*(12), 1440–1451.

*American Psychological Association Presidential Task Force on Evidence-based Practice. (2006). Evidence-based practice in psychology. *American Psychologist, 61,* 271–285.

American School Counselor Association. (2016). *Ethical standards for school counselors.* Alexandria, VA: Author.

Ancis, J. R., & Marshall, D. S. (2010). Using a multicultural framework to assess supervisees' perceptions of culturally competent supervision. *Journal of Counseling & Development, 88*(3), 277–284.

Angus, L., Watson, J. C., Elliott, R., Schneider, K., & Timulak, L. (2015). Humanistic psychotherapy research 1990–2015: From methodological innovations to evidence-supported treatment outcomes and beyond. *Psychotherapy Research, 25*(3), 330–347.

Anthony, K. (2015). Training therapists to work effectively online and offline within digital culture. *British Journal of Guidance & Counselling, 43*(1), 36–42.

Antony, M. M. (2014). Behavior therapy. In D. Wedding & R. J. Corsini (Eds.), *Current psychotherapies* (10th ed., pp. 193–229). Belmont, CA: Brooks/Cole, Cengage Learning.

*Arredondo, P., Toporek, R., Brown, S., Jones, J., Locke, D., Sanchez, J., & Stadler, H. A. (1996). Operationalization of multicultural counseling competencies. *Journal of Multicultural Counseling and Development, 24*(1), 42–78.

Association for Counselor Education and Supervision. (1993, Summer). Ethical guidelines for counseling supervisors. *ACES Spectrum, 53*(4), 3–8.

*Association for Counselor Education and Supervision. (1995). Ethical guidelines for counseling supervisors. *Counselor Education and Supervision, 34*(3), 270–276.

*Association for Counselor Education and Supervision. (2011). *Best practices in clinical supervision*. Retrieved from www.acesonline.net/wp-content/uploads/2011/10/ACES-Best-Practices-in-clinical-supervision-document-FINAL.pdf

*Association for Lesbian, Gay, Bisexual and Transgender Issues in Counseling. (2008). *Competencies for counseling gay, lesbian, bisexual and transgendered (GLBT) clients*. Retrieved from www.algbtic.org/resources/competencies.html

Association for Lesbian, Gay, Bisexual and Transgender Issues in Counseling. (2009). *Competencies for counseling with transgender clients*. Alexandria, VA: Author.

Association for Multicultural Counseling and Development. (2015). *Multicultural and social justice counseling competencies*. Alexandria, VA: American Counseling Association.

Association for Specialists in Group Work. (1999). Principles for diversity-competent group workers. *Journal for Specialists in Group Work, 24*(1), 7–14.

Association for Specialists in Group Work. (2000). Professional standards for the training of group workers. *The Group Worker, 29*(3), 1–10.

Association for Specialists in Group Work. (2008). Best practice guidelines. *Journal for Specialists in Group Work, 33*(2), 111–117.

Association for Specialists in Group Work. (2012). *Multicultural and social justice competence principles for group workers*. Retrieved from www.asgw.org/

Association for Spiritual, Ethical, and Religious Values in Counseling. (2009). *Competencies for addressing spiritual and religious issues in counseling*. Retrieved from www.aservic.org/resources/spiritual-competencies/

Association of State and Provincial Psychology Boards. (2012, July 11). *ASPPB receives licensure portability grant from federal government* [News release]. Retrieved from www.asppb.net/files/public/PLUS%20Documents/NEWS%20RELEASE.pdf

Atkinson, D. R. (2004). *Counseling American minorities* (6th ed.). Boston, MA: McGraw-Hill.

Austin, J., Austin, J., Muratori, M., & Corey, G. (2017). Multiple relationships and multiple roles in higher education: Maintaining multiple roles and relationships in counselor education. In O. Zur (Ed.), *Multiple relationships in psychotherapy and counseling: Unavoidable, common, and mandatory dual relations in therapy* (pp. 165–173). New York, NY: Routledge, Taylor & Francis.

Austin, K. M., Moline, M. M., & Williams, G. T. (1990). *Confronting malpractice: Legal and ethical dilemmas in psychotherapy*. Newbury Park, CA: Sage.

Australian Association of Family Therapy. (2013). *Code of ethics*. Melbourne, Australia: Author.

*Baker, E. K. (2003). *Caring for ourselves: A therapist's guide to personal and professional well-being*. Washington, DC: American Psychological Association.

Barlow, S. H. (2008). Group psychotherapy specialty practice. *Professional Psychology: Research and Practice, 39*(2), 240–244.

*Barnett, J. E. (2007). Psychological wellness: A guide for mental health practitioners. *Ethical Issues in Professional Counseling, 10*(Lesson 2), 9–18.

*Barnett, J. E. (2008). Impaired professionals: Distress, professional impairment, self-care, and psychological wellness. In M. Hersen & A. M. Gross (Eds.), *Handbook of clinical psychology* (pp. 857–884). New York, NY: Wiley.

Barnett, J. E. (2017a). An introduction to boundaries and multiple relationships for psychotherapists: Issue, challenges, and recommendations. In O. Zur (Ed.), *Multiple relationships in psychotherapy and counseling: Unavoidable, common, and mandatory dual relations in therapy* (pp. 17–29). New York, NY: Routledge, Taylor & Francis.

Barnett, J. E. (2017b). Unavoidable incidental contacts and multiple relationships in rural practice. In O. Zur (Ed.), *Multiple relationships in psychotherapy and counseling: Unavoidable, common, and mandatory dual relations in therapy* (pp. 97–107). New York, NY: Routledge, Taylor & Francis.

*Barnett, J. E., Baker, E. K., Elman, N. S., & Schoener, G. R. (2007). In pursuit of wellness: The self-care imperative. *Professional Psychology: Research and Practice, 38*(6), 603–612.

*Barnett, J. E., Cornish, J. A. E., Goodyear, R. K., & Lichtenberg, J. W. (2007). Commentaries on the ethical and effective practice of clinical supervision. *Professional Psychology: Research and Practice, 38*(3), 268–275.

*Barnett, J. E., Doll, B., Younggren, J. N., & Rubin, N. J. (2007). Clinical competence for practicing psychologists: Clearly a work in progress. *Professional Psychology: Research and Practice, 38*(5), 510–517.

Barnett, J. E., Hillard, D., & Lowery, K. (2001). Ethical and legal issues in the treatment of minors. In L. VandeCreek & T. Jackson (Eds.), *Innovations in clinical practice: A source book* (vol. 19, pp. 257–272). Sarasota, FL: Professional Resource Press.

*Barnett, J. E., & Johnson, W. B. (2008). *Ethics desk reference for psychologists*. Washington, DC: American Psychological Association.

Barnett, J. E., & Johnson, W. B. (2011). Integrating spirituality and religion into psychotherapy: Persistent dilemmas, ethical issues, and a proposed decision-making process. *Ethics and Behavior, 21*(2), 147–164.

*Barnett, J. E., & Johnson, W. B. (2015). *Ethics desk reference for counselors* (2nd ed.). Alexandria, VA: American Counseling Association.

*Barnett, J. E., Johnston, L. C., & Hillard, D. (2006). Psychological wellness as an ethical imperative. In L. VandeCreek & J. B. Allen (Eds.), *Innovations in clinical practice: Focus on health and wellness* (pp. 257–271). Sarasota, FL: Professional Resources Press.

*Barnett, J. E., Lazarus, A. A., Vasquez, M. J. T., Moorehead-Slaughter, O., & Johnson, W. B. (2007). Boundary issues and multiple relationships: Fantasy and reality. *Professional Psychology: Research and Practice, 38*(4), 401–410.

*Barnett, J. E., Wise, E. H., Johnson-Greene, D., & Bucky, S. F. (2007). Informed consent: Too much of a good thing or not enough? *Professional Psychology: Research and Practice, 38*(2), 179–186.

Barros-Bailey, M., & Saunders, J. L. (2010). Ethics and the use of technology in rehabilitation counseling. *Rehabilitation Counseling Bulletin, 53*(4), 255–259.

Baxter v. State of Montana, MT 449 (2009).

*Bednar, R. L., Bednar, S. C., Lambert, M. J., & Waite, D. R. (1991). *Psychotherapy with high-risk clients: Legal and professional standards*. Belmont, CA: Brooks/Cole, Cengage Learning.

Behnke, S. H. (2012). Constitutional claims in the context of mental health training: Religion, sexual orientation, and tensions between the first amendment and professional ethics. *Training and Education in Professional Psychology, 6*(4), 189–195.

Bemak, F. (2013). Counselors without borders: Community action in counseling. In J. A. Kottler, M. Englar-Carlson, & J. Carlson (Eds.), *Helping beyond the 50-minute hour: Therapists involved in meaningful social action* (pp. 186–196). New York, NY: Routledge, Taylor & Francis.

*Bemak, F., & Chung, R. C-Y. (2008). New professional roles and advocacy strategies for school counselors: A multicultural/social justice perspective to move beyond the nice counselor syndrome. *Journal of Counseling and Development, 86*(3), 372–382.

Bemak, F., Chung, R. C-Y., Talleyrand, R. M., Jones, H., & Daquin, J. (2011). Implementing multicultural social justice strategies in counselor education training programs. *Journal for Social Action in Counseling and Psychology, 3*(1), 29–43.

Bemak, F., & Chung, R. C-Y. (2015). Critical issues in international group counseling. *Journal for Specialists in Group Work, 40*(1), 6–21.

Bemak, F., & Conyne, R. (Eds.). (2018). *Journeys to professional excellence: Stories of courage, innovation, and risk-taking.* Thousand Oaks, CA: Sage.

Benitez, B. R. (2004). Confidentiality and its exceptions. *The Therapist, 16*(4), 32–36.

*Bennett, B. E., Bricklin, P. M., Harris, E., Knapp, S., VandeCreek, L., & Younggren, J. N. (2006). *Assessing and managing risk in psychological practice: An individualized approach.* Rockville, MD: The Trust.

Bennett, B. E., Bryant, B. K., VandenBos, G. R., & Greenwood, A. (1990). *Professional liability and risk management.* Washington, DC: American Psychological Association.

*Bernard, J. M., & Goodyear, R. K. (2014). *Fundamentals of clinical supervision* (5th ed.). Upper Saddle River, NJ: Pearson.

Bersoff, B. N. (2014). Protecting victims of violent patients while protecting confidentiality. *American Psychologist, 69*(5), 461–467.

Bevacqua, F., & Kurpius, S. E. R. (2013). Counseling students' personal values and attitudes toward euthanasia. *Journal of Mental Health Counseling, 35*(2), 172–188.

Bieschke, K. J., & Mintz, L. B. (2012). Counseling psychology model training values statement addressing diversity: History, current use, and future directions. *Training and Education in Professional Psychology, 6*(4), 196–203.

Birdsall, B., & Hubert, M. (2000, October). Ethical issues in school counseling. *Counseling Today,* pp. 30, 36.

Birrell, P. J., & Bruns, C. M. (2016). Ethics and relationship: From risk management to relational engagement. *Journal of Counseling & Development, 94*(4), 391–397.

*Bitter, J. R. (2014). *Theory and practice of family therapy and counseling* (2nd ed.). Belmont, CA: Brooks/Cole, Cengage Learning.

Blount, A. J., Lambie, G. W., & Kissinger, D. B. (2016). Wellness matters. *Counseling Today, 59*(5), 52–59.

Blumenthal-Barby, J. S. (2014). Psychiatry's new manual (*DSM-5*): Ethical and conceptual dimensions. *Medical Ethics, 40,* 531–536.

Board of Curators of the University of Missouri v. Horowitz, 435 U.S. 78 (1978).

Bohart, A. C., & Wade, A. G. (2013). The client in psychotherapy. In M. J. Lambert (Ed.), *Bergin and Garfield's handbook of psychotherapy and behavior change* (6th ed., pp. 219–257). Hoboken, NJ: Wiley.

Boisvert, C. M., & Faust, D. (2003). Leading researchers' consensus on psychotherapy research findings: Implications for the teaching and conduct of psychotherapy. *Professional Psychology: Research and Practice, 34*(5), 508–513.

Bolen, R. M., & Hall, J. C. (2007). Managed care and evidence-based practice: The untold story. *Journal of Social Work Education, 43*(3), 463–479.

Bonger, B. (2013). *The suicidal patient: Clinical and legal standards of care* (3rd ed.) Washington, DC: American Psychological Association.

Borders, L. D. (1991). A systematic approach to peer group supervision. *Journal of Counseling and Development, 69*(3), 248–252.

Borders, L. D. (2005). Snapshot of clinical supervision in counseling and counselor education: A five-year review. *The Clinical Supervisor, 24*(1/2), 69–113.

Borders, L. D. (2014). Best practices in clinical supervision: Another step in delineating effective supervision practice. *American Journal of Psychotherapy, 68*(2), 151–162.

Bouhoutsos, J., Holroyd, J., Lerman, H., Forer, B. R., & Greenberg, M. (1983). Sexual intimacy between psychotherapists and patients. *Professional Psychology: Research and Practice, 14*(2), 185–196.

Bradford, S., & Rickwood, D. (2014). Adolescent's preferred modes of delivery for mental health services. *Child and Adolescent Mental Health, 19*(1), 39–45.

Bradley Center v. Wessner, 250 Ga. 199, 296 S.E. 2d 693 (1982).

Bradley, J. M., Werth, J. L., Jr., & Hastings, S. L. (2012). Social justice advocacy in rural communities: Practical issues and implications. *The Counseling Psychologist, 40*(3), 363–384.

Bradley, L. J., Hendricks, B., Lock, R., Whiting, P. P., & Parr, G. (2011). E-mail communication: Issues for mental health counselors. *Journal of Mental Health Counseling, 33*(1), 67–79.

Braun, S. A., & Cox, J. A. (2005). Managed mental health care: Intentional misdiagnosis of mental disorders. *Journal of Counseling & Development, 83*, 425–433.

Bray, B. (2016). Counseling in isolation. *Counseling Today, 59*(1), 33–38.

*Brems, C., & Johnson, M. E. (2009). Self-care in the context of threats of violence or self-harm from clients. In J. L. Werth Jr., E. R. Welfel, & G. A. H. Benjamin (Eds.), *The duty to protect: Ethical, legal, and professional considerations for mental health professionals* (pp. 211–227). Washington, DC: American Psychological Association.

Brenes, G. A., Ingram, C. W., & Danhauer, S. C. (2011). Benefits and challenges of conducting psychotherapy by telephone. *Professional Psychology: Research and Practice, 42*(6), 543–549.

Bride, B. E., Kintzle, S., Abraham, A. J., & Roman, P. M. (2012). Counselor attitudes toward and use of evidence-based practices in private substance use disorder treatment centers: A comparison of social workers and non-social workers. *Health & Social Work, 37*(3), 135–145.

British Association for Counselling and Psychotherapy. (2013). *Ethical framework for good practice in counselling and psychotherapy*. Lutterworth, UK: Author.

Brown, A. P., Marquis, A., & Guiffrida, D. A. (2013). Mindfulness-based interventions. *Journal of Counseling & Development, 91*, 86–104.

Brown, L. S. (2010). *Feminist therapy*. Washington, DC: American Psychological Association.

Brown-Rice, K. A., & Furr, S. (2013). Preservice counselors' knowledge of classmates' problems of professional competency. *Journal of Counseling & Development, 91*(2), 224–233.

Bruff v. North Mississippi Health Services, Inc., 244 F.3d 495 (5th Cir. 2001).

Burwell-Pender, L., & Halinski, K. H. (2008). Enhanced awareness of countertransference. *Journal of Professional Counseling: Practice, Theory, and Research, 36*(2), 38–50.

Butler, M. H., Seedall, R. B., & Harper, J. M. (2008). Facilitated disclosure versus clinical accommodation of infidelity secrets: An early pivot point in couple therapy. Part 2: Therapy ethics, pragmatics, and protocol. *American Journal of Family Therapy, 36*, 265–283.

Butler-Byrd, N. M. (2010). An African American supervisor's reflections on multicultural supervision. *Training and Education in Professional Psychology, 4*(1), 11–15.

Cain, D. J. (2016). Toward a research-based integration of optimal practices of humanistic psychotherapies. In D. J. Cain, K. Keenan, & S. Rubin (Eds.). *Humanistic psychotherapies: Handbook of research and practice* (2nd ed., pp. 485–535). Washington, DC: American Psychological Association.

Calfee, B. E. (1997). Lawsuit prevention techniques. In *The Hatherleigh guide to ethics in therapy* (pp. 109–125). New York, NY: Hatherleigh Press.

California Association of Marriage and Family Therapists. (2004b, July/August). Disciplinary actions. *The Therapist, 16*(4), 49.

California Association of Marriage and Family Therapists. (2004c, July/August). Disciplinary actions. *The Therapist, 16*(4), 50.

California Association of Marriage and Family Therapists. (2010). Disciplinary actions. *The Therapist, 22*(4), 47–57.

California Association of Marriage and Family Therapists. (2011a). *CAMFT code of ethics*. Retrieved from www.CAMFT.org

California Association of Marriage and Family Therapists. (2011b). Disciplinary actions. *The Therapist, 23*(2), 37–51.

California Board of Behavioral Sciences. (2017). *BBS Newsletter* (Winter).

California Department of Consumer Affairs. (2011). *Professional therapy never includes sex.* Sacramento, CA: Author.

Campbell, J. C., & Christopher, J. C. (2012). Teaching mindfulness to create effective counselors. *Journal of Mental Health Counseling, 34*(3), 213–226.

Canadian Counselling Association. (2007). *CCA code of ethics.* Ottawa, Canada: Author.

Canadian Psychological Association. (2015). *Canadian code of ethics for psychologists* (4th ed., draft). Ottawa, Canada: Author.

Capodilupo, C. M., & Sue, D. W. (2013). Microaggressions in counseling and psychotherapy. In D. W. Sue & D. Sue, *Counseling the culturally diverse: Theory and practice* (6th ed., pp. 147–173). New York, NY: Wiley.

*Capuzzi, D. (2009). *Suicide prevention in the schools: Guidelines for middle and high school settings* (2nd ed.). Alexandria, VA: American Counseling Association.

Capuzzi, D., & Gross, D. R. (Eds.). (2008). *Youth at risk: A prevention resource for counselors, teachers, and parents* (5th ed.). Alexandria, VA: American Counseling Association.

Cardemil, E. V., & Battle, C. L. (2003). Guess who's coming to therapy? Getting comfortable with conversations about race and ethnicity in psychotherapy. *Professional Psychology: Research and Practice, 34*(3), 278–286.

Carlson, E. B., Garvert, D. W., Macia, K. S., Ruzek, J. I., & Burling, T. A. (2013). Traumatic stressor exposure and post-traumatic symptoms in homeless veterans. *Military Medicine, 178*(9), 970–973.

Cash v. Missouri State University, Case No. 2016-CV.

Cashwell, C. S., & Young, J. S. (2011a). Diagnosis and treatment. In C. S. Cashwell & J. S. Young (Eds.), *Integrating spirituality and religion into counseling: A guide to competent practice* (2nd ed., pp. 163–182). Alexandria, VA: American Counseling Association.

*Cashwell, C. S., & Young, J. S. (Eds.). (2011b). *Integrating spirituality and religion into counseling: A guide to competent practice* (2nd ed.). Alexandria, VA: American Counseling Association.

Casto, C., Caldwell, C., & Salazar, C. F. (2005). Creating mentoring relationships between female faculty and students in counselor education: Guidelines for potential mentees and mentors. *Journal of Counseling and Development, 83*(3), 331–336.

Chambers, A. L., Solomon, A. H., & Gurman, A. S. (2016). Couple therapy. In J. Norcross, G. R. VandenBos, & D. K. Freedheim (Eds.), *APA handbook of clinical psychology* (vol. 3, pp 307–326). Washington, DC: American Psychological Association.

Chapman, R. A., Baker, S. B., Nassar-McMillan, S. C., & Gerler, E. R. (2011). Cybersupervision: Further examination of synchronous and asynchronous modalities in counseling practicum supervision. *Counselor Education & Supervision, 50*(5), 298–313.

Chauvin, J. C., & Remley, T. P. (1996). Responding to allegations of unethical conduct. *Journal of Counseling and Development, 74*(6), 563–568.

Choudhuri, D. D., Santiago-Rivera, A. L., & Garrett, M. T. (2012). *Counseling and diversity.* Belmont, CA: Brooks/Cole, Cengage Learning.

Christopher, J. C., & Maris, J. A. (2010). Integrating mindfulness as self-care into counselling and psychotherapy training. *Counselling & Psychotherapy Research, 10,* 114–125.

Chu, J., Leino, A., Pflum, S., & Sue, S. (2016). A model for the theoretical basis of cultural competency to guide psychotherapy. *Professional Psychology: Research and Practice, 47*(1), 18–29.

Chung, R. C., & Bemak, F. P. (2012). *Social justice counseling: The next steps beyond multiculturalism.* Thousand Oaks, CA: Sage.

Clark, P., & Sims, P. L. (2014). The practice of fee setting and collection: Implications for clinical training programs. *American Journal of Family Therapy, 42*(5), 386–397.

Clement, P. (2013). Practice-based evidence: 45 years of psychotherapy's effectiveness in private practice. *American Journal of Psychotherapy, 67*(1), 23–46.

Cohen, L., & Chehimi, S. (2010). The imperative for primary prevention. In L. Cohen, V. Chávez, & S. Chehimi, *Prevention is primary: Strategies for community well-being* (2nd ed., pp. 291–321). San Francisco, CA: Jossey Bass.

Comas-Diaz, L. (2014). Multicultural theories of psychotherapy. In D. Wedding & R. J. Corsini (Eds.), *Current psychotherapies* (10th ed., pp. 533–567). Belmont, CA: Brooks/Cole, Cengage Learning.

Comas-Diaz, L., & Brown, L. S. (2016). Multicultural theories. In J. Norcross, G. R. VandenBos, & D. K. Freedheim (Eds.), *APA handbook of clinical psychology* (vol. 2, pp. 241–272). Washington, DC: American Psychological Association.

Commission on Rehabilitation Counselor Certification. (2010). *Code of professional ethics for rehabilitation counselors.* Schaumburg, IL: Author.

Committee on Professional Practice and Standards. (2003). Legal issues in the professional practice of psychology. *Professional Psychology: Research and Practice, 34*(6), 595–600.

Corey, G. (2013a). *The art of integrative counseling* (3rd ed.).Belmont, CA: Brooks/Cole, Cengage Learning.

Corey, G. (2013b). *Case approach to counseling and psychotherapy* (8th ed.). Belmont, CA: Brooks/Cole, Cengage Learning.

Corey, G. (2017). *Theory and practice of counseling and psychotherapy* (10th ed.) and *Student manual.* Boston, MA: Cengage Learning.

Corey, G., & Corey, M. (2016). Group psychotherapy. In J. Norcross, G. R. VandenBos, & D. K. Freedheim (Eds.), *APA handbook of clinical psychology* (vol. 3, pp. 289–306). Washington, DC: American Psychological Association.

Corey, G., Corey, M., Callanan, P., & Russell, J. M. (2015). *Group techniques* (4th ed.). Belmont, CA: Brooks/Cole, Cengage Learning.

Corey, G., Corey, M. S., Muratori, M., Austin, J., & Austin, J. (2017). Multiple relationships and multiple roles in higher education: Teaching group counseling with a didactic and experiential focus. In O. Zur (Ed.), *Multiple relationships in psychotherapy and counseling: Unavoidable, common, and mandatory dual relations in therapy* (pp. 174–182). New York, NY: Routledge, Taylor & Francis.

*Corey, G., Haynes, R., Moulton, P., & Muratori, M. (2010). *Clinical supervision in the helping professions: A practical guide* (2nd ed.). Alexandria, VA: American Counseling Association.

*Corey, M., Corey, G., & Corey, C. (2018). *Groups: Process and practice* (10th ed.). Boston, MA: Cengage Learning.

Cosgrove, L., & Krimsky, S. (2012). A comparison of *DSM-IV* and *DSM-5* panel members' financial associations with industry: A pernicious problem persists. *PLoS Medicine, 9*(3), 1–4.

Cosgrove, L., & Wheeler, E. E. (2013). Industry's colonization of psychiatry: Ethical and practical implications of financial conflicts of interest in the *DSM-5. Feminism & Psychology, 23*(1), 93–106.

Cottone, R. R. (2001). A social constructivism model of ethical decision making in counseling. *Journal of Counseling and Development, 79*(1), 39–45.

Cottone, R. R., & Tarvydas, V. M. (2016). *Ethics and decision making in counseling and psychotherapy* (4th ed.). New York, NY: Springer.

Council for Accreditation of Counseling and Related Educational Programs. (2016). *CACREP: The 2016 standards* [Statement]. Alexandria, VA: Author.

Council on Rehabilitation Education. (2009). *CORE history.* Retrieved from www.core-rehab.org

Counselman, E. F., & Weber, R. L. (2004). Organizing and maintaining peer supervision groups. *International Journal of Group Psychotherapy, 54*(2), 125–143.

Crethar, H. C., Torres Rivera, E., & Nash, S. (2008). In search of common threads: Linking multicultural, feminist, and social justice counseling paradigms. *Journal of Counseling and Development, 86*(3), 269–278.

Crethar, H. C., & Winterowd, C. L. (2012). Values and social justice in counseling. *Counseling and Values, 57*(1), 3–9.

Crites-Christoph, P., Gibbons, M. B. C., & Mukherjee, D. (2013). Psychotherapy process-outcome research. In M. J. Lambert (Ed.), *Bergin and Garfield's handbook of psychotherapy and behavior change* (6th ed., pp. 298–340). Hoboken, NJ: Wiley.

Cukrowicz, K. C., White, B. A., Reitzel, L. R., Burns, A. B., Driscoll, K. A., Kemper, T. S., & Joiner, T. E. (2005). Improved treatment outcome associated with the shift to empirically supported treatments in a graduate training clinic. *Professional Psychology: Research and Practice, 36*(3), 330–337.

Custer, G. (1994, November). Can universities be liable for incompetent grads? *APA Monitor, 25*(11), 7.

Dadlani, M. B., Overtree, C., & Perry-Jenkins, M. (2012). Culture at the center: A reformulation of diagnostic assessment. *Professional Psychology: Research and Practice, 43*(3), 175–182.

Dailey, S. F. (2012). Spiritual and/or religious assessment. *Interaction, 11*(3), 3–4.

Dallesasse, S. L. (2010). Managing nonsexual multiple relationships in university counseling centers: Recommendations for graduate assistants and practicum students. *Ethics & Behavior, 20*(6), 419–428.

Davenport, R. (2009). From college counselor to "risk manager": The evolving nature of college counseling on today's campuses. *Journal of American College Health, 58*(2), 181–183.

Davis, D., & Younggren, J. N. (2009). Ethical competence in psychotherapy termination. *Professional Psychology: Research and Practice, 40*(6), 572–578.

Day-Vines, N. L., Wood, S. M., Grothaus, T., Craigen, L., Holman, A. Dotson-Blake, K., & Douglass, M. J. (2007). Broaching the subjects of race, ethnicity, and culture during the counseling process. *Journal of Counseling & Development, 85*, 401–409.

Dearing, R. L., Maddux, J. E., & Tangney, J. P. (2005). Predictors of psychological help seeking in clinical and counseling psychology graduate students. *Professional Psychology: Research and Practice, 36*(3), 323–329.

*Debiak, D. (2007). Attending to diversity in group psychotherapy: An ethical imperative. *International Journal of Group Psychotherapy, 57*(1), 1–12.

Deegear, J., & Lawson, D. M. (2003). The utility of empirically supported treatments. *Professional Psychology: Research and Practice, 34*(3), 271–277.

Delaney, H. D., Miller, W. R., & Bisono, A. M. (2007). Religiosity and spirituality among psychologists: A survey of clinician members of the American Psychological Association. *Professional Psychology: Research and Practice, 38*(5), 538–546.

DeLettre, J. L., & Sobell, L. C. (2010). Keeping psychotherapy notes separate from the patient record. *Clinical Psychology and Psychotherapy, 17*, 160–163.

DeLucia-Waack, J. L., & Donigian, J. (2004). *The practice of multicultural group work: Visions and perspectives from the field.* Belmont, CA: Brooks/Cole, Cengage Learning.

DeMers, S. T., & Siegel, A. M. (2016). Legal and statutory regulations. In J. Norcross, G. R. VandenBos, & D. K. Freedheim (Eds.), *APA handbook of clinical psychology* (vol. 5, pp. 375–394). Washington, DC: American Psychological Association.

Devereaux, R. L., & Gottlieb, M. C. (2012). Record keeping in the cloud: Ethical considerations. *Professional Psychology: Research and Practice, 43*(6), 627–632.

Dickens, K. N., Ebrahim, C. H., & Herlihy, B. (2016). Counselor education doctoral students' experiences with multiple roles and relationships. *Counselor Education & Supervision, 55*(4), 234–249.

Diller, J. V. (2015). *Cultural diversity: A primer for the human services* (5th ed.). Boston, MA: Cengage Learning.

Dobmeier, R. A., & Reiner, S. M. (2012). Spirituality in the counselor education curriculum: A national survey of student perceptions. *Counseling and Values, 57*(1), 47–65.

Drogin, E. Y., Connell, M., Foote, W. E., & Sturm, C. A. (2010). The American Psychological Association's revised "record keeping guidelines": Implications for the practitioner. *Professional Psychology: Research and Practice, 41*(3), 236–243.

Drum, K. B., & Littleton, H. L. (2014). Therapeutic boundaries in telepsychology: Unique issues and best practice recommendations. *Professional Psychology: Research and Practice, 45*(5), 309–315.

Dugger, S. M., & Francis, P. C. (2014). Surviving a lawsuit against a counseling program: Lessons learned from *Ward v. Wilbanks. Journal of Counseling & Development, 92*(2), 135–141.

*Duncan, B. L., Miller, S. D., & Sparks, J. A. (2004). *The heroic client: A revolutionary way to improve effectiveness through client-directed, outcome-informed therapy.* San Francisco, CA: Jossey-Bass.

Duncan, B. L., Miller, S. D., Wampold, B. E., & Hubble, M. A. (2010). *The heart and soul of change: Delivering what works in therapy* (2nd ed.). Washington, DC: American Psychological Association.

Duncan, R. E., Williams, B. J., & Knowles, A. (2013). Adolescents, risk behavior, and confidentiality: When would Australian psychologists breach confidentiality to disclose information to parents? *Australian Psychologist, 48*, 408–419.

Duran, E., Firehammer, J., & Gonzalez, J. (2008). Liberation psychology as a path toward healing cultural soul wounds. *Journal of Counseling and Development, 86*(3), 288–295.

Durodoye, B. A. (2013). Ethical issues in multicultural counseling. In C. C. Lee (Ed.), *Multicultural issues in counseling: New approaches to diversity* (4th ed., pp. 295–308). Alexandria, VA: American Counseling Association.

Eastern Michigan University. (2012). *Julea Ward case information re: American Counseling Association code of ethics.* Retrieved from www.emich.edu/aca_case/

Edwards, J. A., Dattilio, F. M., & Bromley, D. B. (2004). Developing evidence-based practice: The role of case-based research. *Professional Psychology: Research and Practice, 35*(6), 589–597.

Eichenberg, C., Becker-Fischer, M., & Fischer, G. (2010). Sexual assaults in therapeutic relationships: Prevalence, risk factors and consequences. *Health, 2*(9), 1018–1026.

Eisel v. Board of Education, 597 A.2d 447 (Md. 1991).

Elkins, D. N. (2012). Toward a common focus in psychotherapy research. *Psychotherapy, 49*(4), 450–454.

*Elkins, D. N. (2016). *Elements of psychotherapy: A nonmedical model of emotional healing.* Washington, DC: American Psychological Association.

Elliott, R., Greenberg, L. S., Watson, J., Timulak, L., & Freire, E. (2013). Research on humanistic-experiential psychotherapies. In M. J. Lambert (Ed.), *Bergin and Garfield's handbook of psychotherapy and behavior change* (6th ed., pp. 495–538). Hoboken, NJ: Wiley.

*Elman, N. S., & Forrest, L. (2004). Psychotherapy in the remediation of psychology trainees: Exploratory interviews with training directors. *Professional Psychology: Research and Practice, 35*(2), 123–130.

*Elman, N. S., & Forrest, L. (2007). From trainee impairment to professional competence problems: Seeking new terminology that facilitates effective action. *Professional Psychology: Research and Practice, 38*(5), 501–509.

Elmore, A. (2016). Empirically supported treatments: Precept or percept? *Professional Psychology: Research and Practice, 47*(3), 198–205.

Eonta, A. M., Christon, L. M., Hourigan, S. E., Ravindran, N., Vrana, S. R., & Southam-Gerow, M. A. (2011). Using everyday technology to enhance evidence-based treatments. *Professional Psychology: Research and Practice, 42*(6), 513–520.

*Eriksen, K., & Kress, V. E. (2005). *Beyond the DSM story: Ethical quandaries, challenges, and best practices.* Thousand Oaks, CA: Sage.

Evans, R., & Hurrell, C. (2016). The role of schools in children and young people's self-harm and suicide: Systematic review and meta-ethnography of qualitative research. *BMC Public Health, 16*, 1–16.

Everytown for Gun Safety. (2015, October). *215 school shootings in America since 2013.* Retrieved from everytownresearch.org/school-shootings

Ewing v. Goldstein, B163122, 2nd Dist. Div. 8. Cal. App. 4th (2004).

Facebook Newsroom. (2017). *Stats.* Retrieved from http://newsroom.fb.com/company-info/

Falender, C. A. (2017). Multiple relationships and clinical supervision. In O. Zur (Ed.), *Multiple relationships in psychotherapy and counseling: Unavoidable, common, and mandatory dual relations in therapy*(pp. 209–220). New York, NY: Routledge, Taylor & Francis.

Falendar, C. A., & Shafranske, E. P. (2007). Competence in competency-based supervision practice: Construct and application. *Professional Psychology: Research and Practice, 38*(3), 232–240.

Falendar, C. A., & Shafranske, E. P. (2014). Clinical supervision: The state of the art. *Journal of Clinical Psychology, 70*(11), 1030–1041.

Falendar, C. A., Shafranske, E. P., & Falicov, C. (Eds.). (2014). *Multiculturalism and diversity in clinical supervision: A competency-based approach.* Washington, DC: American Psychological Association.

Falendar, C. A., Shafranske, E. P., & Ofek, A. (2014). Competent clinical supervision: Emerging effective practices. *Counselling Psychology Quarterly, 27*(4), 393–408.

Farnsworth, J. K., & Callahan, J. L. (2013). A model for addressing client-clinician value conflict. *Training and Education in Professional Psychology, 7*(3), 205–214.

Fein, A. H., Carlisle, C. S., & Isaacson, N. S. (2008). School shootings and counselor leadership: Four lessons from the field. *Professional School Counseling, 11*(4), 246–252.

Ferguson, A. D. (2016). Cultural issues in counseling lesbians, gays, and bisexuals. In I. Marini & M. A. Stebnicki (Eds.), *The professional counselor's desk reference* (2nd ed., pp. 159–162). New York, NY: Springer.

Fieldsteel, N. D. (2005). When the therapist says goodbye. *International Journal of Group Psychotherapy, 55*(2), 245–279.

Fifield, A. O., & Oliver, K. J. (2016). Enhancing the perceived competence and training of rural mental health practitioners. *Journal of Rural Mental Health, 40*(1), 77–83.

*Fisher, C. D. (2004). Ethical issues in therapy: Therapist self-disclosure of sexual feelings. *Ethics and Behavior, 14*(2), 105–121.

Fisher, M. A. (2008). Protecting confidentiality rights: The need for an ethical practice model. *American Psychologist, 63*(1), 1–13.

Fisher, M. A. (2009). Replacing "Who is the client?" with a different ethical question. *Professional Psychology: Research and Practice, 40*(1), 1–7.

*Fisher, M. A. (2016). *Confidentiality limits in psychotherapy: Ethics checklist for mental health professionals.* Washington, DC: American Psychological Association.

Forester-Miller, H., & Moody, E. E., Jr. (2015). Rural communities: Can dual relationships be avoided? In B. Herlihy & G. Corey (Eds.), *Boundary issues in counseling: Multiple roles and responsibilities* (3rd ed., pp. 251–253). Alexandria, VA: American Counseling Association.

Forester-Miller, H., & Davis, T. E. (2016). *Practitioner's guide to ethical decision making* (Rev. ed.). Retrieved from http://www.counseling.org/docs/default-source/ethics/practioner's-guide-to-ethical-decision-making.pdf

*Forrest, L., Elman, N., Gizara, S., & Vacha-Haase, T. (1999). Trainee impairment: A review of identification, remediation, dismissal, and legal issues. *The Counseling Psychologist, 27*(5), 627–686.

*Frame, M. W. (2003). *Integrating religion and spirituality into counseling: A comprehensive approach.* Belmont, CA: Brooks/Cole, Cengage Learning.

Frame, M. W., & Williams, C. B. (2005). A model of ethical decision making from a multicultural perspective. *Counseling and Values, 49*(3), 165–179.

Francis, P. C. (2014). *Report to the ACA governing council: The revision of the 2005 ACA Code of Ethics.* American Counseling Association, Alexandria, VA.

Francis, P. C. (2016). Religion and spirituality in counseling. In I. Marini & M. A. Stebnicki (Eds.), *The professional counselor's desk reference* (2nd ed., pp. 559–564). New York, NY: Springer.

Francis, P. C., & Dugger, S. M. (2014). Special section: Professionalism, ethics, and value-based conflicts in counseling: An introduction to the special section. *Journal of Counseling & Development, 92*(2), 131–134.

Fried, A. L., & Fisher, C. B. (2016). Moral stress and job burnout among frontline staff conducting clinical research on affective and anxiety disorders. *Professional Psychology: Research and Practice, 47*(3), 171–180.

Gabbard, G. O. (1994). Teetering on the precipice: A commentary on Lazarus's "How certain boundaries and ethics diminish therapeutic effectiveness." *Ethics and Behavior, 4*(3), 283–286.

Galek, K., Flannelly, K. J., Greene, P. B., & Kudler, T. (2011). Burnout, secondary traumatic stress, and social support. *Pastoral Psychology, 60*, 633–649.

Gallardo, M. E., Johnson, J., Parham, T. A., & Carter, J. A. (2009). Ethics and multiculturalism: Advancing cultural and clinical responsiveness. *Professional Psychology: Research and Practice, 40*(5), 425–435.

Gamino, L. A., & Bevins, M. B. (2013). Ethical challenges when counseling clients nearing the end of life. In J. L. Werth Jr. (Ed.), *Counseling clients near the end of life: A practical guide for mental health professionals* (pp. 3–22). New York, NY: Springer.

Gamino, L. A., & Ritter, R. H. (2012). Death competence: An ethical imperative. *Death Studies, 36*, 23–40.

Garcia, J. G., Cartwright, B., Winston, S. M., & Borzuchowska, B. (2003). A transcultural integrative model for ethical decision making in counseling. *Journal of Counseling and Development, 81*(3), 268–277.

Gaubatz, M. D., & Vera, E. M. (2002). Do formalized gatekeeping procedures increase programs' follow-up with deficient trainees? *Counselor Education and Supervision, 41*(4), 294–305.

*Gaubatz, M. D., & Vera, E. M. (2006). Trainee competence in master's level counseling programs: A comparison of counselor educators' and students' views. *Counselor Education and Supervision, 46*(1), 32–43.

Gelso, C. J. (2011). *The real relationship in psychotherapy: The hidden foundation of change*. Washington, DC: American Psychological Association.

Glasheen, K. J., Shochet, I., & Campbell, M. A. (2016). Online counselling in secondary schools: Would students seek help by this medium? *British Journal of Guidance & Counselling, 44*(1), 108–122.

*Glosoff, H. L., Renfro-Michel, E., & Nagarajan, S. (2016). Ethical issues related to the use of technology in clinical supervision. In T. Rousmaniere & E. Renfro-Michel (Eds.), *Using technology to enhance clinical supervision* (pp. 31–46). Alexandria, VA: American Counseling Association.

Godley, S. H., Garner, B. R., Smith, J. E., Meyers, R. J., & Godley, M. D. (2011). A large-scale dissemination and implementation model for evidence-based treatment and continuing care. *Clinical Psychology: Science and Practice, 18*, 67–83.

Gold, S. H., & Hilsenroth, M. J. (2009). Effects of graduate clinicians' personal therapy on therapeutic alliance. *Clinical Psychology and Psychotherapy, 16*(3), 159–171.

*Goldenberg, I., Stanton, M., & Goldenberg, H. (2017). *Family therapy: An overview* (9th ed.). Boston: MA: Cengage Learning.

Goodrich, K. M., & Luke, M. (2012). Problematic students in the experiential group: Professional and ethical challenges for counselor educators. *Journal for Specialists in Group Work, 37*(4), 326–346.

Gordon, C., & Luke, M. (2012). Discursive negotiation of face via email: Professional identity development in school counseling supervision. *Linguistics and Education, 23*, 112–122.

Gottlieb, M. C., & Younggren, J. N. (2009). Is there a slippery slope? Considerations regarding multiple relationships and risk management. *Professional Psychology: Research and Practice, 40*(6), 564–571.

Granello, D. H. (2010). The process of suicide risk assessment: Twelve core principles. *Journal of Counseling & Development, 88*(3), 363–370.

Grenyer, B. F. S., & Lewis, K. L. (2012). Prevalence, prediction, and prevention of psychologist misconduct. *Australian Psychologist, 47*(2), 68–76.

Grossman v. South Shore Public School District, 507 F.3d 1097 (7th Cir. 2007).

Gutheil, T. G., & Brodsky, A. (2008). *Preventing boundary violations in clinical practice*. New York, NY: Guilford Press.

Gutheil, T. G., & Gabbard, G. O. (1993). The concept of boundaries in clinical practice: Theoretical and risk-management dimensions. *American Journal of Psychiatry, 150*(2), 188–196.

Haberl, P., & Peterson, K. (2006). Olympic-sized ethical dilemmas: Issues and challenges for sport psychology consultants on the road and at the Olympic games. *Ethics & Behavior, 16*, 25–40.

Haberstroh, S., Barney, L., Foster, N., & Duffey, T. (2014). The ethical and legal practice of online counseling and psychotherapy: A review of mental health professions. *Journal of Technology in Human Services, 32*(3), 149–157.

Haberstroh, S., & Duffey, T. (2016). Establishing and navigating relationships in online supervision. In T. Rousmaniere & E. Renfro-Michel (Eds.), *Using technology to enhance clinical supervision* (pp. 87–101). Alexandria, VA: American Counseling Association.

Hage, S. M., Mason, M., & Kim, J. (2010). A social justice approach to group counseling. In R. K. Conyne (Ed.), *The Oxford handbook of group counseling* (pp. 102–117). New York, NY: Oxford University Press.

Hagedorn, W. B., & Moorhead, H. J. H. (2011). Counselor self-awareness: Exploring attitudes, beliefs, and values. In C. S. Cashwell & J. S. Young (Eds.), *Integrating spirituality and religion into counseling: A guide to competent practice* (2nd ed., pp. 71–96). Alexandria, VA: American Counseling Association.

Hahn, H. D., & Belt, T. L. (2004). Disability identity and attitudes toward cure in a sample of disabled activities. *Journal of Health and Social Behaviour, 45*(4), 453–464.

Hancock, K. A. (2014). Student beliefs, multiculturalism, and client welfare. *Psychology of Sexual Orientation and Gender Diversity, 1*(1), 4–9.

Handelsman, M. M., Gottlieb, M. C., & Knapp, S. (2005). Training ethical psychologists: An acculturation model. *Professional Psychology: Research and Practice, 36*(1), 59–65.

Handerscheid, R. W., Henderson, M. J., & Chalk, M. (2002). Responding to HIPAA regulations: An update on electronic transaction and privacy requirements. *Family Therapy Magazine, 1*(3), 30–33.

Harris, E., & Younggren, J. N. (2011). Risk management in the digital world. *Professional Psychology: Research and Practice, 42*(6), 412–418.

Harris, S. M., & Harriger, D. J. (2009). Sexual attraction in conjoint therapy. *The American Journal of Family Therapy, 37*, 209–216.

Harris, S. M., & Hays, K. W. (2008). Family therapist comfort with and willingness to discuss client sexuality. *Journal of Marital and Family Therapy, 34*(2), 239–250.

Hartley, M. T., & Cartwright, B. Y. (2015). Analysis of the reported ethical complaints and violations to the Commission on Rehabilitation Counselor Certification, 2006–2013. *Rehabilitation Counseling Bulletin, 58*(3), 154–164.

Harway, M., Kadin, S., Gottlieb, M. C., Nutt, R. L., & Celano, M. (2012). Family psychology and systemic approaches: Working effectively in a variety of contexts. *Professional Psychology: Research and Practice, 43*(4), 315–327.

Hawton, K., Witt, K. G., Salisbury, T. T., Arensman, E., Gunnell, D., Hazell, P., . . . van Heeringen, K. (2016). Psychosocial interventions following self-harm in adults: A systematic review and meta-analysis. *The Lancet Psychiatry, 3*, 740–750. doi:10.1016/S2215-0366(16)30070-0

Hayes, J. A., Gelso, C. J., & Hummel, A. M. (2011). Management of countertransference. In J. C. Norcross (Ed.), *Psychotherapy relationships that work: Evidence-based responsiveness* (2nd ed., pp. 239–258). New York, NY: Oxford University Press.

Hays, D. G., Arredondo, P., Gladding, S. T., & Toporek, R. L. (2010). Integrating social justice in group work: The next decade. *Journal for Specialists in Group Work, 35*(2), 177–206.

*Hecker, L. (Ed.). (2010). *Ethics and professional issues in couple and family therapy*. New York, NY: Routledge.

Hecker, L. L. (2015). Ethical, legal, and professional issues in marriage and family therapy. In J. L. Wetchler & L. L. Hecker (Eds.), *An introduction to marriage and family therapy* (pp. 505–545). New York, NY: Routledge.

Hedlund v. Superior Court, 34 Cal. 3d 695, 669, P.2d 41 (1983).

Helms, J. E. (2008). *A race is a nice thing to have: A guide to being a White person or understanding the White persons in your life* (2nd ed.). Hanover, MA: Microtraining.

*Herlihy, B., & Corey, G. (Eds.). (2015a). *ACA ethical standards casebook* (7th ed.). Alexandria, VA: American Counseling Association.

*Herlihy, B., & Corey, G. (2015b). *Boundary issues in counseling: Multiple roles and responsibilities* (3rd ed.). Alexandria, VA: American Counseling Association.

Herlihy, B., & Dufrene, R. L. (2011, October). Current and emerging ethical issues in counseling: A Delphi study of expert opinions. *Counseling and Values, 56*, 10–24.

Herlihy, B. J., Hermann, M. A., & Greden, L. R. (2014). Legal and ethical implications of using religious beliefs as the basis for refusing to counsel certain clients. *Journal of Counseling & Development, 92*(2), 148–153.

Herlihy, B. R., & Watson, Z. E. P. (2007). Social justice and counseling ethics. In C. C. Lee (Ed.), *Counseling for social justice* (pp. 181–199). Alexandria, VA: American Counseling Association.

*Herlihy, B. R., Watson, Z. E. P., & Patureau-Hatchett, M. P. (2008). Ethical concerns in diagnosing culturally diverse clients. *Ethical Issues in Professional Counseling, 11*(3), 25–34. [Published by the Hatherleigh Company, Hobart, New York]

Hermann, M. A. (2001). *Legal issues in counseling: Incidence, preparation, and consultation.* Doctoral dissertation, University of New Orleans.

Hermann, M. A., & Finn, A. (2002). An ethical and legal perspective on the role of school counselors in preventing violence in schools. *Professional School Counseling, 6*, 46–54.

Hermann, M. A., & Herlihy, B. R. (2006). Legal and ethical implications of refusing to counsel homosexual clients. *Journal of Counseling and Development, 84*(4), 414–418.

Hermann, M. A., & Remley, T. P. (2000). Guns, violence, and schools: The results of school violence—litigation against educators and students shedding more constitutional rights at the school house gate. *Loyola Law Review, 46*(2), 389–439.

Hickson, J., Housley, W., & Wages, D. (2011). Counselors' perception of spirituality in the therapeutic process. *Counseling and Values, 45*, 58–66.

Hogan, M. (2013). *Four skills of cultural diversity competence: A process for understanding and practice* (4th ed.). Belmont, CA: Brooks/Cole, Cengage Learning.

*Hogan-Garcia, M., & Scheinberg, C. (2000). Culturally competent practice principles for planned intervention in organizations and communities. *Practicing Anthropology, 22*(2), 27–30.

Hohenshil, T. H., Amundson, N. E., & Niles, S. G. (Eds.). (2013). *Counseling around the world: An international handbook.* Alexandria, VA: American Counseling Association.

*Hollon, S. D., & Beck, A. T. (2013). Cognitive and cognitive-behavioral therapies. In M. J. Lambert (Ed.), *Bergin and Garfield's handbook of psychotherapy and behavior change* (6th ed., pp. 393–492). Hoboken, NJ: Wiley.

*Homan, M. (2016). *Promoting community change: Making it happen in the real world* (6th ed.). Boston, MA: Cengage Learning.

International Association of Marriage and Family Counselors. (2011). *Ethical code for the International Association of Marriage and Family Counselors.* Alexandria, VA: Author.

Ivey, A. E., D'Andrea, M., & Ivey, M. (2012). *Theories of counseling and psychotherapy: A multicultural perspective* (7th ed.). Thousand Oaks, CA: Sage.

Ivey, A. E., Ivey, M. B., Myers, J., & Sweeney, T. (2005). *Developmental counseling and therapy: Promoting wellness over the lifespan.* Boston, MA: Lashaska Houghton Mifflin.

*Ivey, A. E., Ivey, M. B., & Zalaquett, C. P. (2018). *Intentional interviewing and counseling: Facilitating client development in a multicultural society* (9th ed.). Boston, MA: Cengage Learning.

Jablonski v. United States, 712 F.2d 391 (9th Cir. 1983).

Jackson, J., Thoman, L., Suris, A. M., & North, C. S. (2012). Working with trauma-related mental health problems among combat veterans of the Afghanistan and Iraq conflicts. In I. Marini & M. A. Stebnicki (Eds.), *The psychological and social impact of illness and disability* (6th ed., pp. 307–330). New York, NY: Springer.

Jacobs, S. C., Huprich, S. K., Grus, C. L., Cage, E. A., Elman, N. S., Forrest, L., . . . Kaslow, N. J. (2011). Trainees with professional competency problems: Preparing trainers for difficult but necessary conversations. *Training and Education in Professional Psychology, 5*(3), 175–184.

Jadaszewski, S. (2016). Ethically problematic value change as an outcome of psychotherapeutic interventions. *Ethics & Behavior*, 1–16. doi:10.1080/105 08422.2016.1195739

Jaffee v. Redmond, WL 315 841 (U.S. 1996).

Jensen, D. G. (2003a). HIPAA: How to comply with the transaction standards. *The Therapist, 15*(4), 16–19.

Jensen, D. G. (2003b). HIPAA overview. *The Therapist, 15*(3), 26–27.

Jensen, D. G. (2003c). HIPAA: Overview of the security standards. *The Therapist, 15*(5), 22–24.

Jensen, D. G. (2003d). How to comply with the privacy rule. *The Therapist, 15*(3), 28–37.

Jensen, D. G. (2003e). To be or not to be a covered entity: That is the question. *The Therapist, 15*(2), 14–17.

Jensen, D. G. (2006). The fundamentals of reporting elderly and dependent adult abuse. *The Therapist, 18*(2), 11–17.

Jensen, D. G. (2012). The *Tarasoff* two-step. *The Therapist, 24*(5), 44–51.

Jensen, D. R., Abbott, M. K., Beecher, M. E., Griner, D., Golightly, T. R., & Cannon, J. A. N. (2012). Taking the pulse of the group: The utilization of practice-based evidence in group psychotherapy. *Professional Psychology: Research and Practice, 43*(4), 388–394.

Jobes, D. A., & O'Connor, S. S. (2009). The duty to protect suicidal clients: Ethical, legal, and professional considerations. In J. L. Werth Jr., E. R. Welfel, & G. A. H. Benjamin (Eds.), *The duty to protect: Ethical, legal, and professional considerations for mental health professionals* (pp. 163–180). Washington, DC: American Psychological Association.

Johnson, R. (2013). *Spirituality in counseling and psychotherapy: An integrative approach that empowers clients*. Hoboken, NJ: Wiley.

Johnson, W. B., Barnett, J. E., Elman, N. S., Forrest, L., & Kaslow, N. J. (2012). The competent community: Toward a vital reformulation of professional ethics. *American Psychologist, 67*(7), 557–569.

Johnson, W. B., & Campbell, C. D. (2002). Character and fitness requirements for professional psychologists: Are there any? *Professional Psychology: Research and Practice, 33*(1), 46–53.

Johnson, W. B., & Campbell, C. D. (2004). Character and fitness requirements for professional psychologists: Training directors' perspectives. *Professional Psychology: Research and Practice, 35*(4), 405–411.

*Johnson, W. B., Elman, N. S., Forrest, L., Robiner, W. N., Rodolfa, E., & Schaffer, J. B. (2008). Addressing professional competence problems in trainees: Some ethical considerations. *Professional Psychology: Research and Practice, 39*(6), 589–599.

Johnson, W. B., Grasso, I., & Maslowski, K. (2010). Conflicts between ethics and law for military mental health providers. *Military Medicine, 175*(8), 548–533.

Johnson, W. B., & Johnson, S. J. (2017). Unavoidable and mandated multiple relationships in military settings. In O. Zur (Ed.), *Multiple relationships in psychotherapy and counseling: Unavoidable, common, and mandatory dual relations in therapy* (pp. 49–60). New York, NY: Routledge, Taylor & Francis.

Kaplan, D. M. (2014). Ethical implications of a critical legal case for the counseling profession: *Ward v. Wilbanks. Journal of Counseling & Development, 92*(2), 142–146.

Kaplan, D. M., Francis, P. C., Hermann, M. A., Baca, J. V., Goodnough, G. E., Hodges, S., Spurgeon, S. L., & Wade, M. E. (2017). New concepts in the

2014 ACA Code of Ethics. *Journal of Counseling & Development 95*, 100–120.

Kaslow, N. J., Rubin, N. J., Bebeau, M. J., Leigh, I. W., Lichtenberg, J. W., Nelson, P. D., Portnoy, S. M., & Smith, I. L. (2007). Guiding principles and recommendations for the assessment of competence. *Professional Psychology: Research and Practice, 38*(5), 441–451.

Keenan, K., & Rubin, S. (2016). The good therapist: Evidence regarding the therapist's contribution to psychotherapy. In D. J. Cain, K. Keenan, & S. Rubin (Eds.), *Humanistic psychotherapies: Handbook of research and practice* (2nd ed., pp. 421–454). Washington, DC: American Psychological Association.

Kennedy, P. F., Vandehey, M., Norman, W. B., & Diekhoff, G. M. (2003). Recommendations for risk-management practices. *Professional Psychology: Research and Practice, 34*(3), 309–311.

Kerl, S. B., Garcia, J. L., McCullough, S., & Maxwell, M. E. (2002). Systematic evaluation of professional performance: Legally supported procedure and process. *Counselor Education and Supervision, 41*(4), 321–334.

Kirland, K., Kirkland, K. L., & Reaves, R. P. (2004). On the professional use of disciplinary data. *Professional Psychology: Research and Practice, 35*(2), 179–184.

Kitchener, K. S. (1984). Intuition, critical evaluation and ethical principles: The foundation for ethical decisions in counseling psychology. *The Counseling Psychologist, 12*(3), 43–55.

*Kleespies, P. M. (2004). *Life and death decisions: Psychological and ethical considerations in end-of-life care.* Washington, DC: American Psychological Association.

Kleist, D., & Bitter, J. R. (2014). Virtue, ethics, and legality in family practice. In J. R. Bitter, *Theory and practice of family therapy and counseling* (2nd ed., pp. 71–93). Belmont, CA: Brooks/Cole, Cengage Learning.

*Knapp, S., Gottlieb, M., Berman, J., & Handelsman, M. M. (2007). When law and ethics collide: What should psychologists do? *Professional Psychology: Research and Practice, 38*(1), 54–59.

Knapp, S. J., Gottlieb, M., & Handelsman, M. M. (2015). *Ethical dilemmas in psychotherapy: Positive approaches to decision making.* Washington, DC: American Psychological Association.

Knapp, S., Handelsman, M. M., Gottlieb, M. C., & Vandecreek, L. D. (2013). The dark side of professional ethics. *Professional Psychology: Research and Practice, 44*(6), 371–377.

Knapp, S., & VandeCreek, L. (2007). When values of different cultures conflict: Ethical decision making in a multicultural context. *Professional Psychology: Research and Practice, 38*(6), 660–666.

*Knapp, S. J., & VandeCreek, L. (2012). *Practical ethics for psychologists: A positive approach* (2nd ed.). Washington, DC: American Psychological Association.

Kocet, M. M., & Herlihy, B. J. (2014). Addressing values-based conflicts within the counseling relationship: A decision-making model. *Journal of Counseling & Development, 92*(2), 180–186.

Kolmes, K. (2012). Social media in the future of professional psychology. *Professional Psychology: Research & Practice, 43*(6), 606–612.

Kolmes, K. (2017). Digital and social media multiple relationships on the Internet. In O. Zur (Ed.), *Multiple relationships in psychotherapy and counseling: Unavoidable, common, and mandatory dual relations in therapy* (pp. 185–195). New York, NY: Routledge, Taylor & Francis.

Kolmes, K., & Taube, D. G. (2016). Client discovery of psychotherapist personal information online. *Professional Psychology: Research and Practice, 47*(2), 147–154.

Kottler, J. A., & Balkin, R. (2017). *Relationships in counseling and the counselor's life.* Alexandria, VA: American Counseling Association.

Kottler, J. A., & Carlson, J. (2016). *Therapy over 50: Aging issues in psychotherapy and the therapist's life.* New York, NY: Oxford University Press.

Kottler, J. A., Englar-Carlson, M., & Carlson, J. (Eds.). (2013). *Helping beyond the 50-minute hour: Therapists involved in meaningful social action.* New York, NY: Routledge, Taylor & Francis.

Koocher, G. P., & Campbell, L. F. (2016). Professional ethics in the United States. In J. Norcross, G. R. VandenBos, & D. K. Freedheim (Eds.), *APA handbook of clinical psychology* (vol. 5, pp. 301–338). Washington, DC: American Psychological Association.

*Koocher, G. P., & Keith-Spiegel, P. (2008). *Ethics in psychology and the mental health professions: Standards and cases* (3rd ed.). New York, NY: Oxford University Press.

*Koocher, G. P., & Keith-Spiegel, P. (2016). *Ethics in psychology and the mental health professions: Standards and cases* (4th ed.). New York, NY: Oxford University Press.

Kozlowski, J. M., Pruitt, N. T., DeWalt, T. A., & Knox, S. (2014). Can boundary crossings in clinical supervision be beneficial? *Counselling Psychology Quarterly, 27*(2), 109–126.

Kozlowski, K. A., & Holmes, C. M. (2014). Experiences in online process groups: A qualitative study. *Journal for Specialists in Group Work, 39*(4), 276–300.

Kress, V. E. W., Eriksen, K. P., Rayle, A. D., & Ford, S. J. W. (2005). The *DSM-IV-TR* and culture: Considerations for counselors. *Journal of Counseling and Development, 83*(1), 97–104.

Kress, V. E., Hoffman, R. M., Adamson, N., & Eriksen, K. (2013). Informed consent, confidentiality, diagnosing: Ethical guidelines for counselor practice. *Journal of Mental Health Counseling, 35*(1), 15–28.

Kress, V. E., Newgent, R. A., Whitlock, J., & Mease, L. (2015). Spirituality/religiosity, life satisfaction, and life meaning as protective factors for nonsuicidal self-injury in college students. *Journal of College Counseling,18*(2), 160–174. doi: 10.1002/jocc.12012

Kress, V. E., & Protivnak, J. J. (2009). Professional development plans to remedy problematic counseling students' behaviors. *Counselor Education and Supervision, 48*(3), 154–166.

La Roche, M. J., Fuentes, M. A., & Hinton, D. (2015). A cultural examination of the *DSM-5*: Research and clinical implications for cultural minorities. *Professional Psychology: Research and Practice, 46*(3), 183–189.

Lambert, M. J. (2011). Psychotherapy research and its achievements. In J. C. Norcross, G. R. VandenBos, & D. K. Freedheim (Eds.), *History of psychotherapy* (2nd ed., pp. 299–332). Washington, DC: American Psychological Association.

Lambert, M. J. (2013). The efficacy and effectiveness of psychotherapy. In M. J. Lambert (Ed.), *Bergin and Garfield's handbook of psychotherapy and behavior change* (6th ed., pp. 169–218). Hoboken, NJ: Wiley.

*Lasky, G. B., & Riva, M. T. (2006). Confidentiality and privileged communication in group psychotherapy. *International Journal of Group Psychotherapy, 56*(4), 455–476.

Laughran, W., & Bakken, G. M. (1984). The psychotherapist's responsibility toward third parties under current California law. *Western State University Law Review, 12*(1), 1–33.

Lawrence, G., & Kurpius, S. E. R. (2000). Legal and ethical issues involved when counseling minors in nonschool settings. *Journal of Counseling and Development, 78*(2), 130–136.

Lazarus, A. A. (1998). How do you like these boundaries? *The Clinical Psychologist, 51*(1), 22–25.

Lazarus, A. A. (2001). Not all "dual relationships" are taboo: Some tend to enhance treatment outcomes. *The National Psychologist, 10*(1), 16.

Lazarus, A. A., & Rego, S. A. (2013). What really matters? Learning from, not being limited by empirically supported treatments. *The Behavior Therapist, 36*(3), 67–69.

*Lazarus, A. A., & Zur, O. (Eds.). (2002). *Dual relationships and psychotherapy.* New York, NY: Springer.

Lebow, J. L., & Stroud, C. B. (2016). Family therapy. In J. Norcross, G. R. VandenBos, & D. K. Freedheim (Eds.), *APA handbook of clinical psychology* (vol. 3, pp. 327–349). Washington, DC: American Psychological Association.

Lee, C. C. (2013a). The cross-cultural encounter: Meeting the challenge of culturally competent counseling. In C. C. Lee (Ed.), *Multicultural issues in counseling: New approaches to diversity* (4th ed., pp. 13–19). Alexandria, VA: American Counseling Association.

Lee, C. C. (2013b). Global literacy: The foundation of culturally competent counseling. In C. C. Lee (Ed.), *Multicultural issues in counseling: New approaches to diversity* (4th ed., pp. 309–312). Alexandria, VA: American Counseling Association.

*Lee, C. C. (Ed.). (2013c). *Multicultural issues in counseling: New approaches to diversity* (4th ed.). Alexandria, VA: American Counseling Association.

Lee, C. C., & Hipolito-Delgado, C. P. (2007). Introduction: Counselors as agents of social justice. In C. C. Lee (Ed.), *Counseling for social justice* (2nd ed., pp. xiii–xxviii). Alexandria, VA: American Counseling Association.

Lee, C. C., & Park, D. (2013). A conceptual framework for counseling across cultures. In C. C. Lee (Ed.), *Multicultural issues in counseling: New approaches to diversity* (4th ed., pp. 3–12). Alexandria, VA: American Counseling Association.

Lee, C. C., & Rodgers, R. A. (2009). Counselor advocacy: Affecting systemic change in the public arena. *Journal of Counseling and Development, 87*(3), 284–287.

Lee, J., Lim, N., Yang, E., & Lee, S. M. (2011). Antecedents and consequences of three dimensions of burnout in psychotherapists: A meta-analysis. *Professional Psychology: Research and Practice, 42*(3), 252–258.

Leslie, R. S. (2008). The dangerous patient and confidentiality revisited. *The Therapist, 20*(5), 24–30.

Leslie, R. S. (2010). Treatment of minors without parental consent. *Legal Resources, Avoiding Liability Bulletin.* Retrieved from http://cphins.com/LegalResources/tabid/65/

Leslie, R. S. (2016). Licensing board issues warning to patients who travel out of state! *Avoiding Liability Bulletin.* Retrieved from www.cphins.com/wp-content/uploads/2016/08/ALB-Sept 2016

Letourneau, J. L. H. (2016). A decision-making model for addressing problematic behaviors in counseling students. *Counseling and Values, 61*(2), 206–222.

Levitt, D. H., Farry, T. J., & Mazzarella, J. R. (2015). Counselor ethical reasoning: Decision-making practice versus theory. *Counseling and Values, 60,* 84–99.

Levitt, D. H., & Moorhead, H. J. H. (Eds.). (2013). *Values and ethics in counseling: Real-life ethical decision making.* New York, NY: Routledge, Taylor & Francis.

*Lewis, J. A., Lewis, M. D., Daniels, J. A., & D'Andrea, M. J. (2011). *Community counseling: A multicultural-social justice perspective* (4th ed.). Belmont, CA: Brooks/Cole, Cengage Learning.

Lewis, J. A., Toporek, R. L., & Ratts, M. J. (2010). Advocacy and social justice: Entering the mainstream of the counseling profession. In M. J. Ratts, R. L. Toporek, & J. A. Lewis (Eds.), *ACA advocacy competencies: A social justice framework for counselors* (pp. 239–244). Alexandria, VA: American Counseling Association.

Lewis, S. P., Heath, N. L., Michal, N. J., & Duggan, J. M. (2012). Non-suicidal self-injury, youth, and the Internet: What mental health professionals need to know. *Child and Adolescent Psychiatry and Mental Health, 6*(1), 13. doi: 10.1186/1753-2000-6-13

Linde, L. E. (2016). The *ACA Code of Ethics*: Clarifying values and referrals in counseling. *Counseling Today, 59*(4), 20–21.

Linnerooth, P. J., Mrdjenovich, A. J., & Moore, B. A. (2011). Professional burnout in clinical military psychologists: Recommendations before, during, and after deployment. *Professional Psychology: Research and Practice, 42*(1), 87–93.

Livneh, H. (2012). On the origins of negative attitudes toward people with disabilities. In I. Marini & M. A. Stebnicki (Eds.), *The psychological and social impact of illness and disability* (6th ed., pp. 13–25). New York, NY: Springer.

Luke, M., & Hackney, H. (2007). Group coleadership: A critical review. *Counselor Education and Supervision, 46*(4), 280–293.

Lum, D. (2004). *Social work practice and people of color: A process-stage approach* (5th ed.). Belmont, CA: Brooks/Cole, Cengage Learning.

*Lum, D. (2011). *Culturally competent practice: A framework for understanding diverse groups and justice issues* (4th ed.). Belmont, CA: Brooks/Cole, Cengage Learning.

Lustgarten, S. D. (2015). Emerging ethical threats to client privacy in cloud communication and data storage. *Professional Psychology: Research and Practice, 46*(3), 154–160.

MacKinnon, C. J., Bhatia, M., Sunderani, M., Affleck, W., & Smith, N. G. (2011). Opening the dialogue: Implications of feminist supervision theory with male supervisees. *Professional Psychology: Research and Practice, 42*(2), 130–136.

MacLeod, B. P., & McMullen, J. W. (2016). Raising public awareness of the counseling profession. *Counseling Today, 59*(6), 74–78.

MacNair-Semands, R. R. (2007). Attending to the spirit of social justice as an ethical approach in group therapy. *International Journal of Group Psychotherapy, 57*(1), 61–66.

Mallen, M. J., Vogel, D. L., & Rochlen, A. B. (2005). The practical aspects of online counseling: Ethics, training, technology, and competency. *The Counseling Psychologist, 33*(6), 776–818.

Margolin, G. (1982). Ethical and legal considerations in marital and family therapy. *American Psychologist, 37*(7), 788–801.

Markus, H. R. (2008). Pride, prejudice, and ambivalence: Toward a unified theory of race and ethnicity. *American Psychologist, 63*(8), 651–670.

*Maslach, C. (2003). *Burnout: The cost of caring*. Cambridge, MA: Malor Books.

*McAdams, C. R., & Foster, V. A. (2007). A guide to just and fair remediation of counseling students with professional performance deficiencies. *Counselor Education and Supervision, 47*(1), 2–13.

*McAdams, C. R., Foster, V. A., & Ward, T. J. (2007). Remediation and dismissal policies in counselor education: Lessons learned from a challenge in federal court. *Counselor Education and Supervision, 46*(3), 212–229.

McAdams, C. R., III, & Wyatt, K. L. (2010). The regulation of technology-assisted distance counseling and supervision in the United States: An analysis of current extent, trends, and implications. *Counselor Education & Supervision, 49*, 179–192.

McCarthy, C. J., Falco, L. D., & Villalba, J. (2014). Ethical and professional issues in experiential growth groups: Moving forward. *Journal for Specialists in Group Work, 39*(3), 186–193.

McCarthy, H. (2003). The disability rights movement: Experiences and perspectives of selected leaders in the disability community. *Rehabilitation Counseling Bulletin, 46*, 209–223.

McCloskey, M. S. (2011). Training in empirically supported treatments using alternative learning modalities. *Clinical Psychology: Science and Practice, 18*(1), 84–88.

McGee, T. F. (2003). Observations on the retirement of professional psychologists. *Professional Psychology: Research and Practice, 34*(4), 388–395.

McGeorge, C. R., Carlson, T. S., & Farrell, M. (2016). To refer or not to refer: Exploring family therapists' beliefs and practices related to the referral of lesbian, gay, and bisexual clients. *Journal of Marital and Family Therapy, 42*(3), 466–480. doi:10.1111/jmft.12148

McMurtery, R. F., Webb, T. T., & Arnold, R. D. (2011). Assessing perceptions and attitudes of intimate behaviors in clinical supervision among licensed professional counselors, licensed social workers, and licensed psychologists. *The Researcher: An Interdisciplinary Journal, 24*(2), 57–78.

Meara, N. M., Schmidt, L. D., & Day, J. D. (1996). Principles and virtues: A foundation for ethical decisions, policies, and character. *The Counseling Psychologist, 24*(1), 4–77.

Meyers, L. (2016a). License to deny service. *Counseling Today, 59*(1), 24–31.

Meyers, L. (2016b). The relationship as client. *Counseling Today, 59*(4), 22–31.

Miller, G. M., & Larrabee, M. J. (1995). Sexual intimacy in counselor education and supervision: A national survey. *Counselor Education and Supervision, 34*(4), 332–343.

*Miller, S. D., Duncan, B. L., & Hubble, M. A. (2004). Beyond integration: The triumph of outcome over process in clinical practice. *Psychotherapy in Australia, 10*(2), 2–19.

*Miller, S. D., Hubble, M. A., Duncan, B. L., & Wampold, B. E. (2010). Delivering what works. In B. L. Duncan, S. D. Miller, B. E. Wampold, & M. A. Hubble (Eds.), *The heart and soul of change: Delivering what works in therapy* (2nd ed., pp. 421–429). Washington DC: American Psychological Association.

Miller, S. D., Hubble, M. A., & Seidel, J. (2015). Feedback-informed treatment. In E. Neukrug (Ed.), *The Sage encyclopedia of theory in counseling and psychotherapy* (vol. 1, pp. 401–403). Thousand Oaks, CA: Sage.

Moles, T. A., Petrie, T. A., & Watkins, C. E. (2016). Sex and sport: Attractions and boundary crossings between sport psychology consultants and their client-athletes. *Professional Psychology: Research and Practice, 47*(2), 93–101.

Moleski, S. M., & Kiselica, M. S. (2005). Dual relationships: A continuum ranging from the destructive to the therapeutic. *Journal of Counseling and Development, 83*(1), 3–11.

Monk, G. (2013). Walking the tightrope of change: Building trust and effective practice in a diverse multi-stressed urban community. In J. A. Kottler, M. Englar-Carlson, & J. Carlson (Eds.), *Helping beyond the 50-minute hour: Therapists involved in meaningful social action* (pp. 96–111). New York, NY: Routledge, Taylor & Francis.

Mossman, D. (2009). The imperfection of protection through detection and intervention: Lessons from three decades of research on the psychiatric assessment of violence risk. *The Journal of Legal Medicine, 30*, 109–140.

Moyer, M. S., Sullivan, J. R., & Growcock, D. (2012). When is it ethical to inform administrators about student risk-taking behaviors? Perceptions of school counselors. *Professional School Counseling, 15*(3), 98–109.

Muratori, M. C. (2001). Examining supervisor impairment from the counselor trainee's perspective. *Counselor Education and Supervision, 41*(1), 41–56.

Murphy, J. M., & Pomerantz, A. M. (2016). Informed consent: An adaptable question format for telepsychology. *Professional Psychology: Research and Practice, 47*(5), 330–339.

*Nagy, T. F. (2005). *Ethics in plain English: An illustrative casebook for psychologists* (2nd ed.). Washington, DC: American Psychological Association.

*Nagy, T. F. (2011). *Essential ethics for psychologists: A primer for understanding and mastering core issues.* Washington, DC: American Psychological Association.

National Association of Social Workers. (1994). *Guidelines for clinical social work supervision.* Washington, DC: Author.

*National Association of Social Workers. (2003). Client self-determination in end-of-life decisions. In *Social work speaks: National Association of Social Workers policy statements, 2003–2006* (6th ed., pp. 46–49). Washington, DC: NASW Press.

*National Association of Social Workers. (2004). *NASW standards for social work practice in palliative and end of life care.* Retrieved from www.socialworkers.org/practice/bereavement/standards/default.asp

National Association of Social Workers. (2008). *Code of ethics.* Washington, DC: Author.

National Organization for Human Services. (2000). Ethical standards of human service professionals. *Human Service Education, 20*(1), 61–68.

Neff, K. (2011). *Self-compassion: Stop beating up on yourself and leave insecurity behind.* New York, NY: HarperCollins, William Morrow.

Neimeyer, G. J., Taylor, J. M., & Cox, D. R. (2012). On hope and possibility: Does continuing professional development contribute to ongoing professional competence? *Professional Psychology: Research and Practice, 43*(5), 476–486.

Neukrug, E. S., & Milliken, T. (2011). Counselors' perceptions of ethical behaviors. *Journal of Counseling and Development, 89*(2), 206–216.

Newsome, S., Waldo, M., & Gruszka, C. (2012). Mindfulness group work: Preventing stress and increasing self-compassion among helping professionals in training. *Journal for Specialists in Group Work, 37*(4), 297–311.

Nock, M. K. (Ed.). (2014). *The Oxford handbook of suicide and self-injury.* New York, NY: Oxford University Press.

*Norcross, J. C. (2005). The psychotherapist's own psychotherapy: Educating and developing psychologists. *American Psychologist, 60*(8), 840–850.

Norcross, J. C. (2010). The therapeutic relationship. In B. L. Duncan, S. D. Miller, B. E. Wampold, & M. A. Hubble (Eds.), *The heart & soul of change: Delivering what works in therapy* (2nd ed., pp. 113–141). Washington, DC: American Psychological Association.

Norcross, J. C., Beutler, L. E., & Levant, R. F. (2006). *Evidence-based practices in mental health: Debate and dialogue on the fundamental questions.* Washington, DC: American Psychological Association.

*Norcross, J. C., & Guy, J. D. (2007). *Leaving it at the office: A guide to psychotherapist self-care.* New York, NY: Guilford Press.

*Norcross, J. C., Hogan, T. P., & Koocher, G. P. (2008). *Clinician's guide to evidence-based practices.* New York, NY: Oxford University Press.

Nosek, M. A. (2005). Wellness in the context of disability. In J. Myers & T. Sweeney (Eds.), *Wellness in counseling: Theory, research, and practice* (pp. 139–150). Alexandria, VA: American Counseling Association.

Nystul, M. S. (2016). *Introduction to counseling: An art and science perspective* (5th ed.). Los Angeles, CA: Sage.

O'Morain, P., McAuliffe, G. J., Conroy, K., Johnson, J. M., & Michel, R. E. (2012). Counseling in Ireland. *Journal of Counseling and Development, 90*(3), 367–372.

Oliver, M. N. I., Bernstein, J. H., Anderson, K. G., Blashfield, R. K., & Roberts, M. C. (2004). An exploratory examination of student attitudes toward "impaired" peers in clinical psychology training programs. *Professional Psychology: Research and Practice, 35*(2), 141–147.

Orlinsky, D. E., Geller, J. D., & Norcross, J. C. (2005). Epilogue: The patient psychotherapist, the psychotherapist's psychotherapist, and the therapist as a person. In J. D. Geller, J. C. Norcross, & D. E. Orlinsky (Eds.), *The psychotherapist's own psychotherapy: Patient and clinician perspectives* (pp. 405–415). New York, NY: Oxford University Press.

Orlinsky, D. E., Norcross, J. C., Ronnestad, M. H., & Wiseman, H. (2005). Outcomes and impacts of psychotherapists' personal therapy: A research review. In J. D. Geller, J. C. Norcross, & D. E. Orlinsky (Eds.), *The psychotherapist's own psychotherapy* (pp. 214–230). New York, NY: Oxford University Press.

*Orlinsky, D. E., & Ronnestad, M. H. (2005). *How psychotherapists develop: A study of therapeutic work and professional growth.* Washington, DC: American Psychological Association.

Orlinsky, D. E., Schofield, M. J., Schroder, T., & Kazantzis, N. (2011). Utilization of personal therapy by psychotherapists: A practice-friendly review and a new study. *Journal of Clinical Psychology: In Session, 67*(8), 828–842.

Pack-Brown, S. P., Thomas, T. L., & Seymour, J. M. (2008). Infusing professional ethics into counselor education programs: A multicultural/social justice perspective. *Journal of Counseling and Development, 86*(3), 296–302.

*Parham, T. A., & Caldwell, L. D. (2015). Boundaries in the context of a collective community: An African-centered perspective. In B. Herlihy & G. Corey (Eds.), *Boundary issues in counseling: Multiple roles and responsibilities* (3rd ed., pp. 96–99). Alexandria, VA: American Counseling Association.

Patsiopoulos, A. T., & Buchanan, M. J. (2011). The practice of self-compassion in counseling: A narrative inquiry. *Professional Psychology: Research and Practice, 42*(4), 301–307.

Pedersen, P. (1991). Multiculturalism as a generic approach to counseling. *Journal of Counseling and Development, 70*(1), 6–12.

*Pedersen, P. (2000). *A handbook for developing multicultural awareness* (3rd ed.). Alexandria, VA: American Counseling Association.

Pedersen, P. (2008). Ethics, competence, and professional issues in cross-cultural counseling. In

P. B. Pedersen, J. G. Draguns, W. J. Lonner, & J. E. Trimble (Eds.), *Counseling across cultures* (6th ed., pp. 5–20). Thousand Oaks, CA: Sage.

*Pedersen, P., Crethar, H., & Carlson, J. (2008). *Inclusive cultural empathy: Making relationships central in counseling and psychotherapy.* Washington, DC: APA Press.

Perlin, M. L. (1997). The "duty to protect" others from violence. In *The Hatherleigh guide to ethics in therapy* (pp. 127–146). New York, NY: Hatherleigh Press.

Phan, L. T., Hebert, D. J., & DeMitchell, T. A. (2013). School counselor training with LGBTQ clients: A constitutional conflict. *Journal of LGBT Issues in Counseling, 7*(1), 44–64.

Pickersgill, M. D. (2014). Debating *DSM-5*: Diagnosis and the sociology of critique. *Medical Ethics, 40,* 521–525.

Pipes, R. B., Holstein, J. E., & Aguirre, M. G. (2005). Examining the personal-professional distinction: Ethics codes and the difficulty of drawing a boundary. *American Psychologist, 60,* 325–334.

Plener, P. L., Schumacher, T. S., Munz, L. M., & Groschwitz, R. C. (2015). The longitudinal course of non-suicidal self-injury and deliberate self-harm: A systematic review of the literature. *Borderline Personality Disorder and Emotion, 2*(2). doi:10.1186/s40479-014-0024-3

Polychronis, P. D., & Brown, S. G. (2016). The strict liability standard and clinical supervision. *Professional Psychology: Research and Practice, 47*(2), 139–146.

Pomerantz, A. M., & Handelsman, M. M. (2004). Informed consent revisited: An updated written question format. *Professional Psychology: Research and Practice, 35*(2), 201–205.

Pope, K. S. (2015). Record-keeping controversies: Ethical, legal, and clinical challenges. *Canadian Psychology, 56*(3), 348–356.

Pope, K. S., Keith-Spiegel, P., & Tabachnick, B. G. (1986). Sexual attraction to clients: The human therapist and the (sometimes) inhuman training system. *American Psychologist, 41*(2), 147–158.

Pope, K. S., Sonne, J. L., & Greene, B. (2006). *What therapists don't talk about and why: Understanding taboos that hurt us and our clients.* Washington, DC: American Psychological Association.

*Pope, K. S., Sonne, J. L., & Holroyd, J. (1993). *Sexual feelings in psychotherapy: Explorations for therapists and therapists-in-training.* Washington, DC: American Psychological Association.

*Pope, K. S., & Vasquez, M. J. T. (2016). *Ethics in psychotherapy and counseling: A practical guide for psychologists* (5th ed.). Hoboken, NJ: Wiley.

Pope, K. S., & Wedding, D. (2014). Contemporary challenges and controversies. In D. Wedding & R. J. Corsini (Eds.), *Current psychotherapies* (10th ed., pp. 569–603). Belmont, CA: Brooks/Cole, Cengage Learning.

Rapin, L. S. (2014). Guidelines for ethical and legal practice in counseling and psychotherapy groups. In J. L. DeLucia-Waack, C. R. Kalodner, & M. T. Riva (Eds.), *Handbook of group counseling and psychotherapy* (2nd ed., pp. 71–83). Thousand Oaks, CA: Sage.

Ratts, M. J., & Hutchins, A. M. (2009). ACA Advocacy Competencies: Social justice advocacy at the client/student level. *Journal of Counseling and Development, 87*(3), 269–275.

Ratts, M. J., Singh, A. A., Butler, S. K., Nassar-McMillan, S., & McCullough, J. R. (2016). Multicultural and social justice counseling competencies: Practical applications in counseling. *Counseling Today, 58*(8), 40–45.

*Ratts, M. J., Toporek, R. L., & Lewis, J. A. (2010). *ACA advocacy competencies: A social justice framework for counselors.* Alexandria, VA: American Counseling Association.

Ravis, H. B. (2007). Challenges and special problems in distance counseling: How to respond to them. In J. F. Malone, R. M. Miller, & G. R. Walz (Eds.), *Distance counseling: Expanding the counselor's reach and impact* (pp.119–132). Alexandria, VA: American Counseling Association.

Reamer, F. G. (2013). Social work in a digital age: Ethical and risk management challenges. *Social Work, 58*(2), 163–172.

Reamer, F. G. (2015). Clinical social work in a digital environment: Ethical and risk-management challenges. *Clinical Social Work Journal, 43*, 120–132.

Reamer, F. G. (2017). Multiple relationships in a digital world: Unprecedented ethical and risk management challenges. In O. Zur (Ed.), *Multiple relationships in psychotherapy and counseling: Unavoidable, common, and mandatory dual relations in therapy* (pp. 196–206). New York, NY: Routledge, Taylor & Francis.

Reaves, R. P. (2003). *Avoiding liability in mental health practice.* Montgomery, AL: Association of State and Provincial Psychology Boards.

Reeves, J. (2011). Guidelines for recording the use of physical restraint. *Mental Health Practice, 15*(1), 22–24.

Remley, T. P. (1995). A proposed alternative to the licensing of specialties in counseling. *Journal of Counseling and Development, 74*(2) 126–129.

*Remley, T. P. (2009). Legal challenges in counseling suicidal students. In D. Capuzzi, *Suicide prevention in the schools: Guidelines for middle and high school settings* (2nd ed., pp. 71–83). Alexandria, VA: American Counseling Association.

Remley, T. P. (2017, February). *Legal issues in clinical and administrative supervision.* Presentation given at Law and Ethics Counseling Conference, New Orleans, Louisiana.

*Remley, T. P., & Herlihy, B. (2016). *Ethical, legal, and professional issues in counseling* (5th ed.). Boston, MA: Pearson.

Remley, T. P., & Hermann, M. A. (2000). Legal and ethical issues in school counseling. In J. Wittmer (Ed.), *Managing your school counseling program: K–12 developmental strategies* (pp. 314–329). Minneapolis, MN: Educational Media Corporation.

Remley, T. P., Hulse-Killacky, D., Christensen, T., Gibbs, K., Schaefer, P., Tanigoshi, H., Hermann, M., & Miller, J. (2002, October 18). *Dismissing graduate students for non-academic reasons.* Paper presented at the Association for Counselor Education and Supervision Convention, Park City, Utah.

Renfro-Michel, E., Rousmaniere, T., & Spinella, L. (2016). Technological innovations in clinical supervision: Promises and challenges. In T. Rousmaniere & E. Renfro-Michel (Eds.), *Using technology to enhance clinical supervision* (pp. 3–18). Alexandria, VA: American Counseling Association.

Richards, D. (2013). Developments in technology-delivered psychological interventions. *Universitas Psychologica, 12*(2), 571–579.

Ridley, C. R. (2005). *Overcoming unintentional racism in counseling and therapy: A practitioner's guide to intentional intervention* (2nd ed.). Thousand Oaks, CA: Sage.

Riemersma, M. (2007). Use a "no secrets" policy in couple and family therapy—An interview with Richard S. Leslie. *The Therapist, 19*(5), 32–35.

Riggar, T. F. (2016). Counselor burnout. In I. Marini & M. A. Stebnicki (Eds.), *The professional counselor's desk reference* (2nd ed., pp. 555–558). New York, NY: Springer.

Riva, M. T. (2010). Supervision of group counseling. In R. K. Conyne (Ed.), *The Oxford handbook of group counseling* (pp. 370–382). New York, NY: Oxford University Press.

Riva, M. T. (2014). Supervision of group leaders. In J. DeLucia-Waack, C. R. Kalodner, & M. T. Riva (Eds.), *Handbook of group counseling and psychotherapy* (2nd ed., pp. 146–158). Thousand Oaks, CA: Sage.

Rivas-Vasquez, R. A., Blais, M. A., Rey, G. J., & Rivas-Vazquez, A. A. (2001). A brief reminder about documenting the psychological consultation. *Professional Psychology: Research and Practice, 32*(2), 194–199.

Robertson, L. A., & Young, M. E. (2011). The revised ASERVIC spirituality competencies. In C. S. Cashwell & J. S. Young (Eds.), *Integrating spirituality and religion into counseling: A guide to competent practice* (2nd ed., pp. 25–42). Alexandria, VA: American Counseling Association.

Rogers, C. (1961). *On becoming a person.* Boston, MA: Houghton Mifflin.

Rogers, S. (2014). The moving psychoanalytic frame: Ethical challenges for community practitioners.

International Journal of Applied Psychoanalytic Studies, 11(2), 151–162.

Ronnestad, M. H., Orlinsky, D. E., & Wiseman, H. (2016). Professional development and personal therapy. In J. Norcross, G. R. VandenBos, & D. K. Freedheim (Eds.), *APA handbook of clinical psychology* (vol. 5, pp. 223–235). Washington, DC: American Psychological Association.

Rosenberg, J. I. (1999). Suicide prevention: An integrated training model using affective and action-based interventions. *Professional Psychology: Research and Practice, 30*(1), 83–87.

Rosenfeld, G. W. (2011). Contributions from ethics and research that guide integrating religion into psychotherapy. *Professional Psychology: Research and Practice, 42*(2), 192–199.

Rousmaniere, T., Abbass, A., & Frederickson, J. (2014). New developments in technology-assisted supervision and training: A practical overview. *Journal of Clinical Psychology, 70*(11), 1082–1093.

*Rousmaniere, T., & Renfro-Michel, E. (Eds.). (2016). *Using technology to enhance clinical supervision.* Alexandria, VA: American Counseling Association.

Rousmaniere, T., Renfro-Michel, E., & Huggins, R. (2016). Regulatory and legal issues related to the use of technology in clinical supervision. In T. Rousmaniere & E. Renfro-Michel (Eds.), *Using technology to enhance clinical supervision* (pp. 19–30). Alexandria, VA: American Counseling Association.

Rudow, H. (2012, June 28). Judge throws out counseling student's suit against Augusta State. Counseling Today, Online Exclusives. Retrieved from https://ct.counseling.org/2012/06/judge-throws-out-counseling-students-suit-against-augusta-state/.

Rummell, C. M., & Joyce, N. R. (2010). "So wat do u want to wrk on 2day?" The ethical implications of online counseling. *Ethics & Behavior, 20*(6), 482–496.

Rupert, P. A., Miller, A. O., & Dorociak, K. E. (2015). Preventing burnout: What does the research tell us? *Professional Psychology: Research and Practice, 46*(3), 168–174.

Rupert, P. A., Stevanovic, P., & Hunley, H. A. (2009). Work-family conflict among practicing psychologists. *Professional Psychology: Research and Practice, 40*(1), 54–61.

Russell-Chapin, L. A, & Chapin, T. J. (2012). *Clinical supervision: Theory and practice.* Belmont, CA: Brooks/Cole, Cengage Learning.

Safran, J. D., & Kriss, A. (2014). Psychoanalytic psychotherapies. In D. Wedding & R. J. Corsini (Eds.), *Current psychotherapies* (10th ed., pp. 19–54). Belmont, CA: Brooks/Cole, Cengage Learning.

Sahker, E. (2016). Therapy with the nonreligious: Ethical and clinical considerations. *Professional Psychology: Research and Practice, 47*(4), 295–302.

Schank, J. A., Helbok, C. M., Haldeman, D. C., & Gallardo, M. E. (2010). Challenges and benefits of ethical small-community practice. *Professional Psychology: Research and Practice, 41*(6), 502–510.

*Schank J. A., & Skovholt, T. M. (2006). *Ethical practice in small communities: Challenges and rewards for psychologists.* Washington, DC: American Psychological Association.

Scher, S., & Kozlowska, K. (2012). Thinking, doing, and the ethics of family therapy. *American Journal of Family Therapy, 40*(2), 97–114.

Sells, J. N., & Hagedorn, W. B. (2016). CACREP accreditation, ethics, and the affirmation of both religious and sexual identities: A response to Smith and Okech. *Journal of Counseling & Development, 94*(3), 265–279.

Shafranske, E. P. (2016). Finding a place for spirituality in psychology training: Use of competency-based clinical supervision. *Spirituality in Clinical Practice, 3*(1), 18–21.

Shafranske, E. P., & Falender, C. A. (2016). Clinical supervision. In J. Norcross, G. R. VandenBos, & D. K. Freedheim (Eds.), *APA handbook of clinical psychology* (vol. 5, pp. 175–196). Washington, DC: American Psychological Association.

Shah, S., & Rodolfa, E. (2016). Peer supervision and support. In J. Norcross, G. R. VandenBos, & D. K. Freedheim (Eds.), *APA handbook of clinical psychology* (vol. 5, pp. 197–208). Washington, DC: American Psychological Association.

Shavit, N., & Bucky, S. (2004). Sexual contact between psychologists and their former therapy patients: Psychoanalytic perspectives and professional implications. *The American Journal of Psychoanalysis, 64*(3), 229–248.

Shaw, E. (2015). Ethical practice in couple and family therapy: Negotiating rocky terrain. *Australian & New Zealand Journal of Family Therapy, 36,* 504–517.

*Shaw, H. E., & Shaw, S. F. (2006). Critical ethical issues in online counseling: Assessing current practices with an ethical intent checklist. *Journal of Counseling and Development, 84*(1), 41–53.

Shiles, M. (2009). Discriminatory referrals: Uncovering a potential ethical dilemma facing practitioners. *Ethics & Behavior, 19*(2), 142–155.

Shumaker, D., Ortiz, C., & Brenninkmeyer, L. (2011). Revisiting experiential group training in counselor education: A survey of master's-level programs. *Journal for Specialists in Group Work, 36*(2), 111–128.

Shuman, D. W., & Foote, W. (1999). *Jaffee v. Redmond*'s impact: Life after the Supreme Court's recognition of a psychotherapist-patient privilege. *Professional Psychology: Research and Practice, 30*(5), 479–487.

Sisti, D., Young, M., & Caplan, A. (2013). Defining mental illness: Can values and objectivity get along? *BMC Psychiatry, 13*(346), 1–4.

*Skovholt, T. M. (2012). *Becoming a therapist: On the path to mastery.* Hoboken, NJ: Wiley.

*Skovholt, T. M., & Trotter-Mathison, M. (2016). *The resilient practitioner: Burnout and compassion fatigue prevention and self-care strategies for the helping professions* (3rd ed.). New York, NY: Routledge.

Smart, J. (2016). Counseling individuals with disabilities. In I. Marini & M. A. Stebnicki (Eds.), *The professional counselor's desk reference* (2nd ed., pp. 417–421). New York, NY: Springer.

Smith, J. K. (2011). Setting boundaries: Finding a balance. *The Therapist, 23*(6), 63–65.

Smith, L. C., & Okech, J. E. A. (2016a). Ethical issues raised by CACREP accreditation of programs within institutions that disaffirm or disallow diverse sexual orientations. *Journal of Counseling & Development, 94*(3), 252–264.

Smith, L. C., & Okech, J. E. A. (2016b). Negotiating CACREP accreditation practices, religious diversity, and sexual orientation diversity: A rejoinder to Sells and Hagedorn. *Journal of Counseling & Development, 94*(3), 280–284.

Smith, P. L., & Moss, S. B. (2009). Psychologist impairment: Where is it, how can it be prevented, and what can be done to address it? *Clinical Psychology: Science and Practice, 16,* 1–15.

Smith-Augustine, S. (2011, April). School counselors' comfort and competence with spirituality issues. *Counseling and Values, 55,* 149–156.

Smokowski, P. R., Rose, S. D., & Bacallao, M. L. (2001). Damaging experiences in therapeutic groups: How vulnerable consumers become group casualties. *Small Group Research, 32*(2), 223–251.

Sofronoff, K., Helmes, E., & Pachana, N. (2011). Fitness to practice in the profession of psychology: Should we assess this during clinical training? *Australian Psychologist, 46,* 126–132.

Sommers-Flanagan, J., & Sommers-Flanagan, R. (1995). Intake interviewing with suicidal patients: A systematic approach. *Professional Psychology: Research and Practice, 26*(1), 41–47.

Speight, S. L. (2012). An exploration of boundaries and solidarity in counseling relationships. *The Counseling Psychologist, 40*(1), 133–157.

Sperry, L., & Pies, R. (2010, April). Writing about clients: Ethical considerations and options. *Counseling and Values, 54,* 88–102.

Spotts-De Lazzer, A. (2012). Facebook for therapists: Friend or unfriend? *The Therapist, 24*(5), 19–23.

*Stebnicki, M. A. (2008). *Empathy fatigue: Healing the mind, body, and spirit of professional counselors.* New York, NY: Springer.

Stebnicki, M. A. (2016). Military counseling. In I. Marini & M. A. Stebnicki (Eds.), *The professional* counselor's desk reference (2nd ed., pp. 499–506). New York, NY: Springer.

Steele, J. M. (2008). Preparing counselors to advocate for social justice: A liberation model. *Counselor Education and Supervision, 48*(2), 74–85.

Steele, T. M., Jacokes, D. E., & Stone, C. B. (2014/2015). An examination of the role of online technology in school counseling. *Professional School Counseling, 18*(1), 125–135.

Stevanovic, P., & Rupert, P. A. (2009). Work-family spillover and life satisfaction among professional psychologists. *Professional Psychology: Research and Practice, 40*(1), 62–68.

Stone, C. B., & Dahir, C. A. (2016). *The transformed school counselor* (3rd ed.). Boston, MA: Cengage Learning.

Sude, M. E. (2013). Text messaging and private practice: Ethical challenges and guidelines for developing personal best practices. *Journal of Mental Health Counseling, 35*(3), 211–227.

Sue, D. W. (2005). Racism and the conspiracy of silence: Presidential address. *The Counseling Psychologist, 33*(1), 100–114.

Sue, D. W., Arredondo, P., & McDavis, R. J. (1992). Multicultural counseling competencies and standards: A call to the profession. *Journal of Counseling and Development, 70*(4), 477–486.

Sue, D. W., Bernier, J. E., Durran, A., Feinberg, L., Pedersen, P., Smith, E. J., & Nuttall, E. V. (1982). Position paper: Cross-cultural counseling competencies. *The Counseling Psychologist, 10*(2), 45–52.

*Sue, D. W., Carter, R. T., and colleagues. (1998). *Multicultural counseling competencies: Individual and organizational development.* Thousand Oaks, CA: Sage.

Sue, D. W., & Capodilupo, C. M. (2015). Multicultural and community perspectives on multiple relationships. In B. Herlihy & G. Corey (Eds.), *Boundary issues in counseling: Multiple roles and responsibilities* (3rd ed., pp. 92–95). Alexandria, VA: American Counseling Association.

Sue, D. W., Capodilupo, C. M., Nadal, K. L., & Torino, G. C. (2008, May/June). Racial microaggressions and the power to define reality. *American Psychologist, 63*, 277–279.

Sue, D. W., Capodilupo, C. M., Torino, G. C., Bucceri, J. M., Holder, A. M. B., Nadal, K. L., & Esquilin, M. (2007). Racial microaggressions in everyday life: Implications for clinical practice. *American Psychologist, 62*(4), 271–286.

*Sue, D. W., & Sue, D. (2013). *Counseling the culturally diverse: Theory and practice* (6th ed.). New York, NY: Wiley.

Swank, J. M., & Tyson, L. (2012). School counseling site supervisor training: A web-based approach. *Professional School Counseling, 16*(1), 40–47.

Sweeney, T. J. (1995). Accreditation, credentialing, professionalization: The role of specialties. *Journal of Counseling and Development, 74*(2), 117–125.

Swift, J. K., Greenberg, R. P., Whipple, J. L., & Kominiak, N. (2012). Practice recommendations for reducing premature termination in therapy. *Professional Psychology: Research and Practice, 43*(4), 379–387.

Tarasoff v. Board of Regents of the University of California, 17 Cal. 3d 425, 551 (1976).

Tarvydas, V., Addy, A., & Fleming, A. (2010). Reconciling evidence-based research practice with rehabilitation philosophy, ethics and practice: From dichotomy to dialectic. *Rehabilitation Education, 24*(3&4), 191–204.

Tarvydas, V. M., Hartley, M. T., & Gerald, M. (2016). What practitioners need to know about professional credentialing. In I. Marini & M. A. Stebnicki (Eds.), *The professional counselor's desk reference* (2nd ed., pp. 17–22). New York, NY: Springer.

Thapar, v. Zezulka, 994 S. W. 2d 635 (Tex. 1999).

Taylor, J. M., & Neimeyer, G. J. (2015). The assessment of lifelong learning in psychologists. *Professional Psychology: Research and Practice, 46*(6), 385–390.

Taylor, J. M., & Neimeyer, G. J. (2016). Continuing education and lifelong learning. In J. Norcross, G. R. VandenBos, & D. K. Freedheim (Eds.), *APA handbook of clinical psychology* (vol. 5, pp. 135–152). Washington, DC: American Psychological Association.

Thériault, A., & Gazzola, N. (2005). Feelings of inadequacy, insecurity, and incompetence among experienced therapists. *Counselling & Psychotherapy Research, 5*(1), 11–18.

Thomas, J. L. (2002). Bartering. In A. A. Lazarus & O. Zur (Eds.), *Dual relationships and psychotherapy* (pp. 394–408). New York, NY: Springer.

Toporek, R. L., Lewis, J., & Crethar, H. C. (2009). Promoting systemic change through the ACA advocacy competencies. *Journal of Counseling and Development, 87*(3), 260–269.

Toporek, R. L., Lewis, J. A., & Ratts, M. J. (2010). The ACA advocacy competencies: An overview. In M. J. Ratts, R. L. Toporek, & J. A. Lewis (Eds.), *ACA advocacy competencies: A social justice framework for counselors* (pp. 11–20). Alexandria, VA: American Counseling Association.

Tran-Lien, A. (2012). E-mailing your client: Legal and ethical implications. *The Therapist, 24*(3), 20–22.

Van Brunt, B. (2015). *Harm to others: The assessment and treatment of dangerousness.* Alexandria, VA: American Counseling Association.

Vacha-Haase, T., Davenport, D. S., & Kerewsky, S. D. (2004). Problematic students: Gatekeeping practices of academic professional psychology programs. *Professional Psychology: Research and Practice, 35*(2), 115–122.

VandeCreek, L., & Knapp, S. (2001). *Tarasoff and beyond: Legal and clinical considerations in the treatment of life-endangering patients* (3rd ed.). Sarasota, FL: Professional Resource Press.

Vanheule, S., & Devisch, I. (2014). Mental suffering and the *DSM-5*: A critical review. *Journal of Evaluation in Clinical Practice, 20*, 975–980.

Victor, S. E., Styer, D., & Washburn, J. J. (2015). Characteristics of nonsuicidal self-injury associated with suicidal ideation: Evidence from a clinical sample of youth. *Child & Adolescent Psychiatry & Mental Health, 9*(1), 1–8.

Vilardaga, R., Luoma, J. B., Hayes, S. C., Pistorello, J., Levin, M. E., Hildebrandt, M. J., . . . & Bond, F. (2011). Burnout among the addiction counseling workforce: The differential roles of mindfulness and values-based processes and work-site factors. *Journal of Substance Abuse Treatment, 40*, 323–335.

Vismara, L. A., Young, G. S., Stahmer, A. C., Griffith, E. M., & Rogers, S. J. (2009). Dissemination of evidence-based practice: Can we train therapists from a distance? *Journal of Autism and Developmental Disorders, 39*, 1636–1651.

Walden, S. L. (2015). Inclusion of the client's voice in ethical practice. In B. Herlihy & G. Corey (Eds.), *Boundary issues in counseling: Multiple roles and responsibilities* (3rd ed., pp. 59–62). Alexandria, VA: American Counseling Association.

Walfish, S., Barnett, J. E., Marlyere, K., & Zielke, R. (2010). "Doc, there's something I have to tell you": Patient disclosure to their psychotherapist of unprosecuted murder and other violence. *Ethics & Behavior, 20*(5), 311–323.

Walker, D. F., Gorsuch, R. L., & Tan, S. Y. (2004). Therapists' integration of religion and spirituality in counseling: A meta-analysis. *Counseling and Values, 49*(1), 69–80.

Waller, B. (2013). Real-life social action in the community. In J. A. Kottler, M. Englar-Carlson, & J. Carlson (Eds.), *Helping beyond the 50-minute hour: Therapists involved in meaningful social action* (pp. 86–95). New York, NY: Routledge, Taylor & Francis.

Walsh, B., & Muehlenkamp, J. J. (2013). Managing non-suicidal self-injury in schools: Use of a structured protocol to manage the behavior and prevent social contagion. *School Psychology Forum, 7*(4), 161–171.

Walsh, R. (2011). Lifestyle and mental health. *American Psychologist, 66*, 579–592.

Ward v. Wilbanks, Case No. 09-CV-11237 (E.D. Mich. July 26, 2010).

Watkins, C. E. (1985). Countertransference: Its impact on the counseling situation. *Journal of Counseling and Development, 63*(6), 356–359.

Weiss, A. C., & Rutan, J. S. (2016). The benefits of group therapy observation for therapists-in-training. *International Journal of Group Psychotherapy, 66*(2), 246–260.

Welfel, E. R. (2005). Accepting fallibility: A model for personal responsibility for nonegregious ethics infractions. *Counseling and Values, 49*(2), 120–131.

*Welfel, E. R. (2009). Emerging issues in the duty to protect. In J. L. Werth Jr., E. R. Welfel, & G. A. H. Benjamin (Eds.), *The duty to protect: Ethical, legal, and professional considerations for mental health professionals* (pp. 229–248). Washington, DC: American Psychological Association.

*Welfel, E. R. (2016). *Ethics in counseling and psychotherapy: Standards, research, and emerging issues* (6th ed.).Boston, MA: Cengage Learning.

*Welfel, E. R., Werth, J. L., Jr., & Benjamin, G. A. H. (2009). Introduction to the duty to protect. In J. L. Werth Jr., E. R. Welfel, & G. A. H. Benjamin (Eds.), *The duty to protect: Ethical, legal, and professional considerations for mental health professionals* (pp. 3–8). Washington, DC: American Psychological Association.

Werth, J. L., Jr. (Ed.). (2013a). *Counseling clients near the end of life: A practical guide for mental health professionals.* New York, NY: Springer.

Werth, J. L., Jr. (2013b). Counseling clients who are near the end of life. In J. L. Werth Jr. (Ed.), *Counseling clients near the end of life: A practical guide for mental health professionals* (pp. 101–120). New York, NY: Springer.

*Werth, J. L., Jr., & Blevins, D. (Eds.). (2006). *Psychosocial issues near the end of life: A resource for professional care providers.* Washington, DC: American Psychological Association.

Werth, J. L., Jr., & Crow, L. (2009). End-of-life care: An overview for professional counselors. *Journal of Counseling and Development, 87*(2), 194–202.

*Werth, J. L., Jr., & Holdwick, D. J. (2000). A primer on rational suicide and other forms of hastened death. *The Counseling Psychologist, 28*(4), 511–539.

Werth, J. L., Jr., & Kleespies, P. M. (2006). Ethical considerations in providing psychological services in end-of-life-care. In J. L. Werth Jr. & D. Blevins (Eds.), *Psychosocial issues near the end of life: A resource for professional care providers* (pp. 57–87). Washington, DC: American Psychological Association.

*Werth, J. L., Jr., & Richmond, J. (2009). End-of-life decisions and the duty to protect. In J. L. Werth Jr., E. R. Welfel, & G. A. H. Benjamin (Eds.), *The duty to protect: Ethical, legal, and professional considerations for mental health professionals* (pp. 195–208). Washington, DC: American Psychological Association.

*Werth, J. L., Jr., Welfel, E. R., & Benjamin, G. A. H. (Eds.). (2009). *The duty to protect: Ethical, legal, and professional considerations for mental health professionals.* Washington, DC: American Psychological Association.

Werth, J. L., Jr., Welfel, E. R., Benjamin, G. A. H., & Sales, B. D. (Eds.). (2009). Practice and policy responses to the duty to protect. In J. L. Werth Jr., E. R. Welfel, & G. A. H. Benjamin (Eds.), *The duty to protect: Ethical, legal, and professional considerations for mental health professionals* (pp. 249–261). Washington, DC: American Psychological Association.

Westefeld, J. S. (2009). Supervision in psychotherapy: Models, issues, and recommendations. *The Counseling Psychologist, 37*(2), 296–316.

Wester, K. L. (2009). Ethical issues in counseling clients who self-injure. *Ethical Issues in Professional Counseling, 12*(3), 25–37. [Published by the Hatherleigh Company, Hobart, New York]

Wester, K. L., Ivers, N., Villalba, J. A., Trepal, H. C., & Henson, R. (2016). The relationship between nonsuicidal self-injury and suicidal ideation. *Journal of Counseling & Development, 94*(1), 3–12. doi:10.1002/jcad.12057

*Wheeler, A. M., & Bertram, B. (2015). *The counselor and the law: A guide to legal and ethical practice* (7th ed.). Alexandria, VA: American Counseling Association.

Wheeler, A. M., & Reinhardt. R. (2014). *Private practice preparedness: The health care professional's guide to closing a practice due to retirement, death or disability.* Retrieved from http://www.private-practicepreparedness.com

Whisenhunt, J. L., Stargell, N., & Perjessy, C. (2016). Addressing ethical issues in treating client self-injury. *Counseling Today, 59*(2), 40–46.

Whitlock, J., Muehlenkamp, J., Eckenrode, J., Purington, A., Baral Abrams, G., Barreira, P., & Kress, V. (2013). Nonsuicidal self-injury as a gateway to suicide in young adults. *Journal of Adolescent Health, 52*, 486–492. doi:10.1016/j.jadohealth.2012.09.010

Whitlock, J., Prussien, K., & Pietrusza, C. (2015, August). Predictors of self-injury cessation and subsequent psychological growth: Results of a probability sample survey of students in eight universities and colleges. *Child and Adolescent Psychiatry and Mental Health.* doi:10.1186/s13034-015-0048-5

Widgery, A., & Winterfeld, A. (2013). Warning of potential violence. *State Legislatures, 39*(3), 7.

Wierzbicki, M., Siderits, M. A., & Kuchan, A. M. (2012). Ethical questions addressed by a state psychological association. *Professional Psychology: Research and Practice, 43*(2), 80–85.

Wilcoxon, S. A. (2015). Technology and client care: Therapy considerations in a digital society. *Australian & New Zealand Journal of Family Therapy, 36*, 480–491.

*Wilcoxon, S. A., Remley, T. P., & Gladding, S. T. (2012). *Ethical, legal, and professional issues in the practice of marriage and family therapy* (5th ed.) Upper Saddle River, NJ: Merrill/ Prentice-Hall (Pearson).

Wilkerson, K. (2006). Impaired students: Applying the therapeutic process model to graduate training programs. *Counselor Education and Supervision, 45*(3), 207–217.

Wilson, R. E., Gosling, S. D., & Graham, L. T. (2012). A review of Facebook research in the social sciences. *Perspectives on Psychological Science, 7*(3), 203–220.

Wise, E. H., & Barnett, J. E. (2016). Self-care for psychologists. In J. Norcross, G. R. VandenBos, & D. K. Freedheim (Eds.), *APA handbook of clinical psychology* (vol. 5, pp. 209–222). Washington, DC: American Psychological Association.

Wise, E. H., Bieschke, K. L., Forrest, L., Cohen-Filipic, J., Hathaway, W. L., & Douce, L. A. (2015). Psychology's proactive approach to conscience clause court cases and legislation. *Training and Education in Professional Psychology, 9*, 259–268.

Wise, E. H., Hersh, M. A., & Gibson, C. M. (2011). Ethics and self-care: A developmental lifespan perspective. *Register Report, 37*, 20–29.

Wise, E. H., Hersh, M. A., & Gibson, C. M. (2012). Ethics, self-care and well-being for psychologists: Re-envisioning the stress-distress continuum. *Professional Psychology: Research and Practice, 43*(5), 487–494.

Wise, E. H., Sturm, C. A., Nutt, R. L., Rodolfa, E., Schaffer, J. B., & Webb, C. (2010). Life-long learning for psychologists: Current status and a vision for the future. *Professional Psychology: Research and Practice, 41*(4), 288–297.

Wolitzsky, D. L. (2011). Psychoanalytic theories in psychotherapy. In J. C. Norcross, G. R. Vandenbos, & D. K. Freedheim (Eds.), *History of psychotherapy* (2nd ed., pp. 65–100). Washington, DC: American Psychological Association.

Wood, C., & Rayle, A. D. (2006). A model of school counseling supervision: The Goals, Functions, Roles, and Systems Model. *Counselor Education & Supervision, 45*, 253–266.

*Woody, R. H. (1998). Bartering for psychological services. *Professional Psychology: Research and Practice, 29*(2), 174–178.

Worthington, E. L., Jr. (2011). Integration of spirituality and religion into psychotherapy. In J. C. Norcross, G. R. Vandenbos, & D. K. Freedheim (Eds.), *History of psychotherapy* (2nd ed., pp. 533–544). Washington, DC: American Psychological Association.

Wrenn, C. G. (1962). The culturally encapsulated counselor. *Harvard Educational Review, 32*, 444–449.

Wrenn, C. G. (1985). Afterword: The culturally encapsulated counselor revisited. In P. Pedersen (Ed.), *Handbook of cross-cultural counseling and therapy* (pp. 323–329). Westport, CT: Greenwood Press.

Wright, B. A. (1983). *Physical disability: A psychosocial approach* (2nd ed.). New York, NY: Harper & Row.

Wyke v. Polk County School Board, 129 F. 3d 560 (11th Cir. 1997).

*Yalom, I. D. (1997). *Lying on the couch: A novel.* New York, NY: Perennial.

*Yalom, I. D. (2003). *The gift of therapy.* New York, NY: Perennial.

*Yalom, I., with Leszcz, M. (2005). *The theory and practice of group psychotherapy* (5th ed.). New York, NY: Basic Books.

Yep, R. (2016). A dangerous precedent. *Counseling Today, 58*(11), 7.

Young, J. S., Wiggins-Frame, M., & Cashwell, C. S. (2007). Spirituality and counselor competence: A national survey of American Counseling Association members. *Journal of Counseling and Development, 85*(1), 47–52.

Young, T. L. (2010). Sexuality, boundaries, and ethics. In L. Hecker (Ed.), *Ethics and professional issues in couple and family therapy* (pp. 89–106). New York, NY: Routledge.

Younggren, J. N., Fisher, M. A., Foote, W. E., & Hjelt, S. E. (2011). A legal and ethical review of patient responsibilities and psychotherapist duties. *Professional Psychology: Research and Practice, 42*(2), 160–168.

*Younggren, J. N., & Gottlieb, M. C. (2004). Managing risk when contemplating multiple relationships. *Professional Psychology: Research and Practice, 35*(3), 255–260.

*Younggren, J. N., & Gottlieb, M. C. (2008). Termination and abandonment: History, risk, and risk management. *Professional Psychology: Research and Practice, 39*(5), 498–504.

Younggren, J. N., Harris, E. A., & Martin, J. N. (2016). Malpractice and risk management. In J. Norcross, G. R. VandenBos, & D. K. Freedheim (Eds.), *APA handbook of clinical psychology* (vol. 5, pp. 395–408). Washington, DC: American Psychological Association.

Zalaquett, C. P., Fuerth, K. M., Stein, C., Ivey, A. E., & Ivey, M. B. (2008). Reframing the *DSM-IV-TR* from a multicultural/social justice perspective. *Journal of Counseling and Development, 86*(3), 364–371.

Zeranski, L., & Halgin, R. P. (2011). Ethical issues in elder abuse reporting: A professional psychologist's guide. *Professional Psychology: Research and Practice, 42*(4), 294–300.

*Zur, O. (2007). *Boundaries in psychotherapy: Ethical and clinical explorations.* Washington, DC: American Psychological Association.

*Zur, O. (2008). *Beyond the office walls: Home visits, celebrations, adventure therapy, incidental encounters and other encounters outside the office walls.* Retrieved from www.zurinstitute.com/outofoffice-experiences.html

*Zur, O. (2009). *Self-disclosure and transparency in psychotherapy and counseling.* Retrieved from www.zurinstitute.com/selfdisclosure1.html

Zur, O. (2010). *The risky business of risk management.* Retrieved from www.zurinstitute.com/riskmanagement.html

Zur, O. (2011a). *Bartering in psychotherapy and counseling: Complexities, case studies and guidelines.* Retrieved from www.zurinstitute.com/bartertherapy.html

Zur, O. (2011b). *Gifts in psychotherapy.* Retrieved from www.zurinstitute.com/giftsintherapy.html

Zur, O. (2011c). *Therapist burnout: Facts, causes and prevention.* Retrieved from www.zurinstitute.com/therapeutic_ethics.pdf

Zur, O. (2016). *Telemental health services across state lines.* Retrieved from http://www.zurinstitute.com/telehealth_across_state_lines_zur.html

Zur, O. (Ed.). (2017). *Multiple relationships in psychotherapy and counseling: Unavoidable, common, and mandatory dual relations in therapy.* New York, NY: Routledge.

*Zur, O., & Nordmarken, N. (2009). *To touch or not to touch: Exploring the myth of prohibition on touch in psychotherapy and counseling.* Retrieved from www.zurinstitute.com/touchintherapy.html

Zur, O., & Zur, A. (2011). The Facebook dilemma: To accept or not to accept? Responding to clients' "friend requests" on psychotherapists' social networking sites. *Independent Practitioner, 31*(1), 12–17.

Name Index

Abbass, A., 347–348
Abbott, M., 448
Abraham, A., 389
Adamson, N., 164
Addy, A., 389
Affleck, W., 352
Aguirre, M., 80
Anderson, K., 320
American Association for
   Marriage and Family Ther-
   apy (AAMFT), 33, 62, 76, 123,
   151, 176, 207, 257, 272, 276,
   278, 287–288, 293, 304, 328,
   352–353, 355, 398–401, 405, 417
American Counseling
   Association (ACA), 9, 12,
   15–19, 33–34, 62, 70, 73–74,
   79, 97, 114, 123, 127, 151,
   173, 176, 184, 206, 256, 258,
   272, 276, 278, 287–288, 292,
   304, 314, 320, 328, 340, 354,
   360–361, 385, 417, 426, 430,
   434, 464
American Group Psychotherapy
   Association (AGPA), 33, 442
American Mental Health
   Counselors Association
   (AMHCA), 33, 97, 114, 123,
   151, 165, 170, 175, 207, 257,
   273, 276, 278, 288, 293, 304,
   328, 337, 352, 355, 360, 385,
   438, 456, 461
American Music Therapy
   Association (AMTA), 34
American Psychiatric
   Association, 33, 122, 185, 206,
   224, 288, 304, 328, 355, 373,
   377
American Psychological
   Association (APA), 5, 15–16,
   33, 62, 112, 123, 150, 168,
   170–172, 175, 184, 191, 207,
   212, 226, 256, 258, 272, 276,
   287–289, 292, 304, 314, 320,
   337, 340–342, 347, 349, 355,
   361–362, 385
American Psychological
   Association Presidential Task
   Force, 389, 391

American Psychological
   Association Presidential Task
   Force on Evidence-based
   Practice, 391, 447
American School Counselor
   Association (ASCA), 33, 73,
   114, 173, 185, 207, 212–213,
   216, 258, 273, 276, 304, 328,
   442, 457
Amundson, N., 428
Ancis, J., 342, 350–351
Angus, L., 372, 389, 393
Anthony, K., 313
Antony, M., 389
Arensman, E., 186
Arnold, R., 354
Arredondo, P., 138, 429
Association for Counselor
   Education and Supervision
   (ACES), 337–342, 349–350, 352
Association for Lesbian, Gay,
   Bisexual, and Transgender
   Issues in Counseling
   (ALGBTIC), 124–125
Association for Multicultural
   Counseling and Development
   (AMCD), 112, 138, 430, 449
Association for Specialists in
   Group Work (ASGW), 33,
   424, 426, 428, 430, 440, 449
Association for Spiritual,
   Ethical, and Religious Values
   in Counseling (ASERVIC),
   89, 93
Atkinson, D., 465
Austin, J. A., 353, 358, 425
Austin, J. T., 353, 358, 425
Austin, K., 240–241

Baca, J., 9, 18, 71, 251
Bacallao, M., 439
Baker, S., 347
Bakken, G., 229–230
Balkin, R., 372
Barlow, S., 424
Barnett, J., 8, 13, 18–19, 34,
   42, 45–46, 58, 60, 63, 88–90,
   92, 116, 119, 138, 152, 154,
   182, 189, 191, 210, 216, 228,

241, 246, 48, 251, 260–262,
   267–268, 273–274, 303,
   305–306, 311, 329, 339,
   341–342, 349–350, 353, 386,
   434, 462
Barney, L., 175
Barros-Bailey, M., 220, 347
Battle, C., 428
Baxter v. State of Montana, 94
Bebeau, M., 305
Beck, A., 389
Becker-Fischer, M., 290–291
Bednar, R., 241
Bednar, S., 241
Beecher, M., 448
Behnke, S., 78
Belt, T., 131
Bemak, F., 114–115, 142–143,
   427, 429, 453, 455, 460,
   462–464, 472, 474, 476
Benitez, B., 185, 244, 418
Benjamin, G., 199–200, 225
Bennett, B., 169, 194, 200, 241,
   245, 251
Berman, J., 8
Bernard, J., 324, 340, 342,
   345–346
Bernier, J., 138
Bernstein, J., 320
Bersoff, B., 226, 228
Bertram, B., 13, 18, 22–23,
   152–154, 166, 170, 192–194,
   196–197, 207, 211, 216,
   223–224, 226, 231, 238,
   240–241, 251, 434, 440, 443
Beutler, L., 390–391, 448
Bevacqua, F., 94, 96
Bevins, M., 96
Bhatia, M., 352
Bieschke, K., 69, 79–80
Birdsall, B., 173
Birrell, P., 8, 20
Bisono, A., 88
Bitter, J., 398, 402–403, 410,
   416, 421
Blais, M., 170
Blashfield, R., 320
Blount, A., 63
Blumenthal-Barby, J., 377

Dattilio, F., 389–390
Davenport, D., 320
Davenport, R., 230
Davis, D., 55
Davis, T., 13, 17, 22–23, 34
Day, J., 13–15
Day-Vines, N., 428
Dearing, R., 44
Debiak, D., 428
Deegar, J., 389
Delaney, H., 88
DeLettre, J., 167
DeMers, S., 226
DeMitchell, T., 70, 73
Devereaux, R., 174
Devisch, I., 377
Dewalt, T., 353
Dickens, K., 94, 353
Diekhoff, G., 194, 198
Diller, J., 108
Dobmeier, R., 88, 93
Doll, B., 306
Dorociak, K., 60–61
Dotson-Blake, K., 428
Douce, L., 69, 79–80, 307
Douglass, M., 428
Driscoll, K., 389
Drogin, E., 168, 172
Drum, K., 162
Duffey, T., 175, 347–348
Dufrene, R., 320
Duggan, J., 186
Dugger, S., 69, 321
Duncan, B., 158, 372, 391, 448
Duncan, R., 185
Duran, E., 107, 114, 116–117, 374
Durran, A., 138
Durodoye, B., 385

Eastern Michigan University, 78
Ebrahim, C., 353
Edwards, J., 389–390
Eichenberg, C., 290–291
Eisel v. Board of Education, 236
Elkins, D., 372, 392–393
Elliott, R., 372, 389, 393
Elman, N., 116, 189, 191, 303,
    305–306, 315–316, 320–321,
    324, 329, 342, 462

Elmore, A., 391
Englar-Carlson, M., 472
Eonta, A., 180
Eriksen, K., 164, 386
Esquilin, M., 135
Evans, R., 186, 236
Everytown for Gun Safety, 231
Ewing v. Goldstein, 229

Facebook Newsroom, 444
Falco, L., 425–426
Falender, C., 336–337, 339,
    341–342, 345, 349–350, 353,
    358
Falicov, C., 349–350
Farnsworth, J., 74–75
Farrell, M., 76
Farry, T., 3, 20, 22
Faust, D., 392
Ferguson, A., 123
Fein, A., 234
Feinberg, L., 138
Fieldsteel, N., 446
Fifield, A., 269–270
Finn, A., 233
Firehammer, J., 107, 114,
    116–117, 374
Fischer, G., 290–291
Fisher, C., 60, 286
Fisher, M., 160, 165, 195, 200,
    208–209, 211, 216, 222, 309,
    402
Flannelly, K., 60
Fleming, A., 389
Foote, W., 160, 168, 172, 195,
    211, 309
Ford, S., 386
Forer, B., 290
Forester-Miller, H., 13, 17,
    22–23, 34, 274
Forrest, L., 69, 79–80, 116, 189,
    191, 303, 305–307, 315–316,
    320–321, 324, 329, 342, 462
Foster, N., 175
Foster, V., 326
Frame, M., 13, 19, 21–23, 90
Francis, P., 9, 18, 69, 71, 78,
    88–90, 97, 251, 321
Freire, E., 389

Frederickson, J., 347–348
Fried, A., 60
Fuentes, M., 385–386
Fuerth, K., 374, 379, 383, 385
Furr, S., 316, 321

Gabbard, G., 261, 264
Galek, K., 60
Gallardo, M., 113, 269–270
Gamino, L., 96
Garcia, J., 20, 321, 324–326
Garner, B., 390
Garrett, M., 108–109
Garvert, D., 454
Gaubatz, M., 321–322
Gazzola, N., 306
Geller, J., 314
Gelso, C., 52
Gerald, M., 327
Gerler, E., 347
Gibbons, M., 372
Gibbs, K., 324
Gibson, C., 18, 45, 63
Gizara, S., 324
Gladding, S., 397, 402–403, 417,
    429
Glasheen, K., 177, 312–313
Glosoff, H., 338, 345, 347
Godley, M., 390
Godley, S., 390
Gold, S., 44
Goldenberg, H., 397–398, 402
Goldenberg, I., 397–398, 402
Golightly, T., 448
Gonzalez, J., 107, 114, 116–117,
    374
Goodnough, G., 9, 18, 71, 251
Goodrich, K., 426
Goodyear, R., 324, 340–342,
    345–346, 349
Gordon, C., 347
Gorsuch, R., 88
Gosling, S., 444
Gottlieb, M., 6, 8, 12–13, 63, 152,
    160, 172, 174, 194, 260, 264,
    285, 304, 309, 398, 404
Graham, L., 444
Granello, D., 238, 241–243
Grasso, I., 9

Greenberg, L., 389
Greenberg, M., 290
Greenberg, R., 195, 200
Greene, P., 60
Greenwood, A., 200, 241
Grenyer, B., 289
Griffith, E., 390
Griner, D., 448
Groschwitz, R., 186
Gross, D., 236
Grossman v. South Shore Public School District, 73
Grothaus, T., 428
Growcock, D., 213–214, 233
Grus, C., 306, 316, 342
Gruszka, C., 58
Guiggrida, D., 63–64
Gunnell, D., 186
Gurman, A., 414–415
Gutheil, T., 261, 264, 295
Guy, J., 49

Haberl, P., 263
Haberstroh, S., 175, 347–348
Hackney, H., 432
Hage, S., 428–429
Hagedorn, W., 70, 80, 88
Hahn, H., 131
Hall, J., 390
Handelsman, M., 6, 8, 12–13, 304
Haldeman, D., 269–270
Halgin, R., 245
Halinski, K., 285
Hancock, K., 69–70, 74
Handelsman, M., 63, 152, 155, 160, 165, 285
Handerscheid, R., 224
Harper, J., 418
Harriger, D., 284–285
Harris, E., 169, 179–181, 192, 194, 199, 202, 245, 251
Harris, S., 83, 284–285
Hartley, M., 261–263, 327
Harway, M., 172, 398, 404
Hastings, S., 268
Hathaway, W., 69, 79–80, 307
Hawking, S., 130
Hawton, K., 186

Hayes, J., 52
Hayes, S., 61
Haynes, R., 336, 339, 343–346
Hays, D., 429
Hays, K., 83
Hazell, P., 186
Heath, N., 186
Hebert, D., 70, 73
Hedlund v. Superior Court, 230
Helbok, C., 269–270
Helmes, E., 315
Helms, J., 143
Henderson, M., 224
Hendricks, B., 222
Henson, R., 186
Herlihy, B., 6–7, 11, 34, 71, 127–128, 163–164, 166, 182, 186, 192, 199, 209, 217, 235, 240–241, 256, 259, 264–266, 320, 327, 336, 353, 381–382, 385, 462
Hermann, M., 9, 18, 71, 127–128, 173, 233, 236, 251, 324
Hersh, M., 18, 45, 63
Hickson, J., 93
Hildebrand, M., 61
Hillard, D., 46, 63
Hilsenroth, M., 44
Hinton, D., 385–386
Hipolito-Delgado, C., 464
Hjelt, S., 160, 195, 309
Hodges, S., 9, 18, 71, 251
Hoffman, R., 164
Hogan, M., 117, 460
Hogan, T., 388–389, 391, 447
Hogan-Garcia, M., 468
Hohenshil, T., 428
Holder, A., 135
Holdwick, D., 95
Hollon, S., 389
Holman, A., 428
Holmes, C., 443–444
Holroyd, J., 283–285, 290
Holstein, J., 80
Homan, M., 454, 458, 467–470
Hourigan, S., 180
Housley, W., 93
Hubble, M., 158, 372, 391, 448
Hubert, M., 173

Hulse-Killacky, D., 324
Hummel, A., 52
Hunley, H., 61
Huprich, S., 306, 316, 342
Hurrell, C., 186, 236
Hutchins, A., 464

Ingram, C., 221
International Association of Marriage and Family Counselors, 417
Isaacson, N., 234
Ivers, N., 186
Ivey, A., 115, 122, 138, 374, 379, 383, 385
Ivey, M., 115, 122, 138, 374, 379, 383, 385

Jablonski v. United States, 229
Jackson, J., 129
Jacobs, S., 306, 316, 342
Jacokes, D., 312–313
Jadaszewski, S., 73
Jaffee v. Redmond, 210
Jensen, D., 216, 223–224, 227, 229, 448
Jobes, D., 235
Johnson, B., 70
Johnson, J., 113, 326
Johnson, R., 88–89, 91
Johnson, S., 9, 259, 261
Johnson, W., 8–9, 13, 19, 34, 88–90, 92, 116, 119, 138, 154, 182, 189, 191, 210, 216, 228, 241, 246, 248, 251, 259, 260–261, 273–274, 303, 305–306, 311, 320–321, 329, 339, 350, 353, 386, 462
Johnson-Greene, D., 152, 434
Johnston, L., 46, 63
Joiner, T., 389
Jones, H., 142–143
Jones, J., 138
Joyce, N., 176–177, 221

Kadin, S., 172, 398, 404
Kaplan, D., 18, 71, 74–75, 77, 251
Kaslow, N., 116, 189, 191, 305–306, 316, 329, 342, 462

Kazantzis, N., 46
Keenan, K., 372
Keith-Spiegel, P., 13, 190, 273, 283, 286, 293–294
Kemper, T., 389
Kennedy, P., 194, 198
Kenny, M., 155, 173, 245, 316
Kerewsky, S., 320
Kerl, S., 321, 324–326
Kim, J., 428–429
Kintzle, S., 389
Kirkland, K., 194
Kirkland, K. L., 194
Kiselica, M., 259, 298
Kissinger, D., 63
Kitchener, K., 13, 15
Kleespies, P., 98
Kleist, D., 402, 410, 416
Knapp, S., 6, 8–9, 12–13, 15, 34, 63, 152–153, 160, 163, 166, 169, 192–196, 198, 209, 228–229, 240, 245, 251–252, 285, 304
Knowles, A., 185
Knox, S., 353
Kocet, M., 71
Kolmes, K., 177, 181
Kominiak, N., 195, 200
Koocher, G., 13, 190, 273, 286, 293–294, 388–389, 391, 447
Kottler, J., 372, 472
Kozlowski, K., 353, 404, 443–444
Kress, V., 164, 186, 315, 317, 386
Krimsky, S., 377
Kriss, A., 47, 49
Kuchan, A., 193–194
Kudler, T., 60
Kurpius, S., 94, 96, 182, 185

La Roche, M., 385–386
Lambert, M., 241, 370, 372, 390, 392, 447
Lambie, G., 63
Larrabee, M., 354
Lasky, G., 441
Laughran, W., 229–230
Lawrence, G., 182, 185
Lawson, D., 389

Lazarus, A., 260–261, 264, 266, 389–390
Lebow, J., 397, 410, 415
Lee, C., 108–109, 111, 115, 135, 138, 460, 464
Lee, J., 61
Lee, S., 61
Leigh, I., 305
Leino, A., 138
Lerman, H., 290
Leslie, R., 179, 184, 198, 227, 418–419
Letourneau, J., 316, 320–321
Levant, R., 390–391, 448
Levin, M., 61
Levitt, D., 3, 20, 22, 69
Lewis, J., 109, 431, 458–459, 463–464
Lewis, K., 289
Lewis, M., 458–459
Lewis, S., 186
Lichtenberg, J., 305, 341–342, 349
Lim, N., 61
Linde, L., 75, 307
Linnerooth, P., 59
Littleton, H., 162
Livneh, H., 130
Lock, R., 222
Locke, D., 138
Luke, M., 347, 426, 432
Lum, D., 108, 110
Luoma, J., 61
Lustgarten, S., 221, 224

MacKinnon, C., 352
MacLeod, B., 465, 467, 475
MacNair-Semands, R., 429
Macia, K., 454
Maddux, J., 44
Mallen, M., 175
Margolin, G., 411, 414
Markus, H., 108
Marlyere, K., 228
Marquis, A., 63–64
Marshall, D., 342, 350–351
Martin, J., 192, 194, 199, 202
Maslach, C., 60
Maslowski, K., 9

Mason, M., 428–429
Maxwell, M., 321, 324–326
Mazzarella, J., 3, 20, 22
McAdams, C., 326, 347–348
McAuliffe, G., 326
McCarthy, C., 425–426
McCarthy, H., 131
McCloskey, M., 389–390
McCullough, J., 138
McCullough, S., 321, 324–326
McDavis, R., 138
McGee, T., 161
McGeorge, C., 76
McMullen, J., 465, 467, 475
McMurtery, R., 354
Meara, N., 13–15
Mease, L., 186
Meyers, J., 374
Meyers, L., 79
Meyers, R., 390
Michal, N., 186
Michel, R., 326
Miller, A., 60–61
Miller, G., 354
Miller, J., 324
Miller, S., 158, 372, 391, 448
Miller, W., 88
Milliken, T., 279, 284, 293–296
Mintz, L., 79–80
Moles, T., 263, 284
Moleski, S., 259, 298
Moline, M., 240–241
Monk, G., 118
Moore, B., 59
Moorehead-Slaughter, O., 260–261
Moorhead, H., 69, 88
Moss, S., 60
Mossman, D., 225
Moulton, P., 336, 339, 343–346
Moyer, M., 213–214, 233
Mrdjenovich, A., 59
Muehlenkamp, J., 186
Mukherjee, D., 372
Munz, L., 186
Muratori, M., 336, 339, 343–346, 353, 358, 425
Murphy, J., 162

Seymour, J., 461
Shafranske, E., 337, 341–342, 345, 349–351, 358
Shah, S., 330–331
Shavit, N., 293
Shaw, E., 402, 404, 418, 420
Shaw, H., 178
Shaw, S., 178
Shiles, M., 69, 76
Shochet, I., 177, 312–313
Shumaker, D., 43, 426
Shuman, D., 211
Siderits, M., 193–194
Siegel, A., 226
Sims, P., 159
Singh, A., 138
Sisti, D., 377–378
Skovholt, T., 59–60, 62–63
Smart, J., 129
Smith, E., 138
Smith, I., 305
Smith, J., 262, 390
Smith, L., 70, 89
Smith, N., 352
Smith, P., 60
Smith-Augustine, S., 303
Smokowski, P., 439
Sobell, L., 167
Sofronoff, K., 315
Solomon, A., 414–415
Sommers-Flanagan, J., 241
Sommers-Flanagan, R., 241
Sonne, J., 283–285
Southam-Gerow, M., 180
Sparks, J., 448
Speight, S., 263–264
Sperry, L., 212
Spinella, L., 347
Spotts-De Lazzer, A., 444
Spurgeon, S., 9, 18, 71, 251
Stadler, H., 138
Stahmer, A., 390
Stanton, M., 397–398, 402
Stargell, N., 235, 241
Stebnicki, M., 59, 129
Steele, J., 463
Steele, T., 312–313
Stein, C., 374, 379, 383, 385
Stevanovic, P., 60–61

Stone, C., 212, 216, 312–313, 462–464
Stroud, C., 397, 410, 415
Sturm, C., 168, 172
Styer, D., 186
Sude, M., 220
Sue, D., 108–109, 116, 118, 134, 136, 141, 460
Sue, D. W., 108–110, 116, 118, 134–136, 138, 141, 279, 282, 460
Sue, S., 138
Sullivan, J., 213–214, 233
Sunderani, M., 352
Suris, A., 129
Swank, J., 348–349
Sweeney, T., 326, 374
Swift, J., 195, 200

Tabachnick, B., 283
Talleyrand, R., 142–143
Tan, S., 88
Tangney, J., 44
Tanigoshi, H., 324
Tarasoff v. Board of Regents of the University of California, 226
Tarvydas, V., 13, 327, 389
Taylor, J., 329
Thapar v. Zezulka, 225
Thériault, A., 306
Thoman, L., 129
Thomas, L., 274
Thomas, T., 461
Timulak, L., 372, 389, 393
Toporek, R., 109, 138, 429, 431, 459, 463–464
Torino, G., 110, 135
Torres Rivera, E., 374
Tran-Lien, A., 221–222
Trepal, H., 186
Trotter-Mathison, M., 59–60, 62
Tyson, L., 348–349

Vacha-Haase, T., 320, 324
van Heeringen, K., 186
Vandecreek, L., 12–13, 15, 34, 153, 163, 166, 169, 192–196, 198, 209, 228–229, 240, 245, 251–252, 285

Vandehey, M., 194, 198
VandenBos, G., 200, 241
Vanheule, S., 377
Vasquez, M., 5–6, 60, 154, 241, 260–262, 264
Vera, E., 321–322
Victor, S., 186
Vilardaga, R., 61
Villalba, J., 186, 425–426
Vincenzes, K., 369
Vismara, L., 390
Vogel, D., 175
Vrana, S., 180

Wade, A., 391
Wade, M., 9, 18, 71, 251
Wages, D., 93
Waite, D., 41
Walden, S., 19–20
Waldo, M., 58
Walfish, S., 228
Walker, D., 88
Waller, B., 453
Walsh, B., 186
Walsh, R., 63
Wampold, B., 158, 372, 391, 448
Ward, J., 77
Ward, T., 326
Washburn, J., 186
Watkins, C., 49, 263, 284
Watson, J., 372, 389, 393
Watson, Z., 381–382, 462
Webb, T., 354
Weber, R., 331
Wedding, D., 284, 295, 389–390
Weiss, A., 427
Welfel, E., 5–6, 12–13, 22, 166, 176, 184, 199–200, 225, 228, 245, 362
Werth, J., 95, 97–100, 199–200, 225, 268
Westefeld, J., 345, 350
Wester, K., 186
Wheeler, A., 13, 18, 22–23, 152–154, 161, 166, 170, 175, 192–194, 196–197, 207, 211, 216, 223–224, 226, 231, 238, 240–241, 251, 434, 440, 443
Wheeler, E., 377

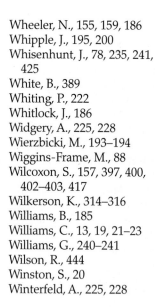

Subject Index

Healthcare, durable power of
attorney for, 95
Hedlund v. Superior Court, 230
Helping relationship, values
and, 67–104
Heterosexism, 123
Hidden agendas, 418
HIV/AIDS-related issues,
confidentiality and,
248–252
Home-based therapy, 112
Homework assignment, 370
Homosexuality, 122
Human development, 458–459

Identified patient, 382, 403
Impairment, 61, 315–316
Imposition, value, 73
Indigenous healing systems,
466
Indigenous support systems,
466
Indirect client services, 459
Indirect community services,
459–460
Individualistic versus
collectivistic cultural values,
116–117
Information, parental right to,
182–183
Informed consent, 79–80,
152–165, 310, 316, 433
and managed care, 155
content, 157–165
couples and family therapy,
402–403
document, 152
educating clients, 153–155
failure to obtain or document,
194
legal aspects, 153
of parents, 183
in private practice and agency
settings, 155–157
process with minors, 184–185
in supervision, 337–338,
344–345
using telecommunication
technology, 162

Institutional racism, 114
Integrity, competence and, 399
Internship, 142
Interruptions in therapy, 161
Interventions, outreach, 465
Interview, clinical, 374
Intimate partner violence,
415–416
Involuntary participation,
437–438
Isms, challenging, 125

Jablonski v. United States,
229–230
Jaffee v. Redmond, 210–211
Justice, as a moral principle, 15,
17, 21

Key terms, ethical decision
making, 11

Law, 7
Law, ethics codes and, 7–9
Learning objectives, 4
client rights and counselor
responsibilities, 148
community and social justice
perspectives, 451
confidentiality, 204
counselor as person and
professional, 37
ethical issues in couples and
family therapy, 395
ethical issues in group work,
422
ethical issues in supervision,
334
introduction to professional
ethics, 1
issues in theory and practice,
365
managing boundaries and
multiple relationships, 254
multicultural perspectives
and diversity issues, 105
professional competence and
training, 301–333
values and helping relationship, 67

Legal aspects of informed
consent, 153
Legal aspects of supervision,
344–347
Legal framework regarding
value discrimination, 77–82
Legal liability, 201
Legal perspective of record
keeping, 170–172
Length of therapy, 159–160
Lesbian, gay, bisexual, and
transgender (LGBT)
people, 123
Levels of ethical practice, 11–13
Liability
direct, 346
strict, 346
vicarious, 346
Licensing, professional, 326–327
Licensure statutes, 327
Life experiences, shared,
133–134
Limitations of codes of ethics,
5–6
Limits to confidentiality, 208,
213, 216–219, 224–248, 345,
402, 440
Live observation, 163
Living will, 95

Malpractice, 192
liability, 191–201
suits, 193–198
Managed care, informed
consent and, 155
Managed care organization, 383
Managed care programs and
record keeping, 172–173
Mandatory ethics, 11
Mandatory participation, 437
Mandatory reporting, 244
Manifestations of
countertransference, 49–51
Marriage, same-sex, 406, 409
Microaggressions, 109, 135–137
Microaggressions, racial, 135–137
Microassault, 136
Microinsults, 136
Microinvalidations, 136

Mindfulness, 64
Minor, 182
Minors
    confidentiality with, 185–188,
        442–443
    informed consent process
        with, 184–185
Misdiagnosis, 196
Mistakes of commission, 177
Mistakes of omission, 176
Model, biomedical, 130
Modeling, 350, 357
Moral principles, in decision
    making, 15–18
Morality, 11
Motivation for becoming
    counselor, 40–41
Multicultural and diversity
    issues in supervision,
    349–352
Multicultural competence, 143,
    430, 458
Multicultural competencies,
    138–141
Multicultural counseling, 108
Multicultural counseling
    competencies, 139–141
Multicultural perspective, 108
Multicultural perspectives and
    diversity issues, 105–147
Multicultural and social justice
    competence, 430–432
Multicultural supervision, 350
Multicultural terminology,
    108–109
Multicultural training, 137–144
Multiculturalism, 108, 428–429
Multiple relationships, 256
    nonsexual, 265–266
    small community, 268–271
Multiple-role relationships in
    supervision, 352

National Child Abuse
    Prevention and Treatment
    Act, 244
Negligence, 192, 196
Neglect, 245
No secrets policy, 418–419

Nonerotic touching, 294–297
Nonmaleficence, as a moral
    principle, 15–17, 21
Nonprofessional relationships,
    256
Nonreligious clients, 90–91
Nonsexist perspective on family
    therapy, 411–414
Nonsexual multiple
    relationships, 265–266
Nonsuicidal self-injury, 235–236
Nonverbal behavior,
    assumptions, 121–122
Notes
    process, 167
    progress, 166
    psychotherapy, 167

Online counseling
    advantages and disadvant-
        ages, 177–178
    emerging issues, 176–177
    ethical issues, 175–182
    legal issues and regulation,
        178–180
    use of smartphones, 180
Online supervision, 347–348
Open groups, 446
Oppressed group, 108
Orientation
    sexual, 74, 77, 122–129
    social justice, 118
Outreach interventions, 465

Parental consent, school
    counseling and, 183–184
Parental right to information,
    182–183
Parents, informed consent of, 183
Participation
    involuntary, 437–438
    mandatory, 437
Peer review, 330
Person-centered therapy, 375
Personal beliefs and values of
    counselors, 91–92
Personal problems and conflicts,
    41
Personal therapy, 42–47, 426

Personal values, 69–70
Physical abuse, 245
Physician-assisted suicide,
    94–95, 97–98
Plan of action, 12
Pluralism, cultural, 108, 110
Policymakers, influencing,
    467–468
Policy standards, professional
    performance review, 326
Populations, diverse client,
    112–113
Positive ethics, 12, 14–15
Postmodern approaches, 376
Power of attorney for
    healthcare, durable, 95
Practice-based evidence,
    448–449
Practice issues, theory and,
    365–394
Practice, professional
    monitoring of, 10
Prevention, suicide, 237,
    240–242
Preventive education programs,
    459
Principle ethics, 13–15
Privacy, 211–212, 443–445
    confidentiality, privileged
        communication, and,
        206–220
    in school setting, 212–215
Privacy issues with
    telecommunications
    devices, 220–222
Privileged communication,
    209–211
    ethical and legal
        ramifications, 215–220
    exceptions, 216–219
    privacy and confidentiality,
        206–220
Pro bono services, 15, 159
Process notes, 167
Professional accountability, 7
Professional competence and
    training, 301–333
Professional impairment, ethics
    codes, 62